Helmut Remschmidt

Myron L. Belfer

Ian Goodyer (Eds.)

Facilitating Pathways

Care, Treatment and Prevention

in Child and Adolescent Mental Health

Helmut Remschmidt
Myron L. Belfer
Ian Goodyer (Eds.)

Facilitating Pathways

Care, Treatment and Prevention
in Child and Adolescent Mental Health

With 9 Figures and 19 Tables

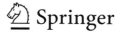 Springer

Prof. Dr. Dr. Helmut Remschmidt
Klinikum der Philipps-Universität Marburg
Klinik für Kinder- und Jugendpsychiatrie
und -psychotherapie
Hans-Sachs-Str. 4 und 6
35033 Marburg, Germany

Prof. Myron L. Belfer, MD, MPH
Harvard Medical School
Department of Social Medicine
641 Huntington Avenue
Boston, MA 02115, USA

Prof. Ian Goodyer, MD
Cambridge University
Douglas House
Developmental Psychiatry
18b Trumpington Road
Cambridge CB2 2AH, United Kingdom

ISBN 3-540-21088-1
Springer Medizin Verlag Berlin Heidelberg New York

Library of Congress Control Number: 2004108431

Springer Medizin Verlag
Part of Springer Science+Business Media

springeronline.com

© Springer-Verlag Berlin Heidelberg 2004
Printed in Germany

Typesetting: K + V Fotosatz, Beerfelden
Cover Design and Layout: deblik Berlin

Printed on acid-free paper   26/3160SM – 5 4 3 2 1 0

Preface

Mental health professionals all over the world are confronted with the necessity to help in very difficult situations and in differing cultural circumstances. Whatever we do and wherever we intervene, our major goal is to change the conditions of the disorders/problems as well as the living conditions in such a way that the child and his family are enabled to better cope with their difficulties and the burden they have to carry. Interventions need to be based on scientific knowledge, clinical experience and psychosocial engagement, and these considerations are expressed in the title of our book »Facilitating pathways« which describes from a multidisciplinary and transcultural perspective the possibilities of care, treatment and prevention. The book is divided into three sections reflecting core concerns in providing care.

Section I describes systems of care and services in selected parts of the world and from all continents with focus on:

- The current status of services in the respective parts of the world
- the major needs and deficits in identifying mental health problems in children and adolescents (awareness and diagnosis)
- the major needs in treatment, care and prevention.

Section II describes on an empirical basis the major principles and strategies for treatment and intervention using a selected number of treatment approaches and treatment settings as examples.

In Section III, the possibilities, strategies and limitations of early detection and prevention are reviewed with a focus on those that can improve the living conditions of children and families in need of mental health support.

The plan for this book emerged in the context of the preparation of the 16th World Congress of the International Association for Child and Adolescent Psychiatry and Allied Professions (IACAPAP) 2004 in Berlin and is in line with the leading principles of this organization: »To improve the study, treatment, care and prevention of mental and emotional disorders and deficiencies of children, adolescents and their families«.

The editors devote this book to IACAPAP, expressing their gratitude to have had the privilege to work many years for this organization and to support its ideals.

This book is the product of the effort of many colleagues, all of them leading experts in their field. We would like to thank them for their valuable contributions and excellence as collaborators. We also thank the staff of Springer Publishers, especially Meike Seeker and Gisela Zech, for outstanding support and cooperation and for the many proposals made to improve the book.

Finally, we hope that our book will find many readers among mental health professionals all over the world and will contribute to the improvement of child mental health by »facilitating the pathways« of many children and their families.

Marburg, Boston, Cambridge (UK), June 2004
Helmut Remschmidt, Myron L. Belfer, Ian Goodyer

Contents

I Systems of Care and Services: A Global Perspective

1 Epidemiology as a Basis for the Conception and Planning of Services 3
Frank C. Verhulst

2 Systems of Care: A Global Perspective . 16
Myron L. Belfer

3 Systems of Care in Europe 27
Per-Anders Rydelius

4 Systems of Care in North America ... 35
Katherine E. Grimes

5 Systems of Care in South America ... 42
Luis Augusto Rohde, Salvador Celia,
Carlos Berganza

6 Systems of Care in Australia 52
Barry Nurcombe

7 Systems of Care in Asia 58
K. Michael Hong, Kosuke Yamazaki,
Cornelio G. Banaag, Du YaSong

8 Systems of Care in Africa 71
Brian Robertson, Custodia Mandlhate,
Amira Seif El Din, Birama Seck

9 Setting Up Services in Difficult
Circumstances 89
Lynne Jones, Mimoza Shahini

II Principles and Strategies of Treatment/Intervention

10 Evidence-Based Psychotherapies
for Children and Adolescents:
Strategies, Strengths, and Limitations . 103
Alan E. Kazdin

11 What Works for Whom? Differential
Indications for Treatment/Intervention . 119
Peter Fonagy, Mary Target

12 Individual and Group Psychotherapies
for Children and Adolescents 140
John R. Weisz, Eunie Jung

13 Family Therapy 164
David Cottrell, Paula Boston, Dawn Walker

14 Innovative Interventions in the
Community 187
Ernesto Caffo, Barbara Forresi, Carlotta
Belaise, Giampaolo Nicolais, Nathaniel
Laor, Leo Wolmer, Helmut Remschmidt

15 Medications 208
Stan Kutcher

16 Outcomes of Treatment 222
Stephen Scott

III Prevention and Early Detection

17 Interventions that are CURRES: Cost-
Effective, Useful, Realistic, Robust,
Evolving, and Sustainable 235
Mary Jane Rotheram-Borus, Diane Flannery,
Naihua Duan

18 Prevention of Risks for Mental Health
Problems: Lessons Learned in
Examining the Prevention of Depression
in Families 245
William R. Beardslee, Tracy R.G. Gladstone

19 Prevention and Early Detection
    of Developmental Disorders   256
    Sophie Willemsen-Swinkels,
    Herman van Engeland

20 Prevention and Early Detection
    of Emotional Disorders   272
    Andreas Dick-Niederhauser,
    Wendy K. Silverman

21 Prevention and Early Detection
    of Conduct Disorder and Delinquency .   287
    David P. Farrington, Brandon C. Welsh

22 Early Detection and Prevention
    of Attention Deficit/Hyperactivity
    Disorders   301
    Eric Taylor

23 Prevention and Intervention in Primary
    Care   313
    Kelly Kelleher

24 Prevention and Intervention in School
    Settings   326
    Amira Seif El Din

Subject Index   335

List of Contributors

Banaag, Cornelio G., Prof. MD
The Medical City
Dept. of Psychiatry, Ortigas Avenue
Pasig City, Metro Manila,
Philippines 1603

Beardslee, William R., MD
Harvard Medical School
Dept. of Psychiatry
Children's Hospital
300 Longwood Avenue
Boston, MA 02115, USA

Belaise, Carlotta, PsyD
University of Modena e Reggio
Emilia
Dept. of Psychiatry and Mental
Health, Largo del Pozzo, 71
41100 Modena, Italy

Belfer, Myron L., Prof. MD, MPA
Harvard Medical School
Dept. of Social Medicine
641 Huntington Avenue
Boston, MA 02115, USA

Berganza, Carlos, Prof. MD
Clinica de Psiquiatría Infantil
Centro Clinico Berganza
San Carlos University School
of Medicine
Avenida La Reforma, 13-70 zona 9
Edificio Real Reforma, Suite 11-B
Guatemala, Guatemala, C.A

Boston, Paula, MSc
School of Psychology
University of Leeds, Leeds LS2 9JT
United Kingdom

Caffo, Ernesto, Prof. MD
University of Modena e Reggio
Emilia, Dept. of Psychiatry and
Mental Health
Chair of Child Neuropsychiatry
Largo del Pozzo, 71
41100 Modena, Italy

Celia, Salvador, Prof. MD
Discipline of Life Cycle
Brazilian Lutheran University
Leo Kanner Clinic
Brazil Rua Castro Alves 1190
ap. 301, Porto Alegre, RS
Brasil, 90430/130

Cottrell, David, Prof.
Acad. Unit of Child & Adolescent
Mental Health, School of Medicine
University of Leeds, 12A
Clarendon Road, Leeds LS2 9NN
United Kingdom

**Dick-Niederhauser,
Andreas, PhD**
Child Anxiety and Phobia Program
Florida International University
University Park, DM 201A
Miami, FL 33199, USA

Duan, Naihua, PhD
UCLA Psychr & Biobehav Sci
Box 956939
1100 Glendon Ave. Ste 850,
Los Angeles, CA 90095-6939, USA

Farrington, David P., Prof. PhD
Institute of Criminology
University of Cambridge
10 West Road, Cambridge CB3 9DZ
United Kingdom

Flannery, Diane M., Mgr.
UCLA, Neuropsychiatric Institute
Box 957051
350 Wilshire Boulevard
Los Angeles, CA 90095-7051, USA

Fonagy, Peter, Prof. PhD
University College London
Psychoanalysis Unit
Sub-Department of Clinical Health
Psychology
Gower Street, London WC1E 6BT
United Kingdom

Forresi, Barbara, PsyD
University of Modena e Reggio
Emilia, Dept. of Psychiatry and
Mental Health, Largo del Pozzo, 71
41100 Modena, Italy

Gladstone, Tracy R.G., PhD
Judge Baker Children's Center
3 Blackfan Circle
Boston MA 02115, USA

Grimes, Katherine E., MD, MPH
MHSPY Medical Director
Cambridge Health Alliance
1493 Cambridge Street
Cambridge, MA 02139, USA

Hong, K. Michael, Prof. MD
Seoul National Univ. Children's
Hospital, Div. of Child & Adolescent
Psychiatry, 28 Yongon-Dong
Chongno-gu, Seoul 110-744
Korea

**Jones, Lynne, OBE, MRC Psych.,
PhD**
Faculty of Social and Political
Sciences, Cambridge University
Free School Lane
Cambridge CB2 3RF, UK

Jung, Eunie, PhD
Dept. of Psychology
Franz Hall, UCLA
405 Hilgard Avenue
Los Angeles, CA 90095-1563, USA

Kazdin, Alan E., Prof. PhD
Child Study Center
Yale University School of Medicine
230 S. Frontage Road
New Haven, CT 06520-7900, USA

Kelleher, Kelly, Prof. MD
The Ohio State University
Columbus Children's Research
Institute, 700 Children's Drive
Columbus, OH 43220, USA

Kutcher, Stan, Prof. MD
Dalhousie University Medical
School, Dept. of Psychiatry
5909 Veterans' Memorial Lane
9th Floor, AJLB
Halifax, Nova Scotia B3H 2E2
Canada

Laor, Nathaniel, Prof. MD, PhD
Tel Aviv Mental Health Center
9 Hat'Tzvi Street, Ramat hatayasim
Tel Aviv 67197, Israel

Loeber, Rolf, Prof. PhD
University of Pittsburgh
Department of Psychiatry
3811 O'Hara Street
Pittsburgh, PA 15213, USA

Mandlhate, Custodia, Dr.
WHO Office for Africa
Parirenyatwa Hospital Medical
School
P.O. Box BE 733
Harare, Zimbabwe

Nicolais, Giampaolo, Dr.
Dept. of Psychology I
University of Rome La Sapienza
Via dei Marsi, 78
00100 Rome, Italy

Nurcombe, Barry, Prof. MD
Child and Adolescent Psychiatry
The University of Queensland
49 Highview Terrace
Brisbane, Queensland 4067
Australia

**Remschmidt, Helmut,
Prof. Dr. Dr.**
Klinikum der Philipps-Universität
Marburg
Klinik für Kinder- und Jugend-
psychiatrie und -psychotherapie
Hans-Sachs-Str. 4 und 6
35033 Marburg, Germany

Robertson, Brian, Prof. MD
Dept. of Psychiatry & Mental
Health, University of Cape Town
Groote Schuur Hospital
Observatory, 7925, Cape Town
Republic of South Africa

**Rohde, Luis Augusto,
Prof. Dr. Dr.**
Division of Child and Adolescent
Psychiatry
Hospital de Clinicas de Porto
Alegre
Servico de Psiquiatria da Infânzia e
Adolescência
Universidade Federal de Rio
Grande do Sul,
Rua Ramiro Barcelos, 2350
Porto Alegre, RS, Brasil, 90035/003

**Rotheram-Borus, Mary Jane,
Prof. PhD**
AIDS Institute, Center for HIV
Identification, Prevention,
and Treatment Services
UCLA, Los Angeles
10920 Wilshire Blvd., Suite #350,
Los Angeles, CA 90024-6521, USA

**Rydelius, Per-Anders,
Prof. MD, PhD**
Korolinska Institutet
Astrid Lindgrens Barnsjukhus
17176 Stockholm, Sweden

Scott, Stephen, Prof. PhD
Institute of Psychiatry
Dept. of Child and Adolescent
Psychiatry, University of London
King's College London
De Crespigny Park
London SE5 8AF, United Kingdom

Seck, Birama, Prof. MD
Centre Hospitalier Universitaire
de Fann, BP 5097
Dakar-Fann, Dakar-Fann, Senegal

Seif El Din, Amira, Prof. MD
Dept. of Community Medicine
Faculty of Medicine
Alexandria University, 36
Moustafa Fahmi Street, Gleem,
Alexandria, Egypt

Shahini, Mimoza, Dr.
Qendra Klinike Universitare
e Kosoves
Klinika e Neuropsikiatrise
Prishtine, Kosove

Silverman, Wendy K., Prof. PhD
Child Anxiety and Phobia Program
Florida International University
University Park, DM 201A
Miami, FL 33199, USA

Target, Mary, PhD
University College London
Psychoanalysis Unit
Sub-Department of Clinical Health
Psychology
Gower Street
London WC1E 6BT
United Kingdom

Taylor, Eric, Prof. MD
Institute of Psychiatry
Dept. of Child and Adolescent
Psychiatry, King's College London
De Crespigny Park
London SE5 8AF, United Kingdom

**van Engeland, Herman,
Prof. MD, PhD**
Dept. of Child & Adol. Psychiatry
Internal postal code B01.324
UMC Utrecht, P.O. Box 85500
3508 GA Utrecht, The Netherlands

Verhulst, Frank C., Prof. MD
Dept. of Child and Adolescent
Psychiatry
Erasmus University Medical Center
Sophia Children's Hospitall
Dr. Molewaterplein 60
3015 GJ Rotterdam
The Netherlands

Walker, Dawn
Leeds Child and Adolescent Mental
Health Service, Willow House
St Mary's Hospital, Greenhill Road
Leeds LS12 3QE, United Kingdom

Weisz, John R., Prof. PhD
Dept. of Psychology
Franz Hall, UCLA
405 Hilgard Avenue, Los Angeles
CA 90095-1563, USA

Welsh, Brandon C., PhD
Dept. of Criminal Justice
University of Massachusetts at
Lowell
870 Broadway, Suite 2
Lowell, MA 01854-3044, USA

**Willemsen-Swinkels, Sophie,
PhD**
Dept. of Psychiatry
Internal post code 333
UMC St Radboud, P.O. Box 9101
6500 HB Nijmegen
The Netherlands

Wolmer, Leo, Prof., MD
Tel Aviv Mental Health Center
9 Hat'Tzvi Street, Ramat hatayasim
Tel Aviv 67197, Israel

**Yamazaki, Kosuke, Prof. MD,
PhD**
Tokai University, Higher Education
Research Institute
Principal Tokai University Sagami
High School
3-33-1 Sounan Sagamihara-Shi Ka-
nagawa 228-8515, Japan

Yasong, Du, Prof., MD
Shanghai Mental Health Center
No. 600 Wan Ping Nan Road
Shanghai, 20030, P.R. China

Systems of Care and Services: A Global Perspective

1 Epidemiology as a Basis for the Conception and Planning of Services 3

Frank C. Verhulst

2 Systems of Care: A Global Perspective 16

Myron L. Belfer

3 Systems of Care in Europe 27

Per-Anders Rydelius

4 Systems of Care in North America 35

Katherine E. Grimes

5   Systems of Care in South America   42

Luis Augusto Rohde, Salvador Celia, Carlos Berganza

6   Systems of Care in Australia   52

Barry Nurcombe

7   Systems of Care in Asia   58

K. Michael Hong, Kosuke Yamazaki, Cornelio G. Banaag, Du Yasong

8   Systems of Care in Africa   71

Brian Robertson, Custodia Mandlhate, Amira Seif El Din, Birama Seck

**9   Setting Up Services
    in Difficult Circumstances**   89

Lynne Jones, Mimoza Shahini

Epidemiology as a Basis for the Conception and Planning of Services

Frank C. Verhulst

1.1 Introduction – 3

1.2 Epidemiological Concepts and Strategies – 3

1.3 Prevalence Studies – 4

1.4 The Referral Pathway to Psychiatric Help – 5

1.5 Methodological Issues of Child Psychiatric Prevalence Studies – 6
1.5.1 Assessment – 6
1.5.2 Multiple Informants – 6
1.5.3 Morbidity Criteria – 7

1.6 Factors Associated with Prevalence – 8
1.6.1 Gender – 8
1.6.2 Age – 8
1.6.3 Socio-economic Status – 8
1.6.4 Degree of Urbanization – 9
1.6.5 Neighborhood Disadvantage – 9
1.6.6 Ethnicity – 9
1.6.7 Historical Trends – 10

1.7 Prospective General Population Studies – 11

1.8 Prospective Studies of Clinical Samples – 11

1.9 Prevention – 12

1.10 Treatment – 13

1.11 Conclusions – 13

References – 13

1.1 Introduction

Epidemiological information is needed for developing public policies to improve children's mental health. (For reasons of brevity we will use »child« to include »adolescent« throughout the text.) In particular, epidemiological research could provide answers to questions such as:

1. How many children in the community have mental health problems;

2. How many children make use of mental health services;

3. What is the distribution of mental health problems and service use across age, sex, and ethnic groups and across levels of socio-economic status, neighborhood disadvantage, and urbanization;

4. Are there historical trends in frequency of child mental health problems;

5. What is the developmental course of mental health problems from childhood into adulthood;

6. What etiological factors can be determined to inform the design of prevention and treatment programs;

7. How cost-effective are child mental health services; and

8. What are the outcomes for children who received services?

Answers to such questions may assist policy-makers in designing strategies for improving mental health in children. After briefly explaining epidemiological concepts and strategies, a selective review of epidemiological research relevant to child mental health policies is given in this chapter.

1.2 Epidemiological Concepts and Strategies

Epidemiology is concerned with the study of the distribution and determinants of disease frequency in human populations. The quantification of the occurrence of a disease (or psychiatric disorder) in populations can be regarded as the central task of epidemiology. Well-known measures of frequency are prevalence (the number of cases in a defined population at a designated time) or incidence (the number of **new** cases in a defined population within a specified period of time). The distribution of disease or disorder involves comparisons between different populations or subpopulations. The examination of factors that are associated with variations in the distribution of psychopathology is essential for testing etiological hypotheses.

Epidemiological studies can be divided into experimental studies such as clinical trials and nonexperimental studies. Nonexperimental studies that test etiologic hypotheses are called analytical; those that are limited to the description of the occurrence of phenomena in populations are called descriptive. Another distinction that can be made in epidemiological research is between prospective and retrospective studies, depending respectively on whether the measurement of exposure to a risk factor was done before or after the disorder occurred. A study in which the presence or absence of a disorder and the presence or absence of associated factors are assessed at the same time is called a cross-sectional study. If the aim of the cross-sectional study is limited to the determination of the prevalence, the study is called prevalence study.

A basic principle in epidemiology is that observations are made on samples of individuals who are selected to be representative of populations. Typically, epidemiological studies are carried out in the general population. However, this is not always the case. General population samples are needed when we want to determine the prevalence of common psychiatric disorders such as anxiety disorders or attention deficit hyperactivity disorder. For other purposes, different populations may be more appropriate, including clinical populations to study rare and severe conditions such as autism or for conducting treatment trials, high-risk populations for testing particular causal hypotheses, and twins or adopted populations to distinguish between genetic and environmental influences on psychopathology.

1.3   Prevalence Studies

Prevalence can be defined as the proportion of a population that has mental health problems at a specific point in time. It is also possible to quantify the number of cases known to have the disorder at any time during a specified period. This so-called period prevalence (e.g., 6-month prevalence or lifetime prevalence) is frequently used in prevalence studies of child psychiatric conditions. Since the majority of child psychiatric conditions do not have a well-de-

marcated onset, incidence as a measure of frequency is used sporadically.

There are two types of studies determining the prevalence of child psychopathology: (a) those that produce prevalence rates of psychiatric diagnoses, usually based on DSM (Diagnostic and Statistical Manual of Mental Disorders) criteria, and (b) those that generate scores on psychiatric symptom rating scales.

Many studies that determined prevalence rates of DSM diagnoses in general population samples of children have been conducted. Roberts, Attkisson and Rosenblatt (1998), Verhulst (1995), Verhulst et al. (1997), and Waddell et al. (2002) provided reviews. Despite huge research efforts and many children involved, comparisons between these studies are seriously hampered by large differences in design and methodology, including differences in sample size, age of children, assessment procedures, case definition, and sampling procedures. Even for studies conducted in countries comparable in language, culture, and availability of services such as Canada, the US, Great Britain, Australia, and New-Zealand, differences in prevalence rates were extremely large and ranged from 10% to 20% (Waddell et al. 2002). It is more likely that these differences reflect variations in methodology than differences in true prevalence. Methodological variations and the lack of standardization among studies seriously limit the value of prevalence figures of categorical diagnoses.

The second approach, the use of rating scales for assessing parent- or self-reported emotional and behavioral problems of children in representative general population samples, is less vulnerable to methodological differences. This approach produces problem scores on continuous scales and does not generate prevalence rates for categorical diagnoses. Often, statistical criteria are used for distinguishing between cases and noncases. Although dividing lines for caseness may be rather arbitrary, there are epidemiological methods for selecting effective cut points. However, prevalence figures will vary with the statistical criterion and cannot be used as absolute population prevalence measures without relating them to similar measures for other populations or subpopulations (see Verhulst 1995 for an overview). In two multicultural prevalence studies, parents' reports and youths' self-reports of problems for children using the Child Behavior Checklist (CBCL) in 12 cultures, and the Youth Self-Report (YSR; Achenbach and Rescorla 2001) in 7 cultures, were compared (Crijnen, Achenbach, and Verhulst

1997, 1999; Verhulst et al. 2003). It was found that when the same standardized assessment procedures are used for assessing children from different cultures, cultural differences per se do not lead to big differences in reported problems. Instead, individual differences within each cultural group are bigger than differences between the average scores obtained in different cultures. Assessment procedures with good cross-cultural track records and appropriate translations that capture individual differences in reliable and valid ways are apt to reflect the mental health needs of children that are robust across cultures.

1.4 The Referral Pathway to Psychiatric Help

Although prevalence rates cannot be reliably compared across studies due to methodological variations, a very robust finding across studies is that the majority of children with psychiatric disorders do not receive specialist mental health services (Angold et al. 1998; Costello et al. 1996; Verhulst and Koot 1992; Zwaanswijk et al. 2003 a, b). General population studies show that only 30% of children with parent-reported and 18% with self-reported significant problems receive help (Verhulst and Van der Ende 1997; Zwaanswijk et al. 2003 a). Understanding which factors are involved in the help-seeking process may facilitate help being provided to those children who need it the most.

The referral pathway to mental health care consists of a sequence of actions that move the individual through different levels. Each level represents a different context, such as the community, primary health care, and specialist psychiatric services (Goldberg and Huxley 1992; Verhulst and Koot 1992). To move from one level to the next, the child has to pass through a »filter.« These filters represent the selection processes that determine for which children help will be sought and at which level treatment will be obtained.

From general population studies that systematically investigated factors involved in receiving professional help, we know that children who are referred are not representative of all those who have psychiatric disorders (Angold et al. 2000; Laitinen-Krispijn et al. 1999; Zwaanswijk et al. 2003 a, b). Referral is affected by many factors besides the children's problems. For example, in a general population sample of 4- to 18-year-olds, it was found that

not only emotional and behavioral problems, but also academic problems and family stress were associated with the likelihood of being referred (Verhulst and Van der Ende 1997). Thus, disordered children who live in families under stress and those who have academic problems are more likely to be referred than those with the same level of emotional and behavioral problems but who live in well-functioning families and do not have academic problems. Also, children who are referred are more likely to have multiple forms of psychopathology (comorbidity) than disordered children are in the general population (Berkson 1946; Caron and Rutter 1991).

In a study among 246 children aged 4–11 years who were selected from general practitioners' (GP) practices for having mental health problems, the GP played a limited role in the process of help-seeking for child psychopathology (Zwaanswijk et al., submitted). A more influential role is played by the school, both in increasing parents' awareness of the need to seek help, as well as in the provision of help and the referral for specialized help.

Factors associated with adolescents' self-reported mental health service need and utilization were studied in 11- to 18-year-olds from the general population (Zwaanswijk et al. 2003 b). It was found that family stress, and adolescents' self-reported behavioral and emotional problems were most strongly related to mental health service need and service utilization. Furthermore, internalizing problems, being a girl, and low educational level were associated with self-perceived unmet need.

Implications of these findings are that (a) adolescents who have problems but who do not recognize them could benefit from interventions focused at providing information about mental health problems; (b) adolescents who report unmet need could be provided with information on how and where professional help may be obtained; (c) adolescents, and especially adolescent girls, with internalizing problems are especially at risk for not effectuating their concerns about their mental health into help; mental health workers and policy makers could focus their efforts to reduce the thresholds for seeking professional help for this group; (d) the importance of school personnel's abilities for detecting and helping children with mental health problems should be recognized and strengthened; and (e) children and adolescents from problem families, those with poor school functioning, and those with comorbidity may be overrepresented in clinical samples. This is especially relevant for studies with clinical samples, because selective factors may lead to conclusions based on these samples that differ from conclusions based on samples of nonreferred children from the general population with the same condition.

1.5 Methodological Issues of Child Psychiatric Prevalence Studies

A number of methodological issues of child psychiatric prevalence studies will be considered for better understanding the results of these studies. Issues that pertain to general epidemiological methodology, such as sampling and data analysis, will not be discussed here. The focus will be on issues that are specific to child psychopathology, such as assessment, diagnostic principles, and morbidity criteria.

1.5.1 Assessment

All assessment procedures are subject to error due to variations in the phenomena being assessed and in the procedures themselves. A way to reduce variations in the data obtained and to improve precision is to use standardized assessment procedures.

Epidemiological researchers in child psychiatry were among the first to use standardized assessment procedures (Rutter et al. 1970). Rating scales were developed because they could easily be applied in a cost effective way in large-scale epidemiological studies, and standardized psychiatric interviews were developed for more in-depth assessments of the prevalence of psychiatric diagnoses. Conversely, epidemiological data are indispensable for obtaining norms and for testing the validity of these instruments (Shaffer et al. 1999). Epidemiological comparisons of normal and disordered children are needed to determine how childhood disorders are actually distributed and for identifying optimal cutoff points for distinguishing between children who will most likely benefit from particular interventions versus those who will not (Fombonne 2002).

There are two main approaches, the **empirical** and the **a priori** approach, to determine the level of psychopathology in individuals. The empirical approach employs multivariate statistical techniques, such as factor analysis and principal components analysis that are used to identify sets of problems that tend to occur together. These co-occurring items constitute empirical syndromes. This approach starts with empirical data derived from informants who describe the behavior of children, without any assumptions about whether these syndromes reflect predetermined diagnostic categories. The empirical-quantitative approach forms the basis of the empirical syndromes of rating scales such as the Child Behavior Checklist (CBCL; Achenbach and Rescorla 2001) or the Conners' Rating Scales (Conners 1997). Prevalence studies using the empirical approach generate quantitative scores reflecting the level of problems of a child. Imposing cut points to the quantitative scores can make categorical distinctions between disordered and normal individuals.

The second approach refers to the diagnostic categories employed by one of the two international nosological systems, the fourth edition of the American Psychiatric Association's (1994) **Diagnostic and Statistical Manual of Mental Disorders (DSM-IV)** or the World Health Organization's (1992) **International Classification of Diseases (ICD)**. This approach starts with assumptions about which disorders exist and about which symptoms define them. Some prevalence studies generating DSM diagnoses for general population samples as discussed above used combinations of both approaches with rating scales for screening the total sample and psychiatric interviews used for assessing a selected subsample of children scoring in the problem range of the rating scales.

1.5.2 Multiple Informants

Many prevalence studies used information from different informants, usually parents, teachers, and the child. The reason for this is because agreement among informants is far from perfect, and because no one informant can substitute for all others. Different informants having different relations to the child and seeing the child under different conditions often vary in their response to the child's behavior. In a meta-analytic study, Achenbach et al. (1987) computed the average correlation between different informants' ratings of problem behaviors in a large number of published samples. The mean correlation between pairs of adult informants who played different roles with respect to the children was 0.28 (e.g., parents versus teachers). The mean correlation between self-reports and reports by parents, teachers, and mental health workers was even lower (0.22). In contrast, the mean correlation between pairs of similar informants (e.g., father and mother, teacher and teacher aide) was 0.60.

The problem that arises is how to combine conflicting information from different informants. As an example, the prevalence of any DSM-III-R diagnosis in a Dutch general population sample of 13- to 18-year-olds based on parent interview information was 21.8%, that based on child interview information was 21.5%. The prevalence based on one informant was strikingly similar to that based on the other. However, when information from both informants was combined by counting individuals as disordered if they met DSM criteria by parent **or** by child information, the prevalence was 35.5%, and if they met DSM criteria by parent **and** by child information, the prevalence was 4%.

Instead of assuming that different procedures should yield the same results, or should be treated in the same fashion, we need to be alerted to similarities as well as differences between different sources of information (Achenbach 1985; Achenbach and McConaughy 1997). Even disagreement among informants can be valuable (Jensen et al. 1999). For example, Ferdinand et al. (2003) studied problem behavior in adolescents from the Dutch general population, aged 15–18 years, across a 4-year period. Initially, parent information was obtained with the Child Behavior Checklist and self-reports with the Youth Self-Report. Signs of poor outcome, including police contacts and drug use, were assessed four years later. Discrepancies between information from parents and adolescents added significantly to the prediction of poor outcome based on information from each informant separately. For instance, scores on the Delinquent Behavior scale based on parent information or on adolescents' self-reports separately did not predict future police contacts. However, if parents reported scores in the deviant range on the Delinquent Behavior scale, while adolescents reported scores in the normal range on this scale, adolescents were at increased risk for later police or judicial contacts. Similarly, high scores on either the CBCL or YSR Aggressive Behavior scale **did not**, but high scores by parents and concurrent low scores by adolescents **did** predict future drug use. In other words, combining the information from both parents **and** adolescents improved prognostic accuracy.

Because there can be many reasons for disagreement among different informants, there are no quick ways or fixed rules to resolve such discrepancies. For reasons of comparability, it is recommended that prevalence studies report prevalence rates based on specific informants separately, and that procedures for combining information from different informants be well documented in ways that can be easily replicated.

1.5.3 Morbidity Criteria

Most problem behaviors in children can best be regarded as quantitative variations rather than present/absent categories. This approach allows for inter-individual differences that are normal. Abnormality can be regarded as the quantitative extreme of the normal distribution. This quantitative approach makes it possible to assess the degree to which an individual child's problems deviate from those that are typical of the individual's age and sex. In order to make such comparisons, we need data on large, representative samples of boys and girls of different ages from the general population. Despite the fact that many psychopathological phenomena in children can best be regarded as quantitative variations, for identifying individuals in the general population with mental health problems we need to dichotomize quantitative information into categories that are defined by cut points for distinguishing between cases and noncases. There is as yet little basis for perfect categorical distinctions between psychopathology and normality. For most problem rating scales this is done by comparing the distribution of scores for noncases with the distribution of scores for cases. In the absence of an ultimate criterion for caseness, the most frequently used morbidity criterion is whether a child has been referred for specialist mental health services. However, caution is needed because this approach is fallible; some children who are not referred may have significant problems, while not all children who are referred really need professional help.

DSM diagnostic criteria can also be used for deciding who is disordered and who is not. These criteria are the result of negotiations among expert panels and often lack firm empirical evidence. Prevalence studies that use DSM diagnostic criteria to define caseness run into the problem that DSM criteria are overinclusive, often resulting in extremely high prevalence rates. For example, Bird et al. (1988) found that 49.5% of children in Puerto Rico met criteria for DSM-III disorders. As a result studies using DSM criteria often combine DSM diagnostic criteria with an impairment measure, for example, the Children's Global Assessment Scale (CGAS; Shaffer et al.

1983). The newest versions of some psychiatric interviews such as the Diagnostic Interview Schedule for Children (DISC) and the Child and Adolescent Psychiatric Assessment (CAPA) have included impairment criteria. Because many children who meet criteria for DSM disorders are not greatly impaired in their everyday functioning, the addition of impairment measures results in a decrease of prevalence rates. In the Dutch prevalence study, for example, the prevalence of 21.8% of children who met criteria for any DSM-III-R disorder based on parent interview information dropped to 5.9% when combined with a CGAS score indicating definite impairment (Verhulst et al. 1997). Conversely there are also many children who can be regarded functionally impaired but do not meet criteria for DSM diagnoses. Some 50% of children attending clinics in the Great Smoky Mountains Study do not reach DSM or ICD criteria for a diagnosis and yet half of these are significantly impaired in their social functioning (Angold et al. 1999). In the Dutch prevalence study, we found that 1.4% of the children in the general population who did not meet criteria for DSM diagnoses could be regarded as definitely impaired based on parent interview information (Verhulst et al. 1997).

1.6 Factors Associated with Prevalence

Of many factors that have been tested for association with prevalence in general population studies, findings for gender, age, socio-economic status (SES), degree of urbanization and neighborhood disadvantage will be discussed here, because those are factors with findings that have been replicated across studies.

1.6.1 Gender

Gender differences in prevalence are very robust across cultures, informants, and types of studies, in particular those that used rating scales and those that used DSM diagnostic criteria. Girls score higher than boys on internalizing psychopathology such as anxiety, depression, and somatic complaints, and boys score higher than girls on externalizing behaviors such as attention and hyperactivity problems and aggressive and delinquent behaviors. These gender differences are found for both parent- and self-reported problems. Despite the range in cultur-

al, economic, political, and genetic differences, there is consistency in population-based findings that boys have more externalizing and girls have more internalizing problems.

1.6.2 Age

From a developmental perspective, the effects of age on levels of psychopathology in individuals can best be studied through longitudinal studies. For public policy purposes, cross-sectional data on prevalence with age can be important for service planning. Age interacts with gender as a factor associated with prevalence. Boys show more problems than girls when they are younger, whereas girls show more problems than boys in adolescence. In a study using survival analyses for investigating lifetime prevalence of DSM-IV mood and anxiety disorders in a general population sample of young adults, Roza et al. (2003) found a steep increase in depression in females from age 14 onwards. The increase of depression in males starts somewhat later and is much less dramatic. The increase of anxiety disorders with age in females starts early (from age 5 onwards), is more gradual and levels off in young adulthood. In the above-cited multicultural study of self-reported problems across 7 countries, both internalizing and externalizing behaviors increased with ages 11–18 years (Verhulst et al. 2003). In the multicultural study of parent-reported problems of children aged 6 through 11 years across 12 countries, and aged 6 through 17 years in 9 countries, externalizing problems decreased and internalizing problems increased with age (Crijnen et al. 1997, 1999). Although parents and adolescents agreed in reporting increases with age of internalizing problems, they disagreed about externalizing problems. Apparently parents are increasingly unaware of their child's externalizing behaviors with increasing age. This is probably caused by a developmental shift in type of externalizing problems, with overt physically aggressive and oppositional behaviors decreasing with age and status violations such as truancy, running away from home, and substance abuse increasing with age (Bongers et al. 2004).

1.6.3 Socio-economic Status

Studies that determined the effect of socio-economic status (SES) on mental health problems reported more problems and lower competencies for lower SES children (Verhulst 1995; Waddell 2002). Although this finding was consistent across studies, the effects were rather small. There are a number of reasons that may be responsible for the finding that children from lower SES are somewhat disadvantaged. Tieman et al. (submitted) compared the effects of parental SES on educational and occupational achievement in biological versus adopted children, 14 years later, when they were young adults. Whereas parental SES was significantly related to educational and professional achievements in biologically related offspring from the general population, there was no effect of parental SES on the adopted children's later achievement. These findings indicate that the relationship between parental SES and the achievements of their children may be largely due to genetic kinship. This study also showed that there were differences in achievement between children born in different countries. Children from South Korea achieved much better than children from Columbia. Selective factors and differences in prenatal and early postnatal environmental factors such as poor antenatal care and malnutrition may be responsible for these differences in level of academic and professional achievement. Other studies showed that factors associated with low SES such as higher rates of stressful life events, poor housing, less adequate parenting, and language delay all may negatively influence children's psychoeducational functioning, though some effects may be the result of gene-environment correlations.

1.6.4 Degree of Urbanization

Most studies investigating differences in prevalence rates between urban and rural populations did not find significant differences (Waddell et al. 2002). Achenbach et al. (1991) conducted a detailed comparison of varying degrees of urbanization while controlling for sex, age, referral status, SES, region, and ethnicity in a US national sample. Children from the most urban areas showed a slight tendency to obtain higher parent-reported problem scores than children from the most rural areas. However, unexpectedly, the greatest contrast in problem scores was found between children in the intermediate categories versus those in the most rural areas, with highest scores for children in the intermediate categories.

1.6.5 Neighborhood Disadvantage

For policy makers, the finding that SES is related to the level of child psychopathology can be important for developing strategies for improving mental health in children such as prevention interventions or improving mental health services. However, risk factors on the individual or family level should be distinguished from risk factors related to the neighborhood context. It is known that neighborhood socio-economic disadvantage (NSD) influences children's mental health (Kalff et al. 2001). It is important to study the effects of NSD while controlling for the effects of SES. Schneiders et al. (2003) investigated whether NSD contributed to emotional and behavioral problems beyond the effect of parental SES in a large community sample of 10–12-year-old children. They found that NSD was associated with parent- and self-reported problems even after controlling for parental SES. They also found that NSD was associated with an increase in problems across a 2-year follow-up period. It was concluded that living in a disadvantaged neighborhood indeed increased the risk of developing emotional and behavioral problems and that NSD may lead to an increase in problems during transition from childhood into adulthood. Possible mechanisms include the exposure in disadvantaged neighborhoods to inappropriate peers and adult role models, low levels of neighborhood cohesion, and lack of informal social control. An implication of these findings is that neighborhood environment should also be taken into account when planning public health interventions for improving children's mental health.

1.6.6 Ethnicity

Multicultural populations containing immigrants and refugees characterize many contemporary societies. It is therefore important to investigate whether the prevalence of mental health problems differs across ethnic groups. When evaluating children of different cultures, it must be determined whether problems merely reflect cultural differences or whether they reflect needs for professional help (e.g., Bengi-Arslan et al. 1997). We therefore need cross-culturally robust instruments for identifying variations in behavioral and emotional problems.

Because many cultures lack well-standardized indigenous instruments for assessing the problems of children, instruments developed in one culture are often translated and adapted for use in other cultures. To apply such instruments to new cultures, they should be tested in various ways to maximize the equivalence of data obtained in the different cultures (Bird 1996; Canino and Bravo 1999).

As an example, Bengi-Arslan et al. (1997) compared parent ratings of children's problems with the CBCL (Achenbach 1991a) in a representative sample of children in The Netherlands, with those obtained for Turkish immigrant children living in The Netherlands, and with ratings obtained for children living in Ankara, Turkey (Bengi-Arslan et al. 1997). It was found that Turkish immigrant children had much higher scores on the CBCL Anxious/Depressed scale than Dutch children. However, Turkish immigrant children living in The Netherlands were very similar in their level and type of problems to those of indigenous children living in Turkey. This kind of information showing variations in problems among cultural groups may have important implications for mental health policies. Higher levels of particular problems in immigrant children versus indigenous children may result from stress factors associated with immigration. This may alert policy makers or mental health professionals to the need for special interventions. However, if the level of problems in immigrant children is comparable to that in children from the home country, the elevated levels of problems in immigrant children over indigenous children may have rather been influenced by cross-cultural differences in the reporting of problems. These cross-cultural differences may result from differences in parental thresholds for reporting particular kinds of problems, from linguistic differences, or from »true« differences in the prevalence of these problems.

Whenever possible, information should be obtained from parents, teachers, and children themselves. As discussed above, this is true for all child psychiatric epidemiological research, but it is especially important when there are cultural differences between mental health professionals or researchers and those who are being assessed. For example, it was found that parent-reported and self-reported problem scores for Moroccan youths were similar or even lower than scores obtained for Turkish youths and for Dutch youths in the Netherlands (Stevens et al. 2003). However, Dutch teachers reported substantially higher levels of externalizing problems for Moroccan youths than for Turkish and Dutch youths. Such findings may alert policy makers or mental health professionals to pay special attention to issues that may be responsible for this

underreporting, such as the parents' lack of awareness of their child's problem behavior outside the home.

1.6.7 Historical Trends

The question is often brought up whether behavioral and emotional functioning in children in our rapidly changing societies is worsening over the last decades. An international group of researchers concluded that there is limited evidence that rates of depression, suicide, and crime as well as substance use are increasing over the last 50 years (Rutter and Smith 1995). However, it is hard to draw firm conclusions due to changing assessment procedures and diagnostic criteria over time and the retrospective nature of the studies.

There are few studies that compared prevalence rates of children's mental health problems assessed in similar ways in comparable samples selected across time intervals long enough for secular changes to take place. A Dutch study compared parent- and teacher-reported problems assessed with the CBCL and TRF in two general population samples selected from the same region, one in 1983 and the other in 1993 (Verhulst et al. 1997). The methodology in 1983 was similar to the one followed in 1993. No significant differences were found between 1983 and 1993 in total problems scores obtained from teachers and parents. On a few syndrome scales, differences were found indicating a slight increase in problems with time. However, the magnitude of these differences was very small. Unlike this study, a comparable study done in the US (Achenbach and Howell 1993), showed that there were significant increases in parent- and teacher-reported problems assessed for samples in 1976 and between 1981 and 1982 respectively, with problems assessed for a sample in 1989. However, new data collected for a sample assessed in 1999 showed a decrease in parent-reported problems, though they remained higher than in 1976 (Achenbach et al. 2003). These studies showed that there were no systematic dramatic increases in mental health problems across intervals ranging from 10 to 23 years.

1.7 Prospective General Population Studies

Prospective longitudinal studies of general population samples can give us information on the natural course of psychiatric disorders in children. Several studies have followed the course of psychopathology in children in general population samples across long periods (Caspi, Moffitt, Newman and Silva 1996; Fergusson, Horwood and Lynskey 1994; Hofstra, Van der Ende and Verhulst 2002). These studies show that there is considerable continuity of mental health problems. Approximately 30% of children and adolescents with high levels of emotional and behavioral problems will continue to have problems as young adults (Hofstra et al. 2000). As we have discussed earlier, there is also a considerable amount of psychopathology arising de novo, especially among adolescent girls who develop affective problems.

From a mental health policy as well as from an individual perspective it is important to know what the detrimental effects are of chronically persisting mental health problems of children on the outcome in adulthood. It may be as Sroufe (1990) suggested, that the more consistently a deviating pathway is followed over time, the more unlikely it becomes that a normal pathway can be reclaimed. Hofstra et al. (2002) determined the impact of different developmental pathways of psychopathological development on adult outcomes in individuals followed from ages 11–18 to 21–28 years. The authors confirmed Sroufe's (1990) hypothesis that an ongoing devious pathway had negative effects on many domains of functioning. These effects on everyday social functioning were much worse than those for the group of individuals who showed comparable levels of psychopathology as adults but who were well-functioning as adolescents. The third group, consisting of individuals who showed high levels of problems in early adolescence but whose level of psychopathology diminished by adulthood, seemed to be as healthy as people who never attained serious levels of psychopathology.

Bongers et al. (2003) used growth curve analyses to compute normative developmental trajectories of problem behaviors as reported by parents at multiple time points. These normative developmental trajectories provide a basis against which deviations from the expected developmental course can be detected. This approach can be used to select groups of children who, on multiple measurements, deviate from the normative developmental trajectory. Children

who are selected through this longitudinal screening approach can be subjected to interventions.

Longitudinal general population studies also make it possible to compare children with a disorder who received treatment with those with the same type and level of psychopathology who did not receive treatment. Ideally, such comparisons could be used to evaluate certain interventions naturally occurring in clinical settings. However, children who receive treatment may differ systematically in the distribution of prognostic factors from children with comparable problems who do not receive treatment. Biases in receipt of treatment may be responsible for the alarming finding that children who received treatment fared worse after a 4-year follow-up than children with comparable levels of problems who had **not** been treated (Koot and Verhulst 1994).

1.8 Prospective Studies of Clinical Samples

The term »clinical course« refers to the evolution of disorders in children who receive mental health care (e.g., Angold et al. 2000; Heijmens Visser, Van der Ende, Koot and Verhulst 1999; Stanger, MacDonald, McConaughy and Achenbach 1996; Steinhausen and Verhulst 1999). This kind of information is important for: (a) identifying risk and protective factors affecting outcome in children who are being treated for mental health problems, and (b) evaluating the quality of services across mental health settings.

In a 6–10-year follow-up of over 2,000 children who had been referred to one child psychiatric service, the prognosis was generally rather poor (Heijmens Visser et al. 2003). Although there was an overall improvement in mean problem scores, the majority still had significant problems at follow-up. They either showed more psychopathology or had more signs of maladjustment than untreated individuals of the same age from the general population. The mediocre outcomes may lead to the conclusion that typical care is not very effective and that much needs to be improved, for example, by adopting beneficial features of research conditions in clinical settings. It may also be concluded that many forms of psychopathology in children represent chronic conditions and that we need to devise cost-effective strategies of long-term or repeated interventions that help people live normal lives.

Knowledge of factors that adversely affect outcomes in clinically treated children can aid in identifying children for whom routine care may need to be adjusted. Although various factors may adversely affect outcomes (e.g., age, gender, baseline severity of symptoms, functional impairment, family dysfunction, previous treatment), only a limited number of factors have been tested so far (Heijmens Visser et al. 2003; Phillips et al. 2000). Many factors considered by experts to affect the success of treatment (e.g., residential instability, abuse, neglect, exposure to community violence) have not been tested in studies investigating treatment outcomes for adolescents with psychiatric problems (Phillips et al. 2000). Conversely, it may be helpful to know which factors positively affect outcome, and to identify which children improve without any help.

The outcomes of clinically referred children can also be compared across settings for testing the functioning of mental health settings. However, this type of comparison can be very problematic due to methodological problems resulting from selection (Phillips et al. 2000). When patients referred to one clinical setting differ systematically in predictive factors from patients in another setting, then the differences between treatment outcomes across clinical settings may be due to differences in these predictive factors as well as to differences in the quality of the treatments patients received. For example, if children referred to clinic A had generally lower IQs than children referred to clinic B, then it would not be surprising if the treatment success for clinic A was worse than that for clinic B. Another example would be if the main reason why children were referred to a particular clinic was that prior treatment attempts in other clinical settings were unsuccessful. In that case it would not be surprising if the treatment success for that clinic was worse than that for the other clinics. Therefore, statistical adjustment of treatment outcomes to account for differences in predictive factors may be needed if we want to compare the outcomes across different services.

1.9   Prevention

Etiologic epidemiological research forms the basis for prevention interventions by developing strategies for reducing the influence of risk factors. Risk factors refer to exposures to factors that increase the probability of psychopathology (Kraemer et al. 1997), for example, the exposure to certain parent and family factors, or peer group, school, or neighborhood characteristics. Exposures that reduce the probability of psychopathology are protective factors. A host of epidemiological studies, especially longitudinal studies, examined relations between risk factors and subsequent psychiatric disorders (Rutter 2002). There is an increasing emphasis on the interaction between various risk factors, especially interactions between genetic and environmental factors (e.g., Caspi et al. 2002).

To quantify the influence of certain factors on the occurrence of a disease or disorder, epidemiologists use measures of effect and measures of association (Rothman and Greenland 1998). Measures of effect (e.g., the risk ratio) are estimates of the amount of change in a population's disease frequency caused by the exposure to a specific factor. To calculate measures of effect, cohort studies are needed, in which a population is divided into those who are exposed versus those who are not exposed to a specific factor. If measures of disease occurrence in two different populations are contrasted (e.g., incidence rates of depression in adolescent males versus females), measures of association are used such as odds ratio.

Knowledge of risk factors, especially causal risk factors, is essential for the prevention of disorders. Ideally, prevention intervention is aimed at decreasing the effects of risk factors (or increasing the effects of protective factors). For example, knowledge about the risks of prenatal and early postnatal environmental influences on the developing child makes it possible to identify high risk mothers who can then be subjected to prevention programs (e.g., Olds et al. 1997).

Prospective cohort studies are indispensable for determining the effects of risk and protective factors on the development of mental health problems. Prospective studies make it possible to disentangle the temporal sequence between risk factor and the later occurrence of mental health problems. For example, childhood disruptive behavior is a strong predictor for negative outcomes such as antisocial behavior, substance abuse, depression, poor school performance, school dropout, and poor job performance (Caspi et al. 1998; Tremblay et al. 1994). Prevention interventions aim to intervene in the development of disruptive behaviors at an early stage, before patterns of disruptive behavior that are present in the home situation become more firmly established in the school environment and peer group.

Discussion of prevention studies are beyond the scope of this chapter, but see section 3 of this book, where the prevention and early detection of mental health problems in children are discussed in detail.

1.10 Treatment

Once mental health problems have emerged and have been recognized, the child may be referred for mental health services. After diagnostic assessment and formulating a diagnosis, the clinician will identify targets for intervention and select the treatment that works best for a particular type of problem. Ideally, the treatment for each type of problem should be selected on the basis of findings from controlled trials (Harrington, Cartwright-Hatton and Stein 2002; Target and Fonagy 1996). A systematic, clinical epidemiological approach to testing the efficacy of particular treatments for particular problems can enhance the assignment of children to the most effective interventions. For more detailed discussion of evidence based treatments, see section 2 of this book.

It is important to determine the outcomes of mental health services in systematic ways, because this may help improve these services by identifying problems in the quality of these services or by identifying individual children for whom treatment strategies need to be changed. To evaluate outcomes of child mental health services, baseline measures obtained at the time of referral can be compared with measures obtained after services have been provided. Outcome evaluations are most useful when they are done at uniform intervals across all cases seen in a particular clinical setting. This makes it easier to draw generalizable conclusions about whether the interventions were effective.

1.11 Conclusions

Since the first child psychiatric epidemiological studies in the 1950s (Lapouse and Monk 1958) and 1960s (Rutter, Tizard and Whitmore 1970), epidemiological research has provided a wealth of empirical findings that may aid policy-makers in developing strategies for improving the mental health outcomes of children. Descriptive epidemiological data on prevalence rates, service use, historical trends, and outcomes of mental health problems can help planning mental health services for children and provide evidence for setting priorities when resources are limited. Etiologic epidemiological research forms the basis for prevention interventions by unraveling the causative mechanisms in the development of psychopathology. Clinical epidemiological strategies are important for more evidence-based approaches to diagnostic assessment and intervention strategies, and outcome research may help improving the quality of mental health services.

Despite these attainments, child psychiatric epidemiology could be made more useful to policy-makers by resolving outstanding issues such as the improvement of comparability across studies. Also, new issues have emerged that need to be tackled such as those related to the multicultural nature of current societies. Finally, more effort should be put into improving partnerships between epidemiological researchers and prevention specialists and between epidemiological researchers and policy-makers for improving strategies for preventing and treating mental health problems in children.

References

Achenbach TM (1985) Assessment and taxonomy of child and adolescent psychopathology. Sage Publications, Beverly Hills, CA.

Achenbach TM (1991 a) Manual for the Child Behavior Checklist 1991 Profile. Burlington, University of Vermont Department of Psychiatry.

Achenbach TM, Howell CT.(1993) Are American children's problems getting worse? A 13-year comparison. Journal of the American Academy of Child & Adolescent Psychiatry, 32, 1145–1154.

Achenbach TM, McConaughy SH (1997) Empirically based assessment of child and adolescent psychopathology, 2nd edition, USA, Thousands Oaks, Sage.

Achenbach TM, Rescorla LA (2001) Manual for the ASEBA school age forms and profiles. Burlington, VT: University of Vermont, Research Center for Children, Youth and Families.

Achenbach TM, McConaughy SH & Howell CT (1987) Child/adolescent behavioral and emotional problems: Implication of cross-informant correlations for situational specificity. Psychological Bulletin, 101, 213–232.

Achenbach TM, Howell CT, Quay HC, Conners CK (1991) National survey of competencies and problems among 4- to 16-year-olds: Parents' reports for normative and clinical samples. Monographs of the Society for Research in Child Development, in press.

American Psychiatric Association (1994) Diagnostic and Statistical Manual of Mental Disorders. (4th edition) Washington DC: American Psychiatric Association.

Angold A, Messer SC, Stangl D, Farmer EMZ, Costello EJ, Burns BJ (1998) Perceived parental burden and service use for child and adolescent psychiatric disorders. American Journal Public Health, 88, 75–80.

Angold A, Costello EJ, Burns BJ, Erkanli A, Farmer EM (2000) Effectiveness of nonresidential specialty mental health services for children and adolescents in the »real world«.

Journal of the American Academy of Child and Adolescent Psychiatry, 39, 154–160.

Bengi-Arslan L, Verhulst FC, van der Ende J, Erol N (1997) Understanding childhood (problem) behaviors from a cultural perspective: comparison of problem behaviors and competencies in Turkish immigrant, Turkish and Dutch children. Soc Psychiatry Psychiatr Epidemiol, 32, 477–484.

Berkson J (1946) Limitations of application of fourfold table analysis to hospital data. Biometrics Bulletin, 2, 47–53.

Bird HR (1996) Epidemiology of childhood disorders in a cross-cultural context. Journal of Child Psychology and Psychiatry, 37, 35–49.

Bird HR, Canino G, Rubio-Stipec M, Gould MS, Ribera J, Sesman M, Woodbury M, Huertas-Goldman S, Pagan A, Sanchez-Lacay A, Moscoso M (1988) Estimates of the prevalence of childhood maladjustment in a community survey in Puerto Rico: the use of combined measures. Archives of General Psychiatry, 45, 1120–1126.

Bongers IL, Koot HM, Van der Ende J, Verhulst FC (2003) The normative development of child and adolescent problem behavior. Journal of Abnormal Psychology, 112, 179–192.

Canino G, Bravo M (1999) The translation and adaptation of diagnostic instruments for cross-cultural us. In: Diagnostic Assessment in Child and Adolescent Psychopathology. Shaffer D, Lucas CP, Richters JE. Eds, New York, Guilford Press, pp. 285–298

Caron C, Rutter M (1991) Co-morbidity in child psychopathology: concepts, issues and research strategies. Journal of Child Psychology and Psychiatry, 32, 1063–1080.

Caspi A, Moffitt TE, Newman DL, Silva PA (1996) Behavioral observations at age 3 years predict adult psychiatric disorders. Archives of General Psychiatry, 53, 1033–1039.

Caspi A, Moffitt TE, Newman DL, Silva PA (1998) Behavioral observations at age 3 years predict adult psychiatric disorders: Longitudinal evidence from a birth cohort. In ME Hertzig, EA Farber (Eds), Annual progress in child psychiatry and child development: 1997. (pp. 319–331) Bristol, PA, USA: Brunner/Mazel, Inc.

Caspi A, McClay J, Moffitt TE, Mill J, Martin J, Craig IW, Taylor A, Poulton R (2002) Role of genotype in the cycle of violence in maltreated children. Science, 297, 851–853.

Conners CK (1999) Conners' Rating Scales – Revised. In ME Maruish: The use of psychological testing for treatment planning and outcomes assessment (2nd edition) Mahwah, NJ: Lawrence Erlbaum associates, publishers

Costello EJ, Angold A, Burns BJ, Stangl D, Tweed D, Erkanli A, Worthman CM (1996) The Great Smoky Mountains study of youth: goals, design, methods, and the prevalence of DSM-III-R disorders. Archives of General Psychiatry, 53, 1129–1136.

Crijnen AAM, Achenbach TM, Verhulst FC (1997) Comparisons of problems reported by parents of children in 12 cultures: total problems, externalizing, and internalizing. J Am Acad Child Adolesc Psychiatry, 36, 1269–1277.

Crijnen AAM, Achenbach TM, Verhulst FC (1999) Problems reported by parents of children in multiple cultures: the Child Behavior Checklist syndrome constructs. Am J Psychiatry, 156, 569–574.

Fergusson DM, Horwood LJ, Lynskey MT (1994) The childhoods of multiple problem adolescents: a 15-year longitudinal study. Journal of Child Psychology and Psychiatry, 35, 1123–1140.

Fombonne E (2002) Case identification in an epidemiological context. In: Child and Adolescent Psychiatry, 4th edition, Rutter M, Taylor E (Eds) Oxford, England, Blackwell, pp 52–69.

Goldberg D, Huxley P (1992) Common mental disorders: a biosocial model. New York, USA, Routledge.

Harrington RC, Cartwright-Hatton S, Stein A (2002) Annotation: Randomised trials. Journal of Child Psychology and Psychiatry, 43, 695–704.

Heijmens Visser J, Van der Ende J, Koot HM, Verhulst FC (1999) Continuity of psychopathology in youths referred to mental health services. Journal of the American Academy of Child and Adolescent Psychiatry, 38, 1560–1568.

Heijmens Visser J, Van der Ende J, Koot HM, Verhulst FC (2003) Predicting change in psychopathology in youth referred to mental health services in childhood or adolescence. Journal of Child Psychology and Psychiatry, 44, 509–519.

Hofstra M, Van der Ende J, Verhulst FC (2002) Child and adolescent problems predict. DSM-IV disorders in adulthood: a 14-year follow-up of a Dutch epidemiological sample. Journal of the American Academy of Child and Adolescent Psychiatry, 41, 182–189.

Hofstra MB, Van der Ende J, Verhulst FC (2000) Continuity and change of psychopathology from childhood into adulthood: a 14-year follow-up study. Journal of the American Academy of Child and Adolescent Psychiatry, 39, 850–858.

Jensen PS, Rubio-Stipec M, Canino G, Bird H, Dulcan M, Schwab-Stone ME, Lahey B (1999) Parent and child contributions to diagnosis of mental disorder: are both informants necessary? Journal of the American Academy of Child and Adolescent Psychiatry, 3, 1569–1579.

Kalff AC, Kroes M, Vles JS et al (2001) Neighbourhood level and individual level SES effects on child problem behaviour: a multilevel analysis. Journal of Epidemiology Community Health, 55, 246–250.

Koot HM, Verhulst FC (1994) Prediction of children's mental health and special education services from earlier adjustment. Journal of Child Psychology and Psychiatry, 33, 717–729.

Kraemer HC, Kazdin AE, Offord DR, Kessler RC, Jensen PS, Kupfer DJ (1997) Coming to terms with the terms of risk. Archives of General Psychiatry, 54, 337–343.

Laitinen-Krispijn S, Van der Ende J, Wierdsma AI, Verhulst FC (1999) Predicting adolescent mental health service use in a prospective record-linkage study. Journal of the American Academy of Child and Adolescent Psychiatry, 38, 1073–1080.

Lapouse R, Monk MA (1958) An epidemiologic study of behavior characteristics in children. American Journal of Public Health, 48, 1134–144.

Olds DL, Eckenrode J, Henderson CR, Kitzman H, Powers J, Cole R, Sidora K, Morris P, Pettitt LM, Luckey D (1997) Long-term effects of home visitation on maternal life course and child abuse and neglect. Fifteen-year follow up of a randomized trial. Journal American Medical Association, 278, 637–643.

Phillips SD, Hargis MB, Kramer TL, Lensing SY, Taylor JL, Burns BJ, Robbins JM (2000) Toward a level playing field: predictive factors for the outcomes of mental health treatment for adolescents. Journal of the American Academy of Child and Adolescent Psychiatry, 39, 1485–1495.

Roberts EE, Attkisson CC, Rosenblatt A (1998) Prevalence of psychopathology among children and adolescents. American Journal of Psychiatry, 155, 715–725.

Rothman KJ, Greenland S (1998) Modern Epidemiology, 2nd edition. Philadelphia, USA, Lippincott-Raven.

Roza SJ, Hofstra MB, Van der Ende J, Verhulst FC (2003) Stable Prediction of Mood and Anxiety Disorders Based on Behavioral and Emotional Problems in Childhood: 14-Year Follow-Up During Childhood, Adolescence, and Young Adulthood. The American Journal of Psychiatry, in press.

Rutter M (2002) Development and psychopathology. In: Child and Adolescent Psychiatry, 4th edition, Rutter M, Taylor E, eds, Oxford, England, Blackwell, pp 309–324.

Rutter M, Smith DJ (1995) Psychosocial disorders in young people: time trends and their causes. Chichester: John Wiley and Sons.

Rutter M, Tizard J, Whitmore K (Eds) (1970) Education, health and behaviour. London: Longman. (Reprinted 1981, Melbourne: Krieger)

Schneiders J, Drukker M, Van der Ende J, Verhulst FC, Van Os J, Nicolson NA (2003) Neighbourhood socioeconomic disadvantage and behavioural problems from late childhood into early adolescence. Journal of Epidemiology Community Health, 57, 699–703.

Shaffer D, Lucas CP, Richters JE (1999) Diagnostic Assessment in Child and Adolescent Psychopathology, New York, Guilford Press.

Sroufe LA (1989) Pathways to adaptation and maladaptation: Psychopathology as developmental deviation. In: Developmental psychopathology: an emerging discipline. Volume 1. Hillsdale, NJ: Erlbaum, pp 13–40.

Stanger C, MacDonald VV, McConaughy SH, Achenbach TM (1996) Predictors of cross-informant syndromes among children and youth referred for mental health services. Journal of Abnormal Child Psychology,24, 597–614.

Steinhausen H-C, Verhulst FC (1999) (Eds) Risks and outcomes in developmental psychopathology. Oxford, Oxford University Press.

Stevens GWJM, Pels T, Bengi-Arslan L, Verhulst FC, Vollebergh WAM, Crijnen AAM (2003) Parent, teacher and self-reported problem behavior in The Netherlands: comparing Moroccan immigrant with Dutch and with Turkish immigrant children and adolescents. Soc Psychiatry Psychiatr Epidemiol, in press.

Target M, Fonagy P (1996) The psychological treatment of child and adolescent psychiatric disorders. In: What Works for Whom? Roth A & Fonaghy P, eds. New York, Guildford Press, pp 263–320.

Tieman W, Tiemeier H, Van der Ende J, Verhulst FC (2003) Nature versus Nurture in Educational Achievement: A 14-years Follow-up Study of Intercountry Adoptees

Tremblay RE, Pihl RO, Vitaro F, Dobkin PL (1994) Predicting early onset of male antisocial behavior from preschool behavior. Archives of General Psychiatry, 51(9), 732–739.

Verhulst FC (1995) A review of community studies. In: FC Verhulst and JM Koot, The Epidemiology of Child and Adolescent Psychopathology. (pp 146–177) Oxford: Oxford University Press.

Verhulst FC, Koot HM (1992) Child Psychiatric Epidemiology: Concepts, Methods and Findings. Newbury Park: Sage

Verhulst FC, Van der Ende J (1997) Factors associated with child mental health service use in the community. Journal of the American Academy of Child and Adolescent Psychiatry, 36, 901–909.

Verhulst FC, Van der Ende J (2002) Rating scales. In: Child and Adolescent Psychiatry, 4th edition, Rutter M, Taylor E, eds, Oxford, England, Blackwell, pp 70–86.

Verhulst FC, Van der Ende J, Ferdinand RF, Kasius MC (1997) The prevalence of DSM-III-R diagnoses in a national sample of Dutch adolescents. Archives of General Psychiatry, 54, 329–336.

Verhulst FC, Van der Ende J, Rietbergen A (1997) Ten-year time trends of psychopathology in Dutch children and adolescents: no evidence for strong trends. Acta Psychiatrica Scandinavica, 96, 7–13.

Verhulst FC, Achenbach TM, Van der Ende J, Erol N, Lambert MC, Leung PWL, Silva MA, Zilber N, Zubrick SR (2003) Comparisons of problems reported by youths from seven countries. American Journal of Psychiatry, 160, 1479–1485.

Waddell C, Offord DR, Shepherd CA, Hua JM, McEwan K (2002) Child psychiatric epidemiology and Canadian public policy-making: the state of the science and the art of the possible. Canadian Journal of Psychiatry, 47, 825–832.

World Health Organization (1992) Mental Disorders: Glossary and guide to their classification in accordance with the Tenth Revision of the International Classification of Diseases (10th edn.) Geneva: Author

Zwaanswijk M, Van der Ende J, Verhaak PFM, Bensing JM, Verhulst FC (2003 a) Factors associated with adolescent mental health service need and utilization. Journal of the American Academy of Child and Adolescent Psychiatry, 42, 692–700.

Zwaanswijk M, Van der Ende J, Verhaak PFM, Bensing JM, Verhulst FC (2003 b) Help seeking for emotional and behavioural problems in children and adolescents: a review of recent literature. European Child and Adolescent Psychiatry, 12, 153–161.

Systems of Care: A Global Perspective

Myron L. Belfer

2.1 Introduction – 16

2.2 Concepts Needed for Mental Health Services Literacy – 17
2.2.1 »System of Care« – 17
2.2.2 »Continuum of Care« and »Wrap-Around Services« – 17
2.2.3 Managed Care and Insurance – 18
2.2.4 Privatization – 18

2.3 Current Situation – 18
2.3.1 Policy for Care – 19
2.3.2 Cultural Understanding in Providing Care – 19
2.3.3 Barriers to Care – 19
2.3.4 Role of Nongovernmental Organizations – 19
2.3.5 Epidemiology – 20
2.3.6 Training for Care – 20

2.4 Current Status of »Systems of Care« – 20
2.4.1 Replication of Services – 20
2.4.2 WHO Role and Areas of Concern in Improving Care – 20

2.5 Research and Evaluation – 21
2.5.1 Status of Services Research – 21
2.5.2 Disability-Adjusted Life Years – 21
2.5.3 Burden of Disease – 22
2.5.4 Cultural Epidemiology – 22

2.6 Current Global Initiatives – 23
2.6.1 ATLAS Project – 23
2.6.2 Child and Adolescent Mental Health Policy Module – 23

2.7 Advocacy for Services – 23
2.7.1 United Nations Convention on the Rights of the Child – 23
2.7.2 Advocacy for Care by Allied Interests – 24

2.8 Systems of Care for Special Populations – 24
2.8.1 Mainstreaming –24
2.8.2 Learning Disabled – 25
2.8.3 Juvenile Delinquents – 25

2.9 Conclusions – 25

References – 26

2.1 Introduction

There are few places in the world and virtually no country that can claim to have a comprehensive »system of care« for children and adolescents with mental disorders. There are excellent comprehensive programs in some jurisdictions and very well-meaning efforts in many, but a »system of care« implying a continuum in which there are services with a set of definable elements that facilitate access to appropriate levels of care and reduce the dependence on ineffective, excessive, or antiquated modes of care are rare. Understanding the current status of the care for children and adolescents with mental disorders and understanding the potential for the development of »systems of care« can serve to provide an impetus for the development of responsive, modern means for the needed care of children worldwide.

It is important to note that not all knowledgeable individuals agree that the focus on »systems of care«, or the associated services concepts often described as comprehensive services networks, wrap-around services or a continuum of care, all of which will be discussed, is desirable from both an economic, administrative, and clinical perspective (Bickman 1997). Some of this dissent comes from a concern with the current inadequacies in the evidence base for the treatment of child and adolescent mental disorders and lack of an outcome benefit. Also, an underlying concern related to the support for the development of modern systems of care is the persistent inability to make an adequate argument that the morbidity and long-term costs to society associated with child and adolescent mental disorders deserve the same attention and resources accorded infectious disease. This chapter will give an overview of key elements related to understanding »systems of care«. These ideas and others will be elaborated in later chapters.

2.2 Concepts Needed for Mental Health Services Literacy

2.2.1 »System of Care«

What do we mean by a »system of care«? In its most rudimentary form it is meant to imply that care is not dependent on only one vehicle for treatment such as an inpatient hospital. A system implies that there is a range of services usually considered from least restrictive (community and family based) to most restrictive (hospital based). The concept of a »system« does not necessarily dictate the theoretical orientation of the therapies involved, nor is it uniform in its implementation in all settings. The geographic area covered by a »system« can be as small as a local community or as large as a metropolitan city or country. The usual way to think about a system is to consider that outpatient therapy is a starting point. However, this form of »outpatient« treatment may vary from being located in a school system, carried out in a home, or taking place in a clinic. The next step may involve partial care, that is, use of a more specialized form of care for daytime treatment, often taking the child out of the classroom setting and often off-site for varying periods of time for both therapy and education. Then there are residential care facilities, followed by stand alone inpatient care facilities. Crisis teams, specialized home consultation, psychopharmacology consultation services, and many forms of outreach can enhance the completeness of a system of care.

In a system it is assumed that there is some form of facilitated transfer of the patient between components of the continuum of care. Ensuring this facilitated flow between components of a system is often the most difficult challenge. Reticence to share records, competition for funds, lack of a systems vision are all impediments to the easy flow of the patient from one component to another. Record sharing, while it may seem easy to those not concerned with confidentiality, is quite complicated. The inappropriate sharing of information can lead to discrimination and in its worst aspect lead to labeling and the denial of the patient to take part in the opportunities to achieve what would otherwise be accorded the individual.

2.2.2 »Continuum of Care« and »Wrap-Around Services«

In the West the concept of a »continuum of care« and »wrap-around services« is very much in vogue. In some instances, these terms are used synonymously with a »system of care«. The intent of these concepts is to emphasize the need for an interconnected »system« of care that allows for as much flexibility as possible in meeting the needs of the child patient and the family. Associated with these concepts is the notion that a child should be treated in the least restrictive environment, preferably in their local community or that support be provided in the home. Another aspect of the emphasis in the continuum of care is to balance the once-lopsided dependence on, and inappropriate use of, hospital-based services for children who perhaps did not need and would not benefit from this level of care.

In a continuum of care the patient may be treated at differing levels of care depending on his or her clinical condition at any particular time. Thus, it is possible that many different services will be utilized in the course of an illness. The advantage of a continuum is that it gives the patient, the clinician, and the family options for care that can lessen the stresses on all for the provision of appropriate care at a given level of acuity. For a suicidal adolescent with a clear history of depression it may be indicated to use in-patient care to be followed by partial care with family support and ultimately outpatient care. In some cases, especially those involving somatic illnesses, the continuum may include the pediatrician and the pediatric hospital in the continuum. It this latter case the child mental health clinician may provide consultation to the pediatric caregiver.

A particular challenge in the development of any system of care with a continuum is the incorporation of services for those with alcohol or substance abuse. The system for the care of those with these problems all too often seems to parallel and not interact with the system of care for those seen as having mental disorders. This separation runs counter to the common knowledge among mental health providers of the co-occurrence of comorbidity, i.e., the presence of mental disorders with substance use disorders. Efforts have been made at cross-training to enhance the capacities in each system for the care of those with these comorbid conditions, but much remains to be done in almost all jurisdictions.

2.2.3 Managed Care and Insurance

Two other Western-initiated components of systems of care that are now being entertained world-wide are the use of »managed care« and the move toward privatization. The negative lessons learned in adopting these strategies in the delivery of care are not as well known as the popularization of the concepts among administrators and politicians who see the use of these two strategies as a way to save money. Managed care, which was at one time considered to be a way to streamline care and provide more accountable and appropriate care has often become distorted into a means to have relatively rigid oversight into how care is delivered to reduce the period of time in which care is offered and to control the costs of care. Thus, disallowance of care, reduced reimbursement for care, and other administrative steps have become a part of what is now the formal aspects of managed care. Disease management, that is, a program of specified care for a particular disorder can also be incorporated in systems of care and usually has a managed care component. The negatives of managed care have been centered on the lack of clinically informed management, and the failure to recognize the needs of more seriously impacted children and their families. This has resulted in multiple short-term hospitalizations or shorter periods of outpatient care leading to rehospitalizations or repeat outpatient care for the same illness. Some believe that these consequences have led to children being seen initially in appropriate care when they are sicker and leading to more chronic illness.

2.2.4 Privatization

Privatization has led to the closing or reduction in scope of many publicly supported forms of care. This has often had an impact on the most needy. Privatization is a way in which governments can reduce their funding for programs and shift responsibility for oversight to others outside the government sphere. Unfortunately, in some settings government has gone too far in abdicating responsibility. Along with privatization often comes the introduction of insurance for the care of the mentally ill. This sometimes is a thinly veiled effort to help governments to reduce their costs for programs and personnel. The insurance schemes, especially in poor countries, are inadequate to support the types of care needed in

this new »private sector« for those who cannot afford to supplement the payments of the insurance program. Unfortunately, the net effect has been in many countries to destroy once effective systems of care and replace them with systems that are only effective for the wealthier segments of society who can either pay directly without the use of insurance or can afford to supplement payments. The introduction of insurance in some countries has had the further negative impact of draining the systems of their most qualified clinicians who now enter the »private sector«.

2.3 Current Situation

The World Health Organization, professional organizations, nongovernmental organizations (NGOs), foundations, and governments have all been concerned with how to infuse existing, too often antiquated, modes of care with new knowledge about treatment and prevention. It is obvious that these efforts will require persistence and resource support because of the inertia to change, and the adherence to philosophies of treatment that no longer are consistent with the science base of child mental health and child mental disorders.

World-wide there are varying levels of available services to treat child and adolescent mental disorders. Some countries have simply added child and adolescent services to their adult mental health services with little attention to the special needs of the population. This has led to inappropriate and sometimes harsh conditions for children and adolescents with mental disorders. Institutional care is often the only mode of care available. At the other end of the spectrum there are some countries whose philosophy of care is so psychoanalytically oriented that more contemporary interventions including the use of medications and behavioral therapies are not part of preferred clinical practice. The case is most often that fragmented services exist with outpatient services, where they exist, not having direct linkage to inpatient services. Other failures of linkage are evident between schools and health services, health and mental health services, the juvenile criminal justice system and mental health services, and the private and public sectors.

2.3.1 Policy for Care

It is evident that when no national policy exists that clearly supports child and adolescent mental health services these services remain particularly vulnerable. Without legislation, funding is often reduced when governments face deficits, diverted with the adoption of unstudied fads, or drawn away from specific mental health programs due to competition among stakeholders. Optimal policy development should integrate health, mental health, and education, and respect the unique dimensions of child and adolescent mental health. However, particular needs of children and adolescents affected by mental disorders are often neglected unless a crisis presents itself, such as the posited linkage between vaccines and autism, lead exposure and mental retardation, or exposure to violence and PTSD. Providing for preventive mental health initiatives and mental health promotion is even more problematic given the usual short-term focus of politicians and the demands for easily identified outcomes linked to expenditures.

2.3.2 Cultural Understanding in Providing Care

A global perspective on care demands that we consider not only modern concepts of care often related to various types of intervention and financing, but to better understand and incorporate the wisdom and effective interventions associated with more traditional, culture-specific forms of care. The latter are not as well known in the West, but are essential to incorporate in considering any system of care that will reach the maximal number of people in the most acceptable manner, especially in developing countries. With surges in migration and immigration becoming the norm, no nation can avoid the need to better understand how to treat its immigrant populations. Thus, there is much to be learned in a sharing of concepts and practices throughout the world. Nonwestern perspectives give us added data about the importance of the religious community in the provision of care, about families and their potential strengths, about communities and their capacity to support the ill or fragile. Essential in many countries to achieve a maximal development of services for children with mental disorders, is the invocation of the guarantees under the United Nations Convention on the Rights of the Child.

The latter is particularly true as countries and caregivers face the need to address the mental health needs of growing populations of HIV/AIDS orphans, repatriated soldiers, and other marginalized groups of youth who have aggregated as a result of urbanization and declining economies.

2.3.3 Barriers to Care

While it is hoped that the focus can always be on the positive aspects of systems development, reality suggests that it is also important to look at the barriers to care in the development of systems of care. An appreciation of the barriers will aid the design of systems with the potential for sustainability. Not all barriers are visible or linked to resources. Of those less visible barriers stigma and lack of political will dominate. Other barriers exist because of ignorance of the etiologies and treatability of child and adolescent mental disorders. In some countries significant strides have been made in reducing more concrete barriers to care, such as transportation. However, it is clear that both visible and attitudinal issues remain a significant factor in all societies limiting access to care. Interestingly, one possibly effective lever to reduce barriers and increase access to care receives relatively little attention in clinical care settings, that is, the provisions of the United Nations Convention on the Rights of the Child, which has legal standing in most countries.

2.3.4 Role of Nongovernmental Organizations

The role of nongovernmental organizations (NGOs), and international organizations are critical in shaping and sustaining care. Whether they work in concert with existing country resources for care to develop systems of care varies widely both in relation to the context of their work and the organization's mandate. Too often the response of NGOs is focused on an emergency situation and little attention is given to sustainability. The emphasis on crisis response and the provision of services during the crisis, while most worthwhile, often raises expectations, distorts the existing infrastructure, and then leaves little behind to provide needed basic services. In some instances, the residue of bad feelings leaves the mental health care system in worse condition than prior to the emergency.

2.3.5 Epidemiology

The absence of consistent methodologically sound epidemiological data has hampered the ability to develop services globally based on actual need. Further, the lack of data combined with the lack of a tradition of local needs assessment to inform program development has led to waste and inefficiency in developing systems of care.

This gap is evident in both developing and developed societies. The World Health Organization and others have recognized the need for better data on mental disorders in children and adolescents. A first step in the effort to gather better data globally for potential use at the country level is the WHO ATLAS project related to child and adolescent mental disorders.

2.3.6 Training for Care

Lastly, there is a critical need to develop the cadre of trained individuals who can implement child and adolescent mental health programs. There is an almost universal lack of appropriately trained individuals. Highly specialized child and adolescent psychiatric care will remain scarce, but there is the opportunity to develop training and retraining initiatives tailored to the needs of countries and populations that can meet this gap in resources. Innovative retraining programs, and programs to train paraprofessionals are among the many efforts designed to find feasible ways in which treatment resources can be expanded. Pediatricians, behavioral pediatricians, psychologists, nurses, social workers, primary care clinicians, teachers, and religious leaders all can serve to provide services in some areas of the world. Peers and parents are now being trained for counseling in some of the most innovative programs.

There is a danger in providing care in the modern era that it will be too limited and/or focused on one disorder. Narrowing the focus of training may be efficient, but it can result in a failure to understand the etiology and complexity of child and adolescent mental disorders. A basic mental health literacy needs to be part of the overall training of those working with children with mental health disorders.

2.4   Current Status of »Systems of Care«

It is evident that certain basic steps must be taken in a country to establish the framework for the development of a system of care. The items are many and include: Educating the public, reducing stigma, developing policy, increasing the manpower for service implementation, providing the appropriate physical structure and access points, harmonizing traditional care with more modern types of intervention, finding the funding for new services, and lastly, establishing mechanisms to sustain the services.

2.4.1 Replication of Services

While much is known about service delivery systems in countries around the world, communication of models that might be replicated remains poor. It is clear that the adoption of models created for one society need modification to meet the needs of the particular society wishing to improve its services. Not only are language and culture issues, but financing, training, transportation, and sustainability are also persistent issues. Increasingly, the transmission of models of care have taken place through the development of treatment algorithms, treatment guidelines, and manualized treatment programs. While all of these efforts represent a significant step forward and embrace the current concern with utilizing an »evidence-based« approach, too often the specific cultural adaptation of a model is lacking.

2.4.2 WHO Role and Areas of Concern in Improving Care

The World Health Organization convened an expert panel to deliberate about the status of care for children and adolescents with mental disorders. The report, Caring for Children and Adolescents with Mental Disorders: Setting WHO Directions (WHO 2003) sets out a framework for understanding the overall scope of the problem in establishing systems of care for the treatment of child and adolescent mental disorders. The report emphasizes the need for the provision of »rational« care, that is, care that respects and addresses the clinical needs of the child and provides the appropriate intervention. It argues against excesses or inappropriate care in particular situations. Thus, therapies intended for stable affluent societies may not be appropriate in crisis situations or jurisdictions where there are limited resources. The reliance on any one form of treatment without a consideration of providing care appropriate to the clinical situation and validated by professional experience and research is inappropriate. Noted was a particular trend of pharmaceutical industry promotion of disease-specific treatment suggestions directly to the public, which can be problematic and potentially distort clinical practice.

The panel highlighted the need to find a way to use a diagnostic nomenclature that is more easily grasped by less well-trained individuals and that would make sense to policymakers who have little education in this specialized field. Thus, a consideration was for there to be a broader definition of some disorders that would capture the essence of a range of closely linked disorders and to convey along with the definition the potential for impairment in varying domains, such as education and health.

The development of a system of care requires a financial investment and the personal commitment of individuals in a community—providers, families, educators, social welfare staff, religious leaders, and politicians. It is often overlooked by planners that the original highly touted systems of care, such as the Ventura Plan in California, USA, required a significant financial and personal investment. Iterations of this plan have tried to accomplish the same goals as the original project without making a financial investment and have failed, or been surprised by the costs. The Robert Wood Johnson Foundation for many years supported an initiative to develop and implement systems of care (Saxe et al. 1998). The reports of program implementation have so far pointed to the complexity of the political structures in which programs are embedded, a concern with sustainability after demonstration funds cease, and the need for the education of providers.

2.5 Research and Evaluation

2.5.1 Status of Services Research

The development of systems of care is not solely the enterprise of clinicians and administrators. There is a need to encourage the involvement of health services researchers. The area of child and adolescent mental health services research is in its infancy with

few studies that provide information necessary for planning or which support advocacy for services based on cost-effectiveness. Earls (2001) notes the significant gap that exists between research and practice in relation to community factors in child mental health. It is helpful for all involved in systems development to have an awareness of the basic concepts currently the subject of services research. Among the most important concepts currently being studied are ones related to social ecology and burden of disease. There are more specific economic analyses related to cost-benefit, effectiveness, managed care, and other areas relevant to specific clinical interventions addressed in other chapters that are not a focus of this global overview.

Saxe (1998), following the evaluation of a major child mental health systems initiative in the United States, offered this cautionary note about models of care. »What is clear is that no single model of care seems better than any other. In part, this result reflects the need for each system to develop in synchrony with local needs and culture, but it also reflects our lack of knowledge of what specific treatments are linked with what kinds of success in outcome.« Another cautionary perspective comes from the United States Fort Bragg demonstration project which attempted to look at issues of cost and access with the implementation of a comprehensive system of care. The program gained wide recognition for its findings. However, Bickman's evaluation (1996, 1997) demonstrated that, while care provided could be dramatically expanded, utilization of hospitalization and residential treatment reduced, and treatment better sustained, the clinical outcomes appeared no different than in usual care. This surprising finding came with a demonstration project cost for services one and a half times greater than that for usual care. A debate about systems of care persists to the present.

2.5.2 Disability-Adjusted Life Years

Researchers in the field and clinicians need to become attuned to such concepts as the »burden of disease« which can help us to understand both costs associated with care and the absence of the provision of care. The commonly used measure of burden – disability-adjusted life years (DALYs; Desjarlais et al. 1995) – underestimates the burden of child and adolescent mental disorders due to its relatively small set of identified diagnoses and lack of account-

2

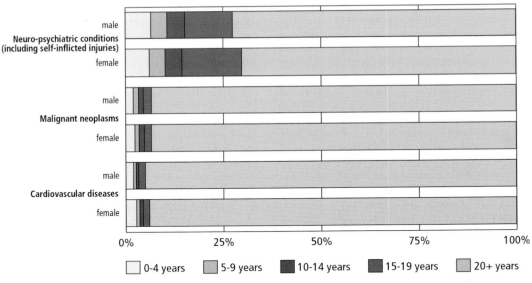

■ **Fig. 2.1.** World: DALYs in 2000 attributable to selected causes by age and sex

ing for longitudinal outcomes. As part of the on-going effort to bring child and adolescent mental health issues to the attention of planners and politicians conceiving of child and adolescent mental health disorders as part of the group of noncommunicable diseases has allowed a new language to develop which gives added weight to concerns with impairment and cost. Thus, understanding mental disorders as noncommunicable diseases is another way to relate the concern for the provision of services to the burden of disease. As noted in ■ Fig. 2.1, the burden in the early years of life associated with child mental disorders including violence is striking compared to other diseases.

2.5.3 Burden of Disease

To support the concern with lifetime costs associated with child and adolescent mental disorders there is a great need for longitudinal studies. Childhood disorders are now known to often be the precursors of adult pathology. Scott (2002) demonstrated the increased costs for care and to society from the childhood diagnosis of conduct disorder. Weissman et al. (1999) demonstrated the poor outcome of adolescent onset depression with associated increased rates of psychiatric and medical hospitalization. Kessler et al. (1995) showed that the early

onset of mental disorders disrupts education and early careers leading to lost productivity (Kessler et al. 1995). An argument can be made that with better data additional support could be accrued for interventions with children and adolescents.

2.5.4 Cultural Epidemiology

Epidemiological study relevant to the provision of services is essential. Such epidemiological data can form the basis of a needs assessment. Needs assessments are too often neglected in the period leading up to the deployment of services. Relying on data from other countries or locales can lead to the development of inappropriate services. Data needs to be locally relevant both in terms of specific services needs and cultural understanding. The recent delineation of »cultural epidemiology« holds the promise of having epidemiological data that truly reflects need by incorporating traditional epidemiological techniques with techniques that capture cultural understandings of disorder/illness (Weiss 2002). Failure to integrate data will lead to a disconnect between the service provided and the needs of the clients. This results in a waste of resources.

2.6 Current Global Initiatives

2.6.1 ATLAS Project

The World Health Organization has embarked on a series of initiatives that should enhance the capacity of countries to develop systems of care for mentally ill children and adolescents. Prime among these initiatives is the ATLAS project. The ATLAS project, Country Resources for Child and Adolescent Mental Health, is one of the first systematic attempts to gather country-wide data on treatment resources for children and adolescents with mental disorders. The survey, using key informants, collects data on demographics, health policy and legislation, mental health financing, mental health services, human resources for care, data collection capacity, care for special populations, and the use of medication. It is not a formal epidemiological study. The database will allow comparisons between countries at differing economic and development levels, but most importantly will inform countries about their own status. The data will be accessible through a web page with materials updated as new information becomes available.

2.6.2 Child and Adolescent Mental Health Policy Module

The ATLAS project is complemented by the Child and Adolescent Mental Health Policy Module of the WHO Mental Health Policy Project. This effort comes with the recognition that there is a virtual world-wide absence of mental health policy for children and adolescents which has hindered service development (Shatkin and Belfer 2004). This document aimed toward Ministers of Health and other policy developers provides precise guidance on policy development to support child and adolescent mental health services. Without policy at the country level there is little guidance for priority setting, financing, and accountability. Further national policy can influence the local utilization of resources. The WHO policy document addresses issues related to the administrative organization for services support at all levels of government and the community. It suggests how a continuum of care can be achieved through specific actions. Most importantly, it provides a guide to developing an accountable system of care. Optimally, national policies will also be in-formed by the needs of populations in the local communities.

2.7 Advocacy for Services

It is a constant challenge to develop and sustain programs to support the care for children and adolescents with mental disorders. Advocacy seeks to keep the needs of these populations on the agenda of nations and communities. Parental advocacy has been a force for the development and maintenance of programs. Professional organizations of all types have also advocated for care, but often advocate in a manner to serve the particular needs of their profession. Competition among the advocates for the mentally has historically been used by less sympathetic legislators and others to thwart program development or resource allocation. Finding common ground among the groups who advocate for those with mental disorders is a priority concern.

2.7.1 United Nations Convention on the Rights of the Child

Not all efforts that improve child and adolescent mental health services relate directly to legislation or specific program initiatives. As mentioned previously, the United Nations Convention on the Rights of the Child is a potentially powerful tool for use with governments to support the development of care for children and adolescents with mental disorders. It gives overall support for children to achieve their maximum potential state of well-being, including mental health, and addresses issues related to stigma and access to care. An instance where the Convention has had a powerful impact is in Brazil. In Brazil there exist Guardianship Councils focused on child well-being. The Guardianship Councils can be seen as a direct outgrowth of the Brazilian governments ratification of the UN Convention of the Rights of the Child. The impact of the Convention was dramatic in its first affects bringing all children, and not just those who violated the law, into the framework of legislation recognizing them as citizens, with their own interests, who should be treated as agents in society and not as passive recipients of philanthropic actions. This first action led to the establishment of Child Rights Councils and Child Guardianship Councils both functioning at the community level, albeit the Rights Council has a macro level view while the Guardianship Council's mission is to ensure that children in need or at risk receive the best possible assistance. Councils can now be found throughout Brazil. It is believed that these Councils have had a positive impact on children's mental health and well-being.

The UN Convention on the Rights of the Child, if implemented by countries that have ratified it, would substantially improve the overall ability of children with mental disorders to be mainstreamed into society, access education, not face incarceration or separation from their families, and receive appropriate treatment. Obviously, in many countries that have adopted the Convention, basic rights are recognized but the full impact of the articles as pertaining to mental health are not appreciated or are seen as secondary to other problems related to exploitation and abuse. Education of advocates, politicians, and administrators is needed to gain the recognition and support for the implementation of those provisions of the Convention that would afford children and adolescents more comprehensive and appropriate mental health care.

2.7.2 Advocacy for Care by Allied Interests

Advocacy for child and adolescent mental health should not be the sole domain of mental health professionals or those impacted by disordered children and adolescents in their families. The health and education sectors have a key role in providing advocacy for child and adolescent mental health services. For the health sector, recognizing the impact of mental disorders on compliance with and adherence to medical regimens, or recognizing the broad range of comorbidities that are likely to be seen in a medical practice should spur on advocacy by the health sector. Likewise, the large number of children who cannot perform or attend school due to child and adolescent mental health disorders should result in the education sector taking a lead in advocating for more and better child and adolescent mental health services. In reality, there are examples in many countries of precisely this type of advocacy taking place.

Child mental health consultation is a routinely and widely dispersed service in Alexandria, Egypt, where the bulk of funding comes from the local education ministry. In Hungary, the Minister of Education plays a major role in the support for child and adolescent mental health services, and in some countries, such as Switzerland, virtually all child

mental health services come under the aegis of the education ministry.

2.8 Systems of Care for Special Populations

In developing and developed countries, caring for special populations presents a particular challenge. With special populations, the intent is to identify individuals such as AIDS orphans, those with physical handicaps, those with chronic medical conditions, and those with learning disabilities who may not have primary mental health problems but whose course is complicated by the presence of a mental disorder continuously or at a point in time. The presence of the mental disorder may impede their full ability to achieve or to maintain their level of functioning.

2.8.1 Mainstreaming

The presence of a mental disorder in a child or adolescent in a special population can further marginalize them. It is important to recognize when a mental disorder becomes manifest in one of these individuals. Failure to recognize the mental disorder and to provide prompt treatment can lead to very serious consequences such as rejection from programs, increased risk of acting out behavior, or suicide. It is new thinking for some to realize that these young people can have more than one problem and, for instance, a retarded individual can become psychotic or a juvenile diabetic can become noncompliant due to depression. The possibility of these dual conditions existing must be appreciated in the evolution of systems of care, both specialized and general.

The focus on care for special populations now emphasizes »participation«, »integration«, and »mainstreaming«. It is recognized by most that it should no longer be acceptable to isolate those with physical handicaps and other disabilities that have in the past resulted in removal from the active participation in society. However, this inclusion remains a global problem. A very current example of the concern can be seen with the growing population of AIDS orphans who are experiencing varying degrees of marginalization depending on the society in which they live. They are denied school access, peers shun them, and sometimes they are even denied basic health care and nutrition.

Though the notion of »mainstreaming« seems intuitively positive, the idea is controversial. Some advocates feel that »mainstreaming« short changes the specific needs of a particular special population. As a counterpoint, others emphasize that failure to »mainstream« a child at the earliest possible time limits the affected child's ability to socialize, and does not give nonaffected peers the opportunity to develop attitudes that can later reduce stigmatization and discrimination.

2.8.2 Learning Disabled

Substantial information is available on how to work with and develop programs for children who present either in the educational system and/or mental health system with a learning disorder and comorbid or primary mental health problem (Fayyad 2001). It is evident that many with learning disorders suffer secondary mental disorders if for no other reason than they become depressed over their lack of achievement or marginalization. However, there is an equal need to recognize those children who present as learning disabled who have a significant primary mental disorder. Failure to recognize the presence of this disorder, possibly a psychosis with minimal behavioral manifestation or an attentional problem, and failure to treat it effectively, can compound the adaptation problems for the child or adolescent. Thus, both educators and mental health clinicians need to improve their literacy about the dimensions of learning disorders to enhance the systems of care needed to maximize the potential of affected children. There are opportunities to develop integrated systems of care for affected children.

2.8.3 Juvenile Delinquents

In countries with a lack of resources, or in countries and locales with a lack of understanding of mental health issues, use of the juvenile justice system as a modality for containment can be excessive. This is particularly the case for children and adolescents whose mental health problems manifest with a range of antisocial or aggressive behavior. In the best of circumstances, entering the juvenile justice system provides the possibility for appropriate diagnostic services for the first time in their lives. However, this salutary outcome is far less common than more usual inappropriate detention or incarceration without an awareness of underlying mental illness. Failure to recognize an underlying or concomitant mental disorder all too frequently results in a worsening of the disorder and a heightened risk of suicide while incarcerated. Certainly the impact of incarceration is rarely, if ever, therapeutic in itself.

There are those children who have evolved into individuals who manifest delinquent behavior not clearly linked to a definable mental disorders. Caring for these children and adolescents judged to be juvenile delinquents is a problem affecting societies throughout the world. Unfortunately, many of those charged with providing care do not have an enlightened attitude toward this population. There is often a failure to recognize the contextual factors leading to the delinquent behavior. The ability to treat these children and adolescents has many obstacles and truly effective programs are relatively rare. However, there is always the need to try to treat because a failure to provide appropriate care leads to recidivism, progression towards ever more serious criminal action, and ultimately societies are deprived of potentially productive individuals. The UN Convention on the Rights of the Child is exercised in some jurisdictions to give these individuals access to care. Finding a way for societies to care for and rehabilitate these youth is a challenge.

2.9 Conclusions

The task of understanding both formal and informal systems of care for children and adolescents with mental disorders is a great challenge. A great deal of research about effective models of care, the financing of care, and the evidence base for treatments must be carried out and the findings disseminated to those responsible for developing services for children and adolescents. While the formal concepts associated with »systems of care« may be controversial, the fact that models are being developed to try to facilitate access and enhance accountability is encouraging. It is evident that negative findings, especially from services initiatives in the West, need to be transmitted to all levels of government and those professionals involved in services development to avoid the consequences which in some instances have not served the best interests of the children and adolescents who are in need. The future offers promise of developing model systems of care adaptable to varying cultures and levels of economic development.

References

Bickman L (1996) A continuum of care: More is not better. American Psychologist, 51:689–701

Bickman L (1997) Resolving issues raised by the Fort Bragg evaluation: New directions for mental health services research. American Psychologist, 52:562–565

Bickman L, Summerfeldt WT, Noser K (1997) Comparative outcomes of emotionally disturbed children and adolescents in a system of services and usual care. Psychiatric Services, 48(12):1543–1548

Carlson M (2001) Child rights and mental health. Child and Adolescent Psychiatric Clinics of North America, 10(4): 825–839

Desjarlais R, Eisenberg L, Good B, et al. (eds) (1995) World Mental Health, New York, Oxford University Press

Earls F (2001) Community factors supporting child mental health. Child and Adolescent Psychiatric Clinics of North America, 10(4):693–709

Fayyad JA, Jahshan CS, Karam EG (2001) Systems development of child mental health services in developing countries in developing countries. Child and Adolescent Psychiatric Clinics of North America, 10(4):745–762

Kessler RC, et al. (1995) Social consequences of psychiatric disorders. I: Educational attainment. American J Psychiatry, 152(7):1026–1032

Saxe L (1998) Evaluating Community-based mental health services for children with serious mental illness: Toward a new paradigm of systems of care. In: Young JG, Ferrari P (eds) Designing Mental Health Services and Systems of Care for Children and Adolescents: A Shrewed Investment Philadelphia, PA, Brunner/Mazel, pp 105–121

Saxe L, Cross TP, Silverman N, et al. (1987) Children's mental health: Problems and services. In: Bickman L, Rog D (eds) Creating a children's mental health service system: Policy, research and evaluation. Durham, NC: Duke University Press

Scott S, Knapp M, Henderson J, et al. (2001) Financial cost of social exclusion: follow-up study of anti-social children into adulthood. Brit Med J, 322:191–195

Shatkin J, Belfer M (In press) The global absence of child and adolescent mental health policy. J Child and Adolescent Mental Health

Weissman MM, Wolk S, Goldstein RB, et al. (1999) Depressed adolescents grown up. JAMA, 281(18):1707–1713

Systems of Care in Europe

Per-Anders Rydelius

3.1   Introduction   – 27

3.2   Roots of the Current Discussion
        About Services   – 27
3.2.1   An Historical Perspective on Services in Europe   – 27
3.2.2   Available Services   – 28

3.3   Methods of Treatment   – 28

3.4   Barriers to Care   – 28

3.5   Disseminating Information   – 28

3.6   Relations with Education   – 29

3.7   Relations with General Psychiatry   – 29

3.8   Relations with Pediatrics   – 30

3.9   Relations with Sociology/Social Work   – 32

3.10   Long-Term Consequences   – 32

3.11   Psychotherapy Versus Treatment Based
        on Biological Psychiatry/Trends   – 32

3.12   Evidence-Based Treatments   – 32

3.13   Conclusions   – 33

        References   – 33

3.1   Introduction

The term »systems of care« refers to two different aspects of caring for children with mental disorders. First, it refers to the structure and organization of the services provided to patients, and second to the ideas and different paradigms that are used to educate the staff to assess, understand, and treat the different child and adolescent psychiatric disorders.

3.2   Roots of the Current Discussion About Services

In May 1992, in Budapest, Hungary the International Association for Child and Adolescent Psychiatry and Allied Professions (IACAPAP) organized a meeting of child and adolescent psychiatrists and allied professionals from the former Soviet Eastern Europe and the West to discuss the current frontiers for child and adolescent psychiatry. While the »Westerners« were eager to present »modern« ideas including neuropsychiatry and genetics, the »Easterners«, »fed up« with neuropsychiatry, were more interested in different alternatives of psychotherapy, social psychiatry, and therapeutic techniques. Some asked for textbooks in psychotherapy and information on the use of Rorschach tests. The ensuing discussions between different schools and paradigms reflecting the complexity of child and adolescent psychiatry and its multidisciplinary origin put much in focus.

3.2.1   An Historical Perspective on Services in Europe

In Europe, services to improve children's mental health have been offered to populations for about 100 years. Both similarities and differences are found when comparing the different countries as described in the volume **Child and Adolescent Psychiatry in Europe, Historical Development, Current Situation and Future Perspectives** edited by Remschmidt and van Engeland. In this book (Remschmidt and van Engeland 1999), authors from 31 different European countries describe child adolescent psychiatry (CAP) in their home countries.

3.2.2 Available Services

Even if there are differences when comparing the European countries to each other and even if the situation in the former Soviet Eastern Europe still lags behind the situation in Western Europe, the following can be stated referring to the structure and organization of the services provided to patients. In the 31 countries described, there are similar kinds of organizations providing CAP services to children, adolescents, parents, and families. There are out- and in-patient departments and day patient services, run by health authorities. In some countries there are special out-patient youth centers, which could be run in collaboration with pediatrics and obstetrics/gynecology departments. There are foster homes and institutions for residential treatment outside hospitals, usually under the supervision or authorization of social welfare authorities and non-governmental organizations. There is also private practice. In the majority of countries there are health insurance systems covering or reducing the costs for CAP care and treatment.

3.3 Methods of Treatment

The treatment programs cover a variety of opportunities for CAP patients ranging from individual treatment based on psychoanalytical and psychodynamic frames of reference to the use of combinations of strategies including individual therapy, group and family therapy, social work, education, occupational therapy, pharmacological treatment, and treatment based on biological psychiatry. In some countries you will find specially designed programs for different disorders and programs to monitor and evaluate treatment effects. Alternatives to hospital-based treatment exist with »home-treatment«.

3.4 Barriers to Care

Although there are some differences, it is quite clear that there is an excellent base for average European children and adolescents to have CAP treatment and there is support for high quality care if needed. Europe is very rich when it comes to research, organizations, structure, and methods in CAP. However, there are also some barriers that need to be broken down in order to fully use the capacity of European

CAP in a way the conditions might allow. In my opinion, for the coming decade the greatest challenge for European CAP is to break down these barriers. As almost all European countries soon will belong to the European Union (EU), European child and adolescent psychiatry will have an excellent chance for a consensus on how the systems of care should be further developed and how barriers should be dealt with. In this respect, the similarities between the different countries may be of special interest, as they reflect the needs of children across countries and over time. Such information may indicate both problems, per se, but also prospects on how the organization and the structure of the services of modern CAP should be developed.

Both problems and prospects are found when analyzing CAP services. There are problems related to the different languages spoken in the countries and the situation of child and adolescent psychiatry in relation to general psychiatry, pediatrics, and behavioral science. In addition, there are issues related to special interests within individual countries, such as juvenile delinquency or autism.

3.5 Disseminating Information

When reading research papers and textbooks on CAP from different countries it is of special interest to analyze the systems of care from the following six perspectives: (a) languages spoken in the countries, (b) trends and relations to education and psychology and relations between CAP and psychiatry, (c) relations between CAP and pediatrics, (d) relations to sociology and social work, (e) psychotherapy versus treatment based on biological psychiatry trends, and (f) questions of special clinical interests The shift to English as the main scientific language after World War II seems to have resulted in a specific problem as major contributions to science from researchers who do not write their papers in English risk being overlooked. The following examples have relevance to CAP. Virtually unrecognized in the English language, the fetal alcohol syndrome (FAS) was described in French (Lemoine et al. 1968) a couple of years before the description of FAS from the United States (Ulleland et al. 1970; Jones et al. 1973). The Asperger syndrome and the similarities/differences between the Asperger and the Kanner syndromes were well described in German CAP text-books more than a decade before Lorna Wing made her publications in English and some 25 years before it appeared in the DSM-system. In the German-speaking countries, there are a number of treatment programs developed, together with instruments and questionnaires to assess CAP problems, to monitor treatment, and to do follow-up, etc. These methods are of a very high quality but not well recognized outside the language area. From this perspective it is rewarding to read German CAP textbooks and the German Journal of Child and Adolescent Psychiatry, **Zeitschrift für Kinder- und Jugendpsychiatrie und Psychotherapie.**

It is a challenge for European CAP to solve the language problem. It may be a barrier for the development of good treatment. There are good examples indicating advantages of having a multilingual situation. In Switzerland, where three different languages are spoken, it is obvious that the development of child and adolescent psychiatry was influenced in a very fruitful way by Italy, France, Austria, and Germany. This is illustrated by the fact that already at the time of World War II a modern textbook in CAP, **Allgemeine Kinderpsychiatrie,** was published by Moritz Tramer and a scientific child psychiatric journal, the **Zeitschrift für Kinderpsychiatrie** was edited, which, under its later name, **Acta Paedopsychiatrica,** was IACAPAP's official organ during the 1960s. **Acta Paedopsychiatrica** illustrated a model to handle the language problem as it was possible to write papers either in English, German, or French with abstracts provided in all three languages. Although expensive and needing difficult editing, such a journal should perhaps be re-established to facilitate information exchange. In 2003, Pierre Ferrari in France presented the idea to launch a »European Textbook of Child and Adolescent Psychiatry«, an initiative that would also reduce a barrier for the development of good treatment.

3.6 Relations with Education

It was found that a specific CAP interest in education appeared, disappeared, and reappeared over time in different countries. A hundred years ago, CAP pioneers in Italy (M. Montessori, S. de Sanctis, G. Montesano), in France (A. Binet), and in Spain (A. Vidal Perera), had an interest in child and adolescent psychopathology, mental retardation, and psychotic behaviors as evidenced by articles in textbooks in our discipline and in efforts to provide children with better services. They were interested in the relationships between the cognitive functioning of the child and the teaching situation, i.e., the relationships between child and adolescent psychiatry, cognitive psychology/education, and psychopathology. As pioneers, they developed systems for CAP care of children.

Other early European examples of fruitful contributions to CAP from education/psychology focused on ways to identify, understand, and treat children having cognitive problems. Among these are the »Vienna School« for developmental psychology, Binet's work on I.Q., and Piaget's work on cognitive psychology. In the »previous« Central Europe, i.e., in Austria, Switzerland and Germany (the German-speaking countries) and in today's Czech Republic, Slovakia, Hungary, and Slovenia, there is an old CAP tradition related to education going back to the »Heilpädagogische« tradition. In Russia and in the Nordic countries you will also find such early interests going back to the late 1800s focusing upon cognitive psychology/education, mental retardation, the relationships between child and adolescent psychiatry, and how children show learning difficulties. As a result, school psychiatry had already developed as a branch of child and adolescent psychiatry in Sweden and Switzerland by the time of World War I. Obviously this early interest in children's cognitive development and the relation between CAP and education disappeared over time until today, when it has reappeared as »cognitive psychology«, »neuropsychology«, »neuropsychiatry«, or as »cognitive science«.

CAP care of children should involve cooperation with education and schools. In many modern European countries, children are spending 12 important years of their lives at school. This gives an opportunity for CAP to develop preventive measures. Important questions include the organization of the school, teaching techniques and how children with learning difficulties should be taught.

3.7 Relations with General Psychiatry

The links and the relationships between CAP and general psychiatry are obvious. In many European countries child and adolescent psychiatry has one of it major roots in hospital psychiatry. One reason was that many children and adolescents with childhood onset pervasive problems traditionally were treated in asylums and mental hospitals. The two disciplines share clinical problems/disorders of different kinds where cooperation is needed, as caring systems overlap each other. Among these clinical entities are children suffering from mental retardation or pervasive developmental disorders, adolescent patients with anorexia nervosa, and adolescents with early onset schizophrenia and bipolar disorders, as these groups need continuous support when they are becoming adults. Cooperation also includes programs for children of psychotic parents and when a parent's disorder affects their children (including traumatic experiences and neglect) or when a depressed mother has committed suicide. Programs are needed to support children of alcoholics, drug abusers, and parents having personality disorders that affect their parenting capacities.

All over Europe, CAP and general psychiatry do cooperate, but from quantitative and qualitative aspects in very different ways. However, important questions need to be addressed.

3.8   Relations with Pediatrics

In some countries, i.e., Austria, Finland, Germany, Italy, and Sweden, the links to disciplines other than psychiatry, such as pediatrics and neurology, are equally strong. In France until 1968, neurology and psychiatry were considered as »neuropsychiatry« and not separated from each other. In some countries, i.e., Sweden, wards for inpatient child psychiatric care developed within children's hospitals while wards for inpatient adolescent psychiatric care developed within hospitals for general psychiatry. In Austria, the pediatrician Professor Hans Asperger was head of the Vienna University Clinic for Pediatrics and of a special unit for Heilpädagogik/curative education, one type of child and adolescent psychiatric service, while a ward for child and adolescent neuropsychiatry was developed within general psychiatry. In Finland, separate specialties for child psychiatry and adolescent psychiatry have been established.

In those countries where CAP has developed in close relation to pediatrics, a true cooperation with mutual benefits has also developed. Besides traditional consultation-liaison work, cooperation and special programs have been developed to support pregnant mothers, newborns suffering from obstetrical/neonatal complications, children with malignant diseases, neglected and abused children, etc. Psychosomatic wards within pediatric clinics led by child and adolescent psychiatrists have been established. In countries where the cooperation has not been extensive, »sub disciplines« of pediatrics, such as »social pediatrics« or »behavioral pedia-

trics« have instead been developed within pediatrics covering CAP aspects.

As is the case with general psychiatry, CAP and pediatrics do share clinical problems/disorders of different kinds where cooperation is needed and where the caring systems overlap each other. Among these clinical entities are children suffering from mental retardation or pervasive developmental disorders, obesity, anorexia nervosa, etc. Together with the pediatricians, child and adolescent psychiatrists have also developed programs to support parents and siblings when children are suffering from chronic diseases, tumors, need transplantation, suffer from severe trauma or are dying. As CAP and pediatrics (especially pediatric endocrinology and neuropediatrics) share a developmental perspective from conception to adolescence, the two disciplines have a unique opportunity to investigate normal and deviant development of cognition, behavior, and the development of psychopathology.

A prospective study by Jonsell in Sweden (Jonsell 1977 a, b; □ Table 3.1) shows the significant relevance of such symptoms in daily pediatric care. Over one year he studied patients at a pediatric outpatient department to test a hypothesis with particular reference to psychological and social background factors among pediatric patients. He found CAP factors in every seventh pediatric patient. Significant CAP problems were found in every twentieth patient. The proportion of such cases increased with age to 17% among the 10–15-year-olds. Compared with the controls, the parents of these patients, the mothers in particular, had a higher frequency of registered sickness for mental-nervous disorders and their families had more frequently been the subject of special social inquiries or assistance. »To a large extent the examining pediatrician was unaware of these background conditions.«

Quite similar to the situation between CAP and general psychiatry, CAP and pediatrics do cooperate all over Europe, but from quantitative and qualitative aspects in very different ways. Within the EU, the two disciplines should try to reach a consensus as to how systems of care should be developed in order to meet the different demands put upon the organizations and as to how prevention should be worked out.

Children with CAP symptoms of somatic origin will show up among general practitioners and/or pediatricians. If there is an excellent cooperation with CAP, these children may be recognized and, if necessary, immediately supported by and cared for by CAP. In this way CAP can develop, in a timely fash-

◻ **Table 3.1.** Summary of Swedish longitudinal prospective studies with relevance to child and adolescent psychiatry

Sample	Discipline	Criminal record	Registered alcohol problems	Followup period
Samples of boys who themselves had shown/been treated for early symptoms of delinquency				
Psychopathic boys treated at the Mellansjö-treatment home	CAP	41%	28%	1928–1968
Delinquent boys treated at the Children's Village SKÅ	CAP	67%	58%	1954–1973 (Andersson et al. 1976)
Young law-breakers	CAP, sociology, psychology, criminology	39%	46%	1960–1972
From the general population				(SOU1973: 25)
Teenage alcoholics	CAP	42%		1964–1985
			58%	1964–1977 (Rydelius 1985)
Samples of boys who had not primarily shown early symptoms of delinquency				
Adopted children with heredity for social problems/alcoholism	CAP	14%	21%	1930–1972 (Bohman 1978)
Children with alcoholic fathers	CAP	42%	35%	1958–1978 (Rydelius 1981)
Samples of CAP patients				
2,164 patients from the Stockholm CAP outpatient service	CAP	23% 3% girls	23% 3% girls	1953–1975 (Nylander 1979)
1,420 patients from CAP in- and out patient services	CAP	50% boys 20% girls		1976–2003 (Enqvist et al. 2004)
Problem-free groups from the general population				
Lundby project	Psychiatry	8%		1947–1987
			10%	1947–1972 (Öjesjö 1983; Fried 1995)
222 boys	CAP	15%	19%	1954–1973 (Andersson et al. 1976)
Controls/»social twins« to children of alcoholic fathers	CAP	25%	20%	1958–1978 (Rydelius 1981)
The Metropolitan project Criminology	Sociology	31%		1963–1979 (Jansson 1975; Wikström 1987)
The Solna Study	Pediatrics CAP Psychology	35%	22%	1955–1988 (Stattin et al. 1989; Bohman et al. 2000)
The IDA project	Psychology	38%		1965–1985
			17%	1965–1980 (Magnusson et al. 1975; Stattin et al. 1989)

ion, prevention programs and offer good care and treatment when needed.

3.9 Relations with Sociology/Social Work

In many European countries, the establishment of CAP was inspired by the US child guidance movement. In some countries, these child guidance clinics did develop as true CAP outpatient departments led by child and adolescent psychiatrists and based on a cooperation within a team consisting of a child and adolescent psychiatrist, a psychologist, a social worker, and a teacher, while in other countries there were departments for guidance to parents by psychologists and social workers with or without the help of a consultant child and adolescent psychiatrist.

One of the ideas behind the child guidance clinics was to prevent and treat antisocial behavior in children and teenagers. The work was based on a multidisciplinary team where CAP, psychology, sociology/social work, and education cooperated.

As a consequence, the work within today's CAP out- and inpatient departments often includes »forensic child and adolescent psychiatry«. The work includes preparing reports to police authorities, to courts, and to social authorities when neglect, child abuse, or child sexual-abuse, etc. is suspected, when parents divorce, or when a person under the age of 18 has committed a serious crime.

3.10 Long-Term Consequences

In reference to CAP, study results indicate that the majority of children seeking advice and help from CAP for behavioral problems are not facing psychiatric disorders as adults, but are at risk for developing criminality and alcohol/drug abuse. Quite clearly, prior and current information support the notion that a multidisciplinary view is needed if CAP is to achieve the objective of engaging in the prevention of delinquency in youth. This is a true challenge for the future of CAP and also has implications for the organization of services.

3.11 Psychotherapy Versus Treatment Based on Biological Psychiatry/Trends

Today's European CAP has adopted an integrated view of biology, behavioral science, and psychodynamics. Thus, a »multidisciplinary« view on how children and adolescents will be assessed and treated is emphasized in Remschmidt's and van Engeland's volume **Child and Adolescent Psychiatry in Europe, Historical Development, Current Situation and Future Perspectives** (edited by Remschmidt and Engeland 1999). The following examples illustrate the current situation. In Austria, work is based on a holistic approach according to »somatic, intellectual, emotional, and social aspects« also using a »psychotherapeutic polypragmasy« where different psychotherapeutic techniques are »linked together«. In France: »The majority of the inpatient and outpatient departments use an eclectic approach with the integration of different methods, including family counseling and family therapy, and also, if indicated, medication.« In Norway, the work is based on a »bio-psycho-social model«. In Germany, this integration of biology and psychodynamics is illustrated by the fact that since 1993 the discipline of CAP has been called »child and adolescent psychiatry and psychotherapy«. It is quite clear that this integration has been very fruitful as treatment programs of different kinds have been developed and provided a base for »evidence based treatment« to be established.

3.12 Evidence-Based Treatments

As discussed above and summarized below, there are some questions of special interest referring to CAP and cooperation with school/education, general psychiatry, and pediatrics that need to be further explored in order to improve the quality of CAP assessment and treatment. Similarly, questions relating to overall prevention for mental health and how to deal with delinquency are of special interest for CAP.

Europe is very rich when it comes to research, organizations, structure, and methods in CAP. The time has come when European CAP should strongly engage in developing evidence-based programs for treatment and prevention. Such efforts are ongoing in some European countries. Local and European guidelines have been developed for certain disorders. However, with a few exceptions, there is a lack of treatment programs that have been scientifically evaluated.

German CAP has taken good initiatives. The efficacy of inpatient vs. home treatment of psychiatrically disturbed children and adolescents (Mattejat et al. 2001) has been evaluated and home treatment was found to have a favorable impact. A reliable and valid method for routine quality assurance and therapy evaluation has been developed using telephone interviews (Mattejat et al. 2003).

European CAP should engage in all kinds of efforts to prevent mental ill health. Educating politicians could be one way to do this. Perhaps a goal for European preventive CAP work could be a future EU committee focused on planning for the needs of children.

3.13 Conclusions

Although, European CAP is very developed when it comes to research, organizations, structure, and methods, there are barriers that need to be »broken down« in order to fully use the available capacity. One such barrier is the lack of a »multilingual« scientific journal. Almost all European countries will soon belong to the European Union. This will give European CAP an excellent opportunity to educate politicians on children's needs and to reach a European CAP consensus on how the systems of care should be further developed.

Another future development should involve cooperation with educators and schools. In many modern European countries, children are spending 12 important years of their lives at school. This important period of a child's life should be used by CAP to develop preventive measures in cooperation with school authorities. Important questions include the organization of the school day, teaching techniques, and programs against bullying and how children with learning difficulties should be taught. A priority for European CAP is the unique opportunity to develop evidence-based treatment. All over Europe, CAP and general psychiatry do cooperate, but from quantitative and qualitative aspects in very different ways. Some important questions need to be solved. One question refers to whether early symptoms/phases of schizophrenia/bipolar disorders exist or not. Children with CAP symptoms of somatic origin will appear before general practitioners and/or pediatricians before they

appear at CAP departments. The development of cooperative arrangements with pediatrics will enhance prevention efforts.

References

Andersson M, Jonsson G, Kälvesten AL (1976) Hur går det för 50-talets Stockholmspojkar. Stockholms Kommuns Monografiserie nr 38, Stockholm [in Swedish]

Bohman M (1978) Some genetic aspects of alcoholism and criminality. Arch Gen Psych 35:19–25.

Bohman M, Wennberg P, Andersson T (2000) Alcohol habits in a suburban male cohort. Scand J Public Health 28(4):275–282.

Emminghaus H (1887) Die Psychischen Störungen des Kindesalters. Laupp, Tübingen

Engqvist U, Rydelius PA (2004) Deaths and suicides among former child and adolescent psychiatric patients. Submitted manuscript

Fried I (1995) The Mellansjö School-Home – Psychopathic children admitted 1928–1940, their social adaptation over 30 years; a longitudinal prospective follow-up. Acta Paediatrica, Suppl 408

Giller H, Hagell A, Rutter M (1998) Antisocial Behavior by Young People, Cambridge University Press

Glück S, Glück ET (1970) Toward a typology of juvenile offenders: Implications for therapy and prevention. Grune & Stratton, New York

Jansson CG (1975) Project Metropolitan, a presentation. Project metropolitan. Research Report No 1. Department of Sociology, University of Stockholm, Stockholm

Jones KL, Smith DW, Ulleland CN, Streissguth P (1973) Pattern of malformation in offspring of chronic alcoholic mothers. Lancet 9:1(7815):1267–1271

Jonsell R (1977a) Patients at a paediatric out-patient clinic. A study with particular reference to psychological and social background factors. I. The problem, material, methods and actual visit. Acta Paediatr Scand 66:6:723–728

Jonsell R (1977b) Patients at a paediatric out-patient clinic. A study with particular reference to psychological and social background factors. II. Earlier contacts with the health service, social background, parents' morbidity, general discussion and recommendations. Acta Paediatr Scand 66:6:729–734

Kanner L (1964) A history of the care and study of the mentally retarded. Springfield, Ill, USA

Lemoine P, Harousseau H, Borteyru JP, Menuet JC (1968) Les enfants de parents alcooliques. Anomalies observées. A propos de 127 cas. Quest Méd 25:476–482

Macfarlane JW (1938) Studies in Child Guidance. I. Methodology of Data Collection and Organization. Monogr Soc Res Child development 3:6

Macfarlane JW, Allen L, Honzik MP (1954) A developmental study of the behavior problems of normal children between twenty-one months and fourteen years. UC Press, LA

Magnusson D, Dunér A, Zetterblom G (1975) Adjustment: A longitudinal study. Wiley, New York

Mattejat F, Hirt BR, Wilken J, Schmidt MH, Remschmidt H (2001) Efficacy of inpatient and home treatment in psychiatrically disturbed children and adolescents. Follow-up assessment of the results of a controlled treatment study. Eur Child Adolesc Psychiatry Suppl I:171–179.

Mattejat F, Hirsch O, Remschmidt H (2003) Value of telephone interview for quality assurance and therapy evaluation in child and adolescent psychiatry. Review of the literature and empirical results of participation quota and possible sampling bias. Z Kinder Jugendpsychiatr Psychother 31:1:17–34

Nicolson R, Rapoport JL (1999) Childhood onset schizophrenia: rare but worth studying. Biological Psychiatry 46: 1418–1428.

Nylander I (1979) A 20-year prospective follow-up study of 2164 cases at the Child Guidance Clinics in Stockholm. Acta Paed Scand, Suppl 276

Öjesjö L (1983) An epidemiological investigation of alcoholism in a total population. The Lundby Study. University of Lund, Lund

Remschmidt H (2002) Early-onset schizophrenia as a progressive-deteriorating developmental disorder: evidence from child psychiatry. J Neural Transm 109:1:101–117 Review

Remschmidt H, van Engeland H (1999) Child and Adolescent Psychiatry in Europe – Historical Development, Current Situation and Future Perspectives. Steinkopff/Springer, Darmstadt/New York

Remschmidt H, Schulz E, Martin M, Warnke A, Trott GE (1994 a) Childhood-onset schizophrenia: history of the concept and recent studies. Schizophr Bull 20:4:727–745

Remschmidt H, Schulz E, Martin M, Fleischhaker C, Trott GE (1994 b) [Early manifestations of schizophrenic psychoses] Z Kinder Jugendpsychiatr 22:4:239–252 [Article in German]

Robins LN (1966) Deviant children grown up: a sociological and psychiatric study of sociopathic personality. Williams & Wilkins, Baltimore

Rydelius PA (1981) Children of Alcoholic Fathers. Their social adjustment and their health status over 20 years. Acta Paediatrica Scand, Suppl 286

Rydelius P-A (1985) Long-term prognosis for the young alcohol abuser. In: Alcohol and the Developing Brain, (Eds U Rydberg, C Alling, J Engel) pp 187–191. Raven Press Books Ltd

Silberg J, Rutter M, D'Onofrio B, Eaves L (2003) Genetic and environmental risk factors in adolescent substance use. J Child Psychol Psychiatry 44:5:664–676

SOU:2 (1999) Steriliseringsfrågor i Sverige 1935–1975 – Ekonomisk ersättning. Delbetänkandet av 1997 års steriliseringsutredning [in Swedish]. The Swedish Government, Stockholm

SOU:20 (2000) Steriliseringsfrågan i Sverige 1935–1975 Historisk belysning – Kartläggning – Intervjuer. Slutbetänkande från 1997 års steriliseringsutredning [in Swedish]. The Swedish Government, Stockholm

SOU:25 (1973) Statens Offentliga Utredningar, Unga Lagöverträdare III. Hem, uppfostran, skola och kamratmiljö i belysning av intervju- och uppföljningsdata. The Swedish Government, Stockholm

Sporn AL, Greenstein DK, Gogtay N, Jeffries NO, Lenane M, Gochman P, Clasen LS, Blumenthal J, Giedd JN, Rapoport JL (2003) Progressive brain volume loss during adolescence in childhood-onset schizophrenia. Am J Psychiatry 160:12:2181–2189

Stattin H, Klackenberg-Larsson I (1989) Delinquency as related to parents' preferences for their child's gender. Reports from the Departments of Psychology, University of Stockholm No 686, Stockholm

Stattin H, Magnusson D, Reichel H (1989) Criminal activity of different ages. A study based on a Swedish longitudinal research population. British Journal of Criminology 29: 4:368–385

Ulleland C, Wennberg RP, Igo RP, Smith NJ (1970) The offspring of alcoholic mothers. Pediat Res 4:474

Wikström POH (1987) Patterns of crime in a birth-cohort. Age, sex and class differences. Project metropolitan. Research Report No 24. Department of Sociology, University of Stockholm, Stockholm

Systems of Care in North America

Katherine E. Grimes

4.1   Introduction – 35

4.2   Systems of Care in the USA – 35
4.2.1   Values and Principles for Systems of Care – 35
4.2.2   Phases of Knowledge Development – 36
4.2.2.1   Phase I: Infrastructure – 36
4.2.2.2   Phase II: Wraparound – 37
4.2.2.3   Phase III: Blended Funding/Shared Governance – 37
4.2.2.4   Phase IV: Integrated Care – 38

4.3   Systems of Care in Canada – 39

4.4   Conclusions – 40

References – 41

4.1   Introduction

Child and adolescent mental health care in North American has historically gotten lost somewhere between pediatrics and psychiatry. Although child mental health clinicians share a population of concern with pediatricians and other primary care providers, child psychiatry is not considered a pediatric medicine specialty area but rather a psychiatric one. The bulk of the psychiatric »business«, however, deals with adults and, therefore, has closer ties to internal medicine than to child psychiatry. This creates a no-man's land organizationally, where service need and responsibility are disconnected (Rae-Grant 1986). Adding to the disconnect are the barriers of stigma (families experiencing shame when their child has a mental illness) and scarcity. (The subspecialty of child psychiatry produces very few doctors compared to other medical specialties, and both the training of psychiatric nurses and that of clinical social workers is focused on adults.)

Even in a child-oriented setting, like the pediatrician's office, a family may be loathe to voice concerns about their child's emotional health, and even if the concern is voiced, the pediatrician may have far greater trouble locating appropriate consultation for evidence of a thought disorder than for evidence of leukemia (AACAP 1999).

4.2   Systems of Care in the USA

4.2.1   Values and Principles for Systems of Care

Additionally, in the USA, medicine has been dominated over the past fifteen years by managed care, with the economic driver being what »benefit package« (or array of services) the employer will agree to buy. Employers, understandably, are concerned with the health of their employees, so benefits (and care) are oriented toward adults, not children or families (Lourie 1996). More recently, the emergence of mental health »carve-outs« (where another entity, usually a for-profit company, takes over the management of mental health benefits for a health plan), has shifted mental health treatment still further away from primary care, leaving pediatrics and child mental health even more isolated from each other (Grimes 2003).

These health care delivery issues combine to exacerbate the fragmentation that accompanies most other service delivery for children and families. It is a common experience for families to find themselves struggling to communicate about their child to schools and mental health, juvenile justice, and social service systems that do not communicate with each other (Koyanagi 1993). Funding for services is often designed along bureaucratically simple but clinically unrealistic lines of mutual exclusivity that can cause delays and increased morbidity for families seeking help (Cole 1993).

Against this backdrop of increasing frustration on the part of family members and providers, as well as alarm voiced by advocates at growing numbers of youths in hospitals or placed out of home, a consensus emerged that there must be a better way to respond to the needs of children and families (Knitzer 1982). Beginning with the federally sponsored Child and Adolescent Service System Program, or CASSP, in 1984 (Stroul 1986), and aided by the Robert Wood Johnson Foundation's Mental Health Services Programs for Youth, or MHSPY, in 1988 (Saxe 1998), multiple initiatives have been launched across the USA to demonstrate the added value of intensively coordinated care, organized around family needs and based on existing strengths. The most successful of these initiatives have been founded on the so-called CASSP Principles (Stroul 1986), outlined below in ◘ Table 4.1. In fact, the degree to which the programs are consistent with these principles appears directly related to their sustainability (Koyanagi 2000).

The knowledge base underpinning child and adolescent systems of care has grown over the 15 years since its inception. There appear to be four related but distinct phases of knowledge development that have contributed to what is now understood as »Child and Adolescent Systems of Care«.

4.2.2 Phases of Knowledge Development

4.2.2.1 Phase I: Infrastructure

Initially, there was the realization, so well articulated by Jane Knitzer, that large numbers of children in need were going without services, and that what services were available were being delivered in isolation from each other. The CASSP movement, supported by generous federal Child Mental Health Service Initiative grant dollars, encouraged better coordination and communication between service providers and

---

◘ **Table 4.1.** Values and principles for the systems of care

Core values

The system-of-care should be child centered and family focused, with the needs of the child and family dictating the types and mix of services provided

The system-of-care should be community based, with the locus of services as well as management and decision making responsibility resting at the community level

The system-of-care should be culturally competent, with agencies, programs, and services that are responsive to the cultural, racial, and ethnic differences of the populations they serve

---

Guidelines

Children with emotional disturbances should have access to a comprehensive array of services that address the child's physical, emotional, social, and educational needs

Children with emotional disturbances should receive individualized services in accordance with the unique needs and potentials of each child and guided by an individualized service plan

Children with emotional disturbances should receive services within the least restrictive, most normative environment that is clinically appropriate

The families and surrogate families of children with emotional disturbances should be full participants in all aspects of the planning and delivery of services

Children with emotional disturbances should receive services that are integrated, with linkages between child-serving agencies and programs and mechanisms for planning, developing and coordinating services

Children with emotional disturbances should be provided with case management or similar mechanisms to ensure that multiple services are delivered in a coordinated and therapeutic manner and that they can move through the system of services in accordance with their changing needs

Early identification and intervention for children with emotional disturbances should be promoted by the system-of-care in order to enhance the likelihood of positive outcomes

Children with emotional disturbances should be ensured smooth transitions to the adult service system as they reach maturity

The rights of children with emotional disturbances should be protected, and effective advocacy efforts for children and youth with emotional disturbances should be promoted

Children with emotional disturbances should receive services without regard to race, religion, national origin, sex, physical disability, or other characteristics, and services should be sensitive and responsive to cultural differences and special needs

related agencies and institutionalized awareness that communities needed a responsive and responsible »infrastructure« within which to provide services. The degree to which grant applicants were consistent with the CASSP principles often guided decisions regarding funding support and subsequent growth and development of community-based infrastructures to deliver services to children and families.

4.2.2.2 Phase II: Wraparound

Overlapping in time with the CASSP initiatives and sharing, as well, an origin in the community psychiatry efforts of a decade earlier, the consumer movement within mental health gained momentum and forever changed how patients and families were viewed by mental health professionals. For children and youths, the emergence of the necessity of »family friendly« interventions contributed to the development of individualized services and supports known as the wraparound process (Vandenberg 1996). The dissemination of this process, which emphasizes identification of **needs** across a set of life domains and the use of child and family **strengths** in building interventions, continues to influence the design of systems of care across the USA. An adaptation of the life domain concept developed by John Vandenberg is displayed in ◘ Fig. 4.1 (Vandenberg 1998).

4.2.2.3 Phase III: Blended Funding/ Shared Governance

The Mental Health Services Program for Youth initiative, privately funded via the Robert Wood Johnson Foundation (RWJF) and the Washington Business Group on Health (WBGH), took the CASSP pilot efforts a step further in an effort to accomplish the development of local systems of care that did not depend on infusions of federal grant dollars. As the CASSP principles and the wraparound process became better known, the idea that existing dollars could be redirected to create and sustain such systems of care was jointly promoted by RWJF and WBGH (Cole 1993). The concept of blended funding across categorically distinct state agencies, which required collaboration and shared commitment to achieve, launched a new series of state and local pilot programs and the beginnings of a research base on cost effectiveness (Saxe 1999). The RWJF MHSPY experience, in turn, influenced the administration of the federally funded CMHS systems of care grant sites for children. Several of these former grant sites now rely on funding from multiple public agencies, including Medicaid; examples include Santa Barbara, Vermont, Stark County, »Wraparound Milwaukee« and Maine (see Koyanagi 2000, for full list). RWJF and the Washington Business Group on Health next chose to fund twelve »MHSPY-replication« sites in 1997. All were to be value-based on CASSP principles, use the wraparound process, develop a blended funding process across child serving agencies and deliver services via managed care (Grimes 2001). Two of these sites have grown and are now sustained via existing state agency budgets: one, the »Dawn Project« in Indiana, after five years of federal CMHS dollars now uses braided funding across several state agencies; the other, »Massachusetts-MHSPY« in Massachusetts, was never funded by CMHS but went directly to blended funding from its five major stakeholder state agencies to create a comprehensive capitation rate (Pires 2002).

◘ Figure 4.2 is a visual representation of the possible areas of responsibility and sources of funding that a child in major difficulties may have. Examples of current ways the dollars may be being spent are included. The clinical care managers within the system-of-care, working closely with the family, may choose to maintain those same services (i.e., hospital) and just pick up the cost, or may choose to reallocate resources (i.e., from individual therapy to an after-school program) depending on the child's

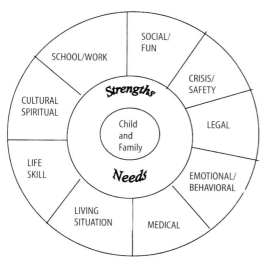

◘ Fig. 4.1. Strengths and needs assessment across child and family life domains. Phase III: Blended Funding/Shared Governance

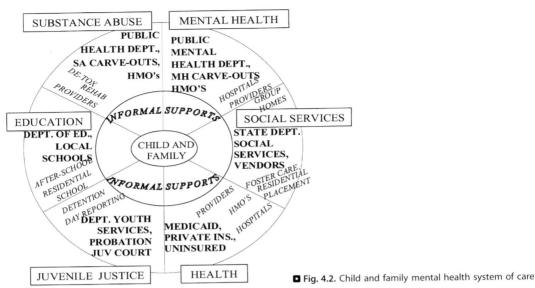

● Fig. 4.2. Child and family mental health system of care

needs. In an ideal scenario, the agencies or stakeholders involved combine resources but retain their mandates and participate in a collaborative, shared governance over the system-of-care that offers the opportunity to influence and inform policy decisions. Together they are able to make more of a difference in a child's life than any single entity, mindful of financial and categorical constraints.

4.2.2.4 Phase IV: Integrated Care

Despite close to twenty years of USA government spending on first CASSP then CMHS grants to promote child mental health systems of care, efforts to evaluate the results have proven controversial (Burns 1990; Bickman 1996; Friedman 1996). It has been necessary to establish distinctions between methodologies suited for individual clinical outcomes versus measures of systemic change. In addition to these issues, health care delivery has shifted repeatedly, first to managed care, then to behavioral health carve-outs, during the same time that these systems of care were being initiated and evaluated. Finding appropriate baseline measurements, as well as relevant comparison populations have both been difficult. Systems were clearly changing, care was being delivered in more »family friendly« ways, but the jury was still out on whether youths were actually clinically benefiting more from the new infrastructure constructs.

However, a unique effort since 1998 by the Mental Health Services Program for Youth in Massachusetts is providing a new level of clinical outcomes information which suggests a direct association between involvement in the system of care and reduced risk of harm to self or others, use of substances and/or being placed out of the community. This system-of-care is the only one to include physical health care within the overall system, resulting in the integration of medical, social, educational, mental health, and substance abuse care. Five years worth of outcomes information indicate that highly coordinated, actively integrated care delivery appears to be providing positive effects at the overall program level, as well as for the majority of individual children. The hypothesized effect modifier is »**continuity of intent**«: an alignment of goals and interventions on behalf of a consistent mission determined by the family and processed using consensus methods within the members of the child's Care Planning Team (Grimes 2003). Crucial to this »continuity of intent« is the resonance of shared mission throughout both administrative and clinical aspects of the system. There is high-level shared governance provided by the stakeholder leadership within the Steering Committee, which determines the system policy and authorizes funding. Next, there is a layer of operational and implementation support provided in the Area Level Operations Team by the local system partners who control immediate resources and supply the referrals into the system. At the front

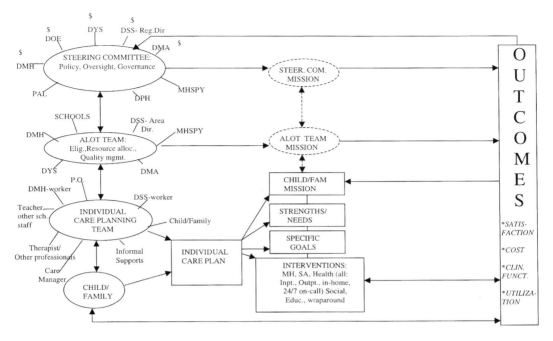

Note: **PAL** = Parent Advocacy League; **DMH** = Department of Mental Health; **DOE** = Department of Education; **DYS** = Juvenile Justice; **DSS** = Child Protection; **DMA** = Medicaid; **DPH** = Department of Public Health; **Schools** = local school districts.

◘ **Fig. 4.3.** Massachusetts MHSPY System of Care

lines, change is mediated by the individual Care Planning Team (CPT), which is formed around the family and includes both professional providers and nonprofessionals chosen by the family. This team first identifies strengths and needs for each child. Next, the CPT builds an individualized mission, determines the goals, based on needs, to support the mission, and builds interventions to support the goals, using existing strengths. Measurement and accountability permeate the entire system and every goal's progress is documented on a monthly basis. Multiple standardized instruments to determine child and family functioning are used, as well as tracking of all expenses and service types. The outcomes, both clinical and administrative, are reported at regular intervals by the system-of-care back to the stakeholders and purchasers of the care, as well as to the consumers and providers. This information supports continuous quality improvement and the opportunity to study the effectiveness of selected interventions at both individual and aggregate levels. An illustration of the way this integrated system-of-care example functions is provided in ◘ Fig. 4.3.

SAMHSA, the U.S. Substance Abuse and Mental Health Services Administration, recently released a report consistent with the findings of the Massachusetts MHSPY program. The SAMHSA 2002 Report to Congress, Chapter Four, addresses the evidence base for an integrated system level approach to co-occurring disorders (substance abuse and mental health), for adults as well as children. It cites growing experience within the USA and Canada regarding the added value of creating **integrated systems**, which the report concludes are superior to solely **integrating services**. The importance of congruent policies, which support more comprehensive sharing of information and existing resources, is stressed along with more coherent use of treatment goals and expectations. Taken together, these system characteristics appear to be associated with improved outcomes (SAMHSA 2002).

4.3   Systems of Care in Canada

While Canada, which has national health insurance, functions very differently from the USA in some ways, such as the federal government has no direct service delivery role and there is universal access to care, health disparities remain (Sin 2003), and children with mental health needs still challenge the system (Zachik 2003). Although for-profit companies have a far more minor role in Canada than in the USA, with managed care not really a factor, recent Canadian studies indicate that inpatient stays at child psychiatric wards have followed very similar declines in lengths of stay to those in the USA (Gloor 1993; Anderson 1997). The need to develop appropriate alternative community-based resources is a shared one throughout North America. The family voice necessary to contribute to the momentum of such community-based delivery systems is less overt in Canada, consistent with the lower profile of the consumer movement overall (Zachik 2003), but providers themselves have taken active advocacy positions urging greater collaboration between the traditionally distinct psychiatric and community health service sectors (Lamontagne 1995). An Ontario study found that coordination and outreach, or »provider initiated proactive comprehensive care«, resulted in enhanced clinical improvements, as well as cost reduction (Browne 2001). In an earlier multisite study with nine sites, »a recurring pattern of equal or better client outcomes and lower expenditures was associated with well-integrated proactive community services when compared to individual, fragmented, reactive community approaches to care« (Browne 1996). Even in Ontario, however, which has the benefit of an integrated provincial ministry in contrast to much of the rest of Canada, collaborative efforts at the local level are fraught with barriers very similar to those faced by system-of-care proponents in the USA. Despite national health insurance which seems so tantalizing to many system-of-care advocates in the USA, Canada struggles with its own multiple bureaucracies. Canadian health policy experts, Wade Junek and Terry Russell, suggest that the three levels of governance (federal, provincial, and territorial) plus the nine different service organization types represent almost insurmountable barriers to implementing a true system-of-care for children and families as envisioned in the CASSP principles (Zachik 2003). Mandates and funding mechanisms are so divided, even with universal access, that parallel systems for treating children with mental health needs exist simultaneously within pediatric settings, adult psychiatric settings, child welfare, young offender (juvenile justice) settings, and local schools. Various pilot attempts to organize services differently for children and families have occurred in several provinces, notably Nova Scotia, Ontario, Manitoba, and British Columbia, but Junek and Russell report that none appear to have had the multilayer administrative and operational support (continuity of intent) necessary for sustainability and subsequent success (Zachik 2003).

4.4   Conclusions

Related institutional and political barriers, in both the USA and Canada, have blunted efforts to address the broader sources of morbidity from a public health perspective, even for adults, and even within traditional medical spheres, such as cardiac outcomes. The compelling concept of »social capital«, with its implications for improving the health of populations, has its advocates in both countries (Lomas 1998; Kawachi 2000). These advocates suggest that by building up the social and financial health of vulnerable families and communities, increasing their political voice and self-efficacy, the physical and mental health status within the population will also be improved. Social capital is a congruent concept with the comprehensive, wraparound approach taken within systems-of-care, where strengths are key to building interventions that will successfully meet needs. Recognizing that some outside of these programs might view this as »pie-in-the-sky« philosophy, systems-of-care advocates urge that scientific measurement be stepped up and given more weight in institutional policy and resource decision making. Across North America and Canada, »usual care« outcomes for children's mental health are understudied and underreported. Governments and policy makers often function in the dark regarding the cost-effectiveness of prevailing treatments and programs, and unified cost accounting, even in Canada, is not available for »episodes of care« that cross designated delivery systems. Yet, as indicated above, multiple studies exist documenting improved clinical outcomes and reduced cost via implementation of truly integrated systems of care. Individual advocates can continue to work on creating more pilots, with varying success in recruiting appropriate authority and an appropriate knowledge base or child mental health stakeholders can work together in a consensus process to establish a clear baseline of current results in »usual care« and actively define desired improvements with specified measures and a process for achieving them. The latter would require sustained political commitment, but would allow significant, large scale system improvements to be made that would be data driven, inherently accountable, clinically and financially, and ultimately bring hope for real change to both providers and the children and families they serve.

References

American Academy of Child and Adolescent Psychiatry (1999) Workforce fact sheet: Critical shortage of child and adolescent psychiatrists. Available on-line at: http://www.aacap.org/training/workforce/htm.

Anderson, G. (1997) Hospital restructuring and the epidemiology of hospital utilization: recent experience in Ontario. Med Care. 35(10 Suppl):OS93–101.

Bickman, L. (1996) A Continuum of care. More is not always better. Am Psychol 51:689–701.

Browne, G. et al (1996) More effective and less expensive: lessons from nine studies examining community approaches to care. Annu Meet Int Soc Technol Assess Health Care 12:21.

Browne, G. et al (2001) When the bough breaks: provider-initiated comprehensive care is more effective and less expensive for sole-support parents on social assistance. Soc Sci Med 53(12):1697–710.

Burns, B. & Friedman, R. (1990) Examining the research base for child mental health services and policy. J Ment Health Adm17(1):87–98.

Cole, R. & Poe, S. (1993) Partnerships for care: Systems of care for children with serious emotional disturbances and their families. Washington, DC: Washington Business Group on Health.

Friedman, R. & Burns, B. (1996) The evaluation of the Fort Bragg Demonstration Project: an alternative interpretation of the findings. J. Ment Health Adm 23:128–136.

Gloor, J. (1993) Appropriateness of hospitalization in a Canadian pediatric hospital. Pediatrics 91(1):70–74.

Grimes, K. (2001) »Massachusetts-Mental Health Services Program for Youth: A Blended Funding Model for Integrated Care«, in Newman, C. (Ed.), Development of a Comprehensive Cost Capture for Children with Severe Emotional Disorders, Research and Training Center for Children's Mental Health, University of South Florida, Tampa, FL.

Grimes, K. (2002) Opportunities for enhanced effectiveness via continuity of intent. In Newman, C., Liberton, C., Kutash, K., Friedman, R. (Eds.), The 15th Annual Research Conference Proceedings, A System-of-care for Children's Mental Health: Expanding the Research Base 83–86. The Louis de la Parte Florida Mental Health Institute, Research and Training Center for Children's Mental Health, University of South Florida, Tampa.

Grimes, K. (2003) »Collaboration with Primary Care: Sharing Risks, Goals, and Outcomes in an Integrated System-of-care«, in (Eds.) Pumariega, AJ & Winters, NC. The Handbook of Child and Adolescent Systems of Care: The New Community Psychiatry. Jossey-Bass, New York.

Kawachi, I. & Berkman, L. (2000) Social Epidemiology. Oxford University Press. Oxford, England.

Knitzer, J. (1982) Unclaimed Children. Washington, DC: Children's Defense Fund.

Koyanagi, C. & Feres-Merchant, D. (2000) »For the long haul: Maintaining systems of care beyond the federal invest-

ment.« Systems of Care: Promising Practices in Children's Mental Health, 2000 Series, Volume III. Washington, DC. Center for Effective Collaboration and Practice, American Institutes for Research.

Koyanagi, C. & Gaines, M. (1993) All systems failure: An examination of the results of neglecting the needs of children with serious emotional disturbance. Washington, DC: National Institute for Mental Health and the Federation of Families for Children's Mental Health.

Lamontagne, Y. (1995) Psychiatric and medical specialties in community health: 2 solitary fields. Can J Comm Ment Health 14 (1):123–127.

Lomas, J. (1998) Social capital and health: implications for public health and epidemiology. Soc Sci Med 47(9):1181–8.

Lourie, I., Howe, S. & Roebuck, L. (1996) Systematic approaches to mental health care in the private sector for children, adolescents and their families: Managed care organizations and service providers. Washington, DC: Georgetown University Child Development Center, National Technical Assistance Center for Child Mental Health.

Pires, S. (2002) Health care reform tracking project: Promising approaches to behavioral health services to children and adolescents and their families in managed care systems – 1: Managed care design and financing. Tampa, Fl: Research and Training Center for Children's Mental Health, Department of Child and Family Studies, Division of State and Local Support, Louis de la Parte Florida Mental Health Institute, University of South Florida.

Rae-Grant, Q. (1986) Child Psychiatrists in the 90's: who will want us, who will need us. Can J Psychiatry 31(6):493–8.

SAMHSA (2002) Report to Congress; Chapter Four, Evidence-based practices for co-occurring disorders: System level approaches. Substance Abuse and Mental Health Services Administration, U.S. Department of Health and Human Services, Washington, DC.

Saxe, L. & Cross, T. (1998) RWJF Anthology 1998: Chapter Nine – The Mental Health Services Program for Youth. http://www.rwjf.org/publications/publicationsPdfs/library/oldhealth/anth998.htm.

Sin, D. et al, (2003) Can universal access to health care eliminate health inequities between children of poor and non-poor families? A case study of childhood asthma in Alberta. Chest 124(1):51–56.

Stroul, B. & Friedman, R. (1986) A system-of-care for children and youth with severe emotional disturbance. Washington, D.C.: Georgetown University Child Development Center, CASSP Technical Assistance Center.

VanDenBerg, J & Grealish, M. (1996) »Individualized services and supports through the wraparound process: Philosophy and procedures.« Journal of Child and Family Studies, 5, 7–21.

VanDenBerg, J. and Grealish, M. (1998) The Wraparound Process: Training Manual. Pittsburgh: Community Partnership Group and Ontario: Lunwood Hall Child and Family Centre.

Zachik, A. et al (2003) »Relationships between systems of care and federal, state and local governments«, in (Eds.) Pumariega, AJ & Winters, NC. The Handbook of Child and Adolescent Systems of Care: The New Community Psychiatry. Jossey-Bass, New York.

Systems of Care in South America

Luis Augusto Rohde, Salvador Celia, Carlos Berganza

5.1 Introduction – 42

5.2 Historical Background – 43

5.3 Epidemiology – 43

5.4 Services of Mental Health – 45

5.5 The Role of the Child Psychiatrist – 47

5.6 Training and Education – 48

5.7 Research Development and Future Perspectives – 49

References – 50

5.1 Introduction

From Rio Bravo to Patagonia, Latin America covers a geographical area of over 22 million square kilometers (Rojas-Malpica 1998), and embraces a population of over 500,000,000 people. It would certainly be erroneous to draw a monolithic conceptualization of the status of child mental health and psychiatry across Latin America, since there is a wide variation of circumstances among different countries within the region. These circumstances include ethnic composition, macro-economic achievements, political structures and stability, social organization and the nature of the government control upon mental health services, degree of urbanization, and political and civil unrest, among other variables.

Latin America is one of the most unfair world regions in terms of income distribution. Some studies have suggested that approximately 10% of the population earns 90% of the total income, while 90% of the population survives with 10% of the total income (UNESCO 1984). Huge economic problems in the last two decades have produced a significant reduction of the middle class and a tremendous decrease in investments in social and health programs in Latin America (Selle 1997). For the most part, La-tin American countries face serious problems of health with infectious diseases and problems of living, such as malnutrition and poverty running rampant among a high percentage of the total population (Belfort 2002). The Pan American Health Organization (2001) has estimated that every year in the Americas more than 250,000 children less than 5 years of age die from illnesses that can be easily prevented, such as acute respiratory infections, diarrhea, and malnutrition.

From the psychosocial point of view, children in Latin America face an enormous number of risk factors. Poverty, forcing a vast number of children to live out in the streets, predisposes these children to become involved very early in their lives in drug use, crime, violence, and unprotected sex, with serious consequences for their health in general and mental health in particular (Inciardi and Surratt 1998). These children clearly demonstrate significantly lower developmental appropriateness, self-esteem and social skills scores than children from poor families that are able to stay home (Rohde et al. 1998).

Another important source of mental suffering for the population in the region has been the social and political unrest, especially in some countries such as Colombia. In this regard, an estimated number of 6,000 to 14,000 children take part in armed conflicts in Latin America and more than 10,000 children are an active part of the army in Paraguay (Belfort 2002). The impact of stress upon the mental health of children exposed to the counter-insurgency policies of some South American governments has been well documented (Hjern et al. 1991).

Any effort to understand systems of care in South America should be understood in this context. First of all, it is important to emphasize that systems of care for children and adolescents include several different domains, such as health, social services, education, and justice/protection of civil rights. This chapter aims to present a critical review of the literature on a specific part of one of these domains, the systems of care for child and adolescent mental health in South America. To accomplish this task, a systematic review of the literature was performed. Three data sets were assessed: PubMed, Psychinfo, and Lilacs (Latin American Literature on Health Science). References were searched using the following words: child psychiatry, child psychiatric services, child psychiatric care, child mental health care, and child mental health services. Only papers describing data from countries in South America (Argentina, Bolivia, Brazil, Chile, Colombia, Equator, Guyana, Paraguay, Peru, Suriname, Uruguay, and Venezuela) were included. We assessed all articles published in Portuguese, English, and Spanish in the last fifteen years. This search resulted in 34 papers; all of them were reviewed. References mentioned in those papers were also reviewed. In addition, some experts from those countries were contacted and asked to provide a brief description on: (a) historical background of the field in their country, (b) epidemiological studies on child mental health disorders in their country, (c) structure, organization, and theoretical orientation of services in their country, and (d) unmet needs. Finally, the manuscript was reviewed by three senior child psychiatrists who are leaders in the field in South America.

5.2   Historical Background

It is important to note that child psychiatry in the majority of South American countries is a very young field and some of the pioneers are still alive and productive. For instance, the first inpatient service for children resembling those seen today was created in Brazil only in 1929. This was a division inside an adult psychiatric hospital in São Paulo, where mainly children with mental retardation were seen (Assumpção 1995). In Peru, the first child neuropsychiatric outpatient facility was created as part of a general hospital in 1918 and an inpatient unit was opened only in 1938 (Mariategui 1990). Thus, the roots of the field in South America, as in some developed countries, are strongly associated with the care of mentally retarded children.

In addition, there was a strong connection between the roots of child psychiatry and mental health disciplines in the continent with pediatrics. For instance, Professor Prego e Silva, one of the pioneers of child psychiatry in South America, developed the medical-psychological polyclinic inside a pediatric hospital in Uruguay during the 1940s (M. Cherro, personal communication).

The most prominent theoretical background for child mental health in South America was psychoanalysis. During the Second World War, several psychoanalysts left Europe and came to South America where they established the roots of child psychoanalysis and child psychoanalytic psychotherapy on the continent (Biermann 1973).

Although psychoanalysis continues to be a relevant framework for child mental health in South America, the last 15 years were marked by the increase of a more integrative model of thinking in several countries where a bio-psycho-social model emerged (Marimon 1999). In this regard, modern concepts of child psychopathology and psychiatric nomenclature, biological psychiatry, family therapy, and cognitive-behavior therapy have been extensively incorporated in the way of understanding child mental health problems at least in University centers (Rohde et al. 1999). Even so, cultural aspects of understanding continue to defy the establishment of a more integrative way of conceptualizing mental disorders and their approach on the continent. For instance, the split between brain and mind tends to be great in Latin cultures. Moreover, families have difficulties accepting any role for brain dysfunction in emotional problems. Thus, it is not surprising that psychopharmacologic interventions are less developed and accepted in our environment (Belfort 2001).

5.3   Epidemiology

As stated by Bird (1996): »One of the principal goals of psychiatric epidemiology is to determine the rates and distribution of child and adolescent psychopathology. Epidemiological data are useful for both administrative and descriptive purpose. These data provide a scientific basis for appropriate mental health planning (p. 35)«.

Unfortunately, we were not able to find studies addressing mental health problems that have taken advantage of representative national samples in any South American country. The few studies found in the literature were conducted with at most regional samples and/or addressed specific mental health problems like Attention Deficit/Hyperactivity Disorder (ADHD; see for example, Bralic et al. 1987 or Rohde et al. 1999). It is important to note that results of studies conducted in school, clinical, or primary care settings should be considered cautiously in South America, where many children do not go to school and the access to health treatment is highly determined by social class. Thus, any conclusion on the global prevalence of child mental health disorders in South American countries should be considered an estimate.

In addition, most of the epidemiological investigations conducted in these countries have used instruments from developed countries without adequate cross-cultural validation. Although some child psychiatric disorders (mainly those with a clear biological basis) may have a similar clinical presentation in cultures from developing countries to the one described in developed countries (Rohde 2002), several child mental disorders suffer the impact of the cross-cultural context (Bird 1996; Berganza et al. 2001; Fleitlich-Bilyk and Goodman 2000). Thus, it is impossible to estimate the prevalence of child mental disorders in South America based on rates from developed countries.

The description of all epidemiological studies with regional samples and/or addressing specific child psychiatric disorders in South America is beyond the scope of this chapter (for a comprehensive review, see Berganza et al. 2003). However, the analysis of the available literature tends to suggest that 10–20% of the child and adolescent population in the continent would be in need of professional child psychiatry services (Berganza et al. 2003). If these numbers reflect the reality, they are very close to what has been reported in developed countries (Bird 1996; Richardson et al. 1996).

It is important to note that very few children and adolescents needing psychiatric care were able to get it in those countries. Recently, a study conducted in Puerto Rico with 1,897 children and adolescents from 4 to 17 years of age documented that only 3.6% of children with ADHD were receiving stimulants and 25% or less of those children received any school-based or psychosocial treatment (Bauermeister et al. 2003). Although the study was conducted in a Latin American country, this reality is probably not different in South American countries.

Recently, a very well-designed study was conducted to assess the prevalence of psychiatric disorders in children and adolescents from 7 to 14 years of age in a medium-sized city and its surrounding rural areas in the state of São Paulo, Brazil (Fleitlich-Bilyk, 2002). In the first part of the study, instruments [for screening: Strengths and Difficulties Questionnaire (SDQ); for diagnoses: Development and Well-Being Assessment (DAWBA). This instrument derives diagnoses according to ICD-10] were extensively evaluated to check their cross-cultural validity. In a second cross-sectional study, a two-stage sampling via school lists was used. A sample comprising 1,251 subjects was assessed, representing 83% of those approached. The overall weighted prevalence rate of psychiatric disorders was 12.5% (95%CI = 9.6%–15.3%). disruptive behavior disorders (oppositional defiant disorder or conduct disorder) were the most prevalent disorders (7%; 95%CI = 5.1%–8.9%), followed by anxiety disorders (5.2%; 95%CI = 3.91%–7.9%). Lower prevalences were detected for both hyperkinetic disorder (1.5%; 95%CI = 0.6%–2.5%), and depressive disorder (1%; 95%CI = 0.2%–1.9%). The overall weighted prevalence of mental disorders was significantly higher than the one found in Britain using comparable measures (9.5%; Fleitlich-Bilyk 2002).

In addition, Fleitlich-Bilyk (2002) documented significant differences in the prevalence of mental disorders according to the type of school (p = 0.005). A higher prevalence was detected in children from urban government-funded schools (serving low and very low-income families), followed by children from rural government-funded schools. The lower prevalence was found in children from urban private schools. These data suggest the importance of the social-economic context as a risk factor for child mental disorders in a developing country like Brazil. This is a neglected area of research in South American countries: the impact of risk and protective factors on prevalence rates of child mental disorders.

In this regard, Graham and Orley (1998), describing the position of the World Health Organization (WHO) on mental health of children, stated: »Children whose parents are isolated, depressed, uninformed or misinformed about health and nutrition, or unskilled in child care, are obviously at much greater risk« (p. 271). In a study conducted in Brazil, the scores on the HOME, an instrument that measures the quality of the family environment, showed a higher impact than socio-economic indexes in a multiple regression model created to explain the variance of child psychiatric morbid scores (Bastos and Almeida Filho 1991). Brook et al. (1998) assessed the pathways to marijuana use among adolescents in a mixed urban-rural sample from three cities in Colombia through a stratified sampling approach. They were able to document that adverse family factors, drug-prone personality characteristics, and deviant peer groups were significantly associated with marijuana use in adolescents. Adverse family factors were associated with the development of drug-prone personality characteristics, which were associated with the selection of deviant friends, which in turn was related to marijuana use.

5.4   Services of Mental Health

There is a scarcity of funding and infrastructure for child mental health services in South American countries. Thus, the majority of them are concentrated in large cities either at University centers or inside the private system. Moreover, few, if any, of the South American countries have an effective national plan or policy for child mental health (Organizacion Panamericana de la Salud 1991). Consequently, initiatives are isolated depending most of the time on personal efforts and preferences (Fleitlich-Bilyk 2002; Langdon et al. 1990). Thus, it is not surprising that an important part of the clinical work in those countries is addressed to severe and rare child mental disorders, or to intervention not supported by the modern »evidence-based medicine«. In addition, government-funded services tend to be quickly created and dissolved based on »who is in charge« at a particular time.

Due to the lack of national policies for child mental health in South American countries, we were not able to find global data on the source of referral, family demographic factors, and diagnoses most frequently seen in child mental health services in those countries. Even so, some isolated reports tend to suggest that the majority of patients seen in those settings were referred either from schools or other health professionals like pediatricians and primary care workers (Linhares et al. 1993). However, a substantial proportion of children are also taken to treatment spontaneously by parents in some settings (Recart et al. 2002). In the few reports on characteristics of patients seen in outpatient services, the most common diagnoses were: ADHD, conduct disorders, adaptive/reactive disorders, and emotional disorders (a category that includes anxiety and depressive disorders; Escobar et al. 1987; Falceto 2003; Recart et al. 2002). Andrade et al. (1998) reported that psychotic disorders including schizophrenia, bipolar disorder, major depression, and pervasive development disorders were the most frequent diagnoses in the child and adolescent inpatient unit at the teaching hospital of the University of São Paulo, Brazil. The main di-

agnoses at discharge for child and adolescent inpatients in the teaching hospital of the Federal University of Rio Grande do Sul, Brazil from 2000 to 2001 were mood disorders, conduct disorders, and eating disorders. The reasons for the difference in the prevalence of the most-seen disorders between these two tertiary care centers in Brazil remain unclear, though it might be related to the specific interests of the team of child psychiatrists working in both settings (psychosis and pervasive development disorders in São Paulo; behavior and eating disorders in Porto Alegre).

Despite the above-mentioned problems, it is important to note that there are some well-organized child psychiatric services based on an integrative conceptual model in some South American countries that might be considered centers of excellence even in developed countries. For instance, the child psychiatric service in the teaching hospital of the Federal University of Rio Grande do Sul (Porto Alegre) has outpatient, day care, and inpatient facilities. Patients initially evaluated in community health centers in the city of Porto Alegre are referred to the screening outpatient program of the service (▶ see ◘ Fig. 5.1). According to the evaluation there, they are referred to one of the outpatient programs: (a) child psychoanalytic psychotherapy, (b) systemic family therapy, (c) cognitive-behavior therapy (specific for ADHD cases), or (d) psychopharmacological interventions. Specific research programs are also available for eating disorders and ADHD. Severe cases might be referred to the day treatment center or the inpatient unit. A team of seven child psychiatrists with diverse theoretical backgrounds coordinates different areas of the service. Taking advantage of this infrastructure, a two-year residency program in child psychiatry is offered. Approximately six child psychiatry residents from different parts of the country enter the program each year. Other examples are two child psychiatric services in Venezuela that are training areas for the graduate course on child psychiatry in the Universidad Central de Venezuela since 1986. The first is a pediatric consultation liaison psychiatric service inside a pediatric hospital and the second is a child psychiatric service inside a general psychiatric hospital that offers integrative outpatient and inpatient facilities (E. Belfort, personal communication). In addition, there is a University child psychiatric service in Uruguay where the integration of care, teaching, and research is also firmly pursued. This service is the base for the graduate course on child psychiatry. A strong emphasis exists on consultation liaison psy-

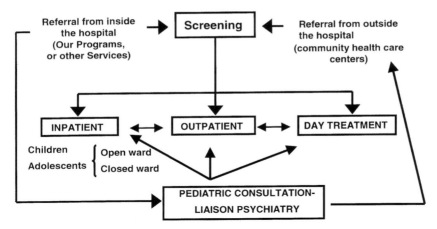

□ Fig. 5.1. Child and Adolescent Psychiatric Unit at the Federal University of Rio Grande do Sul

chiatry with special attention to the community needs (M. Cherro, personal communication).

In a joint effort, the WHO and the Pan-American Health Organization conducted an interinstitutional meeting on child mental health in Washington in 1993. The main objectives were to facilitate exchanges of experiences and to coordinate potential cooperation for the development of a child mental health plan for Latin America. The final document from this meeting highlighted that: »child mental health is a concept that transcends only psychiatric care, presenting its roots on the interplay of psychosocial factors, environment characteristics, economic factors, education, and cultural aspects« (Belfort 2002). Thus, it is important to note that child mental health services are not synonymous with child psychiatric services. In fact, the majority of child mental health services in South America do not have child psychiatrists. Although the description of each of these services is beyond the scope of this chapter, it should be emphasized that isolated child mental health centers addressing specific priority problems can be easily found in South American countries. First, there are several efficient services devoted to the protection of children victimized by violence (e.g., physical or sexual abuse) in hospitals or inside the justice systems. Second, centers to treat juvenile drug abuse or dependence are frequently found. Third, child services to deal with pregnant adolescents are not rare. Finally, nongovernmental organizations or advocacy groups to protect child civil rights can be found in several countries. However, the number of these child mental health care services is much lower than the need on the continent.

In developing countries, models integrating child mental health in the schools and/or primary care settings are very appealing. However, few initiatives in the field are described in the literature. For instance, a school-based program called »Growing Together« was implemented in Chile. This is a primary drug abuse prevention program directed at teachers and teenagers (Langdon et al. 1990). In addition, a program called »The teacher as a mental health worker« was created in Uruguay to train teachers to improve their ability to recognize mental health problems in school-age children (A. Gold, personal communication). Some university settings have also developed isolated school consultation programs where child psychiatrists provide psychoeducational interventions, helping teachers to better recognize, understand, and manage students' mental health problems. In addition, group dynamic concepts are reviewed with the teachers (for a comprehensive discussion of these programs, see Bassols et al. 2003). Unfortunately, no evaluation of the effectiveness of these programs is presented in the literature. Recently, a very simple psychoeducational program to deal with drug problems in elementary school youngsters was developed and tested in 12 schools in the capital of the southernmost state of Brazil (S.P. Ramos, personal communication). The prevalence of tobacco, alcohol, and drug use was measured by a questionnaire developed by the WHO (SMART) in those schools. During 6 months, letters were sent (one every month) to parents from six of these schools addressing the following topics: (a) presentation of the project, the importance of partnership between parents and school to deal with drug problems, general health concepts, (2) the importance of monitoring children and adolescents' life during summer vacation, (3) specific needs and care for these age groups, (4) the role of adults and the importance of setting limits, (5) the identification of problems, at risk students, and signs of alert, (6) the use and abuse of licit and illicit drugs. Two general meetings with parents in these six schools were conducted to discuss doubts and worries at 3 and 6 months. In the other six schools, no intervention was implemented. The prevalence of tobacco, alcohol, and drug use was reassessed at the end of the 6 months in the 12 schools. A significant reduction in the prevalence of tobacco use, and a trend for reduction in the prevalence of other substances were only detected in those schools where the program was implemented.

The high prevalence and the relevant associated repercussions of child mental disorders in the most poor regions of the continent clearly indicate the need to implement child mental health services in primary care settings. These services should give priority to the most frequent child mental disorders, those that might be treatable. The services have to integrate mental health professionals from the community into the team to be effective (Fleitlich and Goodman 2002). In addition, a group of experts in a meeting organized by the Pan-American Health Organization in 1991 emphasized that child mental health services should be created in the context of horizontal community programs as part of traditional general health programs, taking advantage of supportive social networks (Organizacion Panamericana de la Salud 1991). In this regard, De la Barra and Escobar (1987) assessed the prevalence of child psychiatric problems in a sample of children and adolescents from primary care settings in Chile. Appointments having psychiatric problems as the main reason for evaluation represented only 0.02% of the total number of medical visits. Main diagnoses in these settings were ADHD, conduct disorders, emotional disorders, and enuresis. The low prevalence of detected child mental health problems suggests that primary care physicians are not well trained for recognizing mental health problems in children and adolescents.

Taken together, these data seem to demonstrate the need to stimulate trained child psychiatrists to work collaboratively with schools and primary care providers in South American countries. Programs in these settings should aim to: (a) educate professionals (teachers and primary care providers) to recognize and manage most prevalent child psychiatric problems, (b) implement basic crisis management techniques to deal with simple family problems, (c) develop simple school and community programs where children and their parents can discuss issues related to self-esteem and quality of life, (d) provide care for the caretakers (support groups for professionals), and (e) teach professionals when and how to refer the most severe cases. Finally, as described for developed countries, such programs should be frequently assessed for cost-effectiveness of the interventions (Bower et al. 2001; Fleitlich and Goodman 2002).

5.5 The Role of the Child Psychiatrist

According to the WHO, at least two child psychiatrists should work full-time for each 60,000 children and adolescents in the population (Escobar et al. 1987). In South America, there is a scarcity of child psychiatrists. Most of the countries are very distant from this threshold. For example, the estimated number of child psychiatrists in Venezuela was 51 in 1997 (Selle 1997). In Chile, there is an estimated 85 child psychiatrists (Berganza et al. 2003). In addition, the majority of these professionals are working in huge urban areas. Thus, most experts in child psychiatry in South America indicate that either pediatricians, psychologists, or general psychiatrists are caring for the majority of children in need of mental health services.

Child psychiatrists in South American countries are mainly involved in: (a) private clinical and/or psychotherapeutic outpatient work, (b) coordination of multidisciplinary mental health teams, (c) teaching activities in university settings, or (d) consultation for other child medical specialties in inpatient settings. In this latter regard, they are requested to provide mental health assessment and interventions for sick children and/or their families, and support for the medical team (e.g., in neonatal or child intensive care units; Marimon 1999). The work in collaboration with other colleagues is very important in these countries. For instance, the consultation in pregnancy and post-partum clinics can be preventive in the sense that early mother-infant interaction problems can be recognized and managed, and puerperal depression can be early detected, avoiding future impact on child development (Hernandez et al. 2000). In this regard, a longitudinal study following 100 families from child birth to his/her second year of age in Canela, Brazil was able to detect a positive screening score for maternal depression on the Beck scale in 30% of the mothers of this cohort. These findings suggest a high prevalence of maternal depression in some populations from the continent (S. Celia, personal communication).

5.6   Training and Education

For most developed countries in South America, formal child psychiatric training is performed at the local level, mostly in national universities. For those less developed countries, training of most specialists in child psychiatry takes place out of the country either in the United States, Europe, or Mexico.

Argentina, Brazil, Chile, Uruguay, and Venezuela have local university-backed training programs for child psychiatrists. However, as far as we are aware, it is important to note that very few medical schools in South American countries have integrated child psychiatry or, at least, topics on normal child mental development as part of their curriculum. For instance, Assumpção and Barbosa (1997) sent a questionnaire to all Brazilian medical schools in 1993 (72 schools) requesting information on the teaching of child psychiatry. The rate of response was low (33%), probably reflecting the disregard either with the field or with research. From those schools that answered the questionnaire, only one had the discipline of child psychiatry or normal child mental development as part of its curriculum. Eighteen schools had some concepts of child psychiatry discussed as part of other disciplines (e.g., general psychiatry), but the mean length of time dedicated to child psychiatry in the curriculum was only 6.5 hours in those schools. Thus, most students end medical school without any idea of how to differentiate normal child development from child psychopathology. Moreover, they are not even able to conduct simple psychoeducational interventions for mild family or child mental problems. However, there are some exceptions. The medical school at the University of Chile has a well-developed program on child psychiatry as part of its curriculum. Regarding general objectives, at the end of the program, the student should be able to: (a) recognize the psychosocial development according to different aspects, as well as its deviations; (b) recognize the most frequent psychiatric disorders in children and adolescents, (c) have basic knowledge of child psychopharmacology and environmental interventions, (d) rec-

ognize the constant and dynamic somatic-psychic interaction with health and child disorders, and (e) understand the relevance of socio-cultural aspects of child/juvenile mental health with emphasis on the national reality (Comisión de Enlace de Profesores de Psiquiatría 1994). In addition, the Brazilian Lutheran University has been developing an innovative program for undergraduate students in the Medical School since 1996. Besides teaching the life cycle with emphasis on infancy, childhood, and adolescence from the very beginning of the curriculum, each student follows a child and his/her family from birth during the six years of the medical school. The program is based on frequent home visits (Escosteguy and Celia 2003).

The first formal child psychiatric training in Brazil began outside a University setting inside a private clinic (Leo Kanner) in 1968. To give a general sense on the scarcity of formal child psychiatric training inside Universities in South American countries, it is important to note that there were no more than three child psychiatric residency programs in a huge country like Brazil in 2000 (Rohde et al. 2000). However, the majority of child psychiatrists on the continent, especially those in poor regions or situated far from large cities, are trained at local nonuniversity institutions by senior psychiatrists with limited experience in the treatment of children and adolescents. Although this is an intermediate step still needed due to the lack of child psychiatrists on the continent, there are several risks in adopting this training strategy. The differentiation between normal characteristics of some developmental phases and child psychopathology is a very complex task. The knowledge of normal child development is not a regular part of adult/general psychiatric training. In addition, child psychopathology is profoundly influenced by the environment. Thus, the assessment of children and adolescents depends on adequate knowledge about family dynamics, which again is not part of the majority of adult/general psychiatric training. Moreover, children and adolescents tend to express their psychological suffering by nonverbal forms of communication. Thus, their assessment depends on the ability to integrate games, drawings, or dramatizations in the evaluation process. Finally, adult psychiatrist are not used to diagnosing some child psychiatric disorders such as autism or separation anxiety disorders, and, more important, there are several significant differences in the effectiveness between child and adult psychopharmacological interventions (for a more comprehensive discussion, see Rohde et al. 2000).

In those special cases where formal and university-accredited training programs for child psychiatry exist, the academic content and requirements are similar to the training programs in the United States or Europe. Thus, to be admitted to a child psychiatry training program, candidates must have completed at least two years of training in adult or general psychiatry. They have to fulfill an additional two-year residency in child psychiatry to finish their training. The academic content of these programs typically includes issues such as child development, child psychopathology, psychoanalytic psychotherapy, family psychotherapy, and child psychopharmacology (Berganza et al. 2003; Selle 1997).

The clinical training in child and adolescent psychiatry usually includes the rotation of the resident for variable periods of time through treatment centers for specific types of patients, such as outpatient divisions and consultation-liaison services in general hospitals, institutions providing care for serious developmental disorders in specialized settings (e.g., mental retardation and autism), school consultation, and settings holding children with serious criminal behavior, such as those belonging to the juvenile justice system (Berganza et al. 2003).

The tremendous impact of the lack of adequate child psychiatric training in the continent might be demonstrated by a very provocative study conducted in Brazil. Assumpção and Carvalho (1999) revised national data on hospital psychiatric morbidity according to ICD-9 criteria in children and adolescents (0–19 years of age) from 1992 to 1997. They found 2,120 children under 1 year of age with registered diagnoses of schizophrenia.

5.7 Research Development and Future Perspectives

We were able to find just one paper in the assessed literature describing research perspectives in a South American country (Rohde et al. 1999). There are very few well-designed investigations conducted by child psychiatrists on the continent. As the result of this situation, there is a scarcity of papers from South American investigators on topics of child mental health in international journals. The great majority of work published by our child psychiatrists can only be found in local journals tending to concentrate on isolated descriptions of the services provided to children, case reports, and chapters of books that describe theoretical issues related to the field. For instance, most graduate courses on

medicine and those few specific for mental health in Brazil suggest that potential mentors for master degree students should have, besides a doctoral degree, a productivity in research documented by at least one paper published in an international journal indexed by PubMed in the last 35 years. Certainly, no more than 5–10 Brazilian child psychiatrists achieve this threshold.

Although a comprehensive discussion on the reasons for this situation is beyond the scope of this chapter, some considerations might be relevant. First, there is a scarcity of resources for research in the majority of South American countries, making it very difficult to conduct studies on the continent. Second, in general, child psychiatrists are either not trained in concepts of modern evidence-based medicine, or not sufficiently fluent in English (the majority of international journals request papers in English). Third, since there is a scarcity of mentors (senior child psychiatrists doing research) in the field, young child psychiatrists do no have models of identification which are very important to stimulate them to pursue a research career (Rohde et al. 1999).

Regarding future goals to be achieved, eight major tasks deserve to be more comprehensively developed in South America:

1. National policies for child mental health should be implemented in South American countries, based on well-designed national community child epidemiological studies.

2. Diagnostic instruments and child psychopharmacological/psychosocial interventions derived from developed countries should be assessed for cross-cultural validity before their use or implementation.

3. Programs addressing infant mental health that promote community mobilization and/or improvement of social networks are mandatory for the continent. Special attention should be given to scientific analyses of the preventive role of interventions in this population.

4. Child mental health services for special populations like native Indians, children of refugees, street children, pregnant adolescents, abandoned or victimized children should be supported or implemented.

5. Several other centers of excellence in child psychiatry should be created on the continent to allow the development of child psychiatric residency programs based on an integrative framework, instead of being compromised with one theoretical background.

6. The integration of child mental health professionals in school settings and primary care centers providing consultation-liaison for other professionals should be pursued. In this regard, mental health training for pediatricians must be a central part of this process.

7. The exchange of experiences among child mental health professionals from all South American countries should be supported. In this regard, the participation of these professionals in representative institutions like the Latin American Federation of Child and Adolescent Psychiatry and Allied Disciplines (FLAPIA) should be encouraged.

8. An increase in research on different aspects of child psychiatry in the context of evidence-based medicine should be stimulated.

Acknowledgements. The authors wish to thanks the following colleagues for their work in reviewing and making suggestions on the manuscript: Amélia Thereza de Moura Vasconcellos, Ariel Gold, Bacy Fleitlich-Bilyk, Edgar Belfort, Francisco Baptista Assumpção Jr., Maria Lucrécia Zavaschi, Miguel Cherro, and Olga Falceto.

References

Andrade ER, Busse SR, Zanuzzo Z, Assumpção FB (1998) Internação em um serviço de psiquiatria infantil: análise de um modelo. J Bras Psiq 47:337–341

Assumpção FB (1995) Psiquiatria infantil brasileira: Um esboço histórico. Lemos, São Paulo

Assumpção FB, Barbosa GA (1997) Ensino em Psiquiatria Infantil no Brasil. Informação Psiquiátrica 16:147–149.

Assumpção FB, Carvalho LN (1995) Child Psychiatry in Brazil. J Bras Psiq 48:449–452

Bauermeister JJ, Canino G, Bravo M, Ramírez R, Jensen P, Chavez L, Martinez-Taboas A, Ribera J, Alegria M, Garcia P (2003) Stimulant and psychosocial treatment of ADHD in latino/hispanic children. J Am Acad Child Adolesc Psychiatry 42:851–855

Bassols A, Cristovão P, de Santis M, Fortes M, Sukiennik P (2003) Saúde Mental na Escola: Consultoria como estratégia de prevenção. Mediação, Porto Alegre

Bastos ACS, Almeida Filho N (1991) Determinação social da saúde mental infantil: Revisão da literatura epidemiológica. Psic Teor Pesq 4:268–282

Belfort E (2001) Antiepileptic Drugs in Child Neuropsychiatry: A Latin American View. In: Miyoshi K, Shapiro CM, Gaviria M, Morita Y (eds) Contemporary Neuropsychiatry. Springer, Tokyo. pp 397–401

Belfort E (2002) Reflexiones sobre salud mental infantil en el contexto de latinoamerica. Psiquiatria y Salud Integral 2:38–42

Berganza CE, Mezzich JE, Otero-Ojeda AA, Jorge MR, Villaseñor SJ, Rojas-Malpica C (2001) The Latin American Guide for Psychiatric Diagnosis: An overview. Psychiatric Clinics of North America 24:433–446

Berganza C, Rohde LA, Duarte C, Brasil HH (2003) The current status of child psychiatry in Latin America. In: Mezzich JE (ed) Images of psychiatry in Latin America. World Psychiatric Association, New York

Biermann G (1973) Handbuch der Kinderpsychotherapie. Ernst Reinhardt, München

Bird HR (1996) Epidemiology of childhood disorders in a cross-cultural context. J Child Psychol Psychiat 37:35–49

Bower P, Garralda E, Kramer T, Harrington R, Sibbald B (2001) The treatment of child and adolescent mental health problems in primary care: a systematic review. Family Practice 18:373–382

Bralic SE, Seguel X, Montenegro H (1987) Prevalencia de trastornos psíquicos en la población escolar de Santiago de Chile. Acta Psiquiatrica y Psicologica de America Latina 33:316–325

Comision de Enlace de Professores de Psiquiatria (1994) Aspectos psicosociales de la práctica médica: su enseñanza en el curriculo de pregrado de la facultad de medicina de la Universidad de Chile. Rev Psiquiatr Clin 31:69–89

De la Barra F, Escobar MC (1987) Atención de niños con problemas psiquiátricos en el nivel primario. Rev Chil Pediatr 58:169–173

Escobar MC, de la Barra F, Verdugo C, Lérida PL, Olivares E, Grau A (1987) Interconsultas de pediatría a psiquiatría infantil. Rev Chil Pediatr 58:368–373

Escosteguy N, Celia S (2003) Primeiro ano de vida. In: Cataldo A, Gauer GJ, Furtado NR (eds) Psiquiatria para estudantes de medicina. EdiPucrgs, Porto Alegre, pp 205–211

Falceto O (2003) Serviço de Psiquiatria da Infância e Adolescência do Hospital de Clínicas de Porto Alegre: Um modelo integrado. Apresentado no Congresso Brasileiro de Neurologia e Psiquiatria da Infância, Vitória, Brasil

Fleitlich-Bilyk W (2002) The prevalence of psychiatric disorders in 7–14 year olds in South East of Brazil. PhD Thesis, Institute of Psychiatry, University of London, London

Fleitlich-Bilyk W, Goodman R (2000) Epidemiologia. Rev Bras Psiquiatr 22 (Suppl II):2–6

Fleitlich-Bilyk W, Goodman R (2002) Implantação e implementação de serviços de saúde mental comunitários para crianças e adolescentes. Rev Bras Psiquiatr 24:2

Graham P, Orley J (1998) WHO and the mental health of children. World Health Forum 19:268–272

Hernandez G, Kimelman M, Montino O (2000) Salud mental perinatal en la assistencia hospitalaria del parto y puerperio. Rev Med Chile 128:1283–1289

Hjern A, Angel B, Hojer B (1991) Persecution and behavior: a report of refugee children from Chile. Child Abuse and Neglect 15:239–248

Inciardi JA, Surratt HL (1998) Children in the streets of Brazil: Drug use, crime, violence and HIV risks. Substance Use & Misuse 33:1461–1480

Langdon MC, Gazmuri C, Venegas L (1990) Chile: Perspective in school health. Journal of School Health 60:313–317

Linhares MB, Parreira VC, Maturano AC, Sant'anna SC (1993) Caracterização dos motivos de procura de atendimento infantil em um serviço de psicopedagogia clínica. Medicina, Ribeirão Preto 26:148–160

Mariategui J (1990) Dessarollo de la psiquiatria infantil en el Peru. Revista de Neuro-Psiquiatria 53:17–32

Marimon JG (1999) La labor de un Psiquiatra en un servicio de pediatria. Pediatr Py 26:41–43

Organizacion Panamericana de la Salud (1991) Grupo de consulta para la formulacion de un plan de accion regional sobre salud mental del nino. Montevideo, p 21

Pan American Health Organization (2001) About the Healthy Children Goal: Goal 2002 Initiative. Document available by Internet from PAHO Website

Recart C, Castro P, Alvarez H, Bedregal P (2002) Características de niños y adolescentes atendidos en un consultorio psiquiátrico del sistema privado de salud en Chile. Rev Med Chile 130:295–303

Richardson LA, Keller AM, Selby-Harrington ML, Parrish R (1996) Identification and treatment of children's mental health problems by primary care providers: a critical review of the research. Arch Psychiatric Nursing 10:293–303

Rohde LA (2002) ADHD in a developing country: Are DSM-IV criteria suitable for culturally different populations? J Am Acad Child Adolesc Psychiatry 41:1131–1133

Rohde LA, Biederman J, Busnello EA, Zimmermann H, Schmitz M, Martins S, Tramontina S (1999) ADHD in a school sample of Brazilian adolescents: A study of prevalence, comorbid conditions and impairments. J Am Acad Child Adolesc Psychiatry 38:716–722

Rohde LA, Ferreira MH, Zomer A, Forster L (1998) The impact of living on the streets on latency children's friendships. Journal of Public Health 32:273–280

Rohde LA, Eizirik M, Ketzer CR, Michalowski M (1999) Pesquisa em psiquiatria da infância e adolescência. Infanto 7:25–31

Rohde LA, Lima D, Assumpção FB, Barbosa G, Golfeto JH, Zavaschi ML, Reis R (2000) Quem deve tratar crianças e adolescente com transtornos mentais? O espaço da psiquiatria da infância e adolescência em questão. Revista da Associação Brasileira de Psiquiatria 22:2–3

Rojas-Malpica C (1998) La cultura latinoamericana y la salud mental [The Latin American culture and mental health]. Presented at the Latin American Congress of Psychiatry, Havana, Cuba

Selle MS (1997) La pertinencia de los factores psicosociales en la programacion para la formacion de recursos humanos e salud mental. Infanto 5:136–141

UNESCO (1984) The impact of world recession on children. The state of the world's children. New York

Systems of Care in Australia

Barry Nurcombe

6.1   Introduction   – 52

6.2   History   – 52

6.3   Population Distribution   – 53

6.4   Health   – 53

6.5   Health Funding   – 53

6.6   The History and Present Status of Child Mental Health Services   – 53

6.7   The Epidemiology of Child and Adolescent Psychiatry   – 54

6.8   The Spectrum of Mental Health Services   – 54

6.9   Problems   – 54

6.10   Recent Advances   – 55
6.10.1   Training Innovations   – 55
6.10.2   Services   – 55
6.10.3   Promotion and Prevention   – 55
6.10.4   Early Intervention   – 56
6.10.5   Research   – 56

6.11   Conclusion   – 56

References   – 57

6.1   Introduction

In an island roughly the size of the continental United States, Australia has a population of approximately 20,000,000, representing an increase of 13% since 1991. About 4,000,000 (20%) of the inhabitants were born overseas. Between 1995 and 2000, over 400,000 permanent settlers arrived in Australia. Twenty percent of the population speak a language at home other than English, including Chinese (2.1%), Italian (1.9%), and Greek (1.4%) (Yearbook Australia 2001).

Prior to World War II, the Australian population was almost entirely Anglo-Celt. Since then, there have been waves of migration from the UK, Europe, the Middle East, South-East Asia, and New Zealand. Following the dismantling of racist immigration policies in 1970, Australia has attempted to create a multicultural society, and to search for a new identity. This process has not been without controversy.

Australia is an affluent country, rich in natural resources and diversified in agricultural and pastoral production. Its chief trading partners are Japan, South Korea, China, and the USA. As a result of the elimination of tariffs and subsidies during the 1980s, the manufacturing sector is now very efficient: Australia's current annual growth rate (3.2%) exceeds that of any other developed country: the Real Growth Domestic Product Index grew from 90 to 130 in the last ten years.

6.2   History

Prior to the European settlement of Australia, it is estimated that the Aboriginal population was 400,000. After the loss of its American colonies, the UK looked elsewhere for a place to send its unwanted people. Between 1788 and 1840, about 200,000 male and female convicts were transported to settlements in New South Wales, Tasmania, Queensland, and Western Australia. Victoria and South Australia were founded by free settlers.

In 1851, gold was discovered in New South Wales, soon followed by finds in Victoria, Queensland, and Western Australia. As a result, there was a rapid increase in immigration, the population more than doubling over the next 5 years. Between 1800 and 1940, the Aboriginal population dropped to less than 100,000, as a result of dispossession and disease. Following World War II, the trend reversed, and the Aboriginal population has risen to 410,000.

In 1900, the six sovereign states confederated, the Commonwealth of Australia was formed, and the capital city of Canberra was established. By the outbreak of World War I the population was 4,000,000. Australia suffered greatly during the Depression of 1932–1939. During World War II, after the fall of Singapore, the Australian-American alliance was forged. Following 1945, industrial expansion demanded a liberalization of immigration policies. Japan, from having been a mortal enemy 60 years ago, has become Australia's premier trading partner.

6.3 Population Distribution

Most of Australia's population now lives along the eastern, south-eastern, and western seaboards, in cities that serve the productive hinterland. The largest cities are the capitals of the six states: Sydney, Melbourne, Brisbane, Perth, Adelaide, and Hobart, which have populations varying from 4,160,000 to 200,000. Only 40% of the population live outside the capital cities (Yearbook Australia 2002).

6.4 Health

The leading causes of death in Australia are cancer, ischemic heart disease, and cerebrovascular disease. Mental illness causes 13% of the total disease burden, particularly alcohol and drug use disorders in males, and affective disorders in females (Yearbook Australia 2002). The National Mental Health Strategy, formulated in 1992, is now in its third phase (2003–8; Australian Health Ministers 2003). This plan provides a framework for the modernization of public mental health services, and for the monitoring of the progress of the plan, particularly in regard to deinstitutionalization, consumer rights, the linkage of mental health services with allied health services, the promotion of mental health, prevention, primary care, and the evaluation of the quality and effectiveness of services. As a result, mental health services are now provided as part of mainstream health and community care. Particular emphasis has been placed on improved public policy planning, the reduction of risk factors for suicide, improved access to care, deinstitutionalization, community care, Aboriginal mental health, and the improvement of service integration.

6.5 Health Funding

The cost of health care has been reasonably well contained: it now amounts to 8–9% of the Gross National Product. The entire population is covered by Medicare, a public system introduced in 1984 and financed through the Federal Income Tax. About 45% of the population voluntarily supplement Medicare by subscribing to private health insurance for hospitalization and ancillary services (Yearbook Australia 2002). The balance between public and private health care ensures a high level of access to health care for all citizens; however, patients without private insurance may have to wait up to six months for elective surgery. The »gap« between fees charged by doctors and the health benefits paid by combined Medicare and private health insurance is a source of continual complaint.

6.6 The History and Present Status of Child Mental Health Services

Child psychiatry began after 1950, when a number of adult psychiatrists developed an interest in children's mental health. Aside from a University of Queensland research chair in medical psychology to which John Bostock was appointed, there were no academic positions in the field until 1960. Bostock conducted research into psychological factors involved in enuresis and asthma. Winston Rickards developed the Department of Paediatric Psychiatry at the Royal Children's Hospital, Melbourne.

After initially training in general psychiatry in Australia, child psychiatrists originally went overseas to the UK, Canada, or the USA in order to seek specialized training. During the 1960s, Julian Katz and Barry Nurcombe were appointed to academic positions in the Universities of Sydney and New South Wales, and cooperated to design a formal training program under the auspices of the New South Wales Institute of Psychiatry. In Queensland, Bert Phillips developed public community clinics in the only Australian state department which was separate from adult mental health services. Further academic positions were later opened in Melbourne, Adelaide, Brisbane, Perth, and Newcastle. The Universities collaborated with the Royal Australian and New Zealand College of Psychiatry (RANZCP) to establish the Faculty of Child and Adolescent Psychiatry within the RANZCP. The Faculty determines training standards, monitors the quality of each training program and its adherence to accreditation standards, and awards a Certificate of Training to candidates who have completed a formal two-year accredited training program. All child and adolescent psychiatrists who enter specialized training have already completed a two-year general medical internship and four years of training in general psychiatry, qualifying them to sit the examination that will allow them to become Fellows of the Royal Australian and New Zealand College of Psychiatry (FRANZCP).

The recruitment and training of child and adolescent psychiatrists has been relatively slow. As a result, there are now only 350 trained child psychiatrists in the country, for a population of about 5,000,000 under the age of 18 years (approximately 1 : 14,286). Child psychiatrists work in public or private practice. Most private practitioners spend part of their work-week consulting to public child and adolescent inpatient units or community mental health services.

Clinical psychologists, social workers, psychiatric nurses, speech and language pathologists, and occupational therapists work predominantly in community mental health clinics. The greater number have only Bachelor-level training, even though there are excellent programs for the training of clinical psychologists at the doctoral level, particularly in behavioral treatment techniques. Public clinic psychological practice is likely to advance when more highly trained staff become available. Increasingly, psychiatrists, psychologists and social workers are seeking advanced training in such areas as psychoanalysis, infant mental health, family therapy, and group therapy, usually through independent organizations (e.g., the Melbourne Psychoanalytic Institute). Neuropsychologists have become increasingly prominent in collaboration with neurologists, and in the areas of personal injury litigation and rehabilitation following brain injury.

6.7 The Epidemiology of Child and Adolescent Psychiatry

A recent survey has been completed of 4,500 Australian children aged 4–17 years, randomly selected from each state and from rural/urban locations in such a way as to reflect the demographic characteristics of the general population (Sawyer et al. 2001). The total prevalence of mental health problems was 14.1%: 11.2% were diagnosed as having ADHD; 3%

as having Mood Disorder; and 3% as having Conduct Disorder. The more disturbed the child, the greater the adverse impact on family, school performance, and peer relationships, and the more likely the child to be involved in behavior (e.g., suicide, impulsive sexual activity, or drug use) dangerous to health. Only 50% of the most disturbed children had attended any medical, mental health, or educational counseling service in the previous six months, and only 17% had attended a mental health clinician. Family doctors, pediatricians, and school counselors were the most-often-attended practitioners. This study draws attention to the adverse social consequences of mental ill health and serious problems in regard to the availability, accessibility, and coordination of mental health services.

6.8 The Spectrum of Mental Health Services

Mental health services are conceptualized ideally as an integrated spectrum of emergency, inpatient, partial hospital, residential, in-home, outpatient, school-outreach, preventative, and juvenile justice services, coordinated with educational, child protection, pediatric and family practice services. In fact, inpatient services for children and adolescents are patchy in distribution; there are few partial hospital, residential, and in-home services; and the sharing of care with pediatricians and family practitioners (who generally have had little training in child mental health) has only recently begun.

6.9 Problems

Predominant among the problems faced by child and adolescent mental health are the following:
1. Inadequate funding for public mental health services
2. The resistance of adolescents to using mental health services
3. The irrational separation between mental health and alcohol/substance abuse services
4. The disastrous mental health of Aboriginal families
5. A lack of understanding of the needs of children in immigrant families
6. The inadequate training of many nonpsychiatric mental health staff
7. The relatively high prevalence of adolescent suicide

8. Long distances between rural patients and urban mental health services
9. The paucity of emergency, residential, partial hospital, and in-home services
10. Poor coordination with pediatrics, family practice, and educational services
11. Lack of funding for preventative programs
12. The high prevalence of disruptive behavior disorders, anxiety/depression, eating disorders, and trauma spectrum disorders
13. The need to assess the quality and effectiveness of services

6.10   Recent Advances

6.10.1   Training Innovations

The inadequate training of allied mental health staff has been addressed in Queensland by the introduction of the Professional Development Strategy. This manualized, problem-oriented learning program is designed for use in child and adolescent mental health services throughout the State. Training modules have been completed concerning basic clinical problems, advanced clinical problems, consumer involvement, and clinical outreach services. In the modules concerning clinical problems, for example, an extended case history (provided on CD) is divided into four segments. After each of the first three segments, the group of clinician-learners is encouraged by a designated trained facilitator to recognize salient cues, assemble clinical patterns, generate alternative categorical and dynamic explanatory hypotheses, and decide upon the data they would like to collect to confirm or disconfirm the hypotheses. After the fourth segment, the group are asked to formulate a biopsychosocial diagnosis and design a goal-directed treatment plan.

6.10.2   Services

Telemedicine provides an opportunity for the technical skills of diagnosis and treatment planning available in the major coastal cities to be shared with rural services which may be up to 1,500 kilometers distant from their sources of consultation. Each rural center is associated with a central mental health service and a consultant child and adolescent psychiatrist. At regular, scheduled times the rural service presents a problem case via telemedicine screen to the psychiatrist, for consultation concerning diagnosis or treatment. Family therapy has been conducted, as a demonstration, via telemedicine. Since over 150 different telemedicine terminals are dispersed throughout Queensland, for example, this service is readily available to supplement in-person consultation visits.

Concern about the effectiveness of mental health services prompted the preparation of a monograph (Bickman et al. 1999) in which the conceptual basis of outcome measurement is reviewed, the attitude of clinicians and consumers to measurement is surveyed, and existing instruments for outcome measurement are analyzed. Three modules for development were recommended: a Baseline-Follow-up Module (for service effectiveness); a Background Module (for diagnosis); and a Concurrent Module (for the monitoring of treatment progress). Recently, the Commonwealth government has decided to develop Baseline-Follow-up measurement in collaboration with the States, using instruments originally designed in the UK: the Health of the Nation Outcome Scale-Child and Adolescent (HONOSCA; Gowers et al. 2000) and the Strength and Difficulties Questionnaire (SDQ; Goodman 1997).

An innovative telephone counseling service, Kids Help Line, has proven very popular among Australian adolescents. In this service, trained clinicians counsel children who call in crisis. Clients are allowed to remain anonymous if they choose. About 2% of calls are related to suicidal ideation.

6.10.3   Promotion and Prevention

Between 1981 and 1996, the suicide rate among Australian males aged 15–24 years rose from 19.3 to 25.7 per 100,000, placing Australia fifth in order behind New Zealand, Norway, Switzerland, and Canada amongst countries that keep reliable suicide statistics. Suicide rates among females the same age did not increase. The prevalence of suicide among Aboriginal and rural youth, in particular, prompted the design of a National Action Plan for Suicide Prevention (National Advisory Council for Youth Suicide Prevention 1998). Suicide was related to socio-economic disadvantage, limited educational achievement, indigenous communities, rural unemployment, homelessness, hopelessness, loneliness, and clinical depression. The problems has been addressed in a number of ways: raising community awareness; encouraging communities to provide better community facilities for adolescents; controlling the availability of firearms; training school counselors and family practitioners to recognize mood disorder, assess the risk of suicide, and treat or refer children at risk; and improving the link between emergency services and child and youth mental health services.

The National Action Plan for Promotion, Prevention and Early Intervention for Mental Health (Commonwealth Department of Health and Aged Care 2000) defines promotion, prevention, and early intervention. The key strategic sectors for action are identified, outcome and process indicators specified, and linked initiatives identified for infants, toddlers, children, adolescents, and adults. Special attention is paid to rural communities, Aborigines, and Australians from non-English-speaking backgrounds. Consumers, the media, and health professionals are identified as targets for strategic intervention. A national consultation for the promulgation of the Action Plan has been conducted (Parham and Rickwood 2003).

6.10.4   Early Intervention

McGorry and Jackson (1999) have designed a system for the detection of and intervention in early schizophrenia, particularly in young adults. This program is being implemented in all States.

The Australian Early Intervention Network (Davis et al. 1998) has published a stocktaking of national early intervention programs already implemented for infants, children, and adolescents, together with a description of model projects (O'Hanlon et al. 2000) and recommendations for intervention in ADHD, anxiety disorder, and the perinatal period.

6.10.5   Research

Nurcombe et al. (2000) and King et al. (2000) have conducted experimental studies of the effectiveness of cognitive behavior therapy and family therapy in sexually abused children. Martin (e.g., Bergen et al. 2003) studies the association between risk factors and suicidal behavior. McDermott (e.g., McDermott and Palmer 2002; McDermott, Batik, Roberts, and Gibbon 2002) studies children's postdisaster response and eating disorders. Hazell (e.g., Hazell 2003) studies mood disorder and hyperactivity. Tonge (e.g., Tonge 2002) and Einfeld (e.g., Einfeld and Tonge 1996 a, b) have collaborated in research-

ing the prevalence of psychopathology in intellectually disabled children. Sawyer (e.g., Sawyer et al. 2001) conducts epidemiologic studies and investigates the psychopathology of chronic physical illness, building on an earlier epidemiologic survey (Zubrick 2000). Patton et al. (2000) have implemented the Gatehouse Project, aimed at promoting mental health through a mainstream secondary school curriculum.

Spence (e.g., Spence, Sheffield and Donovan 2003), Dadds and Barrett (e.g., Dadds and Barrett 2001) have studied the prevention of anxiety, social phobia, and depression through school-based intervention. Prior (2003) studies autism spectrum disorders, toddler temperament, and the longitudinal predictors of psychological maladjustment in preadolescents (Prior, Smart, Samson and Oberklaid 2001).

6.11   Conclusion

Australia has tackled the tyranny of distance and the paucity of rural consultation services by the intelligent usage of modern information technology. Prominent among the advances are the establishment of a National Mental Health Strategy and an emphasis on promotion, prevention, and early intervention. The vigorous research scene reflects the policies promoted by the National Mental Health Strategy. A national mental health treatment outcome measurement program has commenced.

Serious problems remain. There is a danger that the idealism of the National Mental Health Policy will not be matched by necessary funding. There is a strain between those who advocate prevention and those who favor improving treatment services for existing patients.

Child and adolescent psychiatry has been dominated by adult psychiatry and pediatrics, not always benignly. Clinical psychologists and social workers are largely underskilled: incentives are required for postgraduate training. Alcohol and substance abuse services operate independently of child and adolescent mental health, and are dominated by treatment models designed for adults. Despite the full range of mental health services available in larger metropolitan centers, there are few residential or step-down facilities, outreach and in-home services, or therapeutic foster homes. Though vigorously promoted, the concept of »shared care« with pediatricians, family practitioners, and school counselors is in its infancy. Aboriginal mental health is a scandal of embarrassing proportions.

Australia is a country in transition from being a minor player internationally to becoming a mid-range world power. Increasingly, it turns from Europe to Asia for its trading partners, the immigrants it needs to ensure population increase, and its cuisine. As the old Anglo-Celt traditions become less relevant, Australia struggles to design strategies appropriate for a multicultural society in a complex modern world.

References

Australian Health Ministers (2003). National Mental Health Plan 2003–2008. Australian Government, Canberra.

Bergen HA, Martin G, Richardson AS et al. (2003). Sexual abuse and suicidal behaviour: A model constructed from a large community sample of adolescents. J Am Acad Child Adolesc Psychiatry, 42:1301–1309.

Bickman L, Nurcombe B, Townsend C et al. (2000) Consumer Measurement Systems in Child and Adolescent Mental Health. Department of Health and Family Services, Canberra. (http://www.health.gov.au/hsdd/mentalhe)

Commonwealth Department of Health and Aged Care (2000) National Action Plan for Promotion, Prevention, and Early Intervention for Mental Health. Mental Health and Special Programs Branch, Canberra.

Dadds MR, Barrett PM (2001) Practitioner review: psychological management of anxiety disorders in childhood. J Child Psychol Psychiatry, 42:999–1011.

Davis C, Martin G, Kosky R, O'Hanlon A (1998) National Stocktake of Early Intervention Programs. Glenelg Press: Melrose Park, SA. (http://www.auseinet.flinders.edu.au)

Einfeld S, Tonge BJ (1996 a,b) Population prevalence of psychopathology in children and adolescents with intellectual disability: I Rationale and methods; II Epidemiology. J Intellect Disabil Res, 40:91–98, 99–109.

Goodman R (1997) The strengths and difficulties questionnaire: a research note. J Child Psychol Psychiatry, 38:581–586.

Gowers S, Harrington R, Whitton A et al. (1999) Brief scale for measuring the outcomes of emotional and behavioural disorders in children. Health of the Nation Outcome Scales for Children and Adolescents (HoNOSCA). Brit J Psychiatry, 174:413–417.

Hazell P (2003) Depression in children and adolescents. Clin Evid, Jun (9):356–366.

Kids Help Line: http://kidshelp.com.au.

King NJ, Tonge BJ, Mullen P et al. (2000) Treating sexually abused children with posttraumatic stress symptoms: a randomised clinical trial. J Am Acad Child Adolesc Psychiatry, 39:1347–1355.

McDermott BM, Palmer LJ (2002) Postdisaster emotional distress, depression and event-related variables: findings across child and adolescent developmental stages. Aust NZ J Psychiatry, 36:754–761.

McDermott BM, Batik M, Roberts L, Gibbon P (2002) Parent and child report of family functioning in a clinical child and adolescent eating disorders sample. Aust NZ J Psychiatry, 36:509–514.

McGorry PD, Jackson HJ (1999) The Recognition and Management of Early Psychosis. Cambridge University Press: Cambridge UK.

National Advisory Council for Youth Suicide Prevention (1998) National Action Plan for Suicide Prevention. Commonwealth Department of Health and Aged Care, Canberra.

Nurcombe B (2000) Child sexual abuse: I Psychopathology. Aust NZ J Psychiatry, 34:86–92.

Nurcombe B, Wooding S, Marrington P et al. (2000) Child sexual abuse: II Treatment. Aust NZ J Psychiatry, 34:92–97.

Parham J, Rickwood D (2003) Promotion, Prevention and Early Intervention for Mental Health: National Consultation. The Australian Network for Promotion, Prevention and Early Intervention for Mental Health. (http://www.auseinet.com)

Prior M (2003) Is there an increase in the prevalence of autism spectrum disorders? J Paediatr Child Health, 39:81–82.

Prior M (2003) Toddler temperament, cognition and caregiver interaction predict impulsive functioning. Evid Based Ment Health, 6:20.

Prior M, Smart D, Samson A, Oberklaid F (2001) Longitudinal predictors of behavioural adjustment in pre-adolescent children. Aust NZ J Psychiatry, 35:297–307.

Sawyer MG, Arney FM, Baghurst PA et al. (2001) The mental health of young people in Australia: key findings from the child and adolescent component of the national survey of mental health and well-being. Aust NZ J Psychiatry, 35:806–814.

Spence SH, Sheffield JK, Donovan CL (2003) Preventing adolescent depression: an evaluation of the problem-solving-for-life program. J Consult Clin Psychol, 71:3–13.

Tonge BJ (2002) Autism, autistic spectrum and the need for definition. Med J Aust, 176:412–413.

Year Book Australia (2002) Population and Health. Australian Bureau of Statistics, Canberra.

Zubrick SR, Silburn SR, Burton P, Blair E (2000) Mental health disorders in children and young people: scope, cause and prevention. 34:570–578.

Systems of Care in Asia*

K. Michael Hong, Kosuke Yamazaki, Cornelio G. Banaag, Du Yasong

7.1   Introduction   – 58

7.2   Status and Needs of Child Mental Health/
        Child Psychiatry in Asia: Profiles of Selected
        Countries – 59
7.2.1   China – 59
7.2.1.1 Brief History of Child Mental Health Services
        in China   – 59
7.2.1.2 More and More Mental Health Problems of Children
        and Adolescents Were Demonstrated   – 59
7.2.1.3 Status of Child Mental Health Services   – 60
7.2.2   Japan   – 60
7.2.2.1 The History of Child and Adolescent Psychiatry
        in Japan   – 60
7.2.2.2 Child Psychiatry and Child Mental Health
        Services   – 61
7.2.2.3 Major Mental Health Issues and Child Psychiatric
        Disorders – 61
7.2.3   Korea – 62
7.2.3.1 A Brief History of the Development of Child
        Mental Health Services   – 62
7.2.3.2 Clinical Experiences and Research Data   – 62
7.2.4   The Philippines   – 63
7.2.4.1 Child Mental Health Services of the Philippines –
        A Brief History   – 63
7.2.4.2 Child Psychiatry in the Philippines   – 64
7.2.4.3 Clinical Experiences and Mental Health Issues   – 65

7.3   Common Features and Characteristics of the Status
        and Development of Child Psychiatry/Mental
        Health Services in the Asian Region   – 66

7.4   Developments and Contributions of National/In-
        ternational Professional Organizations in the Asian
        Region   – 68

7.5   Conclusions and Suggestions   – 68

        References   – 70

7.1 Introduction

It is only in recent years that some of the many countries in Asia have begun to actively develop child mental health and psychiatric services. The major reason is likely to be that it has not been long since western medicine, per se, was introduced to the region. It took even longer for the subspecialties like child psychiatry to be recognized as being needed and some adventurous young psychiatrists to go abroad for subspecialty training and come back to begin the service. This does not mean that children's mental health services were not provided in these countries before western medicine was introduced. Professionals were available to intervene in children's emotional and behavioral problems. In fact, pediatricians, family physicians, and other allied professions such as teachers and clergyman delivered services in their own way.

In this chapter, a brief history of the development of child mental health services and the current status of child psychiatry and child mental health services in some selected countries in Asia are described. The availability and activities of the professional organizations are reviewed and recommendations for future development are presented. The selection of the countries included in this chapter was made purely by the availability of the data and information regarding the topics allocated for this chapter. These countries are more visible and somewhat more advanced in their professional activities, and by no means do they represent Asia as a whole. We will try to present the status of the remaining countries by drawing from the commonalities of the countries reported in detail.

---

* For technical reasons no section on Taiwan could be included in this chapter.

7.2 Status and Needs of Child Mental Health/Child Psychiatry in Asia: Profiles of Selected Countries

7.2.1 China

7.2.1.1 Brief History of Child Mental Health Services in China

Child mental health services in China have been developing since the 1920s, after the emergence of the children protection movement. From 1930 to 1949, child mental health services in China almost stopped because of the war with Japan and the civil war. The People's Republic of China was established in 1949 and marked the beginning of the continued growth of child mental health services in China. Although Professor Tao Guotai started child psychiatry in China in the 1930s, the official work began after liberation in 1949 with the opening of the first clinic of child psychiatry in the Nanjing Psychiatric Hospital in Jiangsu province. From 1950 to 1980, other cities began to offer psychiatric outpatient departments for children and adolescents: Shanghai, Beijing, and Changsha in Hunan province; Chengdu in Sichuan province; Guangzhou in Guangdong province; and Shashi in Hubei province. During this time, professional work mainly concentrated on the diagnosis, treatment, and social rehabilitation of children with major psychosis, schizophrenia, manic-depressive disorder, organic psychosis, mental retardation, and Tourette's syndrome. Medication was used to treat both outpatients and inpatients.

During the period of the Cultural Revolution in China, and before the 1980s, medication was the main treatment method in adult psychiatry as well as in child psychiatry, and only a very few child psychiatrists were practicing.

Since the 1980s, child psychiatry in China has been making good progress. The China Mental Health Association (CMHA) was founded in 1986. The Professional Committee of Mental Health for Children (PCMHC) is a branch of the CMHA. The members come from a variety of professions related to child mental health services, such as: child psychiatry, child psychology, education, general medicine, and special education. The PCMHC holds a national meeting every 2 years where participants can present their papers and exchange their experiences.

7.2.1.2 More and More Mental Health Problems of Children and Adolescents Were Demonstrated

Since the end of the 1970s, China has opened and reformed itself for the world. More information has been exchanged with other countries. Psychosis is no longer the only diagnosis and treatment subject, and a variety of mental health problems have become important work for child psychiatrists and mental health workers.

Xin Ren'e et al. (1988–1989) conducted a survey of 24,013 children aged 4–16 in 22 provinces in China using the Achenbach Child Behavior Checklist (CBCL). The results showed that the prevalence of mental health problems was 11–22% (average 12.97%). The main mental health problems were depression, somatic complaints, social withdrawal, and aggression. Around the same time, Professor Li Xuerong (Li 1990) presented his research regarding the incidence of child mental health in the Hunan province. The average incidence of mental disorders was 14.9% (◘ Table 7.1).

In 1992, Xin Ren'e conducted another study, an epidemiological study of 3,000 children in Shanghai aged 4–5. No strong evidence emerged of a distinct psychopathology associated with children from one-child families, although there was a significant correlation between being an only child and having social withdrawal problems. Delinquent behavior and hyperactivity were more frequent among boys, while somatic complaints, schizoid behavior, anxiety, and depression were more frequent among girls. A 4-year follow-up study of 433 children from the original group showed a marked increase in hyperactive syndrome.

Du Yasong et al. (2001) conducted a study on the development of child and adolescent psychiatry from 1986 to 1999 in Shanghai. Mental health problems diagnosed during this 15-year period are as follows, in the order of frequency: attention deficit hyperactivity disorder 50%, mental retardation 11%, learning disorders 9.4%, emotional disorders 5.5%, behavioral disorders 4.8%, tic disorders 4.0%, psychosis 2.1%, autism 1.1%, and multiple diagnoses 4.8%. A study on mental health problems of students in boarding high schools demonstrated that the prevalence of behavioral problems was 11.2% in males and 10.2% in females; the prevalence of emotional problems was 16% in males and 10.5% in females, and learning disabilities were about 10% for the entire group (Du Yasong 1997).

□ Table 7.1. Mental health problems of children aged 4–16 in Hunan province (1990)

	Emotional disorders	Behavioral disorders	Developmental disorders	Psychosomatic disorders
City	1.12	8.34	7.55	0.33
Rural area	0.93	7.70	11.11	0.26
Male	0.67	12.21	10.49	0.24
Female	1.48	3.46	6.97	0.37
45 years	0.96	1.14	7.87	0
6–11 years	0.77	10.68	11.32	0.23
12–16 years	1.45	7.18	5.91	0.49

Although medication has been the most common method of treatment in the past 15 years, in recent years several forms of psychotherapy such as family psychotherapy have been used to treat children and adolescents. The Chinese child and adolescent psychiatry/child mental health services have caught up significantly, as their socio-economic status has improved and their clinical experience has accumulated.

7.2.1.3   Status of Child Mental Health Services

In China, there are only a few child psychiatrists in psychiatric hospitals, mental health centers, and general hospitals. There are 40 million children and adolescents in China, but there are less than 100 child psychiatrists in all. The ratio of children to psychiatrists is 1:1,000,000 in China (1:4,000 in developed countries, such as in the United States). From the 1990s, teachers, pediatricians, and all doctors in child health care have shown an increasing interest in the field of child mental health services. Training courses and seminars have been offered from a variety of professional fields to introduce a range of treatment options. Regional and national continuing medical re-education programs are being offered, but currently only three medical universities (Shanghai, Beijing, and Changsha in the Hunan province) offer a postgraduate degree in child psychiatry.

Compared to 10 years ago, there is a greater awareness of the need for child mental health services among professional health workers and the general population. There is a very large deficit of professional health workers in child mental health services all over the China. The current organization of child mental health services is not enough to meet the needs of the population. Most trained health workers live in the largest cities (Shanghai, Beijing, Nanjing, and Changsha) or are associated with the teaching hospitals affiliated with medical universities. The children and adolescents in rural areas are unable to receive services.

China also lacks a supply of professional journals devoted to the field of child mental health services and research. Currently, there are only two books (**Modern Child Psychiatry**, written by Li Xuerong; and **Child & Adolescent Psychiatry**, written by Tao Guotai) available in Chinese.

7.2.2   Japan

7.2.2.1   The History of Child and Adolescent Psychiatry in Japan

In Japan, efforts to raise public awareness regarding childhood mental disorders and delinquency were already visible in the first two decades of the 1930s. In the 1930s, child guidance clinics were opened in several universities, and child units were established in the National Kohnodai Hospital and Tokyo Metropolitan Umegaoka Hospital in the late 1940s. In the 1950s, a child mental health unit was established in the National Mental Health Institute, and reports on cases of infantile autism and school refusal began to be published in Japan. In 1960, the **Japanese Journal of Child Psychiatry and Allied Professions** was first issued, and the Japanese Society for Child Psychiatry was founded (Founding President: Prof. Hitoshi Murakami); the latter was renamed the Japanese Society for Child and Adolescent Psychiatry in 1983.

In 1962, the Japanese Society became an official member of the International Association of Child and Adolescent Psychiatry and Allied Professions (IACAPAP). And in July 1990, the 12th International Congress of the International Association for Child and Adolescent Psychiatry and Allied Professions (Organizing Committee Chairperson: Dr. Koichiro Shirahashi) was successfully held in Kyoto; it was the first congress of the Association hosted in Asia. Furthermore, the Japanese Society was instrumental in establishing the Asian Society for Child and Adolescent Psychiatry and Allied Professions (Founding President: Prof. Masahisa Nishizono), which held its 1st International Congress in Tokyo in April, 1996.

Movement to establish a chair of child psychiatry in the university medical schools started in the 1970s. Although a proposal for the establishment of a new chair of child psychiatry was put together and submitted to the Science Council of Japan on 18 February 1994, this has yet to be realized. Moreover, in Japan, the term »child psychiatry« has yet to be recognized as an official label for a clinical department.

However, problems related to the minds of children have recently become a social issue in this age of rapid decline in the number of children, which, together with an increase in juvenile crime, has raised the demand for child and adolescent psychiatric care drastically. New child and adolescent psychiatry clinics have begun to be established at university hospitals in the past few years, and programs for training child psychiatrists are becoming increasingly active. In 1998, a system of accreditation of specialists was implemented and 106 candidates have been accredited to date as specialists in child psychiatry, based on strict judgment of case reports, research papers, and contributions to society.

7.2.2.2 Child Psychiatry and Child Mental Health Services

Mental health services for children and adolescents are provided by a variety of professionals including child psychiatrists, general psychiatrists, clinical psychologists, school counselors, pediatricians, school teachers, and social workers. In fact, there are over 2,600 members of the Japanese Society for Child and Adolescent Psychiatry and Allied Professions; 55% of them are physicians, while 45% are paramedical professionals.

However, one of the major problems is the wide difference in competency of child mental health workers. For example, while there are many competent psychologists, there are equally as many incompetent, unqualified psychologists. Even the psychiatrists seeing children and adolescents with mental health problems vary greatly in their level of clinical competency because up until recently there were no formal standardized clinical training programs in child psychiatry. It is only in the past few years that child psychiatry training programs and a qualification accreditation system have been initiated. So far, among the 1,000 psychiatrists who are seeing children and adolescents, 106 have been accredited as child psychiatrists. It appears that critical issues in the field of child psychiatry and child mental health are the lack of standardized, formal clinical training programs and qualification systems of clinical competency; this is also true for most clinical medical specialties and most allied professions as well. Therefore, the establishment of formal child psychiatry training programs at major university medical schools and the institution of a refined accreditation system are urgently needed and are the major tasks of the Japanese Society of Child and Adolescent Psychiatry.

7.2.2.3 Major Mental Health Issues and Child Psychiatric Disorders

Japan is unique in that it is the only developed nation among so many nations in Asia. Japan has suffered from economic depression for the past decade. However, it is still prosperous and enjoys all the benefits of an advanced, modern, high-technology country, but not without concomitant mental health problems, such as juvenile crime, suicide, drug abuse, social withdrawal, school nonattendance, school bullying, child abuse, and parental abuse (violence in the home by children).

Like many developing countries in Asia, major child psychiatric disorders frequently diagnosed include pervasive developmental disorders (particularly high-functioning PDD, Asperger syndrome), learning disorder, ADHD, eating disorder, depression, and reactive attachment disorder, among others.

Much effort has been made by many dedicated child psychiatrists to come up with culture-appropriate treatment methods.

7.2.3   Korea

7.2.3.1   A Brief History of the Development of Child Mental Health Services

The origin of child and adolescent psychiatry and child mental heath services can be traced back to Korean independence from Japan in 1945. A document from that time shows that the juvenile court house requested consultations from a psychiatrist. During and after the Korean Conflict of 1950–1953, the U.S. Military Medical Service introduced modern western medicine to Korea. Psychiatry was one of the areas that benefited; the needs of child psychiatry were advocated by a group of military psychiatrists. In 1958, Judge Kwon opened the Seoul Child Guidance Center, the first one of its kind. A group of psychiatrists, psychologists, educators, and social workers were involved in this center's activities. They imported the model from the United States and were active in providing psychological tests and consultations, parent education, and other needed services. However, the child guidance movement did not continue for long, partly because of the shortage of experts and qualified child psychiatrists on the team. Since then, the educational/school psychologists have carried out most of the psychological services for emotional and behavioral disorders, especially for school-aged children. In 1968, a couple of psychiatrists went abroad to the United States to receive formal child psychiatry training. Meanwhile, a group of psychiatrists were active in research on normal and delinquent adolescents.

Formal child psychiatry services did not begin until 1980, when Professor K. M. Hong returned from the United States after finishing his general and child psychiatry training at the University of Washington, being board certified both in general psychiatry and child and adolescent psychiatry, and having served on the faculty at the University of Minnesota for 6 years. He immediately opened the first child psychiatry clinic and day treatment center for autistic children and established the first division of child psychiatry at the Seoul National University Hospital. He also started the Child Psychiatry Fellowship training program. Since then, many Korean child psychiatrists have traveled abroad for training and some qualified child psychiatrists trained in the United States have returned to run child psychiatric clinics at several university hospitals in Korea.

The Korean Academy of Child and Adolescent Psychiatry was organized in 1983 and has escalated the development of child psychiatry/child mental health services. Currently, there are six child psychiatry fellowship-training centers. In 1996, the Korean Academy of Child and Adolescent Psychiatry set up the first board certification system. Now there are over 77 board-certified child psychiatrists, 48 board eligible, and 18 fellows in training. The Korean Academy holds scientific meetings twice a year. It seems that child psychiatry in Korea is flourishing, most likely due to the availability of formal training centers as well as a board certification system.

In 1990, **the Korean Journal of Child and Adolescent Psychiatry** began publishing its journal twice a year. Korean child psychiatry has done a great job promoting the awareness of child mental health problems, has conducted numerous public lectures, and has stimulated other professions to emerge and develop during the last 20 years. Special education, child psychology, medical social work, speech therapy, and other professions have grown a great deal. Korean child psychiatry has been active and supportive in establishing the Korean Society of Autism and the Korean Association of Child Abuse and Neglect, which has contributed significantly to revise the Child Protection Act in 1999 and set up a nationwide child abuse and neglect prevention centers. The Korean Academy of Child and Adolescent Psychiatry has contributed significantly to the foundation of ASCAPAP (Asian Society of Child and Adolescent Psychiatry and Allied Professions), which was established 1996.

7.2.3.2   Clinical Experience and Research Data

Clinical experience of child psychiatry in Korea has demonstrated the existence of all disorders classified in DSM-IV and ICD-10. An analysis of outpatient visits to a major university revealed a variety of clinical diagnoses although anxiety disorder, ADHD, and pervasive developmental disorder are over-represented (Hong 1982). No systematic epidemiological study for the child population has been carried out. Instead, several prevalence studies were done on several different disorders: ADHD 7.6%, conduct disorder 3.8%, oppositional defiant disorder 4.2% (Cho and Shin 1994), autism 9.2/10,000 (Hong et al. 1999), and dyslexia among 3rd and 4th graders 2.4% (Lee and Hong 1985). Overall, the prevalence of psychiatric morbidity among Korean school adolescents was 31% (Kim et al. 1983). No culture-bound syndrome by strict definition could be delineated, although some of the emotional disorders are noted more in terms of frequency. For example, tic disorder, test anxiety, and severe forms of somatic symptoms are noted very frequently and seem to be related to stress due to a heavy emphasis on scholastic achievement. In lay terms, »senior high disease« indicates that senior high students are victims of this endless pressure to study to get a high grade in order to enter a top-ranked college. One of the most disconcerting problems among adolescents is the high suicide rate (28/100,000) among adolescents; 4.4% of adolescents had a history of attempting suicide (Juon et al. 1994). School bullying, including **wang-ta**, which is a kind of rejection and isolation of a student by peers (similar to **ijime** in Japan), is very high (48%) and the extreme form of school violence is 3% (Kim et al. 2001). Another intriguing form of adolescent violence is parent abuse by adolescents; the prevalence of which is 2.8% (Lee et al. 1997). Some of these adolescents do not have any other problems except they are very quiet and socially isolated, a condition similar to **hikkigomori** in Japan; violence is directed only to their own parents. There is a rapidly growing number of school dropouts and drug abuse cases as well. Most recently, a new form of behavioral addiction has emerged. More than 90% of adolescents are using the Internet and the prevalence of Internet addiction is reportedly 3.5% among Internet users (Whang et al. 2003). Internet addiction seems to serve various functions, such as: experimental relationships, searching for identity, a sexual outlet, and seeking help for depression and social isolation. The Korean Government set up a youth commission to protect adolescents from drug abuse, sexual exploitation, school violence, and obscene media. Many NGOs opened adolescent counseling centers and violence prevention centers.

Another disconcerting problem observed in early developmental years is a sharp increase in the number of autistic-like children referred to child psychiatric clinics for diagnosis. They are definitely related to the lack of appropriate parental care and stimulation for their development; the majority of them meet the diagnostic criteria of reactive attachment disorders or pervasive developmental disorder, not otherwise specified (PDD NOS; Youn and Hong 1995; Hong 1996; Shin et al. 1999). Early detection and intervention of child abuse and neglect and the establishment of nation-wide prevention centers are the significant achievements of a multidisciplinary collaboration.

Many of these problems and issues seem to be related to massive and rapid social changes that have been occurring in Korea for the past 30 years. Korea has gone through phenomenal economic growth, socio-political changes, and various forms of »westernization« (including industrialization, urbanization, democratization, and family nuclearization). These drastic socio-cultural changes have affected every aspect of Korean society and appear to be associated with many reactive, developmental, emotional, and behavioral disorders (Hong 1999).

7.2.4 The Philippines

7.2.4.1 Child Mental Health Services of the Philippines – A Brief History

The history of child mental health services in the Philippines can be traced to the formal establishment of the Philippine Mental Health Association (PMHA) on 15 January 1950. The Philippines, like many Asian nations, was in the process of recovering from the devastation of World War II. Concerned with the impact of this devastation on the mental health of the people, a group of well-meaning professionals organized the first Mental Health Guidance Clinic in the country. They provided clinical services to both individuals and families. The clinic was modeled after the child and youth guidance centers existing in many parts of the United States at the time. Among the first beneficiaries of the guidance clinic were young children and adolescents brought in for help because of various behavioral and emotional disorders. Psychologists and adult psychiatrists saw these young people. There were no child psychiatrists in the country for many years to come.

Complementing the work of the PMHA guidance clinic was a growing group of guidance counselors in grade schools and many high schools in the country. In the late 1960s the Philippine Guidance and Counseling Association was organized, expanding its scope over time to the college level and the work place. In the early years of the Association, many of the guidance counselors in the schools had no formal training in guidance and counseling. They were mostly well-meaning teachers pulled from the ranks because of their interest in the welfare of the youth. Over the years, both organizations have become more professional and nation-wide in range.

The Philippine Mental Health Association has chapters in different parts of the country. They act autonomously and initiate a variety of activities addressing the mental health needs of their communities. Although the initial thrust of the Association was to provide clinical services (through the Mental Health Guidance Clinics), the Association subsequently recognized the primacy of prevention. It organized the Education Information Service to spearhead the new focus of the Association: prevention, education, and information on mental health. This has become the primary program of the Association. As part of its advocacy program, the Association conducts mental health activities throughout the year, addressing mostly the mental health issues of children and adolescents. Among the most significant of these activities are the Youth Life Enrichment Program (YLEP) and the Peer Facilitators Training. The YLEP runs workshop seminars for youth, focusing on enhancement of life skills. The modules that evolved over the years include: »Self-awareness and Interpersonal Relationships«, »Value Inculcation«, »Youth and Health«, »Youth as a Family Facilitator«, and »Life Skills Enhancement and Drug Abuse Prevention«.

In 1992, a National Program for Mental Health was delineated by the Department of Health. Five areas of concern were identified: »Drug Abuse«, »Street Children«, »Overseas Contract Workers«, »Victims of Torture«, »Human Rights Violations and Violence«, and »Victims of Disasters«. These topics are currently included in the YLEP workshops. Also under YLEP, student mental health clubs have been organized in many secondary schools across the country. In metropolitan Manila alone, at present there are 56 active mental health clubs with a membership of about 16,000. Outside Manila, there are 38 such clubs with about 4,000 active members.

Recognizing the need to promote mental health activities at the college level, the PMHA has organized psychological societies in 28 selected colleges and universities in metro Manila, with a current membership of 21,600 students. These members work in partnership with the PMHA in promoting sound mental health among the Filipino youth. Since December 2000, the local college psychological societies have been organized under the Psychological Societies Association on Mental Health (PSAMH).

The Peer Facilitators Training Program consists of a 2-day training workshop involving about 40 youth participants each time. The participants, who are members of the mental health clubs, are provided the necessary knowledge, skills, and attitudes in their roles as peer counselors and assistants to the guidance counselors of their schools. The training utilizes group dynamics, lectures, workshops, and small group discussions focusing on the following models: »Self-awareness«, »Communication«, »Conflict Resolution«, and »Peer Counseling«. The young participants are given hands-on experience with peer counseling.

The Philippine Mental Health Association continues to provide clinical services on an outpatient basis to children, youth, and adults with emotional and behavioral disorders. The range of diagnostic and treatment services include clinical interviews, psychological assessment, play therapy, individual and family counseling, and family support groups, as well as psychiatric treatment and management. Since 2001, the part-time services of a child psychiatrist have been made available. In the past 5 years, some 3,200 young patients with various psychiatric disorders have been seen in the clinics together with family members.

7.2.4.2 Child Psychiatry in the Philippines

Like in many Asian countries, child psychiatry is a relatively recent development in the Philippines. Formal teaching of child psychiatry in the undergraduate and postgraduate medical education began with the arrival of Dr. Cornelio Banaag from the United States in 1970. After finishing his formal training in child and adolescent psychiatry at the Worcester Youth Guidance Center in Worcester, Massachusetts, he returned to the faculty of the University of the Philippines College of Medicine in Manila to pursue the teaching of child psychiatry. Subsequently in 1981, he set up the first child psychiatry training program in the country at the University of the Philippines – Philippine General Hospital. The first graduates of the program completed their training in 1983. In 1990, Banaag set up the second child psychiatry training program at the Philippine Children's Medical Center in Quezon City, metropolitan Manila, producing its first graduate in 1992. The two training programs, the only two in the Philippines at present, have produced 28 of the 34 practicing child psychiatrists in the country. Five candidates are currently undergoing training.

In 1995, the child psychiatrists in the country formed the Child and Adolescent Psychiatrists of the Philippines, Inc. (CAPPI). The organization has since been actively engaged in a mission of promoting mental health among Filipino children and youth, and the prevention of psychiatric illnesses through advocacy and mental health education. CAPPI has organized postgraduate courses in different parts of the Philippines. The themes of the postgraduate courses are varied and attractive to various sectors in the community, including parents and teachers. On 29 January 2004, CAPPI launched a book on parenting (»Parenting: A Special Job for Ordinary People«) authored by several of its members, the first of its kind in Philippine psychiatry. CAPPI is currently making the move to set up a board certification system for child psychiatrists in the Philippines.

7.2.4.3 Clinical Experiences and Mental Health Issues

The clinical experience of the Filipino child psychiatrists confirms the existence in the Philippines of the child psychiatric disorders listed in the DSM-IV and the ICD-10. There is a perceptible increase in the prevalence of emotional and behavioral disorders among Filipino young people posing a heavy challenge to the limited numbers of child psychiatrists in the country. This rising tide of emotional and behavioral problems may be related to the current socio-cultural, economic, and political situation in the country.

The Philippines, like most developing countries, is a country in prolonged transition. It has a population growth that is bigger than its indicators of economic growth. Of the current population of 80 million, about half are young people below the age of 21. These young people are growing up in a complex and very uneven environment. It is an environment that has become unstable and unpredictable; random violence has become common. In many sectors, the adult who should provide protection, security, and love, are psychologically and/or physically unavailable. Three million overseas Filipino workers (not counting long-distance employment of parents within the country) have left many children growing up in single parent homes. Long-distance parenting has become common practice. Add to this the growing number of unstable marriages resulting in separations and annulments of marriages, the consequences of which are more children growing up in circumstances other than the usual family setting. The rapid urbanization taking place in the country has made material goods more accessible to young people, facilitating the shift to more materialistic

values. This urbanization has resulted in congestion, pollution, traffic, and diminishing space for raising children (condominium and townhouses for the middle class, shanties for the poor), with more and more parents coming home late with frayed nerves into limited living space. The explosive growth of information technology has made possible easy access to information, home entertainment, children spending more time at computers (resulting in conflicts between parents and the children, confused parents uncertain how to set limits), TV, video (children have less time for reading, for playing with friends, parents have less time for friends and family gatherings). Mass media (TV, print, movies, Internet) has pushed into children's awareness a lot of information about and powerful images of violence, pornography, sex, rape, incest, teenage pregnancies, accidents, murders vividly reenacted on TV, military rebellion, and corruption perpetrated by people who should be providing protection and role modeling for young people. Children become too aware too early of the dangers in their environment, and lose the illusions of childhood too early. They become skeptical and cynical. They ask questions parents are not prepared for, like a 6-year-old boy who asks »what is rape?« or a 4-year-old who asks »is the world going to be destroyed, are we all going to die?« For many children, the environment in which they are growing has become stressful. They feel unprotected and insecure. They express their fears and insecurities in disturbances of emotions and behavior. Some of the manifestations of disturbances are the children who are stressed and refuse to go to school, or fail in school despite their intelligence. Many children suffer anxiety disorders in various forms, like the 10-year-old boy who gets scared when his mother has to leave, because he saw on TV a mother killed by random violence, or the 15-year-old male tormented by his obsessive counting of numbers in his head and compulsively checking doors and avoiding steps on cracks in the pavement. Many young people suffer depression and associated suicidal thoughts and attempts. A recent survey by the University of the Philippines Population Institute showed a rising trend in adolescent suicide. Not only is the number of drug abusers growing at an alarming rate, but the age of the abusers is also getting younger. It is increasingly common to see a sixth grader smoking, or a 14-year-old drinking beer at parties. The majority of regular users of prohibited substances like marijuana and **shabu** (methamphetamine) are adolescents. An increasing prevalence is also noted in the autistic spectrum disorders, attention deficit hyperactivity disorder, teenage violence, and child abuse in various forms.

The number of disturbed children and adolescents in the Philippines is not known. There is no national survey to tell us the full extent of the problem. An approximation can only be made by looking at the increasing number of children and youth with emotional and behavioral problems seen in the clinics of child psychiatrists, developmental pediatricians, child neurologists, and psychologists. Guidance counselors in schools report increasing case loads. The gap between the demand for services and the number of mental health programs and services is growing. Thirty-four child and adolescent psychiatrists is a small number relative to the population of 80 million, about half of them young people. The challenge to the current group of Filipino child psychiatrists is formidable. To make their chosen specialty viable they need to close ranks, collaborate, and be more assertive in developing training programs and in recruiting potential candidates to the field, and engage in more research activities that will make their practice relevant to the communities they serve.

7.3 Common Features and Characteristics of the Status and Development of Child Psychiatry/Mental Health Services in the Asian Region

In this section, problems and issues of child mental health and child psychiatry shared by most Asian countries will be discussed.

1. **Many countries in the Asian region still face grave problems of general health, and even survival. Normal physical development is threatened.**
   According to the UNICEF report for the year 2002, many Asian countries still belong to a very low socio-economic, poverty-stricken group; they have a high infant mortality rate, and a high prevalence (20–30%) of moderate to severe developmental retardation. Children in these countries are not fed adequately and basic physical health care cannot be provided. At times, it may seem superfluous to discuss the current development of child mental health services in this situation.

2. **Child psychiatry is a newly emerging subspecialty for some countries.**
   While the majority of countries in the Asian region do not have formal child psychiatry services, for some countries like Japan, South Korea, Taiwan, the Philippines, China, India, and Singapore, child psychiatry has begun to emerge recently as a brand new subspecialty in medicine. These countries are the relatively more developed ones in Asia in terms of their socio-economical status and medical-health services. The first task of child psychiatry/child mental health service is to educate the public on the need and importance of child psychiatry/child mental health. Most general psychiatric colleagues and government officials in many countries in the Asian region do not seem to know about child psychiatry services. Therefore, one of the characteristics of child psychiatry in these regions is the variability of development. That is, countries are very different in terms of what is available and what is necessary to prompt the development of child mental health services. In order to establish child psychiatry services in a country, you need one or two pioneering psychiatrists to go abroad to study, receive training, and come back to develop the service system. For many countries in Asia, child psychiatry is still part of general psychiatry, which is inadequate and under-developed itself.

3. **Most disorders classified in DSM-IV and ICD-10 are found in Asian countries.**
   It can be said in general that almost all child psychiatric disorders described in DSM and ICD could be found in any part of Asia if you are a qualified child psychiatrist. There may be differences in terms of frequency and clinical manifestations of the disorders. For example, tic disorders and ADHD may have been considered normal behaviors or some kind of habit and now they are introduced as a disorder; therefore, the public might think they are new kinds of disorder and the clinicians tend to over-diagnose them (Hong et al. 1996). However, it is obvious that they have existed for a long time and yet they had not been recognized as a disorder per se. At the same time, the incidence of certain disorders may have actually increased in relation to rapid social changes, social restructuring, and subsequent increase of stress. It is observed that there are strong **reactive components** in causation and manifestations of certain disorders compared to their counterparts in western

countries. Caution is required when one claims a »culture-bound syndrome«, which usually turns out to be a different manifestation of an existing, already-described disorder in the West.

4. **The breakdown of the traditional family system and reduction in number of children.**
Most countries in the Asian region have undergone drastic changes in their family structure and functions. Traditional family systems are shaken and the nuclear family structure is substituted. On top of these changes, the rise of the divorce rate in this region is very alarming. The number of children in a family has decreased, particularly in several economically advanced countries. Some of them have adopted social and government policies to limit the number of children to one or two. These policies have brought about serious side effects, one of which is the huge imbalance in the male:female ratio of the newly born. For example, the ratio is 120:100 in Korea and 139:100 in China. Because of the nuclear family structure and the reduced number of children, the mother-child relationship has become very close and very intense. It eventually resulted in increased conflicts and power struggles between the two. In addition, parents have become very concerned and anxious to raise their children properly, because they have only one or two children, and therefore, the risks of over-control and over-protection have increased. These kinds of dynamic interactions in the family, together with sustained stress from the pressure and competition for scholastic achievement have put children and adolescents at a higher risk of developing various transient and reactive-emotional and behavioral disorders, suicide, and even psychotic breakdown.

5. **Rising number of working mothers and women's equal right movements.**
In most Asian countries, traditionally women did not work outside the home and were in charge of raising children. Nowadays, an increasing number of women have begun to work outside the home, and in some countries women comprise almost 50% of the work-force. Equal rights movements are underway and successful in some countries, and the women claim their own rights and pursue their careers. The risks are that children may not be taken care of properly and adequately while mothers work since public. Private day care is not adequately provided in many countries. The net result is general child neglect, although it may be a temporary phenomenon.

6. **Confusion and inappropriateness in child rearing practices.**
Many young mothers in highly industrialized countries do not really know how to raise children properly, especially during infancy, partly because they have no skills and knowledge of child rearing, but also because very little support is available while they work because of the breakdown of the extended family system. Many young women do not want to have a baby and even when they have a baby, they do not want to raise the child. This results in an increasing number of child abandonment cases, abuse and neglect, and problems of attachment between the mother and the infant. Many grossly inappropriate child-rearing practices are observed, such as the infant watching TV all day long. These and other forms of gross emotional neglect cannot be unrelated to the sudden increase of developmental disorders, including autistic-like infants and toddlers, which could meet the criteria of reactive attachment disorder (Hong 1996; Shin et al. 1999).

7. **Confusing, often contradictory advice by professionals on child rearing and child behavior management.**
In some advanced Asian countries, the number of professionals in many fields have grown and expanded their roles and professional identities in the last 20 years. This has sometimes created side effects such as territorial fights and difficulties in cooperating with each other. Backgrounds of professionals are different in theory and training experiences. Therefore, they have different ideas and opinions on child rearing and behavior management, which are often not appropriate to the indigenous culture. Also, they try to implement and insist on western styles, and many young mothers are often confused in the end. Professionals as well as parents have not paid enough attention to traditional child rearing methods, which are often downgraded. Rather, they have tried to learn and practice western styles, which may not be appropriate for the Asian culture.

8. **Mental health intervention methods are limited.**
In underdeveloped and developing countries, medication is usually the most frequently used treatment modality for child and adolescent mental health problems, partly because medications are the most popular methods of treatment

in general psychiatry in this region and it is easy to extend downward to children. Another reason could be that psychosocial interventions require more thorough and fuller training in child psychiatry. Health professionals cannot utilize various treatment methods unless they are well and fully trained.

7.4 Developments and Contributions of National/International Professional Organizations in the Asian Region

It is only in recent years that national and international child psychiatry organizations have been established in the Asian region. The first organizations of child and adolescent psychiatry appear to be the Japanese Society of Child and Adolescent Psychiatry and Allied Professions and the Korean Academy of Child and Adolescent Psychiatry in the early 1980s. The ASEAN Forum of Child and Adolescent Psychiatry is being held every 2 years, as a part of the Asian Association of Psychiatry. The ASEAN Forum on Child and Adolescent Psychiatry was first organized in Jakarta, Indonesia in 1978, and the second Forum was held in Manila in 1980. This forum was organized to bring together the few child psychiatrists and mental health professionals then available in the ASEAN region. At that time, ASEAN consisted of five countries: Malaysia, Philippines, Indonesia, Thailand, and Singapore. Since then it has expanded to include Cambodia, Vietnam, Brunei, Laos, and Myanmar. Technically, all child psychiatrists of member countries are members of the Forum. The Forum became subsumed under a bigger organization called the ASEAN Federation for Psychiatry and Allied Professions, founded in 1981. The Forum does not have a set of officers but follows the official leadership of the Federation. The child psychiatrists in the region have been trying to separate from the Federation unsuccessfully because of the limited number of child psychiatrist members of the Federation

The Asian Society of Child and Adolescent Psychiatry and Allied Professions (ASCAPAP) was established in 1996, and the first congress was held successfully in Tokyo. Many child psychiatrists from more than a dozen Asian countries including China, India, Japan, Korea, the Philippines, Taiwan, and Singapore participated in the congress. Professor Nishizono was elected as the first President. The second congress was held in Seoul in 1999 under the leadership of the second President, Prof. K. M. Hong. The third congress was held in Taipei in 2003 under the leadership of Prof. Wei-Tsuen Soong. The fourth congress is scheduled in Manila, Philippines in 2006 and Prof. Cornelio Banaag will be in charge of organizing it. The other main contributors for the development and activities of ASCAPAP are Prof. Yamazaki (Japan), Prof. Malhotra (India), and Dr. Wong (Singapore).

Since the founding of the ASCAPAP, the Taiwanese Society of Child and Adolescent Psychiatry and the Child and Adolescent Psychiatrists of the Philippines, Inc. have been established and there have been definite improvements in child psychiatry professional activities in the region. Some countries have made major progress in setting up training programs, qualification systems, and requirements to be a child psychiatrist. The current status of the known professional organizations in Asia are described in ◘ Table 7.2.

7.5 Conclusions and Suggestions

It is extremely hard to draw certain conclusions regarding the current status of the systems of child mental health/child psychiatry care in the Asian region; mainly because there are so many countries in this region and the levels of development of the service systems are varied from country to country. However, it is also evident that there is a growing recognition of the need for child mental health/child psychiatry services. Many countries are just beginning to develop child psychiatry services, and several countries have taken the initiative and have established a service system rather successfully.

Professional organizations have been founded in recent years and now play a major role in creating and expanding the child mental health care system in Asia. It seems critically important to have a child psychiatry professional organization and some form of training program in order to develop and meet the challenges and growing problems of child and adolescent psychiatry. In order to start a child mental health service program in any country, it is of utmost importance to secure one or two qualified child psychiatrists who will be the pioneers for the development of child psychiatry. They can then train others and develop pertinent service programs, hopefully with the positive assistance from their government. However, there will be a limit to this progress unless more child psychiatrists are pro-

◧ Table 7.2. Current status of professional organizations in the Asian region

Country	Total population (in millions) (2002)	Name of child psychiatry national organization	Year of foundation	Number of qualified child psychiatrists	Requirements for qualification
China	1294	Professional Committee of Mental Health for Children	1986	About 100	NA (3 graduate schools for child psychiatry)
India	1000	NA	NA	24	NA
Indonesia	200	(Section of Indonesian Psychiatry Association)	NA	28	2 years child psychiatry
Japan	127	Japanese Society of Child and Adolescent Psychiatry and Allied Profession	1960	106	5 years clinical practice in child psychiatry, 30 or more case reports, research paper
Korea	47	Korean Academy of Child and Adolescent Psychiatry	1983	145	2 years child psychiatry fellowship or 1 year fellowship + 2 year additional training while practicing
Malaysia	26	(Chapter of Malaysian Psychiatry Association)	NA	13	1 training institution
Philippines	78	Child and Adolescent Psychiatrists of the Philippines, Inc.	1995	34	2 years child psychiatry training
Singapore	4	(Section of Singapore Psychiatry Association)	NA	12	3 years child psychiatry training
Taiwan	20	Taiwanese Society of Child and Adolescent Psychiatry	1998	90	2 years child psychiatry training
Thailand	67	Thai Society of Child Adolescent Psychiatry	NA	25	2 years child psychiatry training

NA = information not available

duced. This means that a training center is needed for every country if possible. This is rather difficult for many countries.

Training people abroad, e.g., in the United States or the United Kingdom, is very time consuming and expensive. It is also limited in terms of the number of trainees and the contents of training, which may not be culturally appropriate since most training centers are located in the western hemisphere. Therefore, it is proposed that several Asian countries seriously consider establishing The Asian Regional Training Center for Child Psychiatry/Child Mental Health and running the center jointly. International societies such as IACAPAP and the American Academy of Child & Adolescent Psychiatry can help the Regional Center by providing lecturers and faculties. This center will be able to produce competent child psychiatrists as well as child mental health workers who are absolutely essential for the development of a child psychiatry service in any country. In the meantime, the few available child psychiatrists/child mental health specialists should continue their lonely struggles to pioneer the field and try their best to educate the public, counsel parents, persuade government officials, and cooperate with those among the allied health professions.

It is hoped that the leading international organizations such as WHO, IACAPAP, and AACAP feel it is their responsibility to assist the establishment of child psychiatry/child mental health services in these developing/underdeveloped countries. In addition, it is strongly recommended that international scientific meetings allocate time and programs to discuss both the many relevant issues in establishing child psychiatry services and clinical problems of those developing countries without adequate child mental health/child psychiatry services.

References

Cho SC, Shin YO (1994) Prevalence of disruptive behavior disorders. Korean J Child & Adol Psychiatry: 141–149

Du Yasong (1999) Child Mental Health Care. Shanghai Science & Technology Press, Shanghai

Hong KM (1982) Developing Child Psychiatry in Korea. J Korean NeuroPsychiatry Assoc 21:183–191

Hong KM (1995) Crisis of child rearing and parental role in Korea. (Korean) Psychotherapy 9 (1):43–55

Hong KM (1996) A follow-up study of 30 preschool children diagnosed as »reactive attachment disorder«. Paper presented at the first Congress of Asian Society of Child and Adolescent Psychiatry, held in Tokyo

Hong KM (1999) Social changes, child rearing and child mental health. Paper presented at the 2nd Congress of Asian Society of Child Adolescent Psychiatry and Allied Professions, held in Seoul

Hong KM, Kim CH, Shin MS, Ahn DH (1996) Evaluations and diagnostic classifications of the patients referred with chief complaints of hyperactivity and distractability. Korean J Child and Adolescent Psychiatry 7 (2):190–202

Hong KM et al. (1999) Prevalence of autistic disorder in a medium size city in Korea (Korean). J Autistic Disorder 1 (1):1–25

Juon HS, Nam JJ, Ensminger M.E (1994) Epidemiology of Suicidal Behaviors among Korean Adolescents. J Child Psychol Psychiat. 35–663–676

Kim KI et al. (1983) A Mental Health Survey among High School Students in Seoul. (1) Findings from Intensive Individual Evaluation. J. Korean Institute of Mental Health, Hanyang University 1

Kim YS et al. (2001) School bullying and Related Psychopathology in Elementary School Students. J Korean NeuroPsychiatry Ass 40 (5):876–884

Lee YS, Hong KM (1985) A preliminary study of dyslexia in Korean 3rd and 4th grade students. J Korean NeuroPsychiatry Assoc 24 (1):103–110

Li Xuerong, Su Linyan, Wan Guobin et al. (1993) Epidemiological study on mental health problems in children aged 4–16 in Human province. Academic Archives of Hunan Medical University 18:43–46

Lee HB, Chun RS, Min SK, Oh KS, Lee SH (1997) Adolescent violence toward parents. Korean J Child & Adolescent Psychiatry 8:199–206

Shin YJ , Lee KS, Min SK, Emde RN (1999) A Korean syndrome of attachment disturbance mimicking symptoms of pervasive developmental disorder. Infant Mental Health Journal 20 (1):60–76

Whang LS, Lee S, Chang G (2003) Internet over-users' psychological profiles: A behavior sampling analysis on internet addiction. Cyber Psychological Behavior 6 (2):143–150

Xin Ren'e, Chen Shoukang, Lin Xiafeng et al. (1992) Behavioral problems among preschool age children in Shanghai: analysis of 3000 cases. Canadian J Psychiatry 37:250–257

Xin Ren'e, Tang Huiqin, Zhang Zhixiong et al. (1992) A survey of mental health problems in 24013 children aged 4–16 in China. Shanghai Archives of Psychiatry 4:47–55

Youn HS, Hong KM (1992) Comparison of psychopathological characteristics of children diagnosed as reactive attachment disorder and those as pervasive developmental disorder. Korean J Child and Adolescent Psychiatry 3 (1):3–13

Systems of Care in Africa

Brian Robertson, Custodia Mandlhate, Amira Seif El Din, Birama Seck

8.1   Introduction   – 71

8.2   **Child and Adolescent Mental Health Care Needs
       in Africa   – 72**
8.2.1 Child and Adolescent Mental Health in Africa   – 72
8.2.2 Major Influences on Child and Adolescent Mental
       Health in Africa   – 75
8.2.3 The Burden of Child and Adolescent Mental Health
       Problems in Africa   – 76

8.3   **Child and Adolescent Mental Health Care Systems
       in Africa   – 77**
8.3.1 Informal Systems of Care   – 78
8.3.2 Formal Systems of Care   – 79
8.3.3 Education and Training   – 81
8.3.4 Research   – 82

8.4   **The Way Forward for Africa   – 83**
8.4.1 Policy Development   – 83
8.4.2 Other Initiatives   – 85
8.4.3 Systems of Care in Africa: The Future   – 85

8.5   **Conclusion   – 86**

       References   – 87

8.1   Introduction

Rapid change against a background of complex diversity is the most prominent feature of Africa today. Threat and promise are engaged in a struggle for supremacy. While nations battle for independence, and revolutionaries cut swathes of instability across the continent, great statesmen rise up to lead the way to peace and prosperity. As countries buckle under poverty and famine, Africa's leaders forge global alliances to secure equitable opportunities for developing regions of the world. Africa, »the slumbering giant«, is stirring.

The divide between the Mediterranean countries and sub-Saharan Africa provides the first level of diversity in Africa. Seven North African countries are members of the Arab League[1]. At the next level, the remaining 46 sub-Saharan countries are diversified according to four European languages of occupation, French (20), English (20), Portuguese (5), and Spanish (1)[2]. The number of indigenous languages and ethnic groups approaches three figures in some countries. Christianity and Islam have made major inroads into traditional African religion and culture. Across the continent and between countries differences with respect to terrain, climate, population density, and rural-urban mix are pronounced. One constant feature is the relative inaccessibility of outlying African villages and settlements, leading to significant isolation of many communities from support structures and resources. Africa, with a total population of close to 800 million, is larger in size than the North American continent, and with as many diverse cultures and languages as Europe. Although sub-Saharan Africa constitutes 11% of the world population, it accounts for only 1.3% of the income (UNDP 2001).

Most countries in Africa fall into the low-income group, with only a scattering of low-middle- or middle-income countries. Of the 40 least wealthy countries in the world, 32 are in Africa (UNDP 2001), with a large proportion living on less than $1 per day. In sub-Saharan Africa, the dependency ratios for the majority of countries range between 108

---

[1] Djibouti, Egypt, Libyan Arab Jamahiriya, Morocco, Somalia, Sudan, Tunisia

[2] **French:** Algeria, Benin, Burkina Faso, Burundi, Cameroon, Central African Republic, Chad, Comoros, Congo, Cote d'Ivoire, Democratic Republic of the Congo, Gabon, Guinea, Madagascar, Mali, Mauritania, Niger, Rwanda, Senegal, Togo. **English:** Botswana, Eritrea, Ethiopia, Gambia, Ghana, Kenya, Lesotho, Liberia, Malawi, Mauritius, Namibia, Nigeria, Seychelles, Sierra Leone, South Africa, Swaziland, Uganda, United Republic of Tanzania, Zambia, Zimbabwe. **Portuguese:** Angola, Cape Verde, Guinea-Bissau, Mozambique, Sao Tome and Principe. **Spanish:** Equatorial Guinea

and 80 per 100, and the percentage of the population that is over 60 years lies between 4% and 7% (World Health Report 2001). Life expectancy at birth is 48 years, and the under-5 mortality rate is 173 for every 1,000 live births (UNICEF 2003). Adult literacy rates are 69% for males and 54% for females (UNICEF 2003).

With regard to mortality rates, all countries except Libya and Tunisia fall into the High Child, High Adult mortality stratum, or the High Child, Very High Adult stratum (World Health Report 2001). The total expenditure on health as a percentage of GDP ranges between 2% and 5% for the majority of countries (World Health Report 2001). Almost a quarter of countries have no national mental health program, while 40% do not have a specified budget for mental health (Atlas 2001). Ninety-five percent of countries have one or less psychiatrist per 100,000 population, and less than half have any epidemiological data or data collection systems. Only 40% of countries have special programs in mental health for children (Atlas 2001). Although the above figures reflect the dire adversities which challenge the development of optimal mental health throughout Africa, there are clearly considerable differences between countries with regard to available mental health services.

The WHO Regional Strategy for Mental Health for Africa (sub-Saharan region) 2000–2010 (WHO undated) summarizes the mental health situation in the following words:

> Populations in the African Region are beset by numerous mental and neurological disorders that are major causes of disability... Increasing poverty, natural disasters, wars and other forms of violence and social unrest are major causes of growing psychosocial problems which include alcohol and drug abuse, prostitution, street children, child abuse and domestic violence. HIV infection has added considerably to the psychosocial problems already being experienced in many countries of the Region, creating a need for extra support and counseling for those affected, and care for their surviving family members, especially children. Many risk factors and social problems are the result of people's lack of mental maturity, self-esteem, and confidence. Strong cultural beliefs about the causes and management of mental disorders also explain the nonutilization of conventional health services as a first choice.

Okasha (2002) highlights particular aspects of the problem, such as the frequency of psychoses resulting from cerebral involvement in infectious diseases, like malaria or HIV infection, which can have chronic consequences if not properly treated. Epilepsy is a major problem, largely due to inadequate care at childbirth, malnutrition, malaria, and parasitic diseases, and is still highly stigmatized. Many African countries are increasingly used as transit points for illicit drug trade, and these drugs are finding their way into the local population. Alcohol and tobacco misuse have free rein, as there are few national policies or controls on their advertising, distribution, and sale.

Opportunities for children to develop their mental health potential are increased or diminished according to the environment in which they live. Many children growing up in Africa are exposed to extremely challenging experiences, as described above. Some experiences are not compatible with physical survival, and seem hardly reconcilable with emotional survival. Yet adversity also breeds resilience, and Africa's children are fortunate to be able to draw on the enormous reserves of spiritual and social capital found in abundance on this continent, and which are a source of encouragement and hope for its future.

The next section analyzes the mental health development and needs of children in Africa in more detail before discussing systems of care.

8.2   Child and Adolescent Mental Health Care Needs in Africa

8.2.1   Child and Adolescent Mental Health in Africa

Child and adolescent mental health can be defined broadly as **the capacity to achieve and maintain optimal psychological functioning and well being** (Policy Guidelines for Child and Adolescent Mental Health 2003). Optimal psychological functioning and well being essentially comprise:

1. A strong sense of identity and self-worth
2. Sound family and peer relationships
3. The ability to be productive in learning and work
4. The capacity to adapt to a changing internal and external environment

Concepts of child and adolescent mental health are shaped by three important realities. Firstly, and most fundamentally, children's development at any age is incomplete. Therefore, mental health is a dynamic, changing capacity, characterized by incremental acquisition of new competencies, appropriate for the specific ages and stages of development, as classically described in the concept of **developmental lines** (Freud 1965) and the **eight ages of man** (Eriksen 1963). Central to this notion of mental health is the capacity of the growing child for turning developmental and environmental challenges into opportunities for further maturation (Sameroff 1975).

Secondly, and of primary significance for any discussion about Africa, notions of psychological functioning and well being are not culture-free. Whereas deficiencies of psychological functioning and well being are evident in all individuals and cultures, **universal** indicators of **optimal** psychological functioning and well being in children and adolescents are more difficult to delineate without sacrificing fundamental individual and cultural differences. No one would dispute the contention that the roots of identity and self worth in African, Arab, Asian, and Caucasian children in Africa arise from differing experiences and world-views, and that notions of childhood and family vary accordingly.

The way in which differing world views translate into cultural practice can be seen in comparative studies of child care. For instance, LeVine et al. (1994) demonstrate that American mothers engage in intense, reciprocal interactions with their infants as the means of developing psychological competence, whereas Gusii mothers in Kenya appear to discourage a strongly dependent relationship with their infant in order to prioritize compliance and adaptability. Comparing the two approaches, Bronfenbrenner (1994) maintains that the hectic pace of contemporary American life undermines the very foundation for the development of psychological competence, in contrast to the situation with the Gusii people, and other traditional African cultures, where the necessary degree of stability is maintained. »This is the lesson from Africa«, he concludes.

An important example of traditional African thought that differs from contemporary European views is the concept enshrined in the Xhosa proverb **umuntu ngumuntu ngabantu**: a person is a person through persons (Shutte 1993). The meaning of the proverb is that persons are defined, not by any natural qualities or set of characteristics, but by the relationships between themselves and others. The Bantu peoples of Southern Africa view the worlds of nature and society as one, in which ac-

tions or attitudes in one part affect the other (Hammond-Tooke 1974). For instance, a failure in health or fortune is thought to be caused by some disruption in social relations, either with regard to the ancestors, or kin or community. Therefore a harmonious social life, and the elimination of discord, are critical to health and well being. This contrasts with contemporary Western thinking, such as that of Erik Eriksen (1963), in which harmony is a lifelong goal to be achieved through the negotiated reconciliation between individuals and within families of opposing drives for self-expression and intimacy.

All Southern African Bantu peoples are patrilineal, with strong emphasis on rank and respect for seniors (Hammond-Tooke 1974). Children are expected to show absolute obedience to parents, and women must respect men. A man's primary loyalty is to his kinsmen, not his wife, and husbands and wives traditionally do not spend their leisure time together. From childhood, the value of reciprocal assistance and cooperation between neighbors is inculcated, not only as a moral imperative, but also to promote the well being of the community, and thereby its individual members. Being familiar with the world views of all cultural groups in Africa, and how they interact with one another, is essential for understanding how culture shapes the development of child and adolescent mental health.

The third important reality shaping child and adolescent mental health is that children are dependent for their optimal physical and psychological development, especially at the beginning of life, on a facilitating environment. The achievement of optimal psychological functioning and well being is relative to the context, or **ecological framework**, into which children are born (Bronfenbrenner 1979). In developing regions of the world in contemporary times, extreme adversity and challenging social contexts threaten the optimal development of children in ways which can hardly be imagined by the inhabitants of more stable, better-resourced societies. Poverty is a pervasive adversity affecting Africa's children, particularly in rural areas. It impacts on, among others, the following basic child rights required for survival and normal development (Biersteker and Robinson 2000)

1. Nutrition
2. Water and sanitation
3. Child and maternal health services
4. Early childhood education and basic education
5. Social welfare developmental services
6. Child protection measures
7. Leisure and cultural activities

The breakdown of traditional African society through contact with colonizers, and through urbanization, has lead to weakening of their traditional values and morals, and their cohesive family and community structures. Until appropriate cultural adaptation has been made, and the social context restabilized, threats to the mental health of children and families will continue to take their toll.

Sadly, war is the only social context some African children have known. Besides its direct effects on children, families, and communities, war »destroys infrastructure, heightens political and economic turmoil, disrupts education, and amplifies poverty« (Wessels and Monteiro 2000). The war in Angola extended over several decades and was a daily social reality for two generations of Angolans:

> Children, who comprise half the population in Angola, shouldered some of the heaviest burdens of war and its aftermath. UNICEF estimated in 1993 that 500,000 child deaths were attributed to war, and 840,000 children were living in especially difficult circumstances. In Luanda, there were large numbers of unaccompanied children, who are particularly vulnerable physically and psychologically. The war devastated the health infrastructure, aggravated already extreme poverty, and ushered in outbreaks of diseases such as measles, malaria, and tetanus. The mortality rate for children under 5 years of age soared to over 300 per 1,000. Malnutrition rates for children under 5 were approximately 15% by 1995. Nearly 60% of children had no regular schooling, and literacy rates for women were under 10%.
> (Wessels and Monteiro 2000)

Well-resourced countries with universal health and social insurance and safe, supportive community living can expect most psychiatric disorders in children and adolescents to arise primarily from interactions between genetic factors and adverse family environments. Although poverty, HIV/AIDS, and acts of violence and terrorism are on the increase globally, they are not yet considered part of the daily reality for the children of well-resourced countries. At most they occur in ghettos, or accidentally involve children unfortunate enough to be in the wrong place at the wrong time. Psychiatry textbooks, which typically emanate from high-income countries, largely reduce such broad environmental hazards to certain Axis 1 disorders, such as Post Traumatic Stress Disorder. Similarly, the range of treatments for psychiatric disorders described by such textbooks is typically confined to interventions directed at individuals, families, schools, and child and family welfare agencies, the implication being that community and society are safe and supportive. This approach does not cater to the majority of the world's children living under difficult circumstances in societies of low- and low-middle-income countries.

The Diagnostic and Statistical Manual of Mental Disorders of the American Psychiatric Association, 4th Edition (DSM-IV, 1994) devotes only two or three sentences to the problems of children living under difficult circumstances. These are found in the discussion of Axis IV: Psychosocial and Environmental Problems, a short 2 pages. Although the DSM-IV allows major psychosocial or environmental problems to be recorded on Axis 1 as **Other Conditions That may be a Focus of Clinical Attention**, the list of **Other Conditions** does not do justice to situations such as those described above in Angola, or such as the effect of the AIDS pandemic on children in Africa. Similar comments can be made with regard to the DSM-IV's marginalizing approach to cultural manifestations of distress and dysfunction. Despite the fact that the majority of the world's population resides in nonwestern countries, DSM-IV disorders essentially are described as they manifest in western cultures.

The World Mental Health Report: Problems and Priorities in Low-Income Countries (Desjarlais et al. 1995) succinctly captures the issues in relation to **disorders** and **difficult circumstances** with the following words:

> The overwhelming conclusion of this report is that formally defined neuropsychiatric disorders are responsible for only a portion of the overall burden of social and psychological morbidity. Alcoholism, drug addiction, suicide and suicide attempts, violence against women, abuse and abandonment of children, forced prostitution, crime and street violence, ethnic warfare and state violence, dislocation and forced migration – all of these constitute a substantial burden in societies of Africa, Asia, Latin America, and the Middle East.

This lesson was clearly demonstrated in Khayelitsha, an informal settlement area of Xhosa-speaking people in Cape Town, South Africa. Whereas a community epidemiological study of children and adolescents in Khayelitsha found that DSM-defined depressive and anxiety disorders were the most prevalent disorders (Robertson et al. 1999), these disorders are the reason for attendance of only a small proportion of the children seen at the community-run mental health center established in the wake of the study. The common mental health needs presenting for care at the center are sexual abuse, antisocial behavior and the effects of HIV/AIDS (WHO 2003).

8.2.2 Major Influences on Child and Adolescent Mental Health in Africa

Poverty and war are not the only major risk factors for child and adolescent mental health in Africa. Children in Africa are all too frequently the victims of **difficult circumstances**, defined as those circumstances in which children are exploited or denied their most basic rights (UNICEF 1990), such as:

1. Armed conflicts and forcible induction as child soldiers
2. Rampant community and domestic violence
3. Child abuse, prostitution, and trafficking
4. Incarceration
5. Street living and homelessness
6. Child labor
7. HIV/AIDS pandemic
8. Societies which do not provide for children's basic needs for access to health care and education
9. Societies which allow discrimination or condone the inhumane treatment of children

Only selected aspects of this veritable assault on children's lives and well being in Africa will be discussed in any detail here, as they are fully described in numerous international publications and reports.

The many horrific forms of domestic, community, and political violence to which children in Africa are regularly exposed are graphically described in the 2002 World Mental Health Day planning kit. The following statement by a 14-year-old girl abducted by the Revolutionary United Front in Sierra Leone poignantly illustrates the plight of child soldiers:

> I've seen people get their hands cut off, a ten-year-old girl raped and die, and so many men and women burned alive... So many times I cried inside my heart because I didn't dare cry out aloud.
> (World Mental Health Day 2002)

Hundreds of children in Africa at this moment are being abducted and tortured by the rebel Lord's Resistance Army and similar plunderers of childhood. Unfortunately, childhood plunderers do not come only from outside the community. HIV/AIDS is a much greater threat to Africa's children, in terms of sheer numbers, than war and armed conflict. According to data provided in the World Mental Health Day global mental health education campaign (2003), of the 36 million people living with AIDS globally, 25.3 million reside in sub-Saharan Africa. Of the world's orphans, 95% live in Africa: 13.2 million children under 15 have lost their mothers to HIV/AIDS since the beginning of the epidemic. Child-headed households are becoming frighteningly common in numerous countries in Africa. Much has been written about the mental health risks facing children and adolescents infected or affected by HIV/AIDS, but estimating the full impact of the AIDS pandemic in Africa on the mental health of children, families, and society is a daunting task, yet to be undertaken.

On a smaller scale, certain traditional child care practices and customs in Africa have come under critical scrutiny for their potentially harmful effect on mental health. In Egypt, despite the banning of corporal punishment in schools in 1971, a substantial proportion of learners, 82% of boys and 62% of girls, continue to incur physical punishment at the hands of their teachers (Youssef et al. 1998). Seif El Din et al. (2002) found that the main reason given by street children for running away from home and for dropping out of school were physical abuse by parents (33%) and maltreatment by teachers (22%).

In Egypt, Sudan, and Somalia female circumcision is very common. A study in Somalia found 100% of women in the study to have been circumcised, despite their relatively high socio-economic status (Dirie and Lindmark 1991). Both excision and infibulation had been performed in 88% of the women. Although female circumcision has been prohibited in Egypt since 1956, the practice is still widespread. Several studies, e.g., Ismail et al. (2002), show that the current prevalence of female circumcision ranges from 76% to 81%. This practice persists because of a belief that circumcision will moderate female sexuality, and will assure marriageability, and because it is sanctioned by religion.

Gender discrimination in many areas of daily living is still entrenched in most countries of Africa. It carries with it an increased risk for women of poverty, poor education, violence, and psychiatric disorder (Desjarlais et al. 1995). Aidoo (1998) found the prevalence of depression among low-income women in Zambia to be 43%. Gender discrimination is clearly a threat to good mothering and child mental health.

Other forms of discrimination also affect child mental health in significant ways. The widening economic gap between high- and low-income countries is a global form of discrimination which has powerful effects on child mental health. Children in low-income countries are 35 times more likely to suffer from epilepsy or mental retardation than their counterparts in high-income countries (Desjarlais et al. 1995). Inaccessibility to cheap medication for the treatment of HIV/AIDS is another example of global discrimination with huge effects on children and families in Africa. Widespread provision of antiretroviral treatment would significantly lengthen the lives of mothers and fathers infected with HIV, and would make an enormous difference to the survival and mental health of children and adolescents.

Stigma associated with mental health problems is common all over the world, including Africa, and accounts for lowered rates of referral for treatment. Stigma is likely to become more entrenched when combined with ignorance. Ignorance about the emotional development and mental health needs of children is prevalent in many parts of Africa, and results in psychiatric disorders like anxiety and depression being regarded as bad behavior or laziness, or due to sinfulness or bewitchment. Ignorance about the psychological principles of good parenting often leads to inappropriate and potentially harmful child care practices.

There are many protective factors to counterbalance the numerous risk factors facing children in Africa. Firstly, it cannot be assumed that all children exposed to risk factors become vulnerable or develop psychiatric disorders. Constant exposure may also have the effect of »steeling« children, and leading to resilience, especially when adult support is available. Furthermore, while Africa does experience its own extreme challenges, it is spared from many of the West's significant challenges, such as **anomie** or global terrorism. Secondly, sustained by their long and rich history, and centuries-old traditions, indigenous Africans have a strong sense of ethnic identity and purpose, which enables them to survive and to adapt to many onslaughts. Thirdly, research has shown that religion can be a significant protective factor in the lives of children. Religious cultures are the most powerful factors that modify an individual's attitudes towards life, death, happiness, and suffering (Bou-Yong Rhi 2001). Despite the persecutory practices of some colonists, indigenous African people continue to maintain strong religious convictions and a deep spirituality. Traditional beliefs provide a dynamic connection between the living, the ancestors, and a supernatural divinity for most indigenous African people, and there is also a strong commitment to other faiths, such as Christianity, Islam, and even Judaism. Finally, strong social support is undoubtedly a significant protective factor for individuals facing the constant challenge of coping with difficult circumstances. Despite the breakdown of the extended family system and traditional family ties in many parts of the continent, supportive family and social relationships and networks remain one of Africa's strengths. These contribute to **social capital**, a source of social trust and cooperation for mutual benefit, which is a powerful mediator of risk factors (Sampson et al. 1997).

8.2.3 The Burden of Child and Adolescent Mental Health Problems in Africa

The World Health Report (2001) comments on the burden of mental health problems in Africa:

> The disability caused by mental and neurological disorders is high in all regions of the world. As a proportion of the total, however, it is comparatively less in the developing countries, mainly because of the large burden of communicable, maternal, perinatal, and nutritional conditions in those regions. Even so, neuropsychiatric disorders cause 17.6% of all years lived with disability in Africa.

When considering the burden of child and adolescent mental health problems in Africa, the first point to note is that 55% of the population of sub-Saharan Africa is under 19 years of age (UNPD 2000). The second critical point has already been addressed extensively, namely that estimates of the burden of mental health problems in children and adolescents in Africa must take into account both psychiatric disorders and the difficult circumstances which constitute their daily social context. Increased vulnerability to mental health problems as a result of a high prevalence of medical and neurological conditions, and intellectual disability, is an important facet of the concept of **difficult circumstances**. Lost opportunities for education is another aspect of difficult circumstances, which needs to be highlighted.

A recent World Health Organization (2003) publication sums up these points in the following statement:

> The magnitude of the burden of disease related to child and adolescent mental disorder is understood by clinicians and parents, but has until recently been difficult to quantify. Now, with worldwide crises involving children impacted by war, exploited for labor and sex, orphaned by AIDS, and forced to migrate for economic and political reasons, the dimensions of the burden of compromised mental health and mental disorders are increasingly evident and quantifiable... Absence from education, underachievement leading to dependency, involvement in criminal activity, the use of illicit drugs, the inability to benefit from rehabilitation, comorbid medical conditions are but some of the very many impacts that have an associated cost. To understand child and adolescent mental health needs it is first necessary to understand the overall dimensions of what are called noncommunicable diseases affecting children, the impact of infectious diseases with direct and indirect impact on the mental health of children, and lastly the available data on diagnosable psychopathology.

The World Health Report (2001) estimates that, from studies in both developed and developing countries, 10–20% of all children have one or more mental or behavioral problems. Regarding the **burden** of mental health problems in children and adolescents, the report concludes that »it would be complex to calculate because many of these disorders can be precursors to much more disabling disorders during later life«.

Although there have been few rigorous, large-scale epidemiological studies involving children and adolescents in Africa like that of Tadesse et al. (1999), many smaller studies have been conducted and some have been published. Discussion of the findings of such studies can be found in international reviews, e.g., Nikapota (1991), reviews of African studies, e.g., Odejide et al. (1989) or of African child and adolescent studies, e.g., Jegede and Olatawura (1982), Robertson and Berger (1994), as well as in journal publications of single studies. Examples of published single studies from a selection of African countries, are: Egypt (Abou Nazel et al. 1991), Ethiopia (Mulatu 1995), Nigeria (Abiodun 1993;

Gureje and Omigbodun 1995), South Africa (Robertson et al. 1999), Senegal (Diop et al. 1982), Sudan (Giel et al. 1981), and Uganda (Minde 1977). Many of the investigators in these epidemiological studies discuss why their prevalence findings cannot simply be compared to international prevalence rates, or even other countries in Africa, citing differing methodologies and the very different social and cultural contexts. Few of these studies include ethnographic approaches, yet ethnographic studies are necessary in order to elicit culture-specific expressions of distress and dysfunction. Reports of culture-bound syndromes have emanated from different countries in Africa, including Nigeria (Prince 1962), Senegal (Seck 1991), South Africa (Ensink and Robertson 1996), and Swaziland (Guinness 1992), as well as in an overview by Ilechukwu (1991).

Current debates question the usefulness of epidemiological studies for planning systems of care to meet the mental health needs of the population (Fayyad et al. 2001). Many epidemiological studies are limited in scope, both in terms of disorders investigated and populations sampled, as well as frequently ignoring the difficult circumstances inherent in the social and cultural context. Also, they do not always measure impairment, or causal relationships between significant factors associated with the mental health problems reported. Epidemiological studies need to »progress« from purely descriptive investigations, to analytic studies which clarify causal relationships, and thence to evaluated intervention studies in order to be useful for the implementation of effective systems of care.

8.3 Child and Adolescent Mental Health Care Systems in Africa

Systems of care for children and adolescents are built upon visions of optimal childhood development. However, it should be recognized that most such visions in the minds of policy makers and planners, even in Africa, derive from psychological knowledge about children in Europe and North America (Kessen 1979). Discussions of systems of care in Africa need to be clear about whose visions of childhood inform them. The influence on concepts of childhood of the world view and moral value system prevailing in their society has been emphasized previously.

Systems of care may be formal or informal. Informal systems will be considered to include those provided by families and their support networks, the services of folk and indigenous healers, and nongovernmental, community, and faith based organizations. Formal systems of care are provided by the private sector or the state. Typically, primary responsibility for state mental health services is taken by health ministries. However systems of care for children and adolescents with mental health problems are also provided by the ministries of education, social services, and justice and prisons/correctional services. This multisectoral provision of care is of critical importance in Africa and other developing regions where health ministries frequently do not provide dedicated systems of child and adolescent mental health care. Only 40% of countries in Africa have special programs in mental health for children (Atlas 2001).

There is a danger that formal and informal systems of care are seen as an either/or option, instead of as complementary systems. For example, there could be an expectation that where formal systems are lacking, the informal sector will take over. Similarly, where formal systems are well-developed, there could be a perception among the users that they should meet every need, without any coresponsibility for service provision by the public. Systems of care that are likely to be the most successful are those where there is active coordination, collaboration, integration and mutual support between the various state sectors, the private sector and the informal sector.

8.3.1 Informal Systems of Care

In Africa, informal systems of care are relatively well developed, whereas formal systems have not developed to the same extent, or have been eroded by poverty or war. The family is the primary system of care. Traditional child care in Africa has many inherent strengths, among them being the social support typical of traditional African families and their close-knit communities. This support is not automatically extended to those outside the community, and where traditional community systems have broken down and become fragmented as a result of colonization or urbanization, newly constituted urban communities may not show the same level of social support as traditional communities. However, one foreign import which has grown and flourished in Africa is ministry to the poor and oppressed, irrespective of whether they belong to the »same« community or not. Literally thousands of community-based organizations, both faith-based and secular, have come into existence to serve every conceivable need and cause in Africa, and continue to develop and multi-

ply. More recently, they include mental health advocacy and consumer movements. The Atlas (2001) lists only four countries in Africa which do not have nongovernmental organizations in mental health.

Nongovernmental organizations may address any or all aspects of care, from promotion and prevention, through to treatment and rehabilitation. Many nongovernmental organizations are supported or even initiated by foreign agencies, but most have been pioneered from within the continent. Their success is due to the incredible energy and creativity generated in Africa in response to the constant challenges facing its inhabitants in their daily lives, supported by the strong spiritual and moral beliefs which characterize the continent.

Numerous examples could be cited of informal systems of care which have arisen in response to the mental health needs of children and adolescents in Africa. Some have been initiated to complement existing formal systems of care, like **Empilweni** in South Africa (WHO 2003), while others have arisen when the needs created by overwhelming catastrophes such as war or the AIDS pandemic have exceeded state resources and required innovative multisectoral efforts (see Box 1 below). Currently, international aid to African countries for HIV/AIDS is enabling governments to set up major interventions to complement or support the programs started by nongovernmental organizations.

Kuhluvuka – Corridor of Hope
Maputo Corridor AIDS Prevention Project, Mozambique

The Foundation for Community Development (FDC), a Mozambican organization, implements a community-based HIV/AIDS prevention and care program in the Maputo transport corridor. The overall project focuses primarily on prevention, but activities to address the needs of orphans and vulnerable children (OVC) are included as an integral part of impact mitigation. The project emphasizes establishing community involvement to identify and address the needs of OVC and mobilizing community leaders to initiate support programs for those infected and affected. The strategy focuses on meeting the needs of OVC in three major areas: education, nutrition, and health. FDC has already raised more than $1 million in private funds.

▼

Key accomplishments include

1. Mapping and identification of OVC
2. Mobilizing communities to register children as citizens, thus enabling free access to education and health care
3. Establishing a vocational training center for youth that particularly targets OVC
4. Information, education, and communication campaigns, particularly targeting OVC – focused primarily on behavior change, both personal and social behavior
5. Sensitizing communities to reduce the stigma associated with HIV/AIDS and ignorance about HIV/AIDS
6. Carrying out research, coordinated with community-based partners and government, on the number and situation of orphaned children, and ensuring that the national strategy for OVC, which is being developed by the Ministry of Women and Social Action, addresses the children's needs and is effectively implemented by the government and partners
USAid Project Profiles –
Children Affected by HIV/AIDS (2003)

Informal systems of care are typically staffed by volunteers or community workers who have undergone training by formally trained mental health workers and, ideally, continue to be supported by them. This complementarity between the two systems increases the likelihood that the service will remain client-centered, evidence-based, and accountable to the community. Informal systems of care have certain advantages over formal systems: they are usually more accessible and affordable, culturally appropriate, and responsive to changing needs. Investing in a cadre of specialized child and adolescent mental health workers is essential for countries of all income levels in order to provide the training, and ongoing education and support which underpin informal systems of care.

Indigenous healers provide an extensive system of care in Africa, both for adults and children. Healers are regularly consulted for mental health problems, even by individuals who are receiving psychiatric treatment. As traditional communities have been disrupted by urbanization or war, controls on good practice in indigenous healing systems have weakened. Current trends are for indigenous healers to organize and regulate themselves nationally and

to become registered as an accredited system of care. Traditional herbs and medicines should be used with due caution regarding appropriate dosage, interactions with other medicaments, and possible toxicity. Collaboration between indigenous healing and other systems of care requires that both fully understand and accept the basis upon which each operates (Bodibe and Sodi 1997). Indigenous healing systems are largely faith-based, with many indigenous healing practices resembling those of ministers of religion rather than of health workers. Accordingly, traditional healers appear to be more successful in intervening with problems of daily living, and illnesses related to interpersonal and existential stresses, than with brain disorders like schizophrenia and bipolar disorder.

8.3.2 Formal Systems of Care

Existing formal systems of care in Africa are largely European in origin, and therefore reflect the national differences found, for instance, between the French and English systems. An example from a francophone African country is given in Box 2. Where formal systems have been eroded by poverty or war, »reforms« and development are currently being promoted and supported by the World Health Organization, the World Bank, and other international agencies. Formal systems of care in Africa, like informal systems, are currently in a state of transition.

Kër Xaleyi – A Pediatric Psychiatry Service in Senegal

In Senegal, children and adolescents with psychiatric problems were seen, between 1971 and 1994, in a small unit called Kër Xaleyi (meaning »Children's Home«). Most of the children were referred because of behavior problems at home or at school.

Over the years the service grew and diversified, and in 1994 an enlarged and beautifully renovated facility called Kër Xaleyi Pediatric Psychiatry Service opened its doors. It is attached to the Centre Hospitalier Universitaire at Fann in Dakar, and is the only public sector university hospital service in Senegal . It is used as a referral center for the entire country and even for other neighboring countries in West Africa. Most of the cases

▼

referred from rural areas are mental disorders due to general medical conditions like epilepsy and encephalopathies, or associated with delayed development and chronic malnutrition. In Dakar, there are frequent school referrals of 8–10-year olds with learning disabilities. Other common problems among children referred in urban areas include enuresis, stuttering, obesity, alopecia, and dermatoses. Juvenile delinquency is a growing problem, related to school dropout and breakdown of traditional value systems.

Kër Xaleyi has a multidisciplinary team of Senegalese professionals: child psychiatrists, psychologists, speech therapists, occupational therapists, social workers, special education teachers, and nurses. Wherever possible, partial rather than full hospitalization is preferred, in order to cope with an increasing demand for services. Community activities are largely preventive in nature, and include mental health training for general health workers, social workers, etc., consultation to schools, and publication of information brochures, e.g., about epilepsy and mental health. In addition, the staff participate in the academic activities of the Faculty of Medicine at the University of Dakar, and conduct research. A number of articles have been published about Kër Xaleyi and the research conducted there, such as Seck et al. 1998.

All health sector reforms advocate the primary health care model. This model incorporates a public health approach, which promotes health through prevention as well as treatment of disease. A comprehensive model of primary care for developing countries is described in a recent publication of the Institute of Medicine, USA (2001). In many African countries, until recently, mental health was not integrated into primary health care. The community mental health movement, which swept through many parts of the world in the 1950s and 1960s, did not reach Africa. Mental health services in Africa remained largely vertical and based in mental hospitals, with all the accompanying isolation, neglect, and stigma that have been described elsewhere. At present, one in five African countries still does not have mental health in primary health care (Atlas 2001).

In Africa, primary health care services are typically provided by nurses, or midlevel medically trained workers such as **clinical officers**. Adequate basic mental health training and ongoing education and support for nurses are essential for sustaining their role as primary health care providers, as well as special regulations to enable them to prescribe medication. Almost half of African countries do not have training facilities for primary care personnel in mental health (Atlas 2001). This is partly due to a shortage of mental health specialists of all disciplines. Only Algeria, South Africa, and Tunisia have more than 1 psychiatrist per 100,000 population, and only Namibia and South Africa have more than 1 psychologist per 100,000 population (Atlas 2001). Few countries have formally trained child psychiatrists, and only South Africa has formal training programs leading to a tertiary qualification in child and adolescent psychiatry.

Dedicated secondary and tertiary psychiatric services for children and adolescents are still to be developed in most countries. Outpatient services have been started in some major centers, but inpatient services are generally lacking except for occasional use of pediatric or general psychiatry wards. The use of general psychiatry wards is of concern, especially as acceptable standards of inpatient psychiatric care for adults have been seriously eroded in many countries in Africa, both with regard to physical facilities and availability of essential medication. Two countries that provide dedicated psychiatric inpatient services for children and adolescents are Senegal and South Africa.

The lack of dedicated psychiatric services for children and adolescents in Africa means that other disciplines and sectors contribute a greater proportion to child mental health services. Pediatrics and maternal and child health departments provide preventive, promotive, and curative interventions to improve the survival, general health, and quality of life of children. These are critical in a continent where medical and neurological conditions have a significant impact on the mental health of children and adolescents. It could be said that the mental health of children and adolescents in Africa is only as good as their medical care.

Although many countries in Africa lack even basic school psychology services, the school itself constitutes the second most important system of care, after the family, for the mental health of children and adolescents. A good education and a positive school experience are almost essential foundations for mental health. Few countries in Africa have special education facilities, such as for children with specific learning disabilities, intellectual disabilities or cerebral palsy, although these children are at increased risk for developing mental health problems. However, nongovernmental organizations make significant contributions to children with special needs in many African countries.

Even access to general education varies greatly. The secondary school enrollment ratio for sub-Saharan Africa is between 20–30%, but there are marked overall and gender differences between countries in education levels. Although adult literacy rates for women are usually lower than those of men, the adult literacy rate in Lesotho for females as a percentage of males is 127 (UNICEF 2003). The AIDS orphan school attendance rate is as low as 35% in some countries (UNICEF 2003). Education sector »reforms« are currently addressing the availability, structure, and standards of education in many countries, and some intersectoral collaborations are emerging, such as the Health-Promoting School initiative (Flisher et al. 2000). There are also an increasing number of nongovernmental initiatives, for instance, the Adolescent Reproductive Health Network, which provides school-based counseling, education, and health promotion in relation to reproductive health in Tanzania and other African countries (Klepp et al. 2000).

Social welfare services provide a potential safety net for the mental health of children and adolescents through, among others, poverty grants, child care grants, disability grants and rehabilitation grants. In addition to budgetary constraints, many African countries have unwieldy administrative requirements and procedures which limit ready access to these welfare benefits when they are offered. Social services often include programs and sometimes residential care for abused children, street children, orphans, or at risk criminal youth, but the pervasive shortage of funds and of social workers, and outdated child protection legislation frequently undermines their effectiveness and sustainability. Nongovernmental organizations make an important contribution in this area.

Ministries of justice and prisons/correctional services have the potential opportunity to provide critical rehabilitation programs for youthful perpetrators of crime and violence, but, as in many other parts of the world, these youth are not yet receiving due attention.

8.3.3 Education and Training

Education of the public and of non-mental health care workers, and training and ongoing education of mental health care workers are essential ingredients of effective systems of care. Before the adoption of the primary care model, mental health education and training in Africa were insufficiently prioritized, frequently Eurocentric, and illness-oriented in their approach, and confined mainly to the health sector. Current primary care-oriented health sector »reforms« are giving much more emphasis to prevention and promotion, but mental health education and training involving other sectors, for instance, the education sector or traditional healers, is still limited. A survey of sub-Saharan African countries in 1991 found that 14 of the 30 countries who responded had revised their undergraduate curricula to include mental health components, 12 had revised postgraduate programs, and 19 had revised the curriculum for training of nurses and social workers (Uznanski and Roos 1997).

It is difficult to develop education and training programs in child and adolescent mental health until they are reasonably well established in general psychiatry and mental health. At this time, few mental health workers in Africa have the necessary knowledge and skills to educate or train others in child and adolescent mental health. Even the World Health Organization, which has traditionally lead the field in producing and disseminating mental health training material, has only recently introduced a child and adolescent mental health component into their Department of Mental Health and Substance Abuse. There is no corresponding initiative yet in their Africa office, although the issue has been discussed there.

Both local and international nongovernmental organizations play an important role in many African countries in promoting child and adolescent mental health through public education. Recent examples of the benefit of international contributions are the many public education activities carried out as part of World Mental Health Day in 2002 (Theme: the effects of trauma and violence on children and adolescents) and 2003 (Theme: emotional and behavioral disorders of children and adolescents), using the excellent educational material disseminated by the World Federation for Mental Health. However, general knowledge among the public in Africa about mental health problems in children and adolescents, and about their emotional development and needs, remains at a low level, especially in rural areas. Olawatura (2001) discusses some of the traditional beliefs that child mental health workers in Nigeria need to take into account when attempting to modify potentially harmful parenting and social practices: the challenge is to »work through and with native ideas in a manner that promotes understanding of sound principles of mental health, while respecting native beliefs and practices… which may conflict with those of the professional… encountered in his or her own childhood…«

For most countries in Africa, transforming existing curricula, e.g., for nurses, to provide adequate training in mental health, requires external donor funding and expertise. The greater challenge lies in **implementing** the new curriculum. Mental health facilities which are less than ideal for training purposes is one such challenge, but even more problematic are the difficulties inherent in recruiting and retaining suitable teachers. Once recruited, they usually have to be sent out of the country for training, either to a neighboring country or overseas. Few return to their home countries, and effective mechanisms for **bonding** and for preventing such attrition have yet to be found.

Brain drain equally affects doctors sent overseas for psychiatric training. The well-resourced psychiatric services of many northern countries are staffed by African psychiatrists whose poor countries of origin struggle to provide basic health care. The current unethical practice of luring health care workers of all disciplines from developing countries to emigrate to high-income countries reinforces the global wealth-poverty differential and increases the illness burden among the poor. Unfortunately, many African psychiatrists who do return to Africa move to countries wealthier than their own. With regard to child psychiatrists, there appear to be less than 40 in the whole continent, of whom more than half are in South Africa. There are even fewer child mental health specialists in other disciplines. This deficiency must be addressed. Fully functioning and effective primary-care-oriented mental health systems of care for children and adolescents cannot be sustained, even in developing countries, without a core multidisciplinary team of child mental health specialists.

South Africa is the only country in Africa with a national child and adolescent psychiatry association, and the only country which offers accredited training in child and adolescent psychiatry. The World Psychiatric Association has been instrumental in reviving the African Association of Psychiatry and Allied Professions, but as yet there is no Child and Adolescent Psychiatry section.

8.3.4 Research

Research-based evidence, and program evaluation skills are critical ingredients of an effective system of care. In developing countries, research programs are difficult to develop and to sustain. The reasons are complex, and were the main theme of an international WHO meeting held in Cape Town in December 2002: Research for Change: Research on Mental Health and Substance Abuse in Developing Countries. The issues are the same for Africa as for other developing areas of the world, and include:

1. Lack of funding
2. Lack of support for research from policy makers, service providers, and even clinicians
3. Lack of research training programs
4. Challenging environments, e.g., poor infrastructure and technology, war
5. Competing clinical demands and few specialist clinicians
6. Brain drain
7. Lack of access to journals, both printed and online
8. Lack of access to regional or international scientific meetings
9. Publication bias against developing countries

Nevertheless, good research is being conducted in Africa, although only some finds its way into publications, and only a small proportion is concerned with children and adolescents. In a review of 2001–2002 indexed mental health publications from developing countries, Saxena and Maulik (2002) found that 15% originated in sub-Saharan Africa, which puts the continent fourth highest among the 6 WHO regions. Not only is there a substantial amount of research which remains unpublished in Africa, there are also many lost opportunities for research which would greatly benefit the development or improvement of systems of care for children and adolescents. For instance, ethnographic studies, and the study and evaluation of existing or new models of clinical or community care, would be of enormous value.

Finally, in concluding this section on systems of care, a number of critical points need to be highlighted. In Africa, and many other developing regions of the world, care outside of health facilities and services arguably makes a greater difference to the mental health of children and adolescents than do formal systems of care. This is so because, even in the most stable countries in Africa, everyday life is no longer the **facilitating environment** it should be for our children, apart from those environments which are positively toxic. It is therefore not realistic to expect that health sector reforms, by themselves, will necessarily enable children and adolescents to attain optimal mental health. The same argument applies to community based interventions, e.g., for HIV/AIDS. Unless poverty is alleviated, education and skill development extended, infrastructure established, and quality of life improved, organizing systems of care may be largely a whitewashing exercise. This is one of the lessons which Africa and other developing regions can contribute to the international community. Wing et al. (1992) reinforce this caveat, in a discussion of quality assurance models for evaluating services, when they maintain that three components are essential for optimal personal and social functioning, namely: optimal treatment and care, optimal social opportunities and environment, and optimal self-attitudes and motivation.

Even the best designed systems of care are only as good as their evaluation finds them to be. Leaf (1998) stresses the need for broad evaluative measures, which include ethnographic and qualitative studies, and which encompass caregivers and community institutions. Implicit in both Wing's and Leaf's approaches is the concept that care is more than treatment. For care to be truly effective, the social context, as well as individual attitudes and motivation, must be actively engaged. Too often good treatment is offered without monitoring and ensuring that it is well utilized. Providing an actively engaged warm, continuous, accessible, nurturing, and personal therapeutic relationship is as essential for systems of care as it is for parenting. Without it, care is as beneficial for its recipients as providing only the material necessities is for children. In mental health, care cannot be separated from the carer.

Current wisdom recognizes that adoption and support by countries of a child and adolescent mental health policy is essential for existing systems of care to be effective and sustainable. Shatkin (2004) conducted an international survey in 2001 to identify countries with child and adolescent mental health policies. Only 7% of countries worldwide were found to have a clearly articulated child and adolescent mental health policy (14 countries, only one of which, South Africa, is situated in Africa), and not a single country was found to have a policy strictly pertaining to children and adolescents alone, according to the criteria used by the investigator. Of the remaining 20 countries with policies having some reference to or impact on children and adoles-

cents, 5 are in Africa (Botswana, Ghana, Mauritius, Mozambique, and Nigeria). The WHO Mental Health Policy Project has recently been established to promote and assist countries to develop and implement policies, and a Child and Adolescent Mental Health Policy Module is expected to be available in 2004.

8.4 The Way Forward for Africa

8.4.1 Policy Development

The way forward for Africa, and all countries, is to develop and adopt mental health and child and adolescent mental health policies as a first priority, in order to ensure implementation and evaluation of strategic plans and programs. For those countries without an existing mental health policy, any child mental health specialists, or a strong NGO lobby for child mental health, it is likely that the impetus for developing a child and adolescent mental health policy will need to come from international development or advocacy organizations such as the World Health Organization, the World Federation for Mental Health, or the World Bank (Institute of Medicine 2001). External consultants will need to be recruited who are able to engage with the national mental health coordinator and local mental health experts to design a country-specific, cost-effective, sustainable, and culturally appropriate policy. This exercise must also build sufficient capacity in key staff to enable the process to be sustained after the consultation has ended.

The recommended content for policies is fully documented in the various modules of the WHO Mental Health Policy Project. Policies should cover the following areas:
1. Planning and budgeting
2. Intersectoral collaboration
3. Advocacy
4. Legislation and human rights
5. Information systems
6. Research and Evaluation of policies and services
7. Quality improvement
8. Organization of services
9. Essential drug procurement and distribution
10. Human resources and training

Adopting a national child and adolescent mental health policy is only the beginning of the process. In many countries, service provision is the responsibility of individual provinces or states, not national government. In such cases, a strategic plan geared towards provincial priorities and circumstances needs to be submitted to provincial government, together with a business or operational plan detailing the proposed programs with their budgets and time lines. In South Africa, national Policy Guidelines for Child and Adolescent Mental Health were adopted in 2003, and within the same year a national meeting was convened in which provincial mental health coordinators were assisted with individual planning of the various steps required to implement programs in their provinces.

There are many potential obstacles to reaching the final stage of implementation, evaluation and quality improvement of child and adolescent mental health programs in countries of Africa and other developing regions (WHO 2003). Besides the availability of sufficient funding, is the issue of capacity. A primary health care oriented system cannot be sustained without specialist input. Child and adolescent primary mental health care programs require for their planning, implementation and evaluation, trainers, clinicians, and researchers skilled in child and adolescent mental health. As most African countries have few mental health specialists, and no child and adolescent mental health specialists, adoption of policies will not lead to effective implementation without redressing this situation (Desjarlais et al. 1995).

Providing training for clinical, research and policy development skills in child and adolescent mental health will, for most countries in Africa, require external funding and expertise. Acquiring these depends equally on local as well as on international interest and initiative. It is important that as much of the training as possible takes place in the country where the trainees will be working, or at least on the continent of Africa, rather than in a foreign environment abroad. Training of health care workers should incorporate local idioms related to mental health, such as »thinking too much« (**kufungisa**) in Zimbabwe (Abas et al. 1994). Within Africa, there is sufficient local expertise to develop and organize, with external support, child and adolescent mental health training centers of excellence for both English and French speaking professionals.

Issues relating to social context in Africa form another constellation of potential obstacles to implementation of policies. Besides disruption due to armed conflicts or epidemics, there are numerous and wide-ranging critical issues like lack of infrastructure, stigma, illiteracy, the rights of women,

and cultural differences (Gureje and Alem 2000; WHO 2003). Solutions need to be found for the organizational problems underlying the poor availability and distribution of essential medications in so many African countries. Stigma associated with mental health is reinforced by the terrible condition and location of most psychiatric facilities in Africa, and keeps many people from coming forward for treatment. Public education should prioritize the use of the radio and television media, to which the majority of the African population was access, despite widespread poverty and high illiteracy rates. As the rights of children are inextricably bound up with the rights of women, having a child and adolescent mental health policy and being a signatory to the Convention on the Rights of the Child needs to be supplemented by policies and plans to ensure that women's rights are guaranteed and their health care and other needs met.

Child and adolescent mental health programs will not be fully utilized or be fully effective unless Western and indigenous African approaches are integrated. Commenting on lessons and insights learned from the Christian Children's Fund Project, invited by the Angolan government to provide postwar psychosocial services, Wessels and Monteiro (2000) state that:

> One of the main insights of the project was that children often benefit most through the integration of indigenous and Western approaches. Since many of children's war-related stresses were spiritual and were grounded in a local belief system, Western approaches by themselves would have been incomplete and ill suited to the local context... At the same time... without sensitization and training, local people typically do not connect their children's problematic behaviors with the children's experience of war and violence. Nor is there typically a comprehensive understanding of children's psychosocial needs. The Western elements of the training seminars enabled people to see their children with new eyes, to understand their children's needs more completely, and to learn a variety of methods for helping children to come to terms with their war experiences and to achieve healthy social integration. No cultural system for understanding and assisting children is complete in itself.

The recent adaptation of interpersonal psychotherapy in a project in rural Uganda is an excellent model of how to integrate western treatment into a local culture to ensure that a good treatment modality becomes good care (Verdeli et al. 2003). **Cultural competence** is as important when working in culturally diverse populations, as it is when introducing western approaches into nonwestern cultures. A culturally competent system of care »acknowledges and incorporates at all levels the importance of culture, the assessment of cross-cultural relations, vigilance towards the dynamics that result from cultural differences, the expansion of cultural knowledge, and the adaptation of services to meet culturally-unique needs« (Ndlela 1995). All staff working in multicultural settings need to be trained in »cultural competence, which is a set of congruent behaviors and attitudes among professionals that enable them to work effectively in cross-cultural situations«. This includes providing services in the local languages.

8.4.2 Other Initiatives

Caring for the mental health needs of children and adolescents cannot be delayed until unique policies and strategic plans have been developed and put in place by the mental health sector. In a great proportion of African countries, due to limited resources, there needs to be a major focus on general health workers, general mental health workers, school personnel, and other nonspecialized workers who will be providing most of the available child mental health services. Developing school mental health programs, and training traditional healers, can be cost-effective ways of increasing access to child mental health services (Seif El Din et al. 1996). Mental health interventions can also be piggy-backed onto those of other sectors which have resources. For instance, in recent years many African countries have received major international funding for programs to combat HIV/AIDS. Interventions targeted at the mental health of orphans and vulnerable children can be included in these programs. Similarly, interventions directed at youth violence, substance abuse, and sexual behavior can join up with school-based programs financed by the Ministry of Education.

Nongovernmental organizations in Africa respond to many mental health needs of children and adolescents, but a mechanism needs to be developed for reducing duplication and fragmentation of services, for sharing best practices, and for reciprocal support and complementarity with the state sector. Similarly, meaningful dialogue and information-sharing needs to take place between the biomedical

and traditional healing systems in order to develop appropriate mutual expectations and collaborations, which are likely to be of greatest benefit to the users.

When the value of their expertise is recognized and used by governments, the academic and professional sectors are able to play a vital role in the development of mental health systems of care for children and adolescents in Africa. Even when not empowered by government, they can make important contributions in training and research, and in designing, conducting, or evaluating interventions. To sustain their activities and necessary self-development, academics and professionals need to organize themselves and network nationally, regionally, and internationally. For many countries in Africa, this is impossible without external funding and support. The World Psychiatric Association recently launched an initiative to organize and provide scientific support for psychiatrists and allied professions in Africa (Okasha 2002), but similar initiatives in the realm of child and adolescent mental health are lacking. The absence of Africans at many international child and adolescent mental health scientific meetings is a loss for both Africa and the international community. The 1996 Declaration of Venice: Principles for Organizing Mental Health Systems for Children and Adolescents needs to be transformed into an international Declaration which reflects the situation in developing as well as industrialized nations (Young and Ferrari 1998).

8.4.3 Systems of Care in Africa: The Future

There is no universal blueprint for child and adolescent mental health care, just as there is no single, universal strategy for preventing mental health problems. Desjarlais et al. (1995) suggest a three-pronged conceptual frame for the organization of action to promote mental health in low-income countries:

1. Through health services and appropriate medical technologies
2. Through a new generation of public health interventions and
3. Through relevant national and international policy innovations

They prioritize seven areas for international concern, all of which are applicable to Africa. The World Health Report (2001) lists the minimum actions across ten fields, which are required for mental

8

health care in countries with low, medium, or high levels of resources. Gureje and Alem (2000) draw attention to the increasing need for mental health programs in Africa, and call for health planners »to rethink the customary ways of viewing the health needs of their communities«. They add that »in many countries, mental health services are placed on the political agenda by a combination of advocacy groups and enlightened citizens«. Such country initiatives are likely to remain vulnerable or limited in scope without international support.

The benefit of international initiatives was borne out by the 2002 WHO Meeting in Cape Town, Research for Change: Research on Mental Health and Substance Abuse in Developing Countries, which resulted in critical insights, important recommendations such as setting up training centers in developing countries, and new north-south research partnerships. Another important WHO initiative was the meeting Caring for Children and Adolescents with Mental Disorders: Setting WHO Directions, convened in Geneva early in 2003, of leading world experts and organizations in the area of child and adolescent psychiatry. The meeting recommended, among others (WHO 2003), that:

1. Due consideration of child and adolescent mental disorders should be incorporated into all WHO initiatives relating to either overall health or specific mental health.
2. A Global Child and Adolescent Mental Health Action Plan should be established within the Department of Mental Health and Substance Abuse.

The future of child and adolescent mental health systems of care in Africa, and other developing regions of the world, is to some extent dependent on international initiatives of this kind, together with concrete support from the international community. However, it is equally true that international interventions of whatever persuasion need to forge ethical, equitable partnerships, which develop and support rather than control or exploit resources and expertise in developing nations.

With reference to **regional** initiatives for child and adolescent mental health care, Dawes and Donald (2000) present some principles for community-based interventions with children in high-risk southern African environments:

1. »Interventions should be informed by a knowledge of developmental pathways and epochs«.
Different risk reduction strategies are appropriate for different ages. Such strategies do not nec-

essarily succeed unless early interventions are supported by later ones. They cannot be expected to succeed in the face of overwhelming poverty, poor nutrition, and substandard schools.
2. »Where possible, interventions should be undertaken at multiple levels«.
Within the limited resource contexts of most southern African countries, the family and the school present the best opportunities for intervention.
3. »Interventions should combine cultural and developmental sensitivity«.
Adults need to be convinced that changing their behavior is necessary for the good of their children.
4. »Interventions should promote community participation«.
Community participation promotes capacity development, and rebuilds fragmented community relationships.
5. »Interventions should build on, and promote, protective factors«.
Interventions can be strengthened by an understanding of whether protective, compensatory, or challenge models of resilience (or all three) are most appropriate to their design.

8.5 Conclusion

For Africa, it is not a choice between medication or psychosocial interventions, prevention or rehabilitation, primary care or specialist care, research or service, poverty alleviation or universal education, psychotherapy or indigenous healing, public health or mental health, but the best balance between all of these that can be achieved, given each country's particular situation, their resources and constraints, and their ability to attract and sustain appropriate international support. We hope we have shown that international support is not a one-way street. Africa is not only rich in minerals, but also in vitality, spirituality, social capital, and many other resources. These riches are waiting to be shared with those with the insight to see how much they stand to gain by partnering with Africa to promote mental health, especially the mental health of its children and adolescents.

References

Abas M, Broadhead J, Mbape P, Khumalo-Sakatukwa G (1994) Defeating depression in the developing world: a Zimbabwean model. British Journal of Psychiatry 164:293–296

Abiodun OA (1993) Emotional illness in a pediatric population in Nigeria. Journal of Tropical Pediatrics 39:49–51

Abou Nazel M, Fahmi S, Seif El Din A (1991) A study of depression among Alexandria preparatory school adolescents. Journal of the Egyptian Health Association 66:69–75

Aidoo M (1998) Explanations for the causes of mental ill-health among low-income women in an urban area: the case of Zambia. Unpublished doctoral thesis, South Bank University, London

Atlas (2001) Mental health resources in the world. World Health Organization, Geneva

Biersteker L, Robinson S (2000) Socio-economic policies: their impact on children in South Africa. In: Donald D, Dawes A, Louw J (eds) Addressing childhood diversity. David Philip, Cape Town, pp 26–59

Bou-Yong Rhi (2001) Culture, spirituality and mental health: the forgotten aspects of religion and health. The Psychiatric Clinics of North America 24:569–579

Bodibe C, Sodi T (1997) Indigenous healing. In: Foster D, Freeman M, Pillay Y (eds) Mental Health Policy Issues for South Africa. Medical Association of South Africa Multimedia Publications, Cape Town, pp 181–192

Bronfenbrenner U (1979) The ecology of human development. Harvard University Press, Cambridge

Bronfenbrenner U (1994) Foreword. In: LeVine A, LeVine S, Leiderman PH, Brazelton TB, Dixon S, Richman A, Keefer CH, Child care and culture: Lessons from Africa. pp xi–xvii

Dawes A, Donald D (2000) Improving children's chances: developmental theory and effective interventions in community contexts. In: Donald D, Dawes A, Louw J (eds) Addressing childhood diversity. David Philip, Cape Town, pp 1–25

Desjarlais R, Eisenberg L, Good B., Kleinman A (1995) World Mental Health: Problems and priorities in low-income countries. Oxford University Press, Oxford.

Diagnostic and Statistical Manual of Mental Disorders of the American Psychiatric Association, 4th edition (1994). American Psychiatric Association, Washington

Diop RC, Gueye M, Harding TW (1982) Diagnosis and symptoms of mental disorder in a rural area of Senegal. African Journal of Medicine 11:95–103

Dirie MA, Lindmark G (1991) Female circumcisions in Somalia and women's motives. Acta Obstetrica Gynaecologica Scandinavica 70:581–585

Ensink K, Robertson B (1996) Indigenous categories of distress and dysfunction in South African Xhosa children and adolescents as described by indigenous healers. Transcultural Psychiatric Research Review 33:137–172

Erikson E (1963) Childhood and society, 2nd edition. WW Norton, New York

Fayyad JA, Jahshan BA, Karam EG (2001) Systems development of child mental health services in developing coun-

tries. Child and Adolescent Psychiatric Clinics of North America 10:745–762

Flisher AJ, Cloete C, Johnson B, Wigton A, Adams R, Joshua P (2000) Health-Promoting schools: lessons from Avondale Primary School. In: Donald D, Dawes A, Louw J (eds) Addressing childhood diversity. David Philip, Cape Town, pp 113–130

Freud A (1965) Normality and pathology in childhood. International Universities Press, New York

Giel R, de Arango MV, Climent CE, Harding TW, Ibrahim HHA, Ladrigo-Ignacio L, Murthy RS, Salazar MC, Wig NN, Younis YOA (1981) Childhood mental disorders in primary health care: results of observations in four countries. Pediatrics 68:677–683

Guinness EA (1992) Patterns of mental illness in the early stages of urbanisation. British Journal of Psychiatry 160 (Suppl 16):42–52

Gureje O, Alem A (2000) Mental Health Policy Development in Africa. Bulletin of the World Health Organization 78:475–482

Gureje O, Omigbodun OO (1995) Children with mental disorders in primary care: functional status and risk factors. Acta Psychiatrica Scandinavica 92:310–314

Hammond-Tooke WD (1974) World-View II: a system of action. In: Hammond-Tooke WD (ed) The Bantu Speaking Peoples of Southern Africa. Routledge and Kegan Paul, New York, pp 344–363

Ilechukwu STC (1991) Psychiatry in Africa: special problems and unique features. Transcultural Psychiatric Research Review 28:169–218

Institute of Medicine (2001) Neurological, Psychiatric and Developmental Disorders: meeting the challenge in the developing world. National Academy Press, Washington

Ismail A, Mostafa S, El Mos Alamany A, Ali A (2002) Female circumcision: factors affecting it, and related knowledge, attitude and practice among the population in Kalyoulia Governorate. Egyptian Journal of Community Medicine 20: 15–29

Jegede RO, Olatawura MO (1982) Child and adolescent psychiatry in Africa: a review. East African Medical Journal 59:435–441

Kessen W (1979) The American child and other cultural inventions. American Psychologist 34:815–820

Klepp K-I, Fuglesang M, Flisher AJ, Leshabari MT, Lie GTH, Mapang KG (2000) Adolescent Reproductive Health Network: health system and health promotion research in Eastern and Southern Africa. East African Medical Journal 77, 6 (Suppl):S38-S42

Leaf PJ (1998) Issues in the evaluation of systems of mental health services: a perspective and recent developments. In: Young GJ, Ferrari P (eds) Designing mental health service systems for children and adolescents: a shrewd investment. Brunner/Mazel, London, pp 95–103

LeVine RA, LeVine S, Leiderman PH, Brazelton TB, Dixon S, Richman A, Keefer CH (1994) Child care and culture: Lessons from Africa. Cambridge University Press, New York

Minde KK (1977) Children in Uganda: rates of behavioral deviations and psychiatric disorders in various schools and clinic populations. Journal of Child Psychology and Psychiatry 18:23–37

Mulatu MS (1995) Prevalence and risk factors of psychopathology in Ethiopian children. Journal of the American Academy of Child and Adolescent Psychiatry 34:100–109

Ndlela J (1995) Some perspectives in caring for culturally diverse populations. University of California, San Francisco

Nikapota AD (1991) Child psychiatry in developing countries. British Journal of Psychiatry 158:743–751

Odejide AO, Oyewunmi LK, Ohaeri JU (1989) Psychiatry in Africa: an overview. American Journal of Psychiatry 146:708–716

Okasha (2002) Mental health in Africa: the role of the WPA. World Psychiatry 1:32–35

Olawatura M (2001) Culture and psychiatric disorders: a Nigerian perspective. The Psychiatric Clinics of North America 24: 497–504

Policy Guidelines for Child and Adolescent Mental Health (2003). National Department of Health, Pretoria, South Africa

Prince RH (1962) Functional symptoms associated with study among Africans. West African Medical Journal 11:198–206

Robertson B, Berger S (1994) Child psychopathology in South Africa. In: Dawes A, Donald D (eds) Childhood and diversity: psychological perspectives from South African research. David Philip, Cape Town, pp 154–176

Robertson BA, Ensink K, Parry CDH, Chalton D (1999) Performance of the Diagnostic Interview Schedule for Children Version 2.3 (DISC-2.3) in an informal settlement area in South Africa. Journal of the American Academy of Child and Adolescent Psychiatry 38:1156–1164

Saxena S, Maulik PK (2002) Review of published literature on mental health from low and middle income group countries: preliminary results. Paper presented at the WHO meeting: Research for Change: Research on Mental Health and Substance Abuse in Developing Countries, Cape Town

Sameroff AJ (1975) Transactional models in early social relations. Human Development 18:65–79

Sampson R, Raudenbush S, Earls F (1997) Neighbourhoods and violent crime: a multi-level study of collective efficacy. Science 277:918–924

Seck B (1991) De l'enfant autiste en occident à l'enfant Nit Ku Bon en Afrique: approches interprétatives en psychopathologie. A propos de cinq cas. Mémoire pour le diplôme universitaire de pédopsychiatrie, Marseille, France

Seck B, Dassa SK, Soulayrol R (1998) Le premier service de pédopsychiatrie de l'Afrique de l'Ouest. Bilan et perspectives d'une première année de fonctionnement après rénovation. Neuropsychiatrie Enfance Adolescence 3:179–186

Seif El Din AG, Kamel FA, Youssef RM, Atta HY (1996) Evaluation of an educational training program for the development

of trainers in child mental health in Alexandria. La Revue de Santé de la Méditerranée orientale 2:482–493

Seif El Din A, Ziady H, Shokeir N, Farghaly N (2002) Study on street children in Alexandria. Part 1. Psychological profile. Alexandria Journal of Pediatrics 16:191–201

Shatkin JP, Belfer ML (2004) The global absence of child and adolescent mental health policy. Journal of Child and Adolescent Mental Health (accepted for publication)

Shutte A (1993) Philosophy for Africa. University of Cape Town Press, Cape Town

Tadesse B, Kebede D, Tegegne T, Alem A (1999) Childhood behavior disorders in Ambo district, western Ethiopia. 1. Prevalence estimates. Acta Psychiatrica Scandinavica 100 (Suppl):92–97

UN Development Program (2001) United Nations, New York

UN Population Data, 2000. United Nations, New York

USAid Project Profiles – children affected by HIV/AIDS (2003). http://www.Synergyaids.com/

UNICEF (1990) Children and development in the 1990s – a UNICEF Sourcebook. On the occasion of the World Summit for Children 29–30 September 1990. United Nations, New York

UNICEF (2003) The state of the world's children 2003. United Nations, New York

Uznanski A, Roos JL (1997) The situation of mental health services of the World Health Organization, African region, in the early 1990s. South African Medical Journal 87:1743–1749

Verdeli H, Clougherty H, Bolton P, Speelman L, Ndogoni L, Bass J, Neugebauer R, Weissman MM (2003) Adapting group interpersonal psychotherapy for a developing country: experience in rural Uganda. World Psychiatry 2:114–120

Wessels M, Monteiro C (2000) Healing wounds of war in Angola. In: Donald D, Dawes A, Louw J (eds) Addressing childhood diversity. David Philip, Cape Town, pp 176–201

Wing J, Brewin CR, Thornicroft G (1992) Defining mental health needs. In: Thornicroft G, Brewin CR, Wing J (eds) Measuring mental health needs. Gaskell, London, pp 1–17

World Health Report (2001) Mental health: new understanding, new hope. World Health Organization, Geneva

WHO (Undated) Regional Strategy for Mental Health 2000–2010. World Health Organization Regional Office for Africa, Brazzaville, Congo

WHO (2003) Caring for children and adolescents with mental disorders: setting WHO directions. World Health Organization, Geneva

Young JG, Ferrari P (eds) (1998) Designing mental health services and systems for children and adolescents. Brunner/Mazel, London

Youssef R, Attia M, Kamel M (1998) Children experiencing violence. II. Prevalence and determinants of corporal punishment in school children. Child Abuse and Neglect 22:975–985

Setting Up Services in Difficult Circumstances

Lynne Jones, Mimoza Shahini

9.1   Introduction   – 89
9.1.1   Beginnings   – 89
9.1.2   Personal Experiences   – 90

9.2   Setting Up the Service   – 92
9.2.1   The Kosovo Mental Health Service   – 92
9.2.1.1 Demography and Epidemiology   – 93
9.2.1.2 Existing Mental Health Services in Kosovo   – 93
9.2.2   The Clinical Services   – 94

9.3   Approach to Care   – 95

9.4   Developing Child Psychiatric Specialists   – 98
9.4.1   The Training Experience   – 98
9.4.2   Training to Support the Family Approach   – 99

9.5   After the NGOs Leave   – 99

9.6   The Future   – 99

         References   – 100

9.1   Introduction

This chapter will give an account of how the child mental health service in Kosovo came to be in the immediate aftermath of NATO air strikes, and detail the practical difficulties encountered in getting the service established. It will describe how the service worked, and the kind of problems that presented. The accounts will provide the perspective of a child psychiatrist working in a humanitarian aid capacity on behalf of a nongovernmental organization and that of a national staff member trained as a psychiatrist and the first member of a new child psychiatry training program in Kosovo. The chapter discusses the issues raised by humanitarian intervention in a complex emergency, the cultural validity of western services, its acceptability with the local population and the methods of intervention adopted. Lastly, the chapter explains what happens when nongovernmental movements and donors withdraw and what are the day-to-day difficulties of sustaining

a new service in the long term. A more personal style is used throughout to convey more clearly and effectively the experience with its dependence on historical circumstances, chance, serendipity, and personal encounters.

9.1.1 Beginnings

The senior author first became involved in Kosovo in 1989. At that time it was a province of Yugoslavia, with a population of 2 million, 90% of whom were Albanians. Since 1974, the province had had an autonomous status almost equivalent to the other republics of the Federal Republic of Yugoslavia. Following the removal of the province's autonomy that year, there ensued 10 years that were extremely difficult for the whole population. Large numbers of Albanians were dismissed from their jobs, in particular within the health service and the university medical school. In response, the Albanians set up parallel structures in the form of private and charitable health facilities, and created a separate university medical school run out of private houses, with only limited access to clinical cases. The State sector also suffered from a lack of resources. Some Albanians were able to keep their jobs within the state sector, particularly in psychiatry (Jones 1993). After the conflict escalated to full-scale war in the summer of 1998, the state health service in rural areas ceased to function, and Albanians from the conflict areas could no longer reach the cities because of security concerns. Most of those with access to the service no longer had health insurance, as they were unemployed, and lacked the means to pay. In October 1998, international negotiation led to an agreement with the government in Belgrade that allowed civilian monitors into the province and humanitarian organizations access to the rural population.

Child Advocacy International (CAI) employed the senior author to become program manager for two emergency mobile primary health care clinics, and to respond to the emergency mental health needs in rural areas providing training for mobile clinic primary health care staff in emergency mental health. The problems encountered ranged from the grief and stress responses engendered by the losses and horrors of the continuing counterinsurgency campaign, to the full range of conventional acute and chronic psychiatric problems of a population unable to access normal health care. In March 1999, after the failure of the talks at Rambouillet, international humanitarian organizations were evacuated from the country and most agencies began to provide services for the expelled Albanian population on the Macedonian and Albanian borders (Mastnak 1999). In June 1999, NATO air strikes ended after Slobodan Milosevic agreed to the withdrawal of Serbian security forces and to allow the province to be administered by the United Nations until the question of its final status was resolved. Some 3,500 people had been killed in the 2 years of violent conflict and some 800,000 expelled from the country. At that point, it was possible to return and try to pursue the original goals.

CAI had almost completely exhausted its funds running emergency pediatric and mental health services on the Albanian border; but still found money to allow for tracking down what had happened to former patients in the most conflict affected areas of the province, to run emergency clinics, and to see if further funding could be found. What follows are edited extracts of the senior author's diary from those first few months.

9.1.2 Personal Experiences

16 June 1999

We left Kukes at 4.30 this morning in a back-to-back queue of tractors and cars waved over the border by Albanians and German NATO soldiers alike. Nine thousand Kosovo Albanians crossed yesterday. They are not listening to UNHCR's suggestions that they wait. They want to get back before any more homes are burnt by departing Serbs, or looted by Kukes bandits. All the way to Prizren we passed shouting, cheering, and flag-waving families. At Suva Reka, an hour south of Prishtina, the scenery changed: burnt and shattered houses and another long convoy of tractors. Only this one looked different. The trailers were loaded with more possessions than people: fridges, washing machines; a young woman stared at me blankly. Opposite her on a substantial sofa, an older one held her head in her hands. »Serbs leaving« Shkumbin, our country director, muttered. These children were not shouting and waving, not even three-fingered gestures of defiance. The most striking thing about Prishtina is its emptiness. The Grand Hotel is stuffed with media, but everywhere else the streets are deserted. All the shops and cafés are either boarded up or trashed.

I got up to go to a World Health Organization meeting on the situation at the hospital. Apparently it is in chaos: very few patients, and only 20% of the Serb staff remain. The Serb director Dr. G. is discussing with lawyers the way previously dismissed Albanians can be integrated back into their jobs – but at the same time we are informed some 25 Serb doctors coming from Belgrade to help! Dr. Afrim, my psychiatric colleague, watched Serb doctors load all the equipment from one Prishtina health care center onto a truck today. They stopped when he called KFOR (the international Kosovo Protection Force). He muttered in my ear that the Albanian doctors have given up negotiating with G. They plan to have a demonstration tomorrow to inform him that he is no longer wanted as director and to take their jobs back.

18 June, Prishtina

It was a very peculiar demonstration. Anxious-looking Serb doctors clustered together in the anteroom of the surgical department eyeing a large crowd of Albanian doctors, who, having discovered that the director was absent, had no clear idea of what they wanted to do. Media hacks pecked at the edges of the crowd, interviewing anyone willing. At one point two KFOR soldiers arrived. An irate Serb grabbed one of them and said »look, these are doctors who lost their jobs 10 years ago and now they have come back. You have to give us security«. Afrim was only sacked 3 days after air strikes began so this was not completely true. More KFOR appeared and put two armed soldiers outside the director's office. Then some kind of a delegation formed itself and a KFOR man said »discussions are ongoing, why don't you all take a bit of fresh air«.

22 June

A soft-spoken American approached me after yet another health meeting: »Apparently President Clinton has made children's mental health a personal priority. Would you be interested in submitting any kind proposal for funding to the Office for Disaster Assistance?« I stared at him in astonishment. I am not often offered money. »Give me 10 days«.

We have no base in Prishtina; the adult psychiatric clinic is not a place to bring children and anyway there is no room. Dialeta, Shkumbin's sister, would allow us to use her old flat as a consultation center. However, no one had been in it since before air strikes. I was worried about booby traps and wanted to get some KFOR people to check it out first, but Dialeta did not want to wait, so a group of us walked across the hot, strangely silent city to explore. The place had been sacked, but once cleared of debris it looked like a beautiful place to have a clinic: quiet, with enough space and a garden.

23 June

It is still not clear who is running Prishtina hospital, let alone Kosovo. In neuropsychiatry last week the Serbian doctors were working alongside the Albanians, but »separately« insisting on seeing their own patients, and doing their own »on call«, until they realized they had not enough cover, so they asked the Albanians for help. The Albanians said fine, but would not accept Serb authority over them. This week all the Serb doctors have gone. Only nurses and patients remain. Professor Bosniaku told me it was their choice. They were welcome to stay, but not in Director positions. And if they cared about Kosovo they would stay. »Their director came into my office 10 years ago and said he was taking it over, but I did not leave. I continued to work here, I insisted. And when people were rude, I still did not go. They leave to make politics and they will say they were driven«.

29 June, Klina

The weekly NGO health coordination meeting has devolved into five sectoral meetings. There are now 60 NGOs attending the mental health meeting so it has split into five working groups. As I am the only person in the child psychiatry working group, I am skipping meetings to write my proposal and carrying on clinics. In Klina today I saw a flat-faced, exhausted boy who survived the summary execution of ten of his friends, a girl with panic attacks whose brother is one of 93 men in the town gone missing, and a family of five almost completely silent children, all under nine. Their thin and exhausted-looking father told me they had just come down from the mountains where they have not done much speaking for 3 months, as he had to tell them to be quiet the whole time for fear they might be found. The children stared wide-eyed at my toys, but were too nervous to touch, just nodding their heads when I asked if they would like me to bring my toys to their house next week.

Then we went to visit a man whom I first saw last week. He had come home to find his house burnt and the skeletons of what he assumed were his extended family, including 11 children, lying among the charred timbers of one of the rooms. Last week he showed us: shoes were still piled up outside the door, a ring of machine-gun bullets round the wall and human skeletal remains among the rubble suggested what had happened. We sat on a rug in the long grass among the apple trees, the garden stinking of death, while he asked how he should tell his own children how their cousins had died. He also wanted me to get hold of a scene of crimes team, so that he could move the bodies and bring the children home. That at least had happened, and I found four small children playing happily in the orchard. Father has decided that after all he is not sure who has died, so for now he has told them nothing. I am always amazed by how we cling to hope. I have two girl patients in another town whose entire family and neighbors were rounded up and shot to pieces around them. They warded off the bullets with their arms and were taken by other soldiers to Prishtina hospital. Arlinda saw blood appear on her 12-year-old cousin's coat, and her brother's head explode. But although her mother was right beside her, she did not actually see her die so she told me she thinks that she might be alive. One of the problems is that burnt and paperless bodies are hard to identify, and the war crimes investigators are not doing this detailed work at present.

7 July, Drenica

I finally seem to have tracked down all my old patients; most of them are well. Some of them are dead. None of them left Drenica. For the most part women and children seem to have been pushed from one village to another in convoys, sometimes being given flour by Serb forces, sometimes being shelled. The boys and men kept moving or hiding or fighting. The other day Illir came hurtling after me on crutches. He has survived 3 months alone in the hospital. Their house is wrecked, and the whole family is in Prishtina. I spent one Sunday playing football with Simon and his sister. The three children are the sole survivors of the massacre of 22 relatives, including their pregnant mother. We did play therapy for 2 months before air strikes, and in spite of a second period of upheaval, they appear remarkably well. Their uncle is already rebuilding their house for the second time. Today, I found Faton and his whole family at home, an empty chair outside the door to indicate mourning, but the whole family welcoming. It seems that the grandfather was one of 18 killed in another massacre. The last mother saw of him was with other men, stripped with his hands against a wall. She and the other women and children were pushed on to Skenderaj. Faton had already escaped out of a window when the tanks came into the village. He spent the next 3 months being extraordinarily resourceful, avoiding one fatal selection by pretending to be disabled and jumping into a line of women, another by running away while a soldier was reloading his gun. Faton was one of my sickest children prior to air strikes. He had seen his father and brothers tortured and killed in front of him and had severe traumatic symptoms. I had been working with him until I was evacuated. Now he told me he was very well, no nightmares, no fear, and only occasional sadness. He thought it was thanks to the fluoxetine I began at the point when I knew I might leave abruptly, but as he had lost the packet in the first onslaught I said it might have more to do with discovering his own abilities and strength.

9.2   Setting Up the Service

Humanitarian intervention, and psychosocial interventions in particular, are currently the subjects of interconnected debates. Briefly summarized, there have been increasing calls for a shift from what is seen as the colonial legacy of humanitarian philanthropy: in which a professional international aid worker elite provide a massive short-term effort to assist a particular country to recover from disaster and then move on. This approach is criticized as paternalistic, sentimental, and inappropriate to today's complex emergencies, which may be chronic or permanent. What is required is long-term, sustainable commitment, detailed political understanding, rights-based agendas that empower local actors rather than patronize them (Slim 1995). Similarly, within the field of psychosocial interventions there have been critiques of the assumptions underpinning trauma programs established in conflict and postconflict regions – in particular that they are based on western criteria for diagnosis and treatment, that may be culturally inappropriate, and that they may pathologize normative responses and undermine local systems of coping (Summerfield 1999). Meanwhile, both critics and advocates of trauma programs have been admonished for neglecting the impact of disabling psychiatric conditions, which have been found in postconflict societies worldwide (Silove, Ekblad et al. 2000).

9.2.1   The Kosovo Mental Health Service

Kosovo in the summer of 1999 presented all the problems of a complex emergency. A large proportion of the population had been exposed to violence, displacement, and massive losses in addition to 10 years of discrimination and human rights abuses. The infrastructure had suffered from decades of neglect. Meanwhile, the complex system of administration, continuing interethnic hostility, and the unresolved political status of the province contributed to continuing insecurity and uncertainty.

In a country emerging from war, where infrastructure and the state structure are in a crisis, it's difficult to set a balance between the needs of an individual and the society. This becomes even more difficult when a balance has to be set up between the approaches of the NGOs and those of the government. The entrance of the NGOs in an uncoordinated way also deepens the crisis in the system of individual and professional values. On many occasions less-skilled individuals or nonprofessionals were being paid to provide assistance because of their language knowledge, while the professionals working within the state system provided assistance for free. Some NGOs provided adequate help, but it was less effective because of very bad coordination. Those NGOs that adapted their philosophy to the needs of the country were more successful than the others.

9.2.1.1 Demography and Epidemiology

The demographic balance in Kosovo is significantly different from the rest of Europe. Approximately 55% of the total population is under 19 years of age, 13% are under 4 and another 23% between 5 and 14 (Albanian health survey report 1999). Kosovo lacked adequate public health data on the mental health needs prior to the conflict but data collected by CAI in the conflict areas prior to air strikes suggested that at least 1–2% of children had serious psychological problems that required skilled professional help.

For example, in the 6-week period during air strikes, working with Kosovar refugees of all ages in Kukes, Northern Albania, CAI accepted 15 cases of acutely disturbed children, a third of whom had previous psychiatric problems that had not been attended to in Kosovo. The smallest family unit in any of these cases was six members, and with each referral it was possible to identify at least one other family member who required clinical help. After air strikes, health houses in rural conflict areas reported seeing two to three children with serious psychological difficulties each day. Many of these children had had psychological difficulties of some kind prior to the period of conflict.

Studies both in developing and developed countries suggest that 10–15% of children suffer from mental health problems, and another 3–4% from varying degree of developmental delay and learning difficulties (Pillay and Lockhat 1997). Thus, even without the effects of conflict and the harsh living conditions of the previous decade, we expected a significant number of children to be in need of mental health services.

9.2.1.2 Existing Mental Health Services in Kosovo

Kosovar psychiatric services, as in the whole of the former Yugoslavia, were predominantly influenced by the Russian system, with resources concentrated on a biological and institutional approach to serious mental disorder in adults. What child mental health services existed were provided by adult psychiatrists with a strong biological orientation. In July 1999, most hospitals in the province lacked a management structure, and mobile teams of expatriate volunteers were still providing most primary health care. Albanian doctors were returning, and WHO planned to take over hospital administration. Although all the Serbian staff had departed, the psychiatric clinic

was functioning and accepting patients. There were 15 adult psychiatrists, but only one with specialist experience with children. The University Department of Psychiatry was reconstituting itself. It had had no psychiatric trainees for 10 years. It now appeared as if it might have at least 20 and there was no one to provide child psychiatry training. A number of NGOs had set up psychosocial programs to provide some training in the identification of psychological disorders in children, but there was no local service to whom children with problems could be referred. The NGO programs gave little attention to serious psychological difficulties.

In discussion with WHO and UNICEF, it was agreed that the best contribution CAI could make was to develop a child and adolescent mental health service, rather than a psycho-trauma service. We hoped from the outset to create a sustainable, culturally appropriate service that met the locally identified mental health needs of children and adolescents throughout Kosovo, and provide a training base for future specialists, as well as residents in general psychiatry. We wished it to be integrated with pediatric and primary health care services, and with adult psychiatric services, which were also being transformed into a community-based service. We wished to attend to severe unaddressed needs and to avoid an overextended role that could arise from treating the whole population as traumatized. Thus, education and support for other health professionals and NGO staff was an essential part of the service.

In the first year, the clinics were located in the flat in Prishtina, which had doubled in size because of the displaced population, and in small towns in two of the most conflict-affected areas. In the second year, these two latter clinics were shifted to four main towns in order to be integrated with the overall development of community-based mental health services in Kosovo, and to provide access to the greatest number of people. This allowed for a more accessible, less stigmatizing service with close connections with primary health care. The residents and nurses also made family and school visits as needed, and some families were seen entirely at home. The service was open to children of all ethnicities up to the age of eighteen, and their parents. We also saw older children in higher education, and in urgent cases where no other psychiatrist was available, adults. In each town in which we worked we informed the local health professionals, schools, and NGOs of our presence, and spent some time explaining what kind of problems with which we could assist. We advertised the service on the local radio and did occasional radio talks on children's mental health problems.

9.2.2 The Clinical Services

In order to provide some means of evaluating the clinical service, the case load was audited at all the clinics over 2 years and data collected on 559 patients (530 aged less than 20 years). The work was conducted under fairly difficult conditions. Frequently during the first year, clinics had to be closed for lack of power or security. Access was sometimes difficult. The assessment and treatment of patients and the residents' training were the priorities. The supervisors and trainees developed the database over the 2 years, thus data was not collected on every patient and not all data categories are complete for all patients. The data provided are a fairly accurate reflection of the range and numbers of cases seen (❑ Tables 9.1, 9.2). However, a proportion of cases with more serious diagnoses still being seen at the end of the second year were not included in the audit because their cases remained open as they were still in therapy.

In the first year, the most common reason for attendance was »exposure to a traumatic event«, even if the child was symptom free, because NGOs (the most common source of referral of this problem) or families were concerned that there might be future problems. Both the international and the general community had »learned« that there might be a reaction, and were concerned. Stress-related disorders were the most common diagnosis, but even so, many of those referred had no psychiatric diagnosis, or any disturbance, and the session was used for education and reassurance.

In the second year, as the number of NGOs in Kosovo declined and the service became better known, self-referrals and referrals from the medical community predominated. Bedwetting (usually primary enuresis) and behavior problems became the most common reasons for attendance. Behavior problems, summed up by the term »Nervoz« in Kosovo, took the form of irritability, or disobedience and aggression. This was often combined with sleep problems, and was distinguished by parents from fear, »Frike«. Learning disability and nonorganic enuresis were the most common diagnoses in the second year. A variety of neuro-developmental difficulties also became more significant. In spite of large numbers presenting with behavior problems, relatively few children met the criteria for conduct dis-

orders. As in the first year, a substantial number did not warrant any psychiatric diagnosis, but benefited from explanation and education and the mobilization of social support.

A psychiatric service can play a significant role in »de-anthologizing« and normalizing in a war-affected society, and in treating minor disturbances. Families might have coped with many of the less serious presenting problems in normal circumstances. However, the difficulties of postwar life – displacement and crowded living conditions – had made them insurmountable. Behavior problems often reflected greater stress in parents, rather than an increase in conduct disturbance. Nocturnal enuresis is much worse a problem when beds are shared, and there are no adequate facilities for washing sheets.

The substantial groups of children with more biologically based problems, and the cluster of older teenagers who presented with serious psychopathology justified the creation of an inclusive mental health service rather than just a psycho-trauma service. However, the large group with stress-related problems and mood disturbances, particularly in the first year, demonstrated that any postconflict mental health service needs the capacity to cope with traumatic reactions and grief and loss. At the same time, we were very aware that many of the cases we saw were a complex mix of social, psychological, and physical difficulties that did not fit easily into diagnostic categories and required long-term, comprehensive interventions sometimes beyond our resources.

Paradoxically, postconflict societies may also offer an opportunity, through access to humanitarian aid. Families who could not previously access help could now do so because of agencies working in remote areas and because of discussions on previously taboo topics. Problems such as domestic violence and sexual abuse that were previously little discussed began to be recognized and to present at the clinic. The ability to identify abuse raised challenges when there were as yet no established mechanisms or facilities for child protection or for dealing with perpetrators.

The most difficult problem was how to provide an adequate response for the large number of children with special needs in the absence of adequate social services and limited educational facilities. The high percentage of children with learning disability, enuresis, and neuro-developmental difficulties resembles findings from developing countries. Poor access to good health services, poor educa-

■ Table 9.1. Reasons given for attending the child and adolescent mental health service, years 1 and 2

Year 1 Reasons	n	%	Year 2 Reasons	n	%
Exposure to traumatic events	32	18.39	Bedwetting	61	15.84
Unspecified	21	12.07	Behavior problems	50	12.99
Behavior problems	17	9.77	Fear	29	7.53
Low mood or tearfulness	11	6.32	Exposure to traumatic events	25	6.49
Bedwetting	10	5.75	Learning difficulties	23	5.97
Somatic complaints	7	4.02	Unspecified	21	5.45
Fear	7	4.02	Nightmares	15	3.90
Learning difficulties	7	4.02	Somatic complaints	15	3.90
Nightmares	6	3.45	Speech problems	15	3.90
Sleep problems	5	2.87	Stuttering	13	3.38
Fits	3	1.72	Developmental delay	12	3.12
Poor appetite	3	1.72	Poor appetite	11	2.86
Strange movements	3	1.72	Fainting	8	2.08
Family difficulties	2	1.15	Fits	8	2.08
Developmental delay	2	1.15	Poor concentration	8	2.08
Forensic assessment	2	1.15	Tearfulness or low mood	8	2.08
Poor communication with others	2	1.15	Assessment for family placement	5	1.30
Poor concentration	2	1.15	Sleep problems	5	1.30
Speech problems	2	1.15	Anger	3	0.78
Stuttering	2	1.15	Mute	3	0.78
Withdrawn	2	1.15	School refusal	3	0.78
Deaf and dumb	1	0.57	Separation difficulties	3	0.78
Fainting	1	0.57	Sleep walking	3	0.78
Head injury	1	0.57	Specific fear	3	0.78
Mute	1	0.57	Strange movements	3	0.78
Overactivity	1	0.57	Medication	2	0.52
Strange behavior	1	0.57	Strange feelings	2	0.52
			Suicidal ideas	2	0.52
			Tremor	2	0.52
			Withdrawal	2	0.52
			Breathing difficulties	1	0.26
			Financial support	1	0.26
			Hair pulling	1	0.26
			Masturbating	1	0.26
			Overactivity	1	0.26
			Poor communication with others	1	0.26
			Poor growth	1	0.26
			Severe mental retardation	1	0.26
			Soiling	1	0.26
			Strange behavior	1	0.26
			Talking to himself	1	0.26
			Tidiness	1	0.26
			Weight loss	1	0.26

tional facilities, and poor obstetric care have all contributed (Pillay and Lockhat 1997; Somasundaram and van de Put 1999). Our aim was to support the family in dealing with the numerous behavioral problems that occurred at home, as well as diagnosing and treating any accompanying mental illness.

9.3 Approach to Care

Integrating all these elements has influenced child mental health services and health policy in Kosovo. Currently, they are divided into day programs and

Table 9.2. ICD-10 diagnoses for patients attending the child and adolescent mental health service, years 1 and 2

ICD-10 code	ICD-10 diagnosis	Males	Females	Total	%	Males	Females	Total	%
F07.02	Postconcussional syndrome	2	0	2	1.30	0	0	0	0.00
F20–23	Schizophrenia, schizotypal and delusional disorders	1	0	0	0.00	3	1	3	0.80
F31–34	Mood disorders	3	6	7	4.55	2	3	5	1.33
F41–42, F44–49.3	Neurotic and somatoform disorders	4	2	9	5.84	5	7	12	3.19
F43.1–43.2	Stress related	21	18	33	21.43	3	12	15	3.99
F50.0	Anorexia nervosa	0	0	1	0.65	0	1	1	0.27
F51	Nonorganic sleep disorders	3	2	5	3.25	8	3	11	2.93
F60	Personality disorders	1	0	0	0.00	1	0	1	0.27
F70–F79	Mental retardation	9	3	10	6.49	29	20	44	11.70
F80	Specific speech and language disorders			1	0.65			4	1.06
F90	Hyperkinetic disorders	0	2	2	1.30	2	2	4	1.06
F91–92.8	Conduct disorders	0	0	0	0.00	6	0	5	1.33
F93–94	Disorders of social and emotional functioning	1	1	2	1.30	1	12	13	3.46
F95–95.2	Tic disorders	2	1	3	1.95	2	0	2	0.53
F98.0	Nonorganic enuresis	6	4	10	6.49	29	19	58	15.43
F98.2	Feeding disorder of infancy and childhood	1	0	1	0.65	0	0	0	0.00
F98.5	Stuttering	1	1	2	1.30	12	3	15	3.99
	Emotional and physical abuse	1	0	1	0.65	0	0	0	0.00
	No psychiatric diagnosis	26	35	53	34.42	174	68	139	36.97
	Assessment not completed	4	3	7	4.55	5	6	11	2.93
	Still attending	0	0	0	0.00	17	16	33	8.78
	Missing data	0	0	5	3.25	0	0	0	0.00

9

parent programs, and there is a close relationship with pediatricians in treatment. Lack of space is one reason for an emphasis on the family as the best means of support for both children and adolescents, and this is likely to continue into the future.

Establishing services that did not exist before the war is quite challenging, especially when local staff have been somewhat confused by the conflicting approaches offered by the international community. We were clear that for the service to meet the needs of the consumers it needed to be based on epidemiological studies and evidence-based medicine. It also needed to have sufficient human and physical resources, be easily accessible, and avoid bureaucracy.

In the situation faced by Kosovo in 1999, there was a need to create short-term solutions which would offer immediate assistance to a particularly needy section of the population, and to create human resources who would be both trainees and service providers. It was particularly important in Kosovo to both define the service as separate and distinct from adult mental health services, and to use the expertise which already existed within the country. Thus, although child psychiatry trainees came from the adult services, we worked most closely with the primary health care system, providing additional training for family practitioners.

As explained above, the child and adolescent psychiatric service at the outset attracted large numbers of families of the children with special needs, who attended out of desperation because of a lack of clinical and educational resources. The new structure of the service encouraged families to take part in the evaluation and educational and developmental process of infants. As the clinical service evolved, parents were encouraged to actively participate in the creation of a new mental health policy for children and adolescents.

In developing a system of care for children and adolescents in Kosovo, the family is seen as the starting point and as the major support for the clinical work. Involving parents in information-seeking and decision-making regarding treatment was a service priority from the outset. Traditionally, doctors were seen as the ones to decide on the treatment of the child and often they were held responsible for cases of treatment failure. The confrontation of Kosovar society with sweeping changes in all aspects of functioning is reflected in families in varying ways, including family structure, the way in which emotions are expressed, communication, and adherence to a system of values. We noticed a

movement from a focus on large families toward one of a focus on nuclear families. This change was included in the approach toward patients. Regarding our own work, our emphasis was on the importance of working together with the family, rather than structured family therapy.

In developing the service, every attempt was made to build a sensitive, culturally competent service that respected the values, beliefs, traditions, and customs of the parents during the intervention. This was reflected in both clinical work and training. At its best when using a family work approach, we noticed on many occasions that the families appeared empowered to take more responsibility for their children rather than handing the problem over to the medical system. Our approach fit organically into a collaborative system of support and care which involved doctors, families, folk doctors, religious persons, extended families, and schools. A balance was achieved between the powerful potential effect of the network and the treatment. Responsibility for improvement was dispersed rather than concentrated on the physician.

A number of cultural variables had to be considered in Kosovo when creating the child and adolescent mental health service. Particularly in rural areas, families are mostly patriarchal, and the oldest male is the most powerful member of the family. When father is dead this may be a brother or older son. Other cultural factors matter: age (the respect for older people); income (there is a well functioning system of mutual assistance, especially involving those working overseas); geographical location (those in rural parts prefer to work within extended families, rather than in institutions); the neighborhood (family decision-making can often be influenced by relatives or by those living close to the client); religion (religious persons such as imams and priests are engaged in the process of assistance and are often open to cooperation, especially when dealing with families); and children with special needs (many families prefer the child to remain within the family, rather than be sent to an asylum or hospital). Another significant factor was the very close relationship between the mother and the child. Particularly because of postwar unemployment, mothers came to play a crucial role when helping the child. Because of the need to take all these cultural aspects into consideration and the fluidity of the situation, flexibility and responsiveness were the key factors in trying to offer a high-quality service.

9.4 Developing Child Psychiatric Specialists

Child psychiatry was a new specialty; though as noted, some child mental health services had existed in the 1990s. Some argued that postconflict situations were not the time to establish services, others that it provided an ideal opportunity for reform. There were understandable tensions between a generation of doctors who had been dismissed from their jobs for over a decade and wanted simply to get back to work in a system with which they were familiar, and a younger generation who had not suffered to the same degree and had many ideas for change. Some feared the specialty would generate more work for those left treating adults; others pointed out that a good service for children would in the long run reduce the burden on adult services.

The work of mental health professionals was very difficult, due to sweeping changes in the political, economic, social, and cultural spheres. Physicians found themselves affected by changes in society as a whole, within the family, and in the individual professional requirements. In countries in transition, lack of clarity regarding the part of policy makers means that individual professionals find their relationships with all aspects of society in flux. A number of particular conditions affected psychiatric work: (a) societies tend to concentrate on basic needs, thus people only come to see the psychiatrist when problems are severe or when a psychiatric diagnosis would bring certain financial benefits, such as a pension; (b) professionals tended to favor contradictory streams in diagnosis, evaluation, and training. Many professionals tried to imitate »western« methods of intervention, driven by a desire for change, and a wish for a new, possibly more efficient approach for both the patient and the family. When these methods were implemented as a »ready-made« recipe they often failed. First, they often failed because they had not adapted to the cultural context and were less acceptable to the population. Second, because although some families grasped new methods, they favored a quick fix. Medication use was often inappropriate with no long-term benefit. Third, there was a lack of a health insurance system which made access to care for all difficult. Finally, methods tailored to the individual were not popular with extended families who favored approaches that engaged them all rather than just one person. For all the above reasons, professional conflicts occurred leading to an inability to

come up with an agreed-upon approach. There was little respect for any collaborative protocols.

A major problem with humanitarian interventions is that high rates of pay and additional training allow foreign NGOs to recruit the best-qualified professionals, thus draining the public sector, but leaving the staff without employment when funding dries up. Much of our time in the first year was taken up with negotiations with the UNMIK administration of the hospital and the Department of Neuropsychiatry to allow CAI to second two psychiatry residents for specialist child psychiatry training from an expatriate consultant child psychiatrist who would remain for at least 3 months at a time. The idea was that the residents would keep their hospital contracts and return to the psychiatry department when their specialist training was over. They would then be in a position to provide specialist services themselves and train others.

The training program began with two full-time residents, one of whom had almost completed her training in Albania and had substantial child psychiatry experience. In the second year, two additional part-time residents were recruited. In addition, four nurses were recruited to assist the clinics and begin training in children's mental health.

The aim from the outset for CAI had been to provide both a clinical service and a training opportunity. Training took the form of supervision and mentoring in the clinics and a regular weekly program of seminars, lectures, and case discussions for all the psychiatry residents. Funding was also used to set up internet access, create a comprehensive library, and provide two residents with the opportunity to study for between 1 and 3 months in the United Kingdom. Because the expatriate consultant supervisors changed every 3 months, the residents were exposed to a wide variety of approaches, and engaged in two-way exchanges as to the appropriateness of western systems of diagnosis and treatment in the Kosovar context.

9.4.1 The Training Experience

In this context, the local doctors, Dr Aferdita Goçi-Uka and Dr. Shahini, were included in the training program of child and adolescent psychiatry provided by CAI. The clinical work was focused in several clinics established throughout Kosovo. Professionals from abroad involved in the CAI project supervised local staff. This provided a formalized clinical training experience. Having experts with different backgrounds was a good experience for the trainees. It was a challenge to integrate the many different approaches, but it afforded the opportunity to test personal abilities and choose the approach that suited us most. Including the local staff in the training offered by an NGO, and providing experts from abroad for the development of the project, in a country in chaos, was very positive.

In the third year, all the residents returned to their hospital posts and the child psychiatry service was taken over by the state health system. CAI engaged in the physical rehabilitation of six outpatient clinics attached to primary health care centers and the running of a 1-year masters level program with international faculty in child and adolescent mental health.

The success of this collaboration became visible after CAI closed its operation. Because many NGOs did not use this strategy, they left nothing behind. CAI left behind a local staff trained in child and adolescent psychiatry. The programs initiated by CAI were further developed by the local staff. The child and adolescent psychiatry clinics continue to function in the six biggest cities in Kosovo, including an outpatient clinic at the University Clinical Center (UCC) of Prishtina. Among the tangible products left behind was a fully equipped library, which provides an excellent opportunity for students to have access to the newest developments in child and adolescent psychiatry. The transition of responsibilities from CAI staff to local staff occurred without any problems because CAI had collaborated well with all the institutions of Kosovo. The leading institutions in Kosovo welcomed the running of the child psychiatry service by the UCC.

9.4.2 Training to Support the Family Approach

To achieve the understanding to be able to implement the family approach there was additional training from different professionals including the University of Prishtina, the Institute of Mental Health and Recovery in Kosovo (IMHRK), the American Family Therapy Academy, the University of Illinois at Chicago, the University of Chicago affiliated Chicago Center for Family Health, Linking Human Systems/The LINC Foundation, and the International Trauma Studies Program of New York University. In order to help in this work, materials were prepared for the parents on various disorders.

This allowed the parents to be more cooperative in the treatment, and at the same time it diffused responsibility for the success of treatment.

9.5 After the NGOs Leave

New staff have had to face many challenges in understanding who was responsible for financing the new service, what the relationship should be between adult psychiatry and child psychiatry, what the position is of child psychiatry in the process of educating physicians, and what is the future of adult and child psychiatry. For the local staff of doctors it was easy to continue working within the state institutions, but many who worked for other NGOs are still trying to find their place within the new mental health services system. They have no clearly defined roles and this is a big challenge for the leaders of the mental health services.

Currently, child psychiatry is under the administration of adult psychiatry. A rapport is slowly being established between adult and child psychiatry; conflicts are gradually being resolved. The child psychiatry service had previously been seen as the property of general psychiatry, and adult psychiatrists were still seeing some patients. This was done, in part, because of the very small number of child psychiatrists. The most important point for sustaining the training program and services is that child psychiatry should be accepted as a specialty in its own right, separate from adult psychiatry. The view of the authors is that, because of the demographics of the population and clearly identified needs, the service should not remain in its current status as a subspecialty. The fact that adult psychiatrists are referring increasing numbers of children to a child psychiatrist bodes well for the future. We also hope that the service can be fully available to families and children of all ethnicities in Kosovo, and that the security fears that prevent many Serbian children from attending the service will diminish.

9.6 The Future

In order to further develop mental health, and because of the increasing needs of children and adolescents for these types of services, it is necessary to create a long-term strategic plan which will open the perspective for further development of this field of medicine.

According to the national strategic plan, the mental health of children and adolescents in the near future is going to be separated from adult psychiatry and it will have its own budget in the department of mental health, within the Ministry of Health. In the Ministry of Health, there will also be an official representative for child mental health.

To support this outcome a multidisciplinary working team was established with the support of the Ministry of Health/Office for Mental Health. This team consists of experts in the field. The working group is addressing:

1. The preparation of a document/strategy for the development of services for the mental health of children and adolescents in Kosovo. This document will be based on international standards.
2. Planning for the development of specialized education, and continuing education of human resources in child and adolescent mental health.
3. Planning and developing a community-based structure for child and adolescent mental health services and for specialized wards for the population.
4. The planning of programs and activities that will be applied in these institutions. Included is the development of criteria for the education of those with mental health problems.
5. Close collaboration with other fields of medicine (family medicine, pediatric wards and services, and other organizations which offer similar services).
6. Collaboration with international organizations and the exchange of experiences.
7. Development of regional community-based services which are easier to access by the population in that region.
8. Establishing a leadership structure that will coordinate all the activities regarding implementation of this strategic plan.

In this national plan it has been decided to expand the service, including the primary health care system, by stressing the importance of their training in the mental health of children and adolescents. At the same time, a system has been proposed to help the country train child and adolescent psychiatrists within a reasonable timeframe. Because of the small number of child psychiatrists, the rural population still has no access to a child psychiatrist, which is why there was a prior focus on the training of family doctors to create sufficient human resources.

A continuing challenge relates to the need to develop services that complement psychiatry, such as social work. This is particularly important, given the increased reporting of child abuse. The other challenge relates to the coordination of the work among professionals in mental health and other professionals engaged in this field.

Acknowledgements. Parts of this chapter are based on articles that previously appeared in the London Review of Books and the British Journal of Psychiatry. The authors would like to thank both publications for permission to reprint the material.

Mental health services for war-affected children: Report of a survey in Kosovo, with A. Rrustemi, M. Shahini, A. Uka, **British Journal of Psychiatry** (December 2004).

Mastnak LL Jr (1999) Why are you leaving? London Review of Books. www.lrb.co.uk.

The CAI child psychiatry program was funded by the Bureau for Population Refugees and Migration, US State Department, from 1999–2002.

The authors would also like to acknowledge: Dr. Partha Banerjea, Dr. Kathy Brooks, Dr. Elisabeth Cormack, Professor Zana Dobroshi, and Dr. Kami Saedi for their help in establishing the service, providing supervision and collecting data; Dr. Naim Fanaj, Dr. Muharem Asllani, and Dr. Aferdita Uka for collecting data; Alban Rrustemi for designing a data base and assisting with data presentation; Shkumbin Dauti and Jeton Beqiri for logistic management of the program; Lume Asllani and Arta Rrustemi for data entry and secretarial assistance.

References

Albanian health survey report (1999) International Rescue Committee Institute of Public Health, World Health Organization, Centres for Disease Control and the Institute of Public Health

Mastnak LJ (1999) Why are you leaving? London Review of Books

Pillay AL, Lockhat MR (1997) Developing community mental health services for children in South Africa. Soc Sci Med 10:1493–1501

Silove D, Ekblad S, et al. (2000) The rights of the severely mentally ill in post-conflict societies. Lancet 355:1548–1549

Slim H (1995) The continuing metamorphosis of the humanitarian practitioner: some new colours for an endangered chameleon. Disasters 19(2):110–126

Somasundaram DJ, van de Put WACM (1999) Mental health care in Cambodia. Bulletin World Health Organization 77(3): 275–277

Summerfield D (1999) A critique of seven assumptions behind psychological trauma programmes in war-affected areas. Soc Sci Med 48:1449–1462

II

Principles and Strategies of Treatment/ Intervention

10 Evidence-Based Psychotherapies for Children and Adolescents: Strategies, Strengths, and Limitations 103

Alan E. Kazdin

11 What Works for Whom? Differential Indications for Treatment/Intervention 119

Peter Fonagy, Mary Target

12 Individual and Group Psychotherapies for Children and Adolescents 140

John R. Weisz, Eunie Jung

13 Family Therapy 164

David Cottrell, Paula Boston, Dawn Walker

14 Innovative Interventions in the Community 187

Ernesto Caffo, Barbara Forresi, Carlotta Belaise, Giampaolo Nicolais, Nathaniel Laor, Leo Wolmer, Helmut Remschmidt

15 Medications 208

Stan Kutcher

16 Outcomes of Treatment 222

Stephen Scott

Evidence-Based Psychotherapies for Children and Adolescents: Strategies, Strengths, and Limitations

Alan E. Kazdin

10.1   Introduction   – 103

10.2   Background and Context: An Overview   – 103
10.2.1   Identifying Effective Treatments   – 104
10.2.1.1   Practice Guidelines   – 104
10.2.1.2   Evidence-Based Treatments   – 105
10.2.2   Challenges to the Research on Evidence-Based Treatments   – 106
10.2.2.1   The Generalizability or Transportability of Results from Research to Clinic Settings   – 106
10.2.2.2   Demonstrating Treatment Efficacy   – 108
10.2.3   Obstacles to Integration of Research Findings into Clinical Work   – 109
10.2.3.1   Disparate Views Among Interested Parties   – 109
10.2.3.2   Training of Therapists   – 110

10.3   Categorization of Treatment   – 110
10.3.1   Refining the Classification of Treatments   – 110
10.3.2   Weak Treatments Can be Wonderful   – 112

10.4   The Psychotherapy Research Agenda: More Attention to Mechanisms of Change   – 113

10.5   Conclusions   – 115

References   – 116

pirically validated treatment, empirically supported treatments, evidence-based practice, and treatments that work. The term evidence-based treatment (EBT) is used in this chapter in keeping with a tradition already established in several other areas (e.g., dentistry, nursing, health care, social work, education, psychiatry, and mental health) where interventions are used to produce change in a particular clientele.

The movement toward EBTs in research, clinical practice, and training of psychotherapists must be applauded because it underscores the scientific basis of treatment and the importance of translating findings of research into improved patient care. At the same time, sources of caution about the treatments and questions about the transportability of EBTs and their likely effectiveness in clinical work reflect serious concerns. This chapter discusses issues critical to the development of effective therapies, strengths and limitations of EBTs, and the need to expand the focus beyond identifying EBTs and testing their effects in clinical settings.

10.1 Introduction

Evidence-based treatments refer to interventions that have empirical research on their behalf. The evidence refers to rigorous tests that the treatments, relative to various control or other treatment conditions, produce therapeutic change. In the context of psychotherapy, there have been separate and somewhat independent efforts to identify evidence-based treatments by different professional organizations and committees spanning different countries (e.g., Evidence Based Mental Health 1998; Nathan and Gorman 2002; Roth and Fonagy 1996; Task Force on Promotion and Dissemination of Psychological Procedures 1995). These efforts have used different terms to delineate such treatments, including em-

10.2 Background and Context: An Overview

Several background and contextual factors played critical roles in heightening current interest in EBTs. First, there has been a longstanding concern about the effects of psychotherapy. Eysenck's (1952) provocative review of psychotherapy research galvanized opinions about the issue and firmly placed psychotherapy into the empirical arena. The review concluded that approximately two thirds of patients who received psychotherapy improved and that this proportion was the same for individuals who did not receive treatment, i.e., no treatment control group. The influence of this review was remarkable in stirring controversy and prompting greater attention to the evidence on behalf of psychotherapy (e.g., see Eysenck 1966). Subsequent reviews of the evidence, including reviews of child therapy (Levitt 1957, 1963) kept the conclusion very much alive, namely, therapy is not very effective if effective at all. The reviews were criticized on several grounds, but the criticisms did not mitigate the impact or concern.

Second, challenges to the effects of therapy were followed by a great deal of empirical research (Bergin and Garfield 1971; Garfield and Bergin 1978). Reviewers using different methods of collating studies (e.g., box score, meta-analyses) concluded that therapy was effective and surpassed the effects of no treatment (e.g., Luborsky, Singer, and Luborsky 1975; Smith and Glass 1977; Smith, Glass, and Miller 1980). Currently, there are scores of meta-analyses of psychotherapy. The conclusions are quite similar across treatments for children, adolescents, and adults, namely, various psychotherapies are effective and surpass the effects of no treatment. This seemingly modest conclusion is important historically. Interest in EBTs is a logical step from years of accumulating research on psychotherapy. There are hundreds of forms of psychotherapy for children, adolescents, and adults (Kazdin 2000; Remschmidt 2001). The vast majority have never been studied empirically. Efforts to identify EBT are designed to focus more specifically on the specific treatments that have generated empirical support.

Third, there has been an enduring hiatus between psychotherapy research and clinical practice (e.g., Hayes, Follette, Dawes, and Grady 1995; Stricker and Keisner 1985). Among the lamentable aspects of this hiatus is the fact that treatment research has had little impact on clinical practice, and clinical practice has had little impact on treatment research (Kazdin, Bass, Ayers, and Rodgers 1990). For example, clinical practice does not rely very heavily on EBTs and indeed has been accused of showing a »blatant disregard of the empirical literature« (Ammerman, Last, and Hersen 1999, p. 4) in deciding what treatments to use. Clinical practice continues to spawn new treatments with no evidence attesting to their efficacy and unclear interest in the evidence [e.g., horticulture therapy as applied to childhood psychiatric disorders (Simson and Straus 1998)]. This dissatisfaction with clinical practice reflects on the research as well. Perhaps the research cannot be drawn on because it is not very relevant to clinical practice. Clinicians are alert to these issues and raise cogent questions about whether treatment research is relevant to clinical practice (e.g., Fensterheim and Raw 1996; Persons and Silberschatz 1998).

Fourth, concerns about the spiraling costs of health care provide an important impetus for the emphasis on EBT. Third party payers (e.g., businesses, insurance companies, government) have led to managed care and concerns about the costs of diagnosis, assessment, and treatment. The challenges question whether a procedure (diagnostic test, treatment) ought to be provided at all, let alone reimbursed. In relation to psychotherapy, managed care emerged to raise questions such as: Why this treatment? Why this number of sessions? When will treatment end? Why is more treatment needed? What effects will it have? This new accountability underscores the important of having evidence about what is needed for treatment.

10.2.1   Identifying Effective Treatments

10.2.1.1   Practice Guidelines

The mental health professions have been responsive and equally concerned about what transpires in clinical practice and the rationale or justification for such practices. Efforts have been made to provide guidelines for clinical practice and standards of clinical care. These guidelines, sometimes referred to as practice guidelines or practice parameters, are based on reviews of the evidence and consensus expert opinions about the status of treatment and what are reasonable treatments to use in clinical work. Various organizations (e.g., the American Psychiatric Association and the American Psychological Association) have proposals for identifying effective treatments as well as practice guidelines for such clinical problems as depression, bipolar disorder, and substance abuse in adults. Within the domain of child and adolescent disorders, practice parameters have been advanced by the American Academy of Child and Adolescent Psychiatry (AACAP) beginning in the late 1980s and continuing to the present (www.aacap.org/clinical/parameters). The guidelines focus on a given disorder or clinical problem (e.g., attention-deficit/hyperactivity disorder, sexual abuse) and what current opinion and evidence suggest as the treatment. The process of developing the guidelines can be lengthy in part because guidelines are adopted on a disorder-by-disorder basis and involve multiple experts and committees.

The guidelines have been based on consensus among experts and have been based on clinical experience to a large extent. As research has progressed, evidence has played an increasingly greater role in the guidelines. As an example, the Columbia Guidelines for Child and Adolescent Mental Health examine psychotherapies and medications on a disorder-by-disorder basis (Wasserman, Ko, and Jensen 2001). The goal is to identify treatments with evidence, those treatments in use that are inconsistent in their effects, and where the gaps in knowledge are. ◘ Table 10.1 provides an illustration for unipolar depression and conveys the status of treatment.

Practice guidelines are designed to be instructive for clinicians. They draw on available evidence but often consider clinical realities that are neglected in research. For example, comorbidity of disorders or family problems that are likely to be associated with various clinical disorders may require decisions and combinations of interventions for which no evidence exists. Practice guidelines attempt to address many demands of treatment beyond selecting this or that single intervention.

10.2.1.2   Evidence-Based Treatments

Efforts to identify EBTs tend to differ slightly from those that focus on clinical practice guidelines. The efforts have been less prescriptive about what ought to be used in practice and somewhat more cautious in drawing conclusions about what treatments produce change. Identification of EBTs usually is accomplished by identifying all of the pertinent controlled treatment trials. The search may begin with a diagnostic category or problem domain (e.g., attention-deficit/hyperactivity disorder, anxiety, conduct problems) and then identifies controlled studies of all treatments related to that clinical focus. Reviews sometime begin with the treatment technique and organize the evidence by problem area.

As I mentioned previously, there are many different efforts to identify EBTs. They are consistent in seeking rigorous scientific data but differ slightly in the criteria that are used to define EBTs. Typically, the criteria include several characteristics (▶ see ◘ Table 10.2). Using these criteria and its variants, several books and articles have identified EBTs for children and adolescents (e.g., Christophersen and Mortweet 2001; Fonagy et al. 2002; Kazdin and Weisz 2003; Lonigan and Elbert 1998).

Many EBTs have been identified; ◘ Table 10.3 lists many to illustrate what can be culled from the various reviews available. A few points are conspicuous from the table. First, there are EBTs for children. Clearly, a child referred for anxiety, for example, ought to receive one of the EBTs as a treatment of choice. Second,

◘ **Table 10.1.** Illustration of Columbia Practice Guidelines: Unipolar depression

Diagnosis	Positive effects, consistent evidence	Positive/ mixed effects, inconsistent evidence
Unipolar depression	Psychosocial Interpersonal psychotherapy for adolescents	Psychosocial Supportive therapy
	Cognitive behavioral therapy	Systemic family therapy
	Cognitive therapy	
	Self-control therapy	
	Coping with depression	
	Medication	Medication (none listed)
	SSRIs (e.g., Fluoxetine [Prozac])	

◘ **Table 10.2.** Criteria to decide whether treatment is evidence based

At least two studies with:
Random assignment of subjects to conditions
Careful specification of the patient population
Use of treatment manuals
Multiple outcome measures (raters, if used, are naïve to conditions)
Statistically significant difference of treatment and comparison group
Replication of outcome effects, especially by an independent investigator or team

the list of EBTs is not that long. The goal of therapy research is not necessarily to identify long lists of effective treatments but rather to develop and identify clear alternatives for a given problem. Third, the list is dominated by cognitive-behavioral treatments. This is no coincidence. Many more studies of child psychotherapy focus on interventions that would fall under this rubric than under more traditional (e.g., talk, play) therapies. Also, to be counted as evidence based, studies must include several methodological features (e.g., use of treatment manuals, random assignment). These characteristics are much more likely among contemporary than past studies. Cog-

▣ **Table 10.3.** Treatments for children and adolescents that are evidence-based for key problem domains

Problem domain	Treatment
Anxiety, fear, phobias	Cognitive behavior therapy Modeling Reinforced practice Systematic desensitization
Depression	Cognitive-behavior therapy Coping with depression course Interpersonal psychotherapy for adolescents
Oppositional and conduct disorder	Anger coping therapy Multisystemic therapy Parent management training Problem-solving skills training
Attention-deficit/hyperactivity	Classroom contingency management Parent management training Psychostimulant medication

Note: The techniques noted here draw from different methods of defining and evaluating evidence-based treatments. The techniques are those that would meet criteria for well-established or probably efficacious (Lonigan and Elbert 1998) or those with randomized controlled trials in their behalf (Nathan and Gorman 2002). Evaluation of treatments and identification of those that meet criteria for empirical support are ongoing and hence the above is an illustrative rather than fixed or exhaustive list. Psychostimulant medication is mentioned because this is the standard treatment for attention-deficit/hyperactivity disorder

nitive-behavioral therapies are more popular in contemporary work and are more likely to use the methodology required for establishing treatment.

Fourth, evidence based does not necessarily mean effective or most effective. For example, for the treatment of attention-deficit/hyperactivity disorder, medication, and parent training are listed (in ▣ Table 10.3) as evidence based. Parent training is not usually viewed as an effective treatment by itself in addressing the core symptoms. Medication is viewed as much better in this regard. Even so, the treatments, alone or combined, do not achieve strong and enduring therapeutic changes. The criteria for establishing treatment as evidence based are those noted in the prior table (▣ Table 10.2) and may not necessarily reflect what is implied, i.e., that x or y is an effective treatment for a particular clinical problem. I shall return to this point shortly. Overall, there clearly has been palpable progress in identifying EBTs.

10.2.2   Challenges to the Research on Evidence-Based Treatments

There are several issues, obstacles, and challenges related to the generality of the findings to clinical

work, the criteria for qualifying as evidence-based, and the obstacles of integrating findings into clinical work.

10.2.2.1   The Generalizability or Transportability of Results from Research to Clinic Settings

The most fundamental and frequently voiced issue is that evidence obtained in well controlled studies may not apply (generalize) to the conditions of clinical settings. In contemporary writings, this concern has been reflected in the distinction of efficacy and effectiveness research (Hoagwood, Hibbs, Brent, and Jensen 1995)[1]. Efficacy research refers to treat-

---

[1] The concern about whether research in controlled settings can be generalized to clinical practice has been an ongoing concern in psychotherapy research. In previous years (e.g., 1960s through the present) other terms used to reflect the concern were analogue versus clinical research and laboratory versus clinical or applied research (see Kazdin 2003). Thus, the issues and concerns about efficacy and effectiveness are not new at all. What is new in contemporary work is an urgency to test treatments in clinical settings to move beyond mere repetition of the concerns in an armchair fashion.

■ Table 10.4. Select dimensions that vary among studies and the degree of resemblance to the clinical situation

Dimension	Identity with or great resemblance	Moderate resemblance	Relatively low resemblance
Target problem	Problem seen in the clinic, intense or disabling	Similar to that in clinic but less severe	Nonproblem behavior or experimental task
Population	Clients in outpatient treatment	College students with nontreatment interest	Infrahuman subjects
Manner of recruitment	Clients who seek treatment	Individuals recruited for available treatment	Captive subjects who serve for course credit
Therapists	Professional therapists	Therapists in training	Nontherapists or non-professionals
Client set	Expect treatment and improvement	Expect »experimental« treatment with unclear effects	Expect experiment with nontreatment focus
Selection of treatment	Client chooses therapist and specific treatment	Client given choice over few alternative procedures in an experiment	Client assigned to treatment with no choice for specific therapist or condition
Specification of treatment	What to do is at the discretion of the therapist	General guidelines, goals, and themes to direct focus of the session	Treatment manual specifies procedures, foci, means, or ends treatment session, including, maybe, even many of the statements of the therapist
Monitoring of treatment	Little or no monitoring of what is done with the client	Case supervision or discussion to review what was done, how it was done, and client progress	Careful assessment of how treatment was delivered (audio, videotape; direct observation, case supervision)
Setting of treatment	Professional treatment facility	University facility that may not regularly offer treatment	Laboratory setting
Variation of treatment	Treatment as usually conducted	Variation to standardize treatment for research	Analogue of the treatment as in infrahuman equivalent of treatment
Assessment methods	Direct unobtrusive measure of the problem that the client originally reported	Assessment on psychological devices that sample behaviors of interest directly	Questionnaire responses about the behaviors that are a problem

ment outcomes obtained in controlled psychotherapy studies that are conducted under laboratory and quasi-laboratory conditions (e.g., subjects are recruited, they may show a narrow range of problems, treatment is specified in manual form, and treatment delivery is closely supervised and monitored). Effectiveness research refers to treatment outcomes obtained in clinic settings where the usual control procedures are not implemented (e.g., patients seek treatment, many present multiple clinical problems).

Efficacy and effectiveness studies can be conceived as a continuum or multiple continua because several dimensions can vary across clinic and laboratory settings that affect generality of the results (Kazdin 2003; Schoenwald and Hoagwood 2001).

■ Table 10.4 conveys many of these dimensions and points on the continuum that vary from a clinical setting (effectiveness type of research) versus laboratory setting (efficacy). A given psychotherapy study can vary along the different dimensions. The closer one moves toward the right side of the table where conditions of the experiment do not resemble very well clinical or applied settings, the greater the ability of the investigator to control facets of the investigation and hence rule out many potential sources of confound, artifact, and bias. Studies characterized by features toward the right of the table are more likely to be labeled as efficacy studies. The closer one moves toward the left side of the table where conditions resemble applied settings, the greater the applicability of the findings, but also the more difficulty in controlling many facets of the study. Studies characterized by features toward the left of the table are more likely to be labeled as effectiveness studies.

The extent to which a study has generalizable results that apply to the clinical setting cannot be decided by merely looking whether the study departs from the left side of the table on various dimensions. Many of the dimensions listed may not influence generality of the findings, even though the study departs from the conditions of applied settings. However, there is the haunting possibility that conclusions obtained from treatment research do not apply to and have no bearing on clinical practice. The calls for more research of treatment outcome in clinical settings emanates from this concern.

10.2.2.2 Demonstrating Treatment Efficacy

The efficacy/effectiveness issue is a challenge to the body of research, namely, can the findings from any/all of the controlled studies be generalized to clinical practice. There is a much more central issue from my perspective that pertains to what counts as evidence at the level of the individual study. More specifically, the criteria for demonstrating treatment efficacy and concluding treatment is »evidence based« are not sufficiently stringent.

At the level of individual studies, the requirement includes demonstrating that treatment is better than no treatment or treatment as usual. The basic criterion is that the treatment, when compared to no treatment, reflects a statistically significant difference. This is not a very difficult obstacle to surmount. Research in adult therapy has shown that any active treatment is better (statistically) than

no treatment. Expectations, attention, and the common factors associated with coming to therapy alone can produce such a difference. Indeed, active »fake« treatments in which the patient engages in some activities not considered on a priori grounds to have therapeutic value can generate such a difference and surpass the effects of no treatment (Grissom 1996). If each of us took the trouble to test our favorite treatment vs. no treatment, the results would likely yield statistically significant differences, with reasonable but perhaps not even excessive statistical power.

Statistical significance alone is an odd or limited criterion to establish whether a treatment ought to be anointed as evidence based. The results of a clinical trial might be evaluated in terms of statistical significance, measures of the magnitude of effect (e.g., effect size), and clinical significance. Statistical significance may have no bearing on the practical impact of treatment on the patient. For example, a statistically significant difference favoring one treatment over another on some measure of anxiety may not reflect genuine differences or improvements on patient anxiety or functioning in everyday life. Similarly, indices of magnitude of effect (e.g., d, r, β) are excellent supplements to statistical significance. Yet, strength of an effect from a statistical standpoint (e.g., in standard deviation units) may have no bearing on the impact of treatment on patients (see Kazdin 2003). Indeed, effect size can be quite large in cases where impact on the patient is nugatory.

Clinical significance, a weighty topic in its own right, refers to a set of measures designed to evaluate whether impact of treatment translates to meaningful changes in the patient (Kendall 1999; Kazdin 2003). For example, a commonly used measure is whether the patient has shown a large enough change so that the level of symptoms or functioning falls within the normative range of individuals not referred for treatment. Such a change is regarded as clinically significant, i.e., important in relation to what was accomplished by the treatment. Measures of clinical significance are not standard criteria for evaluating or establishing EBTs. A treatment that produces a statistically significant difference in relation to a no-treatment control condition or another treatment may qualify as evidence based but not really help patients very much or in ways that make a difference. This is a rather stark qualifier to the evidence and the criteria used to establish EBTs.

It is still the case that EBTs have priority over non-EBTs. These latter treatments may not effect any change or yield harmful effects, as I mention later. However, we also want to reconsider or expand the criteria for evidence based so we have some assurance about the impact of the treatment on individual patients. As researchers we want to be able to say that a given treatment produces change and that the change makes a difference.

In some cases, the outcomes of treatment make clear that the treatment is not only evidence based but also has strong impact on patients. For example, for the treatment of adults with panic attacks, the treatment may eliminate panic for many individuals. The qualitative difference in patient functioning from several to no panic attacks provides a fairly clear verdict on impact. In other areas, statistically significant differences may reflect change (e.g., reductions in aggression or hyperactivity), and we must contend with deciding whether the statistical difference translates in palpable benefits for patients.

10.2.3   Obstacles to Integration of Research Findings into Clinical Work

Assume for a moment that the research issues were resolved, namely, that findings from controlled studies generalize to clinical practice and that statistically significant differences between two treatments or between treatment and control conditions actually make a difference in the lives of patients. There are obstacles to adoption and integration of EBTs. Let me mention two.

10.2.3.1   Disparate Views Among Interested Parties

Different parties or stakeholders in treatment are likely to have quite different views about EBTs, their value and utility. These views may have significant impact on whether, to what extent, or at what speed EBTs are integrated into clinical practice. First, researchers are likely to favor greatly EBTs and their integration into clinical work. Indeed, researchers may well view EBTs as the high moral ground and wonder who could be against use of such treatments or delay their integration.

Second, clinicians are less likely to favor EBTs. The research identifying EBTs is completed in highly controlled settings where the people (patients and therapists) are select and depart from the conditions of clinical practice. Patients recruited in re-

search are less likely to reflect the complexity of conditions (e.g., comorbidity) than the patients seen in practice. Therapists in research, while less experienced (e.g., often graduate students), are highly trained and supervised to carry out the procedures, have small case loads, and do not depend on providing treatment for their income – a very different situation from what transpires in clinical practice. Also, clinicians are less likely to know or to be trained in EBTs because of the cohort in which they were trained. Thus, they are not keen to have imposed on them treatments they have not learned.

Trainees and training directors (of child psychiatry residents, psychology interns, and social work fellows) probably are in favor of EBTs. However, they would be greatly limited in their adoption of such by the resources of the training program. How would one train fellows in these different programs? The supervisors of treatment are often the clinicians (e.g., clinical and volunteer faculty) who have the views and training experiences mentioned previously. One cannot easily integrate new treatments into training programs without pertinent faculty committed to and trained in these treatments.

Agencies responsible for reimbursing treatment (health maintenance organizations, insurance programs, government agencies) are likely to vary in their views of EBT. If an EBT for a given problem can save costs, the agencies are likely to favor the treatment. For example, an outpatient therapy or medication that averted psychiatric hospitalization would be greatly supported. Yet, an EBT might well increase costs, for example, by showing that a condition not previously covered can be treated effectively or that a longer treatment is effective whereas a shorter one is not.

Finally, the public at large probably is neutral, not interested, or too diffuse to have a strong position on EBTs. This is unfortunate because the public may have the greatest potential to exert influence on the quality and type of care. The limitations of the public as a lobbying group begin with the fact that the public does not have a uniform agenda. Indeed, people in everyday life are not likely to be interested in mental health unless directly affected by someone in their own lives. Those who are interested may participate, belong to, or indeed organize a foundation or lobbying group related to the specific disorder or condition with which they have had contact.

The difficulty in mobilizing the public is likely to emerge for other reasons. Adults who have received psychotherapy are generally satisfied with their treatment, independently of the specific treatment they received (Consumers Union 1995). Separate lines of research have shown that satisfaction with treatment is not very related to therapeutic change (e.g., Ankuta and Abeles 1993; Lambert, Salzer, and Bickman 1998; Pekarik and Wolff 1996). Thus, the public with any experience in psychotherapy is likely to be satisfied and unlikely to scream out for more effective, well-established, or EBTs. They are not getting EBTs now and are quite satisfied. This leaves relatively silent an influence that could have some impact on clinical care.

I have referred to different roles of stakeholders in treatment and views likely to be associated with them. I have simplified the views for purposes of presentation. Individuals have different and multiple roles (e.g., a person is a researcher and public citizen) and this increases the variability and complexity. The purpose was merely to convey the point that support for EBTs and their extension to clinical practice is mixed at best. There are challenges to conduct the requisite studies that establish treatment as evidence based. However, these are relatively clear and familiar to those who conduct randomized controlled clinical trials. Much less clear is how to mobilize interest and support for the use of EBTs and their integration in patient care once such treatments are identified. Many seem to be of the view that once EBTs are shown to work in clinical settings, this will create the groundswell of interest and perhaps pressure to integrate such treatments routinely. That would be wonderful but remains to be seen.

10.2.3.2   Training of Therapists

I have mentioned training but a brief additional comment is warranted. An obstacle to extending EBTs to clinical practice is training. Most programs do not have the faculty and staff trained in EBTs to serve as models for trainees. At least for the short-term, clinicians are being trained in ways that may well support business as usual.

There are few resources for trainees in psychiatry, psychology, and social work. Consider one example in the context of child therapy. Parent management training is an intervention that is probably the most well-studied intervention for oppositional defiant and conduct disorder (Kazdin 2004). There are scores of trials spanning decades. It is very unlikely that trainees in most child psychiatry, psychology, and social work programs are exposed to this treatment. At best, the treatment may be mentioned, but there are probably few opportunities for

training. Moving EBTs from the lab to the training programs and to those who eventually will provide clinical services has its own challenges.

A key issue is how to place EBTs at the disposal of those involved in training mental health professionals. Perhaps special training curricula could take advantage of the latest technologies (e.g., Web-based training materials). Otherwise one might expect a great delay between demonstrating that a treatment is suited for clinical work and getting this treatment to individuals in training. Hiring young new faculty (trained in EBTs) for a department is not necessarily a solution if much of supervision and training is in the hands of those who are much further along in their career and trained in less well-studied treatments. I offer no solutions here but merely note that delivery of EBTs to the public raises issues related to training of mental health professionals.

10.3   Categorization of Treatment

10.3.1   Refining the Classification of Treatments

There are many forms of psychotherapy. In child and adolescent therapy alone, leaving aside the much larger area of adult therapy, 550+ psychotherapies are in use (Kazdin 2000). This count is conservative because it omits various combinations of treatments and eclectic hybrids and only draws on interventions that are documented within the English language. Even so, consider the number as a reasonable approximation. EBTs reflect only a small fraction of these treatments.

I believe research and clinical work would be served much better by developing a system that encompasses all treatments and their status in relation to their research base. In particular, treatments that are not evidence based ought to be distinguished. Some treatments are not evidence based but have yet to be studied. We ought to leave open the question of their merit and value. Other treatments have been investigated but shown not to produce change or not produce change very reliably. Still others have been investigated and shown to be harmful. Finally, some treatments fall short of the threshold of evidence based (e.g., too few studies, nonrandomized trials) but still ought to be used in practice.

Consider some examples. Several years ago, hyperactivity (ADHD) was considered to be related to diet and nutrition, including various food additives, excessive sugar (e.g., in breakfast cereal), and chemicals in certain foods (e.g., salicylates found in tomatoes, apples, and other fruits). Evidence from individual studies and literature reviews and panels drawing on the weight of the evidence (e.g., American Medical Association, National Institutes of Health) suggested that there was no strong evidence linking these various ingredients to hyperactivity and that interventions relying on diet or nutrition were not supported (e.g., Kavale and Forness 1993; McGee, Stanton, and Sears 1993; www.kidsource.com). In short, the weight of the evidence indicated that dietary manipulations were not effective. Here is a case where there is considerable evidence that treatment is not effective. Codifying EBTs leaves out cases where we would want to know that some treatments have been tested and ought not to be used except under unusual circumstances.

Some treatments can be harmful (see Dishion, McCord, and Poulin 1999). For example, several years ago, delinquent youths were exposed to adult prisoners who described prison life and conveyed their own untoward life experiences. The purpose was to identify youths early in their delinquent careers and to show them the consequences of criminal behavior. The treatment was designed to intimidate and to scare youths away from criminal activity. Variations of these programs (e.g., referred to as »scared straight« or »stay straight«) have shown deleterious effects. Youths exposed to these programs increased in subsequent rates of arrest in comparison to control youths (e.g., Buckner and Chesney-Lind 1983; Finckenauer 1982). Similarly, therapies in which groups of youths with antisocial behavior are brought together have shown deleterious effects, i.e., increases in deviance and delinquent behavior (e.g., Feldman, Caplinger, and Wodarski 1983; O'Donnell 1992). The interpretation of these deleterious effects is that the various interventions brought delinquent youths together and the peer bonding and friendships among youths in the treatment groups maintained or increased criminal behavior. Bonding with and connections to deviant peers can increase delinquent behavior. Efforts to alter the group structure to facilitate bonding of non-deviant peers appears to mitigate the deleterious effect (Feldman et al. 1983).

Group therapy for antisocial youths is often practiced in hospital settings. Also, in the elementary schools such youth are often grouped together in special classes. Group treatment where individuals with oppositional, aggressive, or antisocial are brought together would seem inadvisable. In any case, group interventions for antisocial youth are not empirically supported. Yet, we might want to say more, namely, that evidence supports deleterious effects for some of these, and one ought to be cautious in using them at all without much further evidence.

Some treatments may not meet rigorous evidential standards for empirically supported treatments but still be the best available or at least worth trying. An example is the behavioral treatment for young autistic children which has on its behalf controlled outcome research (nonrandomized study) with long-term follow-up and clinical application with reports of success (Lovaas 1987; McEachin, Smith, and Lovaas 1993; Sheinkopf and Siegel 1998). The evidence is not sufficient for making this a well-established treatment. Even so, reviewers have concluded this intervention is probably the best treatment available (e.g., Rogers 1998; Smith 1999). We are awaiting an effective intervention, but the absence of one that is firmly established does not place all other treatment options on an equal plane.

I have highlighted treatments that would not be considered evidence based but still worthy of delineating in a more fine-grained way. EBTs also might warrant finer grained analyses. Obviously, not all well-established treatments are necessarily equally effective. We do not merely want well-established treatments, but want to know the best available treatment among empirically established options. Similarly, for a given treatment, a particular dose (e.g., 10 vs. 20 sessions) or version (e.g., parents involved in treatment vs. not involved) may be more effective, even though both are effective and empirically supported.

Rather than evidence based or not evidence based, it might be useful to place all treatments on a continuum that reflects the extent to which they have been evaluated and shown to produce therapeutic change. ◻ Table 10.5 presents a continuum for evaluating and classifying treatments and addresses the special situations I have highlighted (e.g., well-investigated treatments that do not work and hence ought not to be practiced). Also, the status of a given treatment can be better represented by seeing where it would fall on the continuum and in relation to other treatments. Finally, research might progress better if we demanded of ourselves that the next study of a treatment make an advance in relation to the continuum. That is, if we know that treatment is promising, the next studies of that intervention ought to move the knowledge base further along the continuum. A continuum like the one

❏ **Table 10.5.** Ways of categorizing treatments beyond evidence vs. nonevidence based

The system here reflects a continuum to evaluate status and research progress. Each treatment would be evaluated (or classified) in the scale below to identify what can be said in light of the evidence:
1. Not-evaluated
2. Evaluated but unclear effects, no effects, or possibly negative effects at this time
3. Promising (e.g., some evidence in its behalf)
4. Well established (e.g., criteria used by one of the systems cited for identifying evidence-based treatment)
5. Better/best treatments (e.g., studies shown to be more effective than one or more other well-established techniques).

above helps to set a template by which studies and progress can be examined. We can evaluate studies in light of where they fit on the continuum, whether another study is needed in light of the literature for that treatment, and, if so, what question(s) that study might address.

10.3.2   Weak Treatments Can be Wonderful

The classification of treatments as evidence based glosses over another situation we may want to know about. As odd as it may seem at first blush, there is an important role and place for treatments that are relatively ineffective or weak in their effects. By weak, I mean interventions that may influence only a small proportion of individuals to which they are applied and/or might reduce but not eliminate the problem for those individuals or on a large scale (the larger group). Many interventions might be relatively weak but also require minimal effort or cost and the benefits, relative to these costs, would be worthwhile.

One program for cigarette smoking provides an example of what might be a weak treatment. In the USA and more recently worldwide there is an annual »smoke-out day« (www.quit-smoking.net/great-americansmokeout.html; www.cdc.gov/tobacco/research_data) in which organizations at local and national levels delineate a day for people to stop smoking for the day. The delineation of the day publicly through the media is merely to make salient the need for people to stop smoking. Allegedly, more

people give up smoking on that day (for one day or permanently) than on any other day. It is not likely that the intervention is very effective in terms of the proportion of smokers »cured«. On the other hand, this is a relatively low cost intervention (e.g., advertising messages) that reaches millions of people world wide. The percentage of smokers who quit permanently could be very small but still reflect a large number of people given that there are many people (e.g., estimated 47 million in the USA) who smoke cigarettes. This is a very low cost intervention, relative to some individual or group therapy.

As another example, many years ago, the spouse of one of the Presidents in the United States advocated that teenagers »just say no« to drugs and other substances when their peers or others with influence were to induce them to use and perhaps abuse. Of course, an intervention such as this ignores completely the factors related to onset of use and abuse of alcohol drugs as well as evidence about effective treatment and prevention programs (Pagliaro and Pagliaro 1996). At the same time, this is a low cost intervention that actually may help a fraction of youths who wish some slight prompt and bolstering to not begin drugs. Moreover, such a grass roots type of intervention has spawned all sorts of supportive efforts in schools and local communities of many different nations that could have a positive impact. As an intervention one cannot be sure whether this has been tested in randomized controlled trials against appropriate controls to qualify as evidence based or indeed whether there is an effect. Even so, the class of interventions like this that might be weak, easy to implement, and checkered in effects could still have huge impact when applied on a large scale.

EBTs as currently and narrowly defined ignore a pivotal question for public mental health. The issue is not merely what works (EBTs) but what works relative to their costs, scale of applicability, and relative to the scope of the problem. An intervention that can be implemented on a large scale and shown to have some impact might be quite worthwhile.

There are therapies completed by self-help manuals, telephone, mail, Internet and computer, and video tapes. Not all the applications are effective using these media but many of them are. For example, self-help manuals is a genre of do-it-yourself books that make extravagant claims, usually with the complete absence of evidence. However, many self-help manuals have been studied and are effective (e.g., Marrs 1995). Similarly, many examples are available in controlled studies showing use of other media can be quite effective for clinical disorders (e.g., anxiety, depression) as well as stress that emerges in everyday life (e.g., divorce, death of a loved one). Under some circumstances, writing about one's problems in special ways can effect therapeutic change (e.g., Smyth 1998). The use of the mail (e.g., providing feedback, and information) can reduce alcohol consumption among individuals with significant problems with alcohol (Sobell, Sobell, and Agrawal 2002). I am not advocating any particular form of treatment or medium through which services are provided, but rather conveying the importance of cost and disseminability of treatment as a dimension that may complement the criteria used to identify EBTs.

The notion of stepped care has been introduced into psychotherapy to suggest that minimal treatments be used first before one moves to more intensive, time consuming, and costly treatments (Haaga 2000). In relation to EBT, minimal treatments ought to have evidence that they can effect change. Appeals through the mail or self-help manuals under many circumstances are effective. Even if they are effective for a small number of individuals, their ease of dissemination and relatively low cost may make them worthwhile. The focus on EBTs alone, as currently conceived, may miss critical facets of such treatments. That is, mailing letters to individuals to reduce their alcohol consumption may be very weak when compared to intensive individual therapy. Yet use of the mail in this way can effect change. The low cost in relation to the benefit and the ease of dissemination of treatment by mail has enormous utility, even if the changes are not as great as another more intensive treatment. We need a portfolio of interventions that vary in effectiveness, cost, and ease of dissemination.

10.4 The Psychotherapy Research Agenda: More Attention to Mechanisms of Change

The interest in EBT has narrowed the focus of therapy research to address primarily two questions: Is a treatment »efficacious« (effective in controlled settings)? and Can the treatment be transported to clinical settings? We would like to have a broad set of questions answered about therapy. ◻ Table 10.6 lists key questions to reflect what we would like to know about a given psychotherapy

Among the highest priorities is understanding why treatment works, i.e., the mechanisms of change (i.e., question 7, highlighted in the table).

◻ **Table 10.6.** Key questions to guide psychotherapy research

1. What is the impact of treatment relative to no treatment?
2. What components contribute to change?
3. What treatments can be added (combined treatments) to optimize change?
4. What parameters can be varied to influence (improve) outcome?
5. How effective is this treatment relative to other treatments for this problem?
6. What patient, therapist, treatment, and contextual factors influence (moderate) outcome?
7. What processes within or during treatment influence, cause, and are responsible for outcome?
8. To what extent are treatment effects generalizable across problem areas, settings, and other domains?

Note: The highlighted question focuses on mechanisms of change and is identified in the discussion as an especially high priority for research

The study of mechanisms of treatment is probably the best short-term and long-term investment for improving clinical practice and patient care. The role of understanding (theory) and application (real world tests) are complementary and essential. Real world tests are absolutely vital and great progress can be made from such tests. For example, the first airplanes that only flew seconds and minutes were cleverly devised with minimal understanding of the aerodynamics of flight (e.g., fluid flow, skin-friction drag, and aspect-wing ratios and the physics and mathematics that govern the design of current airplanes). On television, we have seen many early attempts of flight often replayed as comically tragic film clips of humans sporting feigned wings and jumping off cliffs and rocks. These film clips show a worst case of what empirical tests can yield where there is minimal to no understanding. Needless to say, applications (i.e., commercial flight) have been enhanced enormously by advances in understanding the underpinnings of flight well outside of real-world application. Parallel gains could readily result from identifying the mechanisms of action or underpinnings of therapy.

It is worthwhile distinguishing cause and mechanisms in relation to therapeutic change. By cause, I mean what led to change – a demonstration that some intervention led to some outcome. By mechanisms, I refer to those processes or events that account for the change.[2] A randomized controlled clinical trial (e.g., comparing treatment vs. no treatment) can establish a causal relation between an intervention and therapeutic change. However, demonstrating a causal relation does not necessarily explain why the relation was obtained. Thus, we may know that the intervention caused the change but not understand why (the basis for the cause or the mechanism) the intervention led to change.

As an example, consider cognitive therapy (CT) as applied to depression among adults. By all counts, this treatment is evidence-based and then some in light of the range of trials, replications, and comparisons (Hollon and Beck 2004). Why does CT work, i.e., through what mechanisms? In fact, little can be stated as to why treatment works. The conceptual model has emphasized changes in various cognitions as the basis for action in treatment. However, it is not obvious, clear, or established that changes in cognitions are the basis for therapeutic change (Burns and Spangler 2001; Ilardi and Craighead 1994; Whisman 1993, 1999). Indeed, suitable studies are rarely done. Designs are needed in which processes and symptom changes are evaluated at multiple points over the course of treatment (see Kazdin, in press). Some studies have demonstrated that changes in cognitions during treatment predict symptom change (e.g., DeRubeis et al. 1990; Kwon and Oei 2003). Yet, it has not been clear in such studies whether symptom change preceded rather than followed changes in cognition. In general, there is a firm basis for stating that CT can change depression but little empirical basis for stating why.

Evaluating mechanisms of therapeutic change is important for several reasons. First, there is an embarrassing wealth of treatments in use. I mentioned previously the 550+ therapies in use for children and adolescents. Presumably some of these produce changes; it is not likely that all of the different treatments produce change for different reasons. Understanding the mechanisms of change can bring order and parsimony to the current status of multiple interventions.

Second, therapy can have quite broad outcome effects, beyond the familiar benefits of reducing social, emotional, and behavioral problems (e.g., suicidal ideation, depression, and panic attacks). In addition, therapy reduces physical ailments (e.g., pain, blood pressure), improves recovery from surgery or illness, and increases the quality of life (see Kazdin 2000). How do these effects come about? Understanding how therapy produces change in such a diverse array of outcomes would be important. Some effects may be direct (i.e., altered directly through the process of change in therapy) and others may be concomitant effects that result from improvements in symptoms or impairment. Revealing the mechanisms of therapy will clarify the connections between what is done (treatment) and what happens (outcomes).

Third, an obvious goal of treatment is to optimize therapeutic change. By understanding the processes that account for therapeutic change one ought to be better able to foster and maximize patient improvements. Consider the development and use of treatment manuals to convey the point. Treatment manuals consist of descriptions of procedures used in therapy. The manuals codify what is done, by whom, and when. Manuals vary from explicit statements and transcripts of the therapist's presentations on a session-by-session basis to broad principles that guide the clinician in how to make decisions about what to do in treatment. The advance that treatment manuals represent is not at all in question here. However, without knowing how therapy works and what the necessary, sufficient, and facilitative ingredients are and within what »dose« range, it is difficult to develop optimally effective treatment. Most treatment manuals probably include the following components:

1. Low doses of effective practices (i.e., factors that genuinely make a difference);
2. Ancillary but important facets that make delivery more palatable (e.g., the spoonful of sugar that makes the medicine go down);
3. Superstitious behavior on the part of those of us who develop manuals (e.g., factors that we believe make a difference or that we like); and
4. Factors that impede or merely fail to optimize therapeutic change.

The difficulty is that without understanding how treatment works, which element in a manual falls into which of these categories is a matter of surmise. If we wish to optimize therapeutic change, understanding the critical ingredients and processes through which they operate are essential.

---

[2] Mediator is often used as the term intended to signify a cause or mechanism of change and distinguished from moderator, as evident in the now classic paper by Baron and Kenny (1986). For this discussion, I will retain mechanism as the term. Mediator analyses raises multiple issues and may identify factors that do not explain why treatment works, a topic beyond the scope of this chapter (see Kraemer, Stice, Kazdin, Offord, and Kupfer 2001; Kraemer et al. 2002).

Fourth, understanding how therapy works can help identify moderators of treatment, i.e., variables on which the effectiveness of a given treatment may depend. There are an unlimited number of moderators that can plausibly influence outcome. Understanding the processes through which treatment operates can help sort through those facets that might be particularly influential in treatment outcome. For example, if changes in cognitive processes account for therapeutic change, this finding might draw attention to characteristics of these processes or their underpinnings at pretreatment. Pretreatment status of cognitive processes (abstract reasoning, problem-solving, attributions), stages of cognitive development, and neurological or neuropsychological characteristics on which these cognitions might depend are just some of the moderators that might be especially worth studying, depending on the specific processes shown to mediate treatment effects. Other promising moderators that influence treatment might be proposed on theoretical grounds once the mechanisms of therapy are known.

Fifth, understanding the mechanisms through which change takes place is important beyond the context of psychotherapy because of its broader relation to social and behavioral science. There are many therapeutic processes in everyday life. By therapeutic, I refer to interventions or experiences that improve adjustment and adaptive functioning, ameliorate problems of mental and physical health, help people manage and cope with stress and crises, and more generally navigate the shoals of life. As examples, participating in religion, chatting with friends, exercising, undergoing hypnosis, and writing about sources of stress all have evidence on their behalf. Therapy research is not merely about techniques but rather about the broader question, namely, how does one intervene to change affect, cognition, and behavior. Mechanisms that elaborate how therapy works might have generality for understanding human functioning more generally. The other side is also true. Mechanisms that explain how other change methods work might well inform therapy. Basic psychological processes (e.g., learning, memory, perception, persuasion, social interaction) and their biological pathways (e.g., changes in neurotransmitters, responsiveness of receptors to transmitters) may be common to many types of interventions, including psychotherapy.

A priority of contemporary treatment research is to extend treatment to clinic settings [e.g., National Advisory Mental Health Council (NAMHC) 1999; NAMHC Workgroup on Child and Adolescent Mental Health Intervention Development and Deployment (NAMHC-W) 2001]. Diverse terms have been introduced to describe these extensions, including translational research, transportability, and tests of effectiveness (in contrast to efficacy), to mention a few. The terms refer to a common question, namely, will treatments work in »real world« settings? Obviously, we wish to extend findings from research to practice. Less obvious is that doing so without understanding how treatment works is quite problematic.

Extension and evaluation of treatment in clinic settings has all sorts of challenges related to execution of the study. Many of these challenges will be reflected in increased variability (»error«) and reduce the ability to demonstrate therapeutic change, even if the treatment is effective (Kazdin 2003). We enter the clinical arena with one hand tied beyond our back if we apply an unspecified and possibly low dose of some treatment that we do not understand. To optimize the generality of treatment effects from research to practice we would like to know the critical ingredients. Specifically, we want to know what is needed to make treatment work, what are the optimal conditions, and what we ought to worry about or not as some components get diluted when treatment is moved from the lab to clinical practice.

10.5   Conclusions

I have raised issues and concerns about EBTs, what they mean, and how treatments are established as evidence based. Let me end by underscoring a few key points. There are now several EBTs. This is a decided advance in research in part because in the not-too-distant past, it was not clear that treatments had any solid evidence in their behalf.

Second, the criteria for establishing treatment as evidence based are probably too lenient. It is useful to have criteria, but merely showing a statistically significant difference in group comparisons of treatment versus some other condition is not very demanding. In clinical work, we care about patient change. Measures of the impact of treatment on day-to-day functioning, either by assessing domains that are relevant (e.g., measures of impairment or adaptive functioning, presence of symptoms that affect functioning in everyday life) or the magnitude of change (clinically significant change) need to be incorporated into the criteria. Given the current criteria in use, it is possible in principle and practice to have treatment that qualifies as an EBT but does not help patients in a way that makes a difference in their lives.

Third, a high priority for professional organizations and funding agencies is extending treatment from controlled settings to clinical services. This is obviously worthwhile but has enormous challenges for training of therapists, supervising ongoing treatment, and demonstrating effects. The diversity of therapists, therapist skills, and patient characteristics and the integrity of treatment and the intratherapist and intertherapist consistency can serve to increase variability in the study of treatment in clinical settings and make demonstration of an effect much more difficult. This is one reason why it is so important to understand what is critical to the intervention.

Fourth and related to the prior point, research attention is needed on why treatment works. Understanding how treatment works is the best investment in extending treatment to clinics. The reasons why a given treatment works is often discussed. However, there are few tests of mechanisms, and controlled trials are routinely designed in a way that will not permit demonstration of the mechanisms of therapeutic change (see Kazdin, in press; Kazdin and Nock 2003).

Fifth, an important focus will be to move EBTs into training programs for residents, fellows, and graduate students in the mental health professions. As I have noted previously, this is not easy to do. Those involved in supervision of trainees are usually from a generation in which EBTs were not trained. Supervisors would need to learn EBTs—not a minor challenge.

I have expressed misgivings about the movement, research, and findings about EBTs. That said, there is a message that ought to be stated clearly. For any clinician in practice, it would be difficult to justify using a non-EBT as the first line of attack if there is an available EBT. If the EBT treatment fails, switching to another treatment ought to be noncontroversial. Clearly an EBT treatment is the place to begin. It is one thing to say the strong evidence from controlled trials may not apply to clinical settings. That really does require empirical attention. However, it is quite a leap to use this as a justification for applying an intervention invented by the therapist (some eclectic treatment) or some treatment as usual that does not have evidence on its behalf.

EBTs, whether medical or psychological, are not likely to work for everyone. Perhaps even more important than use of EBT is the integration of assessment and evaluation in clinical practice. Many interventions might work or fail with a given patient. Systematic and user-friendly assessment could greatly inform decisions for individual patients, and the information could be accumulated to contribute to the knowledge base. EBTs raise concerns about extending treatments to clinical practice. In addition, some of the methods of research could be extended as well to enhance clinical care. More systematic assessment in practice is one of these (e.g., Clement 1999; Kazdin 1993). Use of materials to aid therapists so they deliver treatment consistently (e.g., abbreviated manuals) and supervision/feedback opportunities may be critical to the effects of treatment. Research may have to change to be more relevant to clinical practice. Perhaps there are parallel changes that clinical practice ought to make to improve patient care.

Acknowledgements. Completion of this chapter was facilitated by support from the National Institute of Mental Health (MH59029). Correspondence concerning this chapter should be directed to: Alan E. Kazdin, Child Study Center, 230 South Frontage Road, Yale University School of Medicine, New Haven, Connecticut, USA 06520-7900.

References

Ammerman, R.T., Last, C.G., and Hersen, M. (Eds.) (1999). Handbook of prescriptive treatments for children and adolescents (2nd ed.) Needham Heights, MA: Allyn and Bacon.

Ankuta, G.Y., and Abeles, N. (1993) Client satisfaction, clinical significance, and meaningful change in psychotherapy. Professional Psychology: Research and Practice, 24, 70–74.

Baron, R.M., and Kenny, D.A. (1986) The moderator-mediator variable distinction in social psychological research: Conceptual, strategic, and statistical considerations. Journal of Personality and Social Psychology, 51, 1173–1182.

Bergin, A.E., and Garfield, S.L. (Eds.) (1971) Handbook of psychotherapy and behavior change: An empirical analysis. New York: Wiley and Sons.

Buckner, J.C., & Chesney-Lind, M. (1983) Dramatic cures for juvenile crime: An evaluation of a prisoner-run delinquency prevention program. Criminal Justice and Behavior, 10, 227–247.

Burns, D.D., & Spangler, D.L. (2001) Do changes in dysfunctional attitudes mediate changes in depression and anxiety in cognitive behavioral therapy. Behavior Therapy, 32, 337–369.

Christophersen, E.R., & Mortweet, S.L. (2001) Treatments that work with children: Empirically supported strategies for managing childhood problems. Washington, DC: American Psychological Association.

Clement, P.W. (1999) Outcomes and incomes: How to evaluate, improve, and market your practice by measuring outcomes in psychotherapy. New York: Guilford.

Consumers Union. (1995) Mental health: Does therapy help? Consumer Reports, 60 (November), 734–739.

DeRubeis, R.J., Evans, M.D., Hollon, S.D., Garvey, M.J., Grove, W.M., & Tuason, V.B. (1990) How does cognitive therapy work? Cognitive change and symptom change in cognitive therapy and pharmacotherapy for depression. Journal of Consulting and Clinical Psychology, 58, 862–869.

Dishion, T.J., McCord, J., & Poulin, F. (1999) When interventions harm: Peer groups and problem behavior. American Psychologist, 54, 755–764.

Evidence-Based Mental Health (1998) (A journal devoted to evidence-based treatments and linking research to practice.) Vol 1, no 1.

Eysenck, H.J. (1952) The effects of psychotherapy: An evaluation. Journal of Consulting Psychology, 16, 319–324.

Eysenck, H.J. (1966) The effects of psychotherapy (with commentaries) New York: International Science Press.

Feldman, R.A., Caplinger, T.E., & Wodarski, J.S. (1983) The St. Louis conundrum: The effective treatment of antisocial youths. Englewood Cliffs, NJ: Prentice-Hall.

Fensterheim, H., & Raw, S.D. (1996) Psychotherapy research is not psychotherapy practice. Clinical Psychology: Science and Practice, 3, 168–171.

Finckenauer, J.O. (1982) Scared straight! and the panacea phenomenon. Englewood Cliffs, NJ: Prentice-Hall.

Fonagy, P., Target, M., Cottrell, D., Phillips, J., & Kurtz, Z. (2002) What works for whom? A critical review of treatments for children and adolescents. New York: Guilford.

Garfield, S.L., & Bergin, A.E. (Eds.) Handbook of psychotherapy and behavior change: An empirical analysis (2nd ed.) New York: Wiley & Sons.

Grissom, R.J. (1996) The magical number .7 +/– .2: Meta-meta-analysis of the probability of superior outcome in comparisons involving therapy, placebo, and control. Journal of Consulting and Clinical Psychology, 64, 973–982.

Haaga, D.A.F. (2000) Introduction to the special section on stepped-care models in psychotherapy. Journal of Consulting and Clinical Psychology, 68, 547–548.

Hayes, S.C., Follette, V.M., Dawes, R.M., & Grady, K.E. (1995) Scientific standards of psychological practice. Issues and recommendations. Reno, NV: Context Press.

Hoagwood, K., Hibbs, E., Brent, & Jensen, P.J. (1995) Efficacy and effectiveness in studies of child and adolescent psychotherapy. Journal of Consulting and Clinical Psychology, 63, 683–687.

Hollon, S.D., & Beck, A.T. (2004) Cognitive and cognitive behavioral therapies. In M.J. Lambert (Ed.), Bergin and Garfield's handbook of psychotherapy and behavior change (5th ed., pp. 447–492). New York: Wiley & Sons.

Ilardi, S.S., & Craighead, W.E. (1994) The role of nonspecific factors in cognitive-behavior therapy for depression. Clinical Psychology: Science and Practice, 1, 138–156.

Kavale, K.A., & Forness, S.R. (1993) Hyperactivity and diet treatment: A meta-analysis of the Feingold hypothesis. Journal of Learning Disabilities, 16, 324–330.

Kazdin, A.E. (1993) Evaluation in clinical practice: Clinically sensitive and systematic methods of treatment delivery. Behavior Therapy, 24, 11–45.

Kazdin, A.E. (2000) Psychotherapy for children and adolescents: Directions for research and practice. New York: Oxford University Press.

Kazdin, A.E. (2003) Research design in clinical psychology (4th ed.) Needham Heights, MA: Allyn & Bacon.

Kazdin, A.E. (2004) Psychotherapy for children and adolescents. In M. Lambert (Ed.) Bergin and Garfield's handbook of psychotherapy and behavior change (5th ed., pp. 543–589). New York: Wiley & Sons.

Kazdin, A.E. (in press) Mechanisms of change in psychotherapy: Advances, breakthroughs, and cutting-edge research (do not yet exist). In R.R. Bootzin (Ed.) Festschrift in honor of Lee Sechrest. Washington, DC: American Psychological Association.

Kazdin, A.E., & Nock, M.K. (2003) Delineating mechanisms of change in child and adolescent therapy: Methodological issues and research recommendations. Journal of Child Psychology and Psychiatry, 44, 1116–1129.

Kazdin, A.E., & Weisz, J.R. (Eds.) (2003) Evidence-based psychotherapies for children and adolescents. New York: Guilford Press.

Kazdin, A.E., Bass, D., Ayers, W.A., & Rodgers, A. (1990) The empirical and clinical focus of child and adolescent psychotherapy research. Journal of Consulting and Clinical Psychology, 58, 729–740.

Kendall, P.C. (Ed.) (1999) Special section: Clinical significance. Journal of Consulting and Clinical Psychology, 67, 283–339.

Kraemer, H.C., Stice, E., Kazdin, A.E., Offord, D.R., & Kupfer, D.J. (2001) How do risk factors work together? Mediators, moderators, independent, overlapping, and proxy-risk factors. American Journal of Psychiatry, 158, 848–856.

Kraemer, H.C., Wilson, G.T., Fairburn, C.G., & Agras, W.S. (2002) Mediators and moderators of treatment effects in randomized clinical trials. Archives of General Psychiatry, 59, 877–883.

Kwon, S., & Oei, T.P.S. (2003) Cognitive processes in a group cognitive behavior therapy of depression. Journal of Behavior Therapy and Experimental Psychiatry, 34, 73–85.

Lambert, W., Salzer, M.S., & Bickman, L. (1998) Clinical outcome, consumer satisfaction, and ad hoc ratings of improvement in children's mental health. Journal of Consulting and Clinical Psychology, 66, 270–279.

Levitt, E.E. (1957) The results of psychotherapy with children: An evaluation. Journal of Consulting Psychology, 21, 189–196.

Levitt, E.E. (1963) Psychotherapy with children: A further evaluation. Behaviour Research and Therapy, 60, 326–329.

10

Lonigan, C.J., & Elbert, J.C. (1998) Special issue on empirically supported psychosocial interventions for children. Journal of Clinical Child Psychology, 27, 138–226.

Lovaas, O.I. (1987) Behavioral treatment and normal educational/intellectual functioning in young autistic children. Journal of Consulting and Clinical Psychology, 55, 3–9.

Luborsky, L., Singer, B., & Luborsky, L. (1975) Comparative studies of psychotherapies: Is it true that »everyone has won and all must have prizes«? Archives of General Psychiatry, 32, 995–1008.

Lunnen, K.M., & Ogles, B.M. (1998) A multiperspective, multivariable evaluation of reliable change. Journal of Consulting and Clinical Psychology, 66, 400–410.

Marrs, R.W. (1995) A meta-analysis of bibliotherapy studies. American Journal of Community Psychology, 23, 843–870.

McEachin, J.J., Smith, T., & Lovaas, O.I. (1993) Outcome in adolescence of autistic children receiving early intensive behavioral treatment. American Journal of Mental Retardation, 97, 359–372.

McGee, R., Stanton, W.R., & Sears, M.R. (1993) Allergic disorders and attention deficit disorder in children. Journal of Abnormal Child Psychology, 21, 79–88.

Nathan, P.E., & Gorman, J.M. (Eds.) (2002) Treatments that work (2nd ed.). New York: Oxford University Press.

National Advisory Mental Health Council (NAMHC) (1999) Bridging science and service (NIH Publication No. 99-4353). Washington, DC: NIH.

National Advisory Mental Health Council Workgroup on Child and Adolescent Mental Health Intervention Development and Deployment (NAMHC-W) (2001) Blueprint for change: Research on child and adolescent mental health. Washington, DC: NIH.

O'Donnell, C.R. (1992) The interplay of theory and practice in delinquency prevention: From behavior modification to activity settings. In J. McCord & R.E. Tremblay (Eds.), Preventing antisocial behavior (pp. 209–232). New York: Guilford.

Pagliaro, A.M., & Pagliaro, L.A. (1996) Substance use among children and adolescents: Its nature, extent, and effects from conception to adulthood. New York: Wiley & Sons.

Pekarik, G., & Wolff, C.B. (1996) Relationship of satisfaction to symptom change, follow-up adjustment, and clinical significance. Professional Psychology: Research and Practice, 27, 202–208.

Persons, J.B., & Silberschatz, G. (1998) Are results of randomized controlled clinical trials useful to psychotherapists? Journal of Consulting and Clinical Psychology, 66, 126–135.

Remschmidt, H. (Ed.) (2001) Psychotherapy with children and adolescents. Cambridge: Cambridge University Press.

Rogers, S.J. (1998) Empirically supported treatment for young children with autism. Journal of Clinical Child Psychology, 27, 168–179.

Roth, A., & Fonagy, P. (1996) What works for whom: A critical review of psychotherapy research. New York: Guilford.

Schoenwald, S.K., & Hoagwood, K. (2001) Effectiveness, transportability, and dissemination of interventions: What matters when? Psychiatric Services, 52, 1190–1197.

Sheinkopf, S.J., & Siegel, B. (1998) Home based behavioral treatment of young children with autism. Journal of Autism and Developmental Disabilities, 28, 15–23.

Simson, S.P., & Straus, M.C. (Eds.) (1998) Horticulture as therapy: Principles and practice. Binghamton, NY: Hayworth Press.

Smith, M.L., & Glass, G.V. (1977) Meta-analysis of psychotherapy outcome studies. American Psychologist, 32, 752–760.

Smith, M.L., Glass, G.V., & Miller, T.L. (1980) The benefits of psychotherapy. Baltimore: Johns Hopkins University Press.

Smith, T. (1999) Outcome of early intervention for children with autism. Clinical Psychology: Science and Practice, 6, 33–49.

Smyth, J.M. (1998) Written emotional expression: Effect sizes, outcome types, and moderating variables. Journal of Consulting and Clinical Psychology, 66, 174–184.

Sobell, L.C., Sobell, M.B., & Agrawal, S. (2002) Self-change and dual recoveries among individuals with alcohol and tobacco problems: Current knowledge and future directions alcoholism. Alcoholism: Clinical and Experimental Research, 26, 1936–1938.

Stricker, G., & Keisner, R.H. (Eds.) (1985) From research to clinical practice: The implications of social and developmental research for psychotherapy. New York: Plenum.

Task Force on Promotion and Dissemination of Psychological Procedures (1995) Training in and dissemination of empirically validated psychological treatments: Report and recommendations. The Clinical Psychologist, 48 (1), 3–23.

Wasserman, G.A., Ko, S.J., & Jensen, P.S. (2001) Columbia guidelines for child and adolescent mental health referral. Report on Emotional and Behavioral Disorders in Youth, 2 (1), 9–14, 23.

Whisman, M.A. (1993) Mediators and moderators of change in cognitive therapy of depression. Psychological Bulletin, 114, 248–265.

Whisman, M.A. (1999) The importance of the cognitive theory of change in cognitive therapy of depression. Clinical Psychology: Science and Practice, 6, 300–304.

www.aacap.org/clinical/parameters.

www.cdc.gov/tobacco/research_data.

www.kidsource.com/kidsource/content3/ific/ific.hyper.foods.

www.quit-smoking.net/greatamericansmokeout.

What Works for Whom? Differential Indications for Treatment/Intervention

Peter Fonagy, Mary Target

11.1   **Introduction**   – 119

11.2   **Differential Indications**   – 120
11.2.1   Anxiety   – 120
11.2.2   Post-traumatic Stress Disorder   – 121
11.2.3   Depression   – 122
11.2.4   Conduct Problems   – 123
11.2.4.1   Psychosocial Treatment Interventions
　　　　for Preadolescents with ODD and CD   – 123
11.2.5   Attention Deficit/Hyperactivity Disorder   – 125
11.2.6   Tourette Syndrome   – 127
11.2.7   Schizophrenia and Other Psychoses   – 127
11.2.7.1   Schizophrenia   – 127
11.2.7.2   Mania and Bipolar Disorders   – 127
11.2.8   Autism   – 128
11.2.9   Eating Disorders   – 128
11.2.10   Deliberate Self-Harm   – 129
11.2.11   Specific Developmental Disorders   – 130

11.3   **Conclusion**   – 130

　　　References   – 131

11.1   Introduction

The desirability of replacing clinical opinion with reliable, empirically sound observation, ideally based in randomized controlled trials, took hold in an increasing number of areas of medicine throughout the late 1980s and early 1990s. Studies of psychological therapies suddenly became the essential basis for the viability of widely-offered procedures and indeed entire professions. In response to this demand, reviews of »the evidence base« have almost become a cottage industry, whether or not the authors fully understand the limitations of the research on which their reviews are based (Roth and Parry 1997). In this respect it is helpful that carefully framed and consensually developed national policy guidance is emerging in the United Kingdom. As examples, evidence-based psychologi-cal therapy services have been identified as a national goal (NHS Executive 1996), and there is now clear guidance regarding referral for major mental health conditions (Department of Health 2001).

We have recently reviewed the effectiveness of psychosocial interventions for all major forms of mental health problems (including depression, phobias, obsessive compulsive disorder, PTSD, eating disorders, schizophrenia, bipolar disorder, personality disorder, and substance abuse (Fonagy et al. 2002; Roth and Fonagy 1996; Roth and Fonagy, in press; Target and Fonagy, in press) and this will form the basis of this chapter. The chapter covers many of the most important diagnostic categories.

Our work is largely – but not solely – based on systematic reviews of randomized controlled trials; we judged that an exclusive focus on this methodology would be inappropriate. In line with the scientist-practitioner model, many innovations in psychological therapy develop along a hierarchy of designs from clinical observation backed by and linked to clinical theory, which lead first to experimentation on a small scale; results are then tested in open trials and in turn are exposed to full scientific scrutiny in randomized trials. On this basis we were keen to include well-conducted, clinically relevant research, maintaining a balance in our inclusion criteria between research rigor and clinical relevance. A major and regrettable limitation of our review is restriction to the English-language literature. Summarizing all our conclusions in this presentation would be inappropriate and impractical, but by focusing on a few disorders we can give a flavor of our findings and indicate lessons we have learned and offer hints about a profitable future.

11.2   Differential Indications

11.2.1   Anxiety

Anxiety disorders commonly present as part of a more complex picture, frequently including other disorders (e.g., Strauss and Last 1993), and difficulties in adaptation such as shyness, academic underachievement and unhappiness (e.g., Quay and LaGreca 1986). Fears and worries are, of course, very common in normal development (e.g., Bell-Dolan et al. 1990; Muris et al. 1998), and only become diagnosable where a persistent and disabling pattern has become established. Nevertheless, it has been shown that, for children starting school, anxiety symptoms that do not meet diagnostic criteria are associated with academic impairment over the following years (Ialongo et al. 1994, 1995). Here we are concerned with treatments for symptoms that do meet the thresholds for at least one diagnosis.

Anxiety disorders in children and adolescents include the syndromes described for the adult population, so for DSM-IV the following categories can be applied to children: generalized anxiety disorder (GAD), obsessive-compulsive disorder (OCD), agoraphobia, panic disorder, specific phobia, social phobia, and anxiety states due to either medical disorder or substance use. In addition, separation anxiety disorder (SAD) can be diagnosed in children.

Anxiety disorders are very common, but most cases go untreated. Different disorders have different prognoses, but moderate to severe cases are not likely to remit spontaneously, and when they do remit, it is quite common for other disorders to take their places (Flament et al. 1990; Kovacs and Devlin 1998; Pollack et al. 1996). Anxiety disorders commonly evolve into other anxiety or depressive syndromes. Persistent anxiety disorders cause pervasive and lasting impairments. The high placebo response observed in child and adolescent patients makes demonstration of efficacy of all treatments problematic.

Behavioral techniques are often effective in the treatment of children with circumscribed phobias, especially younger children (King et al. 2001; Ollendick and King 1998). OCD can be improved in some cases, though generally not eliminated, by a cognitive-behavioral therapy (CBT) approach (March 1995; March et al. 2001; March and Leonard 1996; March and Mulle 1995). This approach has so far mostly been evaluated with concurrent medication, but there is some evidence that CBT makes a distinc-

tive contribution (DeVeaugh-Geiss et al. 1992; March et al. 1994). Bolton and colleagues (1983) reported results from an open series of 15 adolescents with moderate to severe, entrenched OCD treated primarily with response prevention, with family therapy used to support this (focusing mainly on obstacles to the response prevention approach). Sometimes other treatments were required for associated symptoms (five patients received clomipramine to ease depression or anxiety, with mixed effects on the OCD symptoms). Treatment lasted for up to 4 years. In 8 of the 15 cases, symptoms were completely relieved at the end of treatment; six of these cases remained well at follow-up (between 1 and 4 years later), while the other two had relapsed quite severely. Three cases showed no response to treatment lasting between 5 months and 4 years, and the remaining four showed partial improvement. The authors offered a useful discussion of the factors that appeared to affect response to treatment. Poor motivation, primary obsessional ruminations, conduct disorder, and obsessional slowness were associated with the bad outcomes.

Certain CBT packages have been shown to be effective in the treatment of generalized and other anxiety disorders and, for those who improve, the gains can be maintained (Barrett et al. 1996; Kendall et al. 1997; Toren et al. 2000; Tracey et al. 1999). In a small open trial of parent-child group CBT for preadolescent children with anxiety disorders (Toren et al. 2000) the children whose mothers met criteria for an anxiety disorder (half the sample) did better than those whose mothers were not anxious, even though the anxious mothers' own anxiety levels were not reduced during treatment. This small study strongly justifies extension and clarification, as it involved a relatively brief and low-cost treatment which appears to have been helpful with a challenging group: clinically-referred children, most with comorbid diagnoses and half of whose mothers had similar symptoms.

Exposure has been assumed to be a central aspect of the efficacy of CBT, but two recent well-designed studies of the treatment of school phobia found that therapeutic support without exposure was equally effective (Last et al. 1998; Silverman et al. 1999). Where exposure treatment is used, it may well be more effective as well as humane to use a gradual, rather than a »flooding« approach (King et al. 1998). There is accumulating evidence that CBT for childhood anxiety disorders can be delivered in a group as successfully as in an individual format (Flannery-Schroeder and Kendall 2000; Manassis et al. 2002). Adding a family component to CBT may well be beneficial for younger children, or for families where parental anxiety is also high (Barrett et al. 1996; Cobham et al. 1998; Howard and Kendall 1996).

There is preliminary evidence that psychodynamic psychotherapy may be effective in the treatment of anxiety disorders (Target and Fonagy 1994a). Children with anxiety disorders (with or without comorbidity) showed greater improvements than those with other conditions, and greater improvements than would have been expected on the basis of studies of untreated outcome. Over 85% of 299 children with anxiety and depressive disorders no longer suffered any diagnosable emotional disorder after an average of 2 years' treatment. Looking in more detail at specific diagnostic groups, it was found that phobias ($n = 48$), separation anxiety disorders ($n = 58$) and overanxious disorder ($n = 145$) were resolved in around 86% of cases. OCD was more resistant, ceasing to meet diagnostic criteria in only 70% of cases. There are serious limitations to a retrospective study, and there was no control group or follow-up; however, these rates of improvement appear to be above the level expected from longitudinal studies. A further finding was that children with severe or pervasive symptomatology, such as GAD, or multiple comorbid disorders, required more frequent therapy sessions, whereas more circumscribed symptoms – such as phobias – even if quite severe, improved comparably with once or twice weekly sessions. These findings justify an RCT in which difficult cases, perhaps those which have not improved with briefer treatments, are treated with a manualized psychodynamic approach and assessed using appropriate outcome measures.

No studies have so far examined the effectiveness of family therapy for childhood anxiety disorders, other than CBT delivered in a family format.

A number of studies have examined predictors of improvement in groups of treated children. Berman and colleagues (2000) studied 106 children aged 6–17 years with various anxiety disorders, who were given exposure-based treatment. Children did less well if they were also depressed or had trait anxiety, or whose parents had more psychopathology (this was most important in younger children). Southam-Gerow and colleagues (2001) evaluated predictors of response to individual CBT in a similar group of anxious children. Here, predictors of poor outcome were more severe internalizing problems, more maternal depression, and the child being older. Kendall and colleagues (2001) examined the importance of comorbidity in predicting the outcome

of CBT for 173 children given 16–20 weeks of treatment. Comorbidity was found to be associated with greater pretreatment severity but not with worse outcome. This is consistent with a number of previous findings including from the Southam-Gerow study (2001). Layne and colleagues (2003) examined predictors of outcome in a group of 41 adolescents, all of whom had diagnoses of both anxiety and depression. Worse outcome was associated with worse school attendance at baseline, more SAD and avoidant disorder, and female gender.

Crawford and Manassis (2001) explored the importance of family factors in child anxiety outcome. These authors found that the outcome of either individual or group CBT, with parallel parent training, was heavily mediated by family stress; specifically, clinician-rated child outcome was strongly predicted by the child's rating (before treatment) of family dysfunction and of parental frustration. Greater dysfunction and frustration predicted worse treatment outcome.

11.2.2   Post-traumatic Stress Disorder

Trauma of various kinds is strongly associated with psychopathology, particularly emotional (e.g., Kliewer et al. 1998) and behavioral (e.g., Farrell and Bruce 1997) problems as well as developmental delay (e.g., Delaney-Black et al. 2002). Children who have subthreshold post-traumatic stress disorder (PTSD) have similar problems to those who meet full diagnostic criteria (Carrion et al. 2002). For example, follow-up studies of sexually abused children have identified both short-term and long-term effects, including depression, anxiety, and eating disorders (Beitchman et al. 1991, 1992; Trowell et al. 1999).

The published literature of the treatment of PTSD in children is at an early phase. There is evidence of a number of promising, brief treatments for children with relatively chronic PTSD symptoms as well as treatments that may be applied at an early stage following the trauma. Trauma-specific CBT has emerged from several studies as effective in improving PTSD symptoms and associated depression and anxiety (Cohen and Mannarino 1996, 1998; Deblinger et al. 1999, 2001; March et al. 1998). There is some indication of benefit to social functioning (Cohen and Mannarino 1998). One trial of CBT (Deblinger et al. 1996, 1999) focusing on PTSD and other emotional problems in 100 school-age children with a history of CSA contrasted child-focused, mother-focused, mother and child, and standard community care (TAU) control. All three active treatments were superior to TAU and improvements were maintained at 2-year follow-up. However, treatment continued during the follow-up period and attrition was high. Inclusion of parents resulted in greater improvement in the child's depression and included children benefited more in terms of PTSD symptoms. This suggests that the inclusion of both parents and children is essential for good outcome.

Non-CBT psychotherapeutic approaches have also been tested and are showing promise in both single trauma and chronic or multiple trauma related conditions (Chemtob et al. 2002; Goenjian et al. 1997; Layne et al. 2001; Salloum et al. 2001; Saltzman et al. 2001; Soberman et al. 2002; Trowell et al. 2002). The evidence here is less strong, with no randomized controlled trial showing superiority to an active control group. However, pre-post effect sizes are impressive and the range of benefits include prosocial behaviors (Layne et al. 2001; Soberman et al. 2002) and school performance (Saltzman et al. 2001). Several studies demonstrated powerful effects from relatively brief (4–6 sessions) interventions with individuals with quite chronic PTSD symptoms identified in community cohorts (Chemtob et al. 2002). The status of eye movement desensitization and reprocessing (EMDR) as an adjunct to other trauma-related treatments is as yet uncertain (Chemtob et al. 2002; Rubin et al. 2001; Soberman et al. 2002).

11.2.3   Depression

In children and teenagers, a diagnosis of major depressive disorder (MDD) requires a minimum 2 week period of pervasive mood change towards sadness or irritability, and loss of interest or pleasure (American Psychiatric Association 1994). The symptoms must not be explicable by other influences such as other illnesses, substance abuse, or recent bereavement. Diagnosis also requires some biological characteristics, such as loss of appetite, insomnia, reduced energy, or libido in adolescents. Children and adolescents may show more anxiety and anger, fewer vegetative symptoms and less verbalization of hopelessness than adults (American Academy of Child and Adolescent Psychiatry 1998). Dysthymic disorder (DD) is a chronic condition with depressed and/or irritable mood, present most of the time for at least a year. At least two other symptoms of MDD must be present (American Psychiatric Association 1994).

Treatment of depression in children has generally been approached by adapting approaches used with adult patients, particularly medication and cognitive-behavioral therapy. CBT appears to be effective, whether provided individually (Brent et al. 1998; Kroll et al. 1996; Wood et al. 1996) or in a group (Clarke et al. 1999; Lewinsohn et al. 1984, 1994, 1996; Stark et al. 1987). Reinecke and colleagues (Reinecke et al. 1998) carried out a meta-analysis of studies of CBT for adolescent depression, and found a robust effect size of 1.02 at termination and 0.61 at follow-up. Harrington and colleagues (Harrington et al. 1998) have also carried out a very useful systematic review of all methodologically sound CBT outcome studies ($n = 6$) for childhood depressive disorder. Their pooled odds ratio was 3.2, with children receiving CBT significantly more likely to be in remission by the end of treatment. This odds ratio fell to 2.2 if a (very conservative) intent to treat analysis was applied (in which all dropouts from the control groups were counted as having remitted, and all those from the CBT groups as not having remitted). However, CBT has mainly been tested with mildly-moderately impaired adolescents, rather than with either severe cases or (preadolescent) children. In a trial of CBT including 96 depressed adolescents (Lewinsohn et al. 1994, 1996) adolescents with less severe symptoms and better initial adaptation tended to benefit more from the treatment.

CBT may be particularly effective for adolescents with comorbid anxiety (Brent et al. 1998). Family factors such as maternal depression and family discord can reduce treatment response (e.g., Brent et al. 1998). CBT is not more effective in cases where there are greater cognitive distortions, and its benefits are apparently not explained by a reduction in such cognitions (Brent et al. 1997; Lewinsohn et al. 1990). Providing longer courses of CBT (or booster sessions) in cases of nonresponse to a standard length of treatment seems to hasten recovery (Clarke et al. 1999). CBT seems to be more effective than tricyclic medication (Reinecke et al. 1998). However, it is less likely to be effective in more severe cases. Recent studies have confirmed that referred, depressed adolescents are more difficult than recruited cases to treat successfully, even when severity is comparable (Birmaher et al. 2000; Brent et al. 1998, 1999). As studies of the effectiveness of tricyclic medication for childhood depression have generally involved more severely impaired cases than have the studies of CBT, the apparent superiority of CBT might be partly accounted for by the selection of milder cases.

Rohde and colleagues (2001) have analyzed the data from the combined Oregon cohorts (Clarke et al. 1999; Lewinsohn et al. 1990), to examine the influence of comorbidity on outcomes for CBT. Almost 40% of the sample of the 151 adolescents had had another lifetime diagnosis (in addition to the depressive disorder at intake). Contrary to expectations, although comorbidity was associated with greater impairment at intake, it did not predict poorer outcome (in fact comorbidity with anxiety was a positive factor), nor did it predict slower recovery, with the exception of substance abuse, which did seem to delay improvement.

Interpersonal psychotherapy, adapted for adolescents (IPT-A), appears promising for treatment of adolescent depression (Moreau et al. 1991; Mufson et al. 1994, 1999). Family therapy, or parent work in parallel with individual treatment for the child, has been included as a condition in four RCTs (e.g., Brent et al. 1997). Neither approach has been convincingly shown to be more effective than general support, or routine care, but family therapy in particular needs to be manualized. Social skills training and individual child psychotherapy have not yet been shown to be effective treatments. A chart review study of 763 patients who had been in psychoanalytic therapy (Target and Fonagy 1994b) included 65 children and adolescents with dysthymia and/or major depression, who had been treated for an average of two years. By the end of therapy, over 75% showed reliable improvement in functioning and no depressive symptoms. However, the episodic course of depression means that these pre-post findings with no control group or follow-up cannot be taken as evidence of efficacy. A clearer finding was that children and adolescents with depressive disorders appeared to benefit more from intensive therapy (4–5 sessions per week) than from nonintensive therapy (1–2 sessions per week), after controlling for length of treatment and level of impairment at referral. This is of some interest given that the depressed cases were mostly adolescents, who generally did not gain additional benefit from frequent sessions.

As in outcome studies for many other disorders, outcome of the treatment of depression has generally been defined in terms of symptoms and diagnostic status, whereas other impairments, such as deficient social adaptation and academic performance, are also central.

11.2.4 Conduct Problems

Conduct problems include conduct disorder (CD) and oppositional defiant disorder (ODD). According to DSM-IV, ODD must include a repetitive pattern of defiance and disobedience and a negative and hostile attitude towards authority figures of at least 6 months' duration. Although ODD and CD overlap in definition, CD, unlike ODD, entails the violations of the basic rights of others or of age-appropriate societal norms or rules. Conduct disorder with onset before puberty is generally considered more severe and more likely to entail neuropsychological deficits than adolescent onset antisocial behavior, which may have peer influence as a major part of causation (Moffitt et al. 1996).

11.2.4.1 Psychosocial Treatment Interventions for Preadolescents with ODD and CD

11.2.4.1.1 Parent Training

The parent training model is based on the assumption that ODD and CD reflect parental difficulty in adequately reinforcing socially appropriate forms of conduct as well as a tendency to maintain inappropriate forms through coercive interactions (Kazdin 1995; Miller and Prinz 1990; Patterson 1982). This 6–8 week intervention is conducted with the parents with limited therapist-child contact. Parents are encouraged to refocus on prosocial behaviors rather than on the elimination of conduct problems. The training component of the program is based on behavioral management principles drawn from social learning theory. Although programs vary in terms of the exact syllabus and the methods of delivering these contents, in all programs dyadic instruction is accompanied by other aids to learning, such as role playing, behavioral rehearsal, and structured homework exercises. Evidence that changing families' interaction patterns has the power to alter the child's behavior is very strong (Ducharme et al. 2000; Forehand and Long 1988; Long et al. 1994; Nixon et al. 2003; Nye et al. 1995; Patterson and Chamberlain 1988; Schuhmann et al. 1998; Webster-Stratton and Hammond 1997; Webster-Stratton and Reid 2003). There is accumulating evidence that parent training programs generally may be applied in a wide range of conduct problems and effectively delivered in various settings, including clinical populations (Bradley et al. 1999; Cunningham et al. 1995; Scott et al. 2001).

Larger effects (fewer dropouts, greater gains, and better maintenance) tend to be found for parent training when the children are younger; there is less comorbidity, the disturbance of conduct is less severe, there is less socioeconomic disadvantage in the family (Holden et al. 1990; Kazdin et al. 1992; McMahon et al. 1981), the parents are together (Dumas and Albin 1986; Farmer et al. 2002), parental discord and stress is low (Dadds et al. 1987; Dumas and Albin 1986; Kazdin et al. 1992; McMahon et al. 1981; Webster-Stratton 1996), social support is high, and there is no parental history of antisocial behavior. Failure to benefit from the program may be associated with parental disadvantage, lack of parental perception of a need for intervention, marital discord (Dadds et al. 1987; Nye et al. 1995), parental drug or alcohol problems (Nye et al. 1995), psychiatric difficulties (drug and alcohol problems, depression, personality difficulties), more severe and chronic antisocial behavior and comorbidity in the child (Kazdin 1995; Ruma et al. 1996). However, inattention, impulsivity, and hyperactivity problems increase the size of the response (Hartman et al. 2003). Maternal psychopathology, in particular depression and life events, has been found to reduce the effectiveness of parent training (Dumas and Albin 1986; Kazdin et al. 1992; McMahon et al. 1981; Webster-Stratton 1996). There are also findings which indicate that single parent status (Dumas and Albin 1986), only one parent attending (Farmer et al. 2002), and maternal insecurity of attachment (Routh et al. 1995) may undermine progress, but these associations are not sufficiently consistent across studies. In the case of violent families, consequence procedures normally included in parent training packages can result in confrontation between the parent and the oppositional child which could provoke more serious aversive interactions in parents prone to child abuse (Lutzker 1996). »Errorless« compliance training offers an alternative to the use of physical consequence for noncompliance (Ducharme et al. 2000). Parent training can have quite limited effects when parents themselves did not seek treatment (Barkley et al. 2000; Webster-Stratton and Hammond 1997).

11.2.4.1.2   Child-Oriented Interventions

Psychodynamic treatments have not been shown to be effective for children with conduct problems relative to an untreated or alternative treatment control group. Mild conduct problems are ameliorated with the help of social skills and anger management coping skills training (see Quinn et al. 1999 for a review). In a school-based coping skills intervention (Lochman et al. 1993) children rated aggressive and rejected benefited from this package in terms of reduced aggression (ES = .85) and social acceptance (ES = .89) while those who were aggressive but not socially rejected did not. Attrition was, however, high at 45%. There is no evidence for the use of social skills and anger management coping skills training approaches on their own with more chronic and severe cases (Fonagy et al. 2002). Problem-solving skills training is the most rigorously investigated singular approach to the cognitive-behavioral treatment of conduct problems. Its effectiveness in combination with parent training has been demonstrated by two independent studies (Kazdin et al. 1992; Kazdin and Wasser 2000) and seems to be the treatment of choice for conduct problems in school-aged children (8–12). In a trial contrasting relationship therapy (RT) with (a) PSST, and (b) PSST and in vivo practice outside the treatment setting, PSST produced improvements with the outpatient, milder or moderate severity group, as well as the inpatient group. Children with more severe disturbance of conduct (either in terms of frequency or intensity) were more likely to drop out or have negative outcomes (Kazdin et al. 1994). There is some indication that ethnic minority status may be associated with relatively poorer outcomes (Kazdin 1996).

Of 242 children aged 3–14 years (mean age 8 1/2) who had been referred to a specialist outpatient unit for treatment for oppositional, aggressive, and antisocial behavior, 39.9% dropped out (Kazdin et al. 1997). These families were more likely to be from minority groups, from single-parent families, on public assistance, to have adverse child-rearing practices, to be of low SES, and to have a child with a history of antisocial behavior. Families who dropped out had higher levels of stressors and obstacles which competed with treatment, including conflict with a significant other about coming to treatment, problems with other children, and treatment being seen as adding to other stressors. Those terminating early also perceived the treatment as less relevant to the child's problems and appeared to have poorer relationships with the therapist.

These conclusions were supported by an uncontrolled study of 250 children and families treated with PSST and PMT (Kazdin and Wasser 2000). The combination of these treatments administered to children referred to a community-based University Clinic was found to be quite effective in causing change over an average of 22 weeks of treatment. The greater the severity of the child's dysfunction and the higher the perceived barriers, the smaller the observed changes in the child's problems associated with treatment. Helping parents deal with stress independently improves the outcome of already potent combinations of PMT and PSST (Kazdin and Whitley 2003).

11.2.4.1.3 Classroom Behavior-Focused Interventions

Classroom contingency management methods are demonstrated to be effective in controlling the behavior of children with conduct problems in that setting (e.g., Deitz 1985; Walker et al. 1984), but they have not yet been convincingly shown to generalize beyond the classroom situation or beyond the termination of the programs (Barkley et al. 2000). Parent-administered reinforcements may enhance classroom contingency management in universal or selective prevention programs (Ayllon et al. 1975; Kahle and Kelley 1994). Where children have behavior problems in the classroom, the addition of contingency behavior management programs in the classroom should be considered, in addition to family based treatments.

11.2.4.1.4 Psychosocial Treatment Interventions for Adolescents

In general, the strongest evidence is for those multi-level, relatively intensive, community-based, highly structured and well-integrated programs focusing on goals proximal to offending behavior (for example, family monitoring and supervision of the adolescent). Functional Family Therapy has been shown to be effective in reducing recidivism in adolescents who have multiply offended (Barton et al. 1985; Gordon et al. 1988, 1995). It is a promising treatment which has not yet been widely applied. Structural family therapy has been shown to be effective in Hispanic youths with conduct problems (Santiseban et al. 2003). Several studies have shown that integrating a training program for carefully selected foster parents with problem-solving skills and anger management skills training for delinquent adolescents is a powerful approach, reducing behavior problems as well as recidivism (Chamberlain and Reid 1998; Chamberlain and Rozicky 1995). Multisystemic therapy (MST) is the most effective treatment for delinquent adolescents in reducing recidivism and improving individual and family pathology (Borduin 1999; Henggeler et al. 1986, 1992, 1993,

1996). It is substantially more effective than individual treatment even for quite troubled and disorganized families. MST shares a particular strength with other systemic family approaches in reducing attrition rates in this highly volatile group (Henggeler et al. 1996). A number of treatment packages combining a range of individual skills-oriented techniques appear promising (Feindler et al. 1984; Guerra and Slaby 1990; Huey and Rank 1984), but the most effective combination of specific techniques has not yet been identified and results on long-term outcomes are equivocal.

The effectiveness of parent training has been assessed in adolescents; while trials show statistically significant gains associated with these programs, these gains are of low clinical significance (Bank et al. 1991; Dishion and Andrews 1995; Raue and Spence 1985). Group treatments of conduct-disordered adolescents appear to carry a risk of worsening rather than improving the individual's behavior problems (Dishion and Andrews 1995). Social skills and social problem-solving approaches lead to desirable short-term changes, but do not generalize well across settings or engender lasting improvements (Feindler et al. 1984; Guerra and Slaby 1990; Huey and Rank 1984). Anger management is a promising treatment approach, but the evidence for its efficacy is quite limited (Feindler et al. 1984). School-based approaches have considerable potential, but studies to date have failed to demonstrate powerful effects on delinquency (Esbensen and Osgood 1999; Gottfredson and Gottfredson 1992). The evidence for community-wide implementation of psychosocial treatment programs is inadequate and the results are mixed, although family preservation and systemic family therapy implementations appear most promising (Nugent et al. 1993).

Individual treatment approaches appear to be less effective than family-based approaches, but if individual approaches are implemented, these should focus on proximal causes for delinquent behavior rather than more distal underlying problems. The programs for these adolescents should be skills oriented wherever possible, identifying the skills deficits.

11.2.5 Attention Deficit/ Hyperactivity Disorder

The characteristics of ADHD are reduced levels of concentration or attention, impulsivity and over-activity or restlessness. There is no clear demarcation between extremes of normality and truly abnormal degrees of these behaviors. Findings from several factor analytic studies, such as the study by Lahey and Carlson (1992), suggest two separate dimensions in ADHD: the impulsive hyperactive, and the inattentive disorganized dimension. DSM-IV describes three types of ADHD: predominantly inattentive, predominantly hyperactive, and combined (both sets of symptoms).

Systematic reviews of extended treatment studies underscore the unique value of stimulant medication (Farmer et al. 2002; Schachar et al. 2002). 75% of children with ADHD show normalization of inattention, hyperactivity, and impulsivity when treated with stimulants. It is not possible to predict with certainty who will show a good response. Attention and output during academic tasks improve by 70% with stimulant medication. Efficiency and accuracy show approximately 50% improvement but there is little evidence for improved academic performance in the long term. Prosocial behaviors do not improve substantially although there is evidence that these benefit from the additional use of clonidine (Hazell and Stuart 2003). Despite improvement, behavior is not normalized with medication in all cases (MTA 1999).

A number of psychosocial treatments have been shown to be effective in ADHD compared to wait list controls (e.g., Anastopoulos et al. 1993; Hoath and Sanders 2002; Sonuga-Barke et al. 2001). Compared to medication, the adjunctive effects of psychosocial treatment is unclear, with some studies showing little or no benefit from adding psychosocial interventions to well-administered medication treatments (Horn et al. 1991; Ialongo et al. 1993) and other studies suggesting that the appropriate psychosocial intervention can help attain desired responses with lower doses of medication (Abikoff and Hechtman 1996; Satterfield et al. 1981, 1987; Vitiello et al. 2001). It is possible that the presence of comorbid anxiety (Jensen et al. 2001; The MTA Cooperative Group 1999) and high parental education (Pisterman et al. 1992; Rieppi et al. 2002) indicate greater benefit from intensive behavioral psychosocial treatment. Behavior therapy on its own is less effective than stimulant medication, but it can perhaps prevent a need for higher doses of medication (Vitiello et al. 2001). It improves task behavior and reduces disruptive behavior, but there is little evidence of generalization across settings so far.

Most of these observations are derived from the MTA study, which is a 5-year multimodal treatment study set up by the National Institute of Mental Health (Richters et al. 1995). A sample of 579 children with attention deficit/hyperactivity disorder were randomly allocated to 14 months of treatment into one of three experimental groups or a control group: (a) medication, (b) intensive behavioral management with the parents, child, and school with therapist input reduced over time, (c) the two »optimally« combined, or (d) standard care chosen by families obtained from community providers. In the presence of comorbid anxiety (present in 34% of the sample) there was a trend towards a better response to the combined treatment than to medication on its own, and behavioral intervention alone was better than the standard community care: the presence of comorbid anxiety reduced the relative advantage of medication over the other treatments, but it did not reduce the rate of response to medication (March et al. 2000). ADHD only and ADHD with comorbid conduct or oppositional defiant disorder subjects responded only to treatments that included medication. If comorbidity included anxiety as well as conduct syndromes, the combined treatment group fared best. Combined treatments were more effective for better-educated families and yielded greater patient satisfaction (Rieppi et al. 2002). Treatments involving medication were more likely to assure normalization in the absence of parental depression and less severe initial presentation (Owens et al. 2003). Beneficial effects of the behavioral treatment appeared to remain several months after the treatment had ceased, supporting the notion that combining treatments may allow earlier discontinuation of medication. Further, parental disciplinary practices consistently predicted changes in child outcome at school (Hinshaw et al. 2000; Wells et al. 2000).

Multimodal treatments have not yet consistently demonstrated superiority. There is no good evidence that cognitive-behavioral therapy is effective on its own (e.g., Abikoff et al. 1988; Abikoff and Gittelman 1985; Brown et al. 1986) and its effective component may be the behavioral one. Parent training is effective in improving compliance with instructions (Pisterman et al. 1992, 1989) but not all families are able to persist with the approach. Parent training is more likely to be effective if participating mothers have low levels of ADHD symptoms (Rieppi et al. 2002; Sonuga-Barke et al. 2002; unrelated to other aspects of maternal health or child functioning). Parental ADHD may require treatment before PMT is likely to be effective for younger children with ADHD. Drop-out rates are higher among less-educated parents (Pisterman et al. 1992), suggesting that greater efforts are required to involve this needy group of parents as further parent training courses are developed. Parent training is best carried out when the children are prepubertal (Anastopoulos et al. 1996). There is no evidence that social skills intervention leads to an improvement in poor relationships (Cousins and Weiss 1993). There is no evidence either for or against the effectiveness of systemic or psychodynamic therapy. However, the studies are generally short-term and under-represent female patients relative to the normal duration and gender mix of ADHD clinics. Mediator and moderator analyses indicated clinically relevant person-by-treatment interactions (Jensen et al. 2001).

11.2.6   Tourette Syndrome

Tourette syndrome is a common childhood onset disorder with unknown neurobiological etiology (Comings and Comings 1985). It presents with motor and vocal tics.

Behavioral treatments have been found to be beneficial with such interventions as habit-reversal (performing a movement which is opposite to the tic in question) and relaxation (Azrin and Peterson 1990). This requires approximately a year's course of monthly behavioral treatments but it is not beneficial for all children with Tourette's. Other techniques such as massed negative practice, where the child performs the tic as quickly and forcefully as they can, have had uncertain results (Azrin and Peterson 1988). Leckman and Cohen (1994) found that families generally report only short-term benefits from these interventions.

Leckman and Cohen (1994) report that psychotherapy may be useful in helping children and families cope with this distressing illness, but there have been no controlled studies of its use. Similarly, although not clinically evaluated, studies have suggested that supportive interventions with the family and with the school are beneficial.

There is no one ideal drug treatment for Tourette syndrome either in isolation or in the presence of comorbid disorder(s). In the absence of comorbid problems, the current treatments of choice are haloperidol or clonidine, with little to choose between them.

11.2.7   Schizophrenia and Other Psychoses

11.2.7.1   Schizophrenia

There are very few evaluations of psychosocial treatments for children and young people with schizophrenia. One trial of behavioral family intervention (Linszen et al. 1996) is noteworthy because of the relatively large number of participants. The program consisted of a 3 months inpatient and 12 months outpatient phase. Seventy six patients were randomly assigned to an individual-orientated psychosocial intervention program or to an identical psychosocial program plus a behavioral family intervention. Overall relapse rates during the outpatient interventions were low (16%). Adding family intervention to the psychosocial intervention did not affect the relapse rate. Patients in low expressed emotion (EE) families relapsed slightly more often during the psychosocial plus family intervention. Additional family intervention may increase stress in low EE families, thus affecting relapse in their children. Five-year follow-up of this group found no differential treatment effects with regard to the course of the illness but there was a significant benefit from family therapy in terms of the number of days spent in psychiatric institutions (Lenior et al. 2001).

Practitioner reviews emphasize the need for a range of psychosocial interventions: clear, accurate, and developmentally appropriate information to be made available to patients and their families; psychological interventions for the patient aimed at improving social skills, self-care, and problem solving; family-based interventions to improve family functioning and coping skills (McClellan and Werry 1997). However, there is little empirical evidence for these approaches and some suggestion that extrapolation from studies of adults is not always justified. Asarnow and colleagues (1994) did not find high levels of expressed emotion in the families of children with schizophrenia, suggesting interventions aimed at reducing expressed emotion may not be justified.

11.2.7.2   Mania and Bipolar Disorders

Comprehensive multimodal treatment programs which combine psychoeducation, supportive therapy for child and family, attention to comorbid conditions, and so on are recommended by most authorities but no research evidence supports these recommendations. Miklowitz and colleagues (1988) report that family factors such as expressed emotion and affective style do predict relapse in adult manic bipolar patients, suggesting a possible way forward.

Current best practice suggests a variety of other psychosocial interventions aimed at reducing social disruption, enabling developmental tasks to be seen through, supporting education, and reducing distress (Kafantaris 1995; McClellan and Werry 1997).

11.2.8   Autism

The definition of autism covers problems in three main areas of functioning, with onset in the first three years of life: (a) qualitative impairments in social interactions that may be apparent as failure to comprehend that others have feelings, lack of interest in imitative or social play, and inability to seek friendships or comfort from others; (b) qualitative impairments in verbal and nonverbal communication; (c) restriction of interests and a resistance to change, which may be expressed as an insistence on certain routines or a desire to take part in only a narrow range of interests or activities.

Physical treatments are sometimes required if behavioral therapies are insufficient. However, only a small number of drugs have so far been found to be effective in double-blind studies. Psychostimulants are promising drugs for hyperactivity in children with pervasive developmental disorders and there is an insignificant risk of serious adverse reactions (Birmaher et al. 1988). Haloperidol may reduce aggression, hyperactivity, and preoccupations but there is a risk of tardive dyskinesias and other side effects (Anderson et al. 1984; Campbell et al. 1978; Locascio et al. 1991). Naltrexone has been reported in two controlled studies to improve hyperactivity and disruptive behavior. In one controlled study, clomipramine was superior to placebo in reducing autistic withdrawal, preoccupations, hyperactivity, and oppositionality, and it was certainly more effective than desipramine (Gordon et al. 1993).

Effective behavioral treatments have been shown to reduce some of the secondary problems associated with autism (Anderson et al. 1987; Eikeseth et al. 2002; Howlin and Rutter 1987; Lovaas 1987; McEachin et al. 1993), but social and communicative abnormalities have so far proved more resistant to intervention (Howlin and Rutter 1987). The interventions need to provide a behavior program at home and at school, incorporating parent and teacher training. Expected benefits include persisting gains in IQ, improvements in daily living skills, communication and the ability to socialize, and a decrease of behavior problems. Studies have tended to focus on children under the age of 4 years at the time of commencing treatment, but it is unclear whether early commencement of treatment is a necessary condition for successful treatment. All the studies of behavioral interventions in autistic children have included a parent training approach and have been extended to community and school settings. There is emerging evidence that the behavioral component rather than intensity is responsible for change (Eikeseth et al. 2002). Despite a variety of approaches, there is no good evidence that individual social skills training significantly benefits autistic individuals (Campbell et al. 1996; Matson and Swiezy 1994). Play groups appear to be effective in promoting communication skills in children with autism (Cogher 1999) and improvements appear to generalize to settings outside the play group (Kohler et al. 1995), but there is inadequate evidence for the sustainability of these gains (Kok et al. 2002). A new promising line of studies is exploring interventions related to specific deficits of social cognition assumed to underpin many other behavioral dysfunctions, including the difficulty in engaging in a teaching-learning process (Hadwin et al. 1996, 1997; Howlin et al. 1999; Silver and Oakes 2001; Whalen and Schreibman 2003). Parent training and computer-aided training are both being explored in this area (Drew et al. 2002; Silver and Oakes 2001), and the field seems ripe for a large-scale, comprehensive treatment trial including parent and peer training components focused on social cognitive, rather than behavioral, deficits.

11.2.9   Eating Disorders

Anorexia nervosa is characterized by deliberate refusal to maintain body weight above a level that is 15% **below** that expected for the individual's age and height. The diagnostic criteria also include intense fear of becoming fat even though underweight; severe restriction of food intake, often with excessive exercising, distorted perception of body image and shape, and cessation of menstruation in postmenarchal women.

In children below the age of 15, Bryant-Waugh and Lask (1995) point out that about 25% of referrals to their clinic in London present disturbances of eating that do not fit the existing diagnostic

DSM-IV categories. The variants include selective eating, food-avoidance emotional disorder, and pervasive refusal syndrome. Studies in children and adolescents have led to the suggestion that anorexia nervosa and bulimia nervosa may be different symptom patterns of one basic eating disorder, in which preoccupation with food and a disturbed body image are core symptoms (van der Ham et al. 1994). However, there are no reports of prepubertal bulimia nervosa. Until very recently, very few cases with onset below the age of 14 have been noted (Schmidt et al. 1992).

Most behavioral approaches to anorexia nervosa combine operant techniques for weight gain with other treatment techniques aiming to alter irrational beliefs, disturbance of body image, anxiety, poor interpersonal skills, and dysfunctional eating behavior, and have been shown to be effective in short-term weight gain (Bemis 1987; Lacey 1983; Lee and Rush 1986; Wolchik et al. 1986). No particular benefit has been found of cognitive-behavioral treatments over other forms of brief psychotherapy (Fairburn et al. 1991). There is clinical consensus that multifaceted treatment programs are effective, but there has been little evaluation of the effects of different components of treatment for different patients.

There have been no published studies applying cognitive-behavioral therapy to bulimic children and adolescents, but, as with anorexia, it is likely that this approach may be effective with children and adolescents (typically by age 14 or 15) who have developed the level of cognitive skills and the ability to (a) think abstractly regarding attitudes and beliefs about the meaning of weight, shape, and appearance; (b) entertain alternative possible explanations to the one currently held; (c) be prepared to test out alternative hypotheses through practical exercises (Lewandowski et al. 1997; Turk 1993).

At 5-year follow-up, family therapy has been shown to be more successful than individual therapy in anorectic patients with onset before the age of 19 years and whose illness is not chronic (Robin et al. 1995; Russell et al. 1987). Family change may not be necessary to achieve individual change (Dare et al. 1990, 1994) and individual change appears to result in some family change (Robin et al. 1994, 1999). A controlled trial has compared family therapy with individual supportive therapy in cases of anorexia and bulimia nervosa (Russell et al. 1987). In older patients, individual supportive therapy tended to be more effective than family therapy in terms of weight gain, but the improvement fell short of recovery in most patients.

Steinhausen (1995) cautions that individual psychotherapy is unlikely to be of use in a young person with anorexia nervosa unless they have intact cognitions and sufficient motivation to undertake therapy. These are likely to be absent where the child is emaciated, when severe depression is present, when the course of the illness is chronic, when there is severe intellectual limitation, when the family sabotages therapeutic efforts, or with a very young preadolescent. Individual therapy shows benefit in those with late-onset anorexia and may contribute to the prevention of relapses after discharge from hospital treatment (Robin et al. 1995). The evidence for the efficacy of family therapy in bulimia is equivocal (Dodge et al. 1995; Russell et al. 1987). As yet there is no evidence for the efficacy of cognitive-behavioral treatment of bulimia in children and adolescents.

11.2.10 Deliberate Self-Harm

The definition of deliberate self-harm includes nonfatal or attempted suicide, but also life-threatening behaviors such as self-poisoning where the young person does not necessarily intend to take his or her own life. Diekstra and colleagues (1995) define parasuicide as »the term originally proposed by Kreitman (1977) to cover behaviors that can vary from what are sometimes called ›suicidal gestures‹ or ›manipulative attempts‹ to serious but unsuccessful attempts to kill oneself.«

There is some evidence that forms of brief intervention (problem solving) with the families of adolescents following a suicide attempt can improve adolescents' feelings of depression and suicidality and positive maternal attitudes towards treatment, thus enabling supportive family involvement and further compliance with specialist programs (Piacentini et al. 1995; Rotheram-Borus et al. 1996). Brief forms of intervention are only likely to be effective in subjects without major depression, who tend to have less severe forms of suicidal behavior, and studies of more intensive forms of family intervention are required to determine whether they are more effective in leading to better outcomes for the child (Harrington et al. 2000).

Rotheram-Borus (1999) reports a 6-month follow-up by structured telephone interview of 66 adolescents (13–17 years) hospitalized on an adolescent psychiatry inpatient unit with significant suicidal thoughts, intent, or behaviors. Compliance with recommended medication (66.7%) and individual therapy (50.8%) was better than compliance with parent guidance/family therapy sessions (33.3%). The most dysfunctional families and those with the least involved/affectionate father-adolescent relationships had the poorest follow-through with parent guidance/family therapy.

The only RCT on the treatment of repeated deliberate self-harm in adolescence was by Wood (2001). Randomization into a routine care or group therapy arm was successful for 63 (75% of eligible) referrals. Group therapy consisted of a »developmental« intervention focusing on age specific difficulties (e.g., relationships, school and family problems, anger management) incorporating CBT, dialectical behavior therapy (DBT), and psychodynamic group therapy techniques. Six acute group sessions were followed by long-term group (median = 8 sessions) sometimes augmented by individual sessions at times of crisis (median = 2.5). The risk of being a repeater after randomization was significantly reduced in group treatment (6% vs. 32%). This is equivalent to a number needed to treat (NNT) of 4% or average risk reduction of 26%. However, the group treatment was too brief and did not significantly reduce levels of depression or suicidal thinking. The follow-up of 7 months after baseline might be too brief to judge true treatment effects.

The evidence for effective approaches to the prevention of further suicide attempts in young people is extremely limited, although there is suggestive value from issuing an emergency room card allowing continuing ready access to skilled advice and help, following initial assessment and hospital admission (Cotgrove et al. 1995). Round-the-clock »hot-line« services have not been shown to reduce the incidence of suicide attempts among the populations served (Dew et al. 1987; Miller et al. 1984).

11.2.11 Specific Developmental Disorders

Specific developmental disorders involve delays or abnormalities affecting capacities that would normally have appeared by the age that the child has reached. These disorders cover communication (expressive and/or receptive language, or articulation), motor skills, and learning (reading, mathematics, written expression, or other academic skills).

The only traditional mental health treatment that has been evaluated for an specific developmental disorder (SDD) is psychoanalytic psychotherapy (Heinicke 1965; Heinicke and Ramsey-Klee 1986). In both studies, more intensive treatment (four sessions per week versus one session per week), for at least part of the therapy period, had a more lasting beneficial effect.

Psychological approaches are based on cognitive, cognitive-behavioral, task-analytic, neuropsychological, and constructivist models, although these approaches in fact overlap, with differences largely in emphasis (Hallahan et al. 1996). No single teaching method, treatment intervention, or combination of methods has been found to yield clinically significant, long-term gains (Lyon and Cutting 1998, p. 479).

Psychotherapeutic or other psychological therapies (such as social skills training) may be helpful in managing associated problems, such as demoralization, poor social skills, or social avoidance. It may be important, particularly in severe cases, for the material and activities used in therapy to be adapted to the SDD, with less reliance on verbal activity than might be usual. Support groups for children with SDDs may be helpful (Falik 1995).

11.3 Conclusion

Finally, a word about science and scientism in psychotherapy research. We all have a need for certainty and experience discomfort with not knowing and risk anxious retreat from ignorance into pseudo knowledge (so characteristic of the early years of medicine). A scientific approach has obviously been incredibly helpful and has saved many millions of lives. To argue against it is not just churlish, it is clearly unethical and destructive. But to argue for a mechanical reading of evidence, as some clinical psychologists have done (Chambless and Hollon 1998; Chambless et al. 1996) equally skirts the risk of doing harm.

Research evidence collected as part of the present initiative will need to be carefully weighed. Multiple channels for evaluation are needed and they need to be kept open and actively maintained. No self-respecting clinician will change their practice overnight. They would be unwise to do so. Evidence has to be read and evaluated, placed into the context of what is possible, desirable, and fits with existing opportunities. It should be remembered that in mental health at least, but also probably in most areas of clinical treatment, method accounts for a relatively small proportion of the variance in outcome relative to the nature of the patient's problem (Weisz et al. 1992, 1995), which may well interact with the skills of the attending clinician. This latter form of variance is to be cherished, not only because that is where the art of medicine lies, but also because it is in the study of that variability that future major advances in health care may be made, as long as we can submit these to empirical scrutiny.

References

Abikoff, H.B., and Gittelman, R. (1985) Hyperactive children treated with stimulants. Is cognitive training a useful adjunct? Arch Gen Psychiatry, 42(10), 953–961.

Abikoff, H.B., and Hechtman, L. (1996) Multimodal therapy and stimulants in the treatment of children with attention deficit hyperactivity disorder. In P.S. Jensen and E. D. Hibbs (Eds.), Psychosocial treatments for child and adolescent disorders: Empirically-based strategies for clinical practice (pp. 341–369) Washington, DC: American Psychological Association.

Abikoff, H., Ganeles, D., Reiter, G., Blum, C., Foley, C., and Klein, G. R. (1988) Cognitive training in academically deficient ADDH boys receiving stimulant medication. Journal of Abnormal Child Psychology, 16, 411–432.

American Academy of Child and Adolescent Psychiatry. (1998) Practice parameters for the assessment and treatment of children and adolescents with depressive disorders. Journal of the American Academy of Child and Adolescent Psychiatry, 37 (10 suppl.), 63S–83S.

American Psychiatric Association. (1994) Diagnostic and Statistical Manual of Mental Disorders (DSM-IV) (4 ed.). Washington, DC: American Psychiatric Association.

Anastopoulos, A.D., Shelton, T.L., DuPaul, G.J., and Guevremont, D.C. (1993) Parent training for attention-deficit hyperactivity disorder: Its impact on parent functioning. Journal of Abnormal Child Psychology, 21, 581–596.

Anastopoulos, A.D., Barkley, R.A., and Shelton, T.L. (1996) Family-based treatment: Psychosocial intervention for children and adolescents with attention deficit hyperactivity disorder. In E.D. Hibbs and P.S. Jensen (Eds.), Psychosocial treatments for child and adolescent disorders: Empirically-based strategies for clinical practice (pp. 267–284). Washington, DC: American Psychological Association.

Anderson, L.T., Campbell, M., Grega, D.M., Perry, R., Small, A. M., and Green, W.H. (1984) Haloperidol in the treatment of infantile autism: Effects on learning and behavioral symptoms. American Journal of Psychiatry, 141, 1195–1202.

Anderson, S.R., Avery, D.L., DiPietro, E.K., Edwards, G.L., and Christian, W.P. (1987) Intensive home based early intervention with autistic children. Education and Treatment of Children, 10, 352–366.

Asarnow, J.R., Tompson, M., Hamilton, E.B., Goldstein, M.J., and Guthrie, D. (1994) Family-expressed emotion, childhood-onset depression, and childhood-onset schizophrenia spectrum disorders: is expressed emotion a nonspecific correlate of child psychopathology or a specific risk factor for depression? J Abnorm Child Psychol, 22(2), 129–146.

Ayllon, T., Garber, S., and Pisor, K. (1975) The elimination of discipline problems through a combined school-home motivational system. Behavior Therapy, 6, 616–626.

Azrin, N.H., and Peterson, A.L. (1988) Habit reversal for the treatment of Tourette syndrome. Behavior Research and Therapy, 11, 347–355.

Azrin, N.H., and Peterson, A.L. (1990) Treatment of Tourette syndrome by Habit Reversal: A waiting-list control group comparison. Behavior Therapy, 21, 305–318.

Bank, L., Marlowe, J.H., Reid, J.B., Patterson, G.R., and Weinrott, M. R. (1991) A comparative evaluation of parent-training interventions for families of chronic delinquents. Journal of Abnormal Child Psychology, 19, 15–33.

Barkley, R.A., Shelton, T.L., Crosswait, C.C., Moorehouse, M., Fletcher, K., Barrett, S., et al. (2000) Multi-method psycho-educational intervention for preschool children with disruptive behavior: Preliminary results at post-treatment. Journal of Child Psychology and Psychiatry, 41, 319–332.

Barrett, P.M., Dadds, M.R., and Rapee, R.M. (1996) Family treatment for childhood anxiety: A controlled trial. Journal of Consulting and Clinical Psychology, 64, 333–342.

Barton, C., Alexander, J.F., Waldron, H., Turner, C.W., and Warburton, J. (1985) Generalizing treatment effects of Functional Family Therapy: Three replications. American Journal of Family Therapy, 13, 16–26.

Beitchman, J.H., Zucker, K.J., Hood, J.E., daCosta, G.A., and Akman, D. (1991) A review of the short-term effects of child sexual abuse. Child Abuse and Neglect, 15, 537–556.

Beitchman, J.H., Zucker, K.J., Hood, J.E., daCosta, G.A., Akman, D., and Cassavia, E. (1992) A review of the long-term effects of child sexual abuse. Child Abuse and Neglect, 16, 101–118.

Bell-Dolan, D.J., Last, C.G., and Strauss, C.C. (1990) Symptoms of anxiety disorders in normal children. Journal of the American Academy of Child Psychiatry, 29, 759–765.

Bemis, K.M. (1987) The present status of operant conditioning for the treatment of anorexia nervosa. Behavior Modification, 11, 432–463.

Berman, S.R., Weems, C., Silverman, W., and Kurtines, W. (2000) Predictors of outcome in exposure-based cognitive and behavioral treatments for phobic and anxiety disorders in children. Behavior Therapy, 31, 713–731.

Birmaher, B., Quintana, H., and Greenhill, L.L. (1988) Methylphenidate treatment of hyperactive autistic children. Journal of the American Academy of Child and Adolescent Psychiatry, 27, 248–251.

Birmaher, B., Brent, D.A., Kolko, D., Baugher, M., Bridge, J., Holder, D., et al. (2000) Clinical outcome after short-term psychotherapy for adolescents with major depressive disorder. Arch Gen Psychiatry, 57(1), 29–36.

Bolton, D., Collins, S., and Steinberg, D. (1983) The treatment of obsessive-compulsive disorder in adolescence: A report of fifteen cases. British Journal of Psychiatry, 142, 456–464.

Borduin, C.M. (1999) Multisystemic treatment of criminality and violence in adolescents. Journal of the American Academy for Child and Adolescent Psychiatry, 38, 242–249.

Bradley, S., Brody, J., Landy, S., Tallett, S., Watson, W., Shea, B., et al. (1999) Brief psychoeducational parenting program: An evaluation. Paper presented at the 46th Annual Meeting of the American Academy of Child and Adolescent Psychiatry, Chicago.

Brent, D.A., Holder, D., Kolko, D., Birmaher, B., Baugher, M., Roth, C., et al. (1997) A clinical psychotherapy trial for adolescent depression comparing cognitive, family and supportive therapy. Archives of General Psychiatry, 54, 877–885.

Brent, D.A., Kolko, D., Birmaher, B., Baugher, M., Bridge, J., Roth, C., et al. (1998) Predictors of treatment efficacy in a clinical trial of three psychosocial treatments for adolescent depression. Journal of the American Academy of Child and Adolescent Psychiatry, 37, 906–914.

Brent, D.A., Kolko, D., Birmaher, B., Baugher, M., and Bridge, J. (1999) A clinical trial for adolescent depression: Predictors of additional treatment in the acute and followup phases of the trial. Journal of the American Academy of Child and Adolescent Psychiatry, 38, 263–270.

Brown, R.T., Wynne, M.E., Borden, K.A., Clingerman, S.R., Geniesse, R., and Spunt, A.L. (1986) Methylphenidate and cognitive therapy in children with attention deficit disorder: a double-blind trial. J Dev Behav Pediatr, 7(3), 163–174.

Bryant-Waugh, R., and Lask, B. (1995) Annotation: Eating disorders in children. Journal of Child Psychology and Psychiatry, 36(2), 191–202.

Campbell, M., Schopler, E., Cueva, J.E., and Hallin, A. (1996) Treatment of autistic disorder. Journal of the American Academy of Child and Adolescent Psychiatry, 35, 134–143.

Campbell, M., Anderson, L.T., Meier, M., Cohen, I.L., Small, A.M., Samit, C., et al. (1978) A comparison of haloperidol and behavior therapy and their interaction in autistic children. Journal of the American Academy of Child and Adolescent Psychiatry, 17, 640–655.

Carrion, V.G., Weems, C.F., Ray, R., and Reiss, A.L. (2002) Toward an empirical definition of pediatric PTSD: the phenomenology of PTSD symptoms in youth. J Am Acad Child Adolesc Psychiatry, 41(2), 166–173.

Chamberlain, P., and Reid, J.B. (1998) Comparison of two community alternatives to incarceration for chronic juvenile offenders. Journal of Consulting and Clinical Psychology, 66, 624–633.

Chamberlain, P., and Rozicky, J.G. (1995) The effectiveness of family therapy in the treatment of adolescents with conduct disorders and delinquency. Journal of Marital and Family Therapy, 21, 441–459.

Chambless, D.L., and Hollon, S. (1998) Defining empirically supported therapies. Journal of Consulting and Clinical Psychology, 66, 7–18.

Chambless, D.L., Sanderson, W.C., Shoham, V., Johnson, S.B., Pope, K.S., Crits-Christoph, P., et al. (1996) An update on clinically validated therapies. The Clinical Psychologist, 49, 5–18.

Chemtob, C.M., Nakashima, J.P., and Carlson, J.G. (2002) Brief treatment for elementary school children with disaster-related posttraumatic stress disorder: a field study. J Clin Psychol, 58(1), 99–112.

Chemtob, C.M., Nakashima, J.P., and Hamada, R.S. (2002) Psychosocial intervention for postdisaster trauma symptoms in elementary school children: a controlled community field study. Arch Pediatr Adolesc Med, 156(3), 211–216.

Clarke, G.N., Rohde, P., Lewinsohn, P.M., Hops, H., and Seeley, J.R. (1999) Cognitive-behavioral treatment of adolescent depression: Efficacy of acute group treatment and booster sessions. Journal of the American Academy of Child and Adolescent Psychiatry, 38, 272–279.

Cobham, V.E., Dadds, M.R., and Spence, S.H. (1998) The role of parental anxiety in the treatment of childhood anxiety. Journal of Consulting and Clinical Psychology, 66, 893–905.

Cogher, L. (1999) The use of non-directive play in speech and language therapy. Child Language Teaching and Therapy, 15(1), 7–15.

Cohen, J.A., and Mannarino, A.P. (1996) A treatment outcome study for sexually abused preschool children: initial findings. J Am Acad Child Adolesc Psychiatry, 35(1), 42–50.

Cohen, J.A., and Mannarino, A.P. (1998) Interventions for sexually abused children: Initial treatment outcome findings. Child Maltreatment: Journal of the American Professional Society on the Abuse of Children, 3(1), 17–26.

Comings, D.E., and Comings, B.G. (1985) Tourette Syndrome: Clinical and psychological aspects of 250 cases. American Journal of Human Genetics, 37, 435–450.

Cotgrove, A.J., Zirinsky, L., Black, D., and Weston, D. (1995) Secondary prevention of attempted suicide in adolescence. Journal of Adolescence, 18, 569–577.

Cousins, L.S., and Weiss, G. (1993) Parent training and social skills training for children with attention-deficit hyperactivity disorder. How can they be combined for greater effectiveness? Canadian Journal of Psychiatry. Revue Canadienne de Psychiatrie, 38, 449–457.

Crawford, A.M., and Manassis, K. (2001) Familial predictors of treatment outcome in childhood anxiety disorders. Journal of the American Academy Child and Adolescent Psychiatry, 40, 1182–1189.

Cunningham, C.E., Bremner, R., and Boyle, M. (1995) Large group community-based parenting programs for family of preschoolers at risk for disruptive behavior disorders: Utilization, cost-effectiveness and outcome. Journal of Child Psychology and Psychiatry, 36, 1141–1159.

Dadds, M.R., Schwartz, S., and Sanders, M.R. (1987) Marital discord and treatment outcome in behavioral treatment of child conduct disorders. Journal of Consulting and Clinical Psychology, 55, 396–403.

Dare, C., Eisler, I., Russell, G., and Szmukler, G. (1990) The clinical and theoretical impact of a controlled trial of family therapy in anorexia nervosa. Journal of Marital and Family Therapy, 16, 39–57.

Dare, C., Le Grange, D., Eisler, I., and Rutherford, J. (1994) Redefining the psychosomatic family: Family process of 26 eating disorder families. International Journal of Eating Disorder, 16(3), 211–226.

Deblinger, E., Lippmann, J., and Steer, R. (1996) Sexually abused children suffering post traumatic stress symptoms. Child Maltreatment, 1, 310–321.

Deblinger, E., Steer, R. A., and Lippmann, J. (1999) Two-year followup study of cognitive behavioral therapy for sexually abused children suffering post-traumatic stress symptoms. Child Abuse Negl, 23(12), 1371–1378.

Deblinger, E., Stauffer, L. B., and Steer, R. A. (2001) Comparative efficacies of supportive and cognitive behavioral group therapies for young children who have been sexually abused and their nonoffending mothers. Child Maltreatment: Journal of the American Professional Society on the Abuse of Children, 6(4), 332–343.

Deitz, S. M. (1985) Good Behavior Game. In A. S. Bellack and M. Hersen (Eds.), Dictionary of behavior therapy techniques (pp. 131–132). New York: Pergamon Press.

Delaney-Black, V., Covington, C., Ondersma, S. J., Nordstrom-Klee, B., Templin, T., Ager, J., et al. (2002) Violence exposure, trauma, and IQ and/or reading deficits among urban children. Arch Pediatr Adolesc Med, 156(3), 280–285.

Department of Health (2001) Treatment choice in psychological therapies and counselling: Evidence based clinical practice guideline. London: Department of Health.

DeVeaugh-Geiss, J., Moroz, G., Biederman, J., Cantwell, D. P., Fontaine, R., Greist, J. H., et al. (1992) Clomipramine in child and adolescent obsessive-compulsive disorder: A multicenter trial. Journal of the American Academy of Child and Adolescent Psychiatry, 31, 45–49.

Dew, M. A., Bromet, E. J., Brent, D., and Greenhouse, J. B. (1987) A quantitative literature review of the effectiveness of suicide prevention centers. Journal of Consulting and Clinical Psychology, 55, 239–244.

Diekstra, R. F. W., Kienhorst, C. W. M., and de Wilde, E. J. (1995) Suicide and suicidal behavior among adolescents. In M. Rutter and D. J. Smith (Eds.), Psychosocial Disorders in Young People: Time Trends and their Causes (pp. 686–761). Chichester: Wiley.

Dishion, T. J., and Andrews, D. W. (1995) Preventing escalation in problem behaviors with high-risk young adolescents: Immediate and 1-year outcomes. Journal of Consulting and Clinical Psychology, 63, 538–548.

Dodge, E., Hodes, M., Eisler, I., and Dare, C. (1995) Family therapy for bulimia nervosa in adolescents: An exploratory study. Journal of Family Therapy, 17, 59–77.

Drew, A., Baird, G., Baron-Cohen, S., Cox, A., Slonims, V., Wheelwright, S., et al. (2002) A pilot randomized control trial of a parent training intervention for pre-school children with autism. Preliminary findings and methodological challenges. Eur Child Adolesc Psychiatry, 11(6), 266–272.

Ducharme, J. M., Atkinson, L., and Poulton, L. (2000) Success-based, noncoercive treatment of oppositional behavior in children from violent homes. J Am Acad Child Adolesc Psychiatry, 39(8), 995–1004.

Dumas, J. E., and Albin, J. B. (1986) Parent training outcome: Does active parental involvement matter? Behavior Research and Therapy, 24, 227–230.

Eikeseth, S., Smith, T., Jahr, E., and Eldevik, S. (2002) Intensive behavioral treatment at school for 4- to 7-year-old children with autism: A 1-year comparison controlled study. Behavior Modification, 26(1), 49–68.

Esbensen, F. A., and Osgood, D. W. (1999) Gang resistance education and training (GREAT): Results from the national evaluation. Journal of Research in Crime and Delinquency, 36, 194–225.

Fairburn, C. G., Jones, R., Peveler, R. C., Carr, S. J., Solomon, R. A., O'Connor, M. E., et al. (1991) Three psychological treatments for bulimia nervosa: A comparative trial. Archives of General Psychiatry, 48, 463–469.

Falik, L. H. (1995) Family patterns of reaction to a child with a learning disability: A mediational perspective. Journal of Learning Disabilities, 28, 335–341.

Farmer, E. M., Compton, S. N., Bums, B. J., and Robertson, E. (2002) Review of the evidence base for treatment of childhood psychopathology: externalizing disorders. J Consult Clin Psychol, 70(6), 1267–1302.

Farrell, A. D., and Bruce, S. E. (1997) Impact of exposure to community violence on violent behavior and emotional distress among urban adolescents. J Clin Child Psychol, 26(1), 2–14.

Feindler, E. L., Marriott, S. A., and Iwata, M. (1984) Group anger control training for junior high school delinquents. Cognitive Therapy and Research, 8, 299–311.

Flament, M. F., Koby, E., Rapoport, J. L., Berg, C. J., Zahn, T., Cox, C., et al. (1990) Childhood compulsive disorder: A prospective followup study. Journal of Child Psychology and Psychiatry, 31, 363–380.

Flannery-Schroeder, E. C., and Kendall, P. C. (2000) Group and individual cognitive-behavioral treatments for youth with anxiety disorders: A randomized controlled trial. Cognitive Therapy and Research, 24(3), 251–2781.

Fonagy, P., Target, M., Cottrell, D., Phillips, J., and Kurtz, Z. (2002) What Works For Whom? A Critical Review of Treatments for Children and Adolescents. New York: Guilford.

Forehand, R., and Long, N. (1988) Outpatient treatment of the acting out child: Procedures, long-term followup data, and clinical problems. Advances in Behavior Research and Therapy, 10, 129–177.

Goenjian, A. K., Karayan, I., Pynoos, R. S., Minassian, D., Najarian, L. M., Steinberg, A. M., et al. (1997) Outcome of psychotherapy among early adolescents after trauma. Am J Psychiatry, 154(4), 536–542.

Gordon, C. T., State, R. C., Nelson, J. E., Hamburger, S. D., and Rapoport, J. L. (1993) A double-blind comparison of clomipramine, desipramine, and placebo in the treatment of autistic disorder. Archives of General Psychiatry, 50, 441–447.

Gordon, D. A., Arbuthnot, J., Gustafson, K. E., and McGreen, P. (1988) Home-based systems-systems family therapy with disadvantaged juvenile delinquents. American Journal of Family Therapy, 16, 243–255.

Gordon, D. A., Graves, K., and Arbuthnot, J. (1995) The effect of Functional Family Therapy for delinquents on adult criminal behavior. Criminal Justice and Behavior, 22, 60–73.

Gottfredson, D. C., and Gottfredson, G. D. (1992) Theory-guided investigation: Three field experiments. In J. McCord and R. E. Tremblay (Eds.), Preventing antisocial behavior: Interventions from birth through adolescence (pp. 311–329). New York: Guilford.

Guerra, N., and Slaby, R. G. (1990) Cognitive mediators of aggression in adolescent offenders: II. Intervention. Developmental Psychology, 26, 269–277.

Hadwin, J., Baron Cohen, S., Howlin, P., and Hill, K. (1996) Can we teach children with autism to understand emotions, belief, or pretence? Development and Psychopathology, 8(2), 345–365.

Hadwin, J., Baron-Cohen, S., Howlin, P., and Hill, K. (1997) Does teaching theory of mind have an effect on the ability to develop conversation in children with autism? J Autism Dev Disord, 27(5), 519–537.

Hallahan, D. P., Kauffman, J., and Lloyd, J. (1996) Introduction to Learning Disabilities. Needham Heights, MA: Allyn and Bacon.

Harrington, R., Whittaker, J., Shoebridge, P., and Campbell, F. (1998) Systematic review of efficacy of cognitive behavior therapies in childhood and adolescent depressive disorder. British Medical Journal, 316, 1559–1563.

Harrington, R., Kerfoot, M., Dyer, E., McNiven, F., Gill, J., Harrington, V., et al. (2000) Deliberate self-poisoning in adolescence: Why does a brief family intervention work in some cases and not others? Journal of Adolescence, 23, 13–20.

Hartman, R. R., Stage, S. A., and Webster-Stratton, C. (2003) A growth curve analysis of parent training outcomes: examining the influence of child risk factors (inattention, impulsivity, and hyperactivity problems), parental and family risk factors. J Child Psychol Psychiatry, 44(3), 388–398.

Hazell, P. L., and Stuart, J. E. (2003) A randomized controlled trial of clonidine added to psychostimulant medication for hyperactive and aggressive children. J Am Acad Child Adolesc Psychiatry, 42(8), 886–894.

Heinicke, C. M. (1965) Frequency of psychotherapeutic session as a factor affecting the child's developmental status. The Psychoanalytic Study of the Child 20, 42–98.

Heinicke, C. M., and Ramsey-Klee, D. M. (1986) Outcome of child psychotherapy as a function of frequency of sessions. Journal of the American Academy of Child Psychiatry, 25, 247–253.

Henggeler, S. W., Rodick, J., Borduin, C. M., Hanson, C., Watson, S., and Urey, J. (1986) Multisystemic treatment of juvenile offenders: Effects on adolescent behavior and family interaction. Developmental Psychology, 22, 132–141.

Henggeler, S. W., Melton, G. B., and Smith, L. A. (1992) Family preservation using multisystemic therapy: An effective alternative to incarcerating serious juvenile offenders. Journal of Consulting and Clinical Psychology, 60, 953–961.

Henggeler, S. W., Melton, G. B., Smith, L. A., Schoenwald, S. K., and Hanley, J. H. (1993) Family preservation using multisystemic treatment: Long-term followup to a clinical trial with serious juvenile offenders. Journal of Child and Family Studies, 2, 283–293.

Henggeler, S. W., Cunningham, P. B., Pickrel, S. G., Schoenwald, S. K., and Brondino, M. J. (1996) Multisystemic therapy: An effective violence prevention approach for serious juvenile offenders. Journal of Adolescence, 19, 47–61.

Henggeler, S. W., Pickrel, S. G., Brondino, M. J., and Crouch, J. L. (1996) Eliminating (almost) treatment dropout of substance abusing or dependent delinquents through home-based multisystemic therapy. American Journal of Psychiatry, 153, 427–428.

Hinshaw, S. P., Owens, E. B., Wells, K. C., Kraemer, H. C., Abikoff, H. B., Arnold, L. E., et al. (2000) Family processes and treatment outcome in the MTA: negative/ineffective parenting practices in relation to multimodal treatment. J Abnorm Child Psychol, 28(6), 555–568.

Hoath, F., and Sanders, M. (2002) A feasibility study of Enhanced Group Triple P – Positive parenting program for parents of children with attention-deficit/hyperactivity disorder. Behavior Change 19, 191–206.

Holden, G. W., Lavigne, V. V., and Cameron, A. M. (1990) Probing the continuum of effectiveness in parent training: Characteristics of parents and preschoolers. Journal of Clinical Child Psychology, 19, 2–8.

Horn, W. F., Ialongo, N. S., Pascoe, J. M., Greenberg, G., Packard, T., Lopez, M., et al. (1991) Additive effects of psychostimulants, parent training, and self-control therapy with ADHD children. J Am Acad Child Adolesc Psychiatry, 30(2), 233–240.

Howard, B. L., and Kendall, P. C. (1996) Cognitive-behavioral family therapy for anxiety-disordered children: A multiple-baseline evaluation. Cognitive Therapy and Research, 20, 423–443.

Howlin, P., and Rutter, M. (1987) Treatment of Autistic Children. Chichester: Wiley.

Howlin, P., Baron-Cohen, S., and Hadwin, J. (1999) Teaching children with autism to mind-read: A practical guide. Chichester: Wiley.

Huey, W. C., and Rank, R. C. (1984) Effects of counselor and peer-led group assertiveness training on black adolescent aggression. Journal of Counseling Psychology, 31, 95–98.

Ialongo, N. S., Horn, W. F., Pascoe, J. M., Greenberg, G., Packard, T., Lopez, M., et al. (1993) The effects of a multimodal intervention with attention-deficit hyperactivity disorder children: a 9-month followup. J Am Acad Child Adolesc Psychiatry, 32(1), 182–189.

Ialongo, N. S., Edelsohn, G., Werthamer-Larsson, L., Crockett, L., and Kellam, S. (1994) The significance of self-reported anxious symptoms in first-grade children. Journal of Abnormal Child Psychology, 22, 441–455.

Ialongo, N. S., Edelsohn, G., Werthamer-Larsson, L., Crockett, L., and Kellam, S. (1995) The significance of self-reported anxious symptoms in first-grade children: Prediction to anxious symptoms and adaptive functioning in fifth grade. Journal of Child Psychology and Psychiatry, 36, 427–437.

Jensen, P. S., Hinshaw, S. P., Kraemer, H. C., Lenora, N., Newcorn, J. H., Abikoff, H. B., et al. (2001) ADHD comorbidity findings from the MTA study: comparing comorbid sub-groups. J Am Acad Child Adolesc Psychiatry, 40(2), 147–158.

Kafantaris, V. (1995) Treatment of bipolar disorder in children and adolescents. Journal of the American Academy of Child and Adolescent Psychiatry, 34, 732–741.

Kahle, A. L., and Kelley, M. L. (1994) Children's homework problems: A comparison of goal setting and parent training. Behavior Therapy, 25, 275–290.

Kazdin, A. E. (1995) Child, parent, and family dysfunction as predictors of outcome in cognitive-behavioral treatment of antisocial children. Behavioral Research and Therapy, 33, 271–281.

Kazdin, A. E. (1995) Conduct disorder in childhood and adolescence (2 ed.). Thousand Oaks, CA: Sage.

Kazdin, A. E. (1996) Problem solving and parent management in treating aggressive and antisocial behavior. In E.S. Hibbs and P.S. Jensen (Eds.), Psychosocial treatments for child and adolescent disorders: Empirically based strategies for clinical practice (pp. 377–408). Washington, DC: American Psychological Association.

Kazdin, A. E., and Wasser, G. (2000) Therapeutic changes in children, parents and families resulting from treatment of children with conduct problems. Journal of the American Academy of Child and Adolescent Psychiatry, 39(4), 414–420.

Kazdin, A. E., and Whitley, M. K. (2003) Treatment of parental stress to enhance therapeutic change among children referred for aggressive and antisocial behavior. J Consult Clin Psychol, 71(3), 504–515.

Kazdin, A. E., Siegel, T. C., and Bass, D. (1992) Cognitive problem-solving skills training and parent management training in the treatment of antisocial behavior in children. Journal of Consulting and Clinical Psychology, 60, 733–747.

Kazdin, A. E., Mazurick, J. L., and Siegel, T. C. (1994) Treatment outcome among children with externalising disorder who terminate prematurely versus those who complete psychotherapy. Journal of the American Academy of Child and Adolescent Psychiatry, 33, 549–557.

Kazdin, A. E., Holland, L., and Crowley, M. (1997) Family experience of barriers to treatment and premature termination from child therapy. Journal of Consulting and Clinical Psychology, 65, 453–463.

Kendall, P. C., Flannery-Schroeder, E., Panichelli-Mindel, S. M., Southam-Gerow, M. A., Henin, A., and Warman, M. (1997) Therapy for youths with anxiety disorders: A second randomized clinical trial. Journal of Consulting and Clinical Psychology, 65, 366–380.

Kendall, P. C., Brady, E., and Verduin, T. (2001) Comorbidity in childhod anxiety disorders and treatment outcome. Journal of the American Academy Child and Adolescent Psychiatry, 40, 787–794.

King, N., Tonge, B. J., Heyne, D., Turner, S. M., Pritchard, M. D. Y., et al. (2001) Cognitive-behavioral treatment of school-refusing children: maintenance of improvement at 3- to 5-year followup. Scandinavian Journal of Behavior Therapy, 30, 85–89.

King, N. J., Tonge, B. J., Heyne, D., Pritchard, M., Rollings, S., Young, D., et al. (1998) Cognitive-behavioral treatment of school-refusing children: A controlled evaluation. Journal of the American Academy of Child and Adolescent Psychiatry, 37, 395–403.

Kliewer, W., Lepore, S. J., Oskin, D., and Johnson, P. D. (1998) The role of social and cognitive processes in children's adjustment to community violence. J Consult Clin Psychol, 66(1), 199–209.

Kohler, F. W., Strain, P. S., Hoyson, M., Davis, L., Donina, W. M., and Rapp, N. (1995) Using a group-oriented contingency to increase social interactions between children with autism and their peers. Behavior Modification, 19, 10–32.

Kok, A. J., Kong, T. Y., and Bernard-Opitz, V. (2002) A comparison of the effects of structured play and facilitated play approaches on preschoolers with autism. A case study. Autism, 6(2), 181–196.

Kovacs, M., and Devlin, B. (1998) Internalizing disorders in childhood. Journal of Child Psychology and Psychiatry, 39, 47–63.

Kreitman, N. (1977) Parasuicide. London: Wiley.

Kroll, L., Harrington, R., Jayson, D., Fraser, J., and Gowers, S. (1996) Pilot study of continuation cognitive-behavioral therapy for major depression in adolescent psychiatric patients. Journal of the American Academy of Child and Adolescent Psychiatry, 35, 1156–1161.

Lacey, J. H. (1983) Bulimia nervosa, binge eating and psychogenic vomiting: A controlled treatment study and long-term outcome. British Medical Journal, 286, 1609–1613.

Lahey, B. B., and Carlson, C. (1992) Validity of the diagnostic category of attention deficit disorder without hyperactivity: a review of the literature. In S. E. Shaywitz and B. A. Shaywitz (Eds.), Attention Deficit Disorder Comes of Age: Toward the Twenty- First Century (pp. 119–144). Austin, TX: Pro-ed.

Last, C. G., Hansen, C., and Franco, N. (1998) Cognitive-behavioral treatment of school phobia. Journal of the American Academy of Child and Adolescent Psychiatry, 37, 404–411.

Layne, A. E., Bernstein, G. A., Egan, E. A., and Kushner, M. G. (2003) Predictors of treatment response in anxious-depressed adolescents with school refusal. Journal of the American Academy Child and Adolescent Psychiatry, 42, 319–326.

Layne, C. M., Pynoos, R. S., Saltzman, W. R., Arslanagic, B., Black, M., Savjak, N., et al. (2001) Trauma/grief-focused group psychotherapy: School-based postwar intervention with traumatized Bosnian adolescents. Group Dynamics, 5(4), 277–290.

Leckman, J. F., and Cohen, D. J. (1994) Tic Disorders. In M. Rutter, E. Taylor and L. Hersov (Eds.), Child and Adolescent Psychiatry; Modern approaches. (pp. 455–466). Oxford: Blackwell Scientific Publications.

Lee, N. F., and Rush, A. J. (1986) Cognitive-behavioral group therapy for bulimia. International Journal of Eating Disorders, 5(4), 599–615.

Lenior, M. E., Dingemans, P. M. A. J., Linszen, D. H., de Haan, L., and Schene, A. H. (2001) Social functioning and the course of early-onset schizophrenia: Five-year followup of a psychosocial intervention. British Journal of Psychiatry, 179, 53–58.

Lewandowski, L.M., Gebing, T.A., Anthony, J.L., and O'Brien, W.H. (1997) Meta-analysis of cognitive-behavioral treatment studies for bulimia. Clinical Psychology Review, 17, 703–718.

Lewinsohn, P.M., Antonuccio, D.O., Steinmetz-Breckenridge, J., and Teri, L. (1984) The coping with depression course: A psychoeducational intervention for unipolar depression. Eugene, OR: Castalia Press.

Lewinsohn, P.M., Clarke, G.N., Hops, H., and Andrews, J. (1990) Cognitive-behavioral treatment for depressed adolescents. Behavior Therapy, 21, 385–401.

Lewinsohn, P.M., Clarke, G.N., and Rohde, P. (1994) Psychological approaches to the treatment of depression in adolescents. In W.M. Reynolds and H.F. Johnston (Eds.), Handbook of depression in children and adolescents (pp. 309–344). New York: Plenum Press.

Linszen, D., Dingemans, P., Van der Does, J.W., Nugter, A., Scholte, P., Lenior, R., et al. (1996) Treatment, expressed emotion and relapse in recent onset schizophrenic disorders. Psychol Med, 26(2), 333–342.

Locascio, J.L., Malone, R.P., Small, A.M., Kafantaris, V., Ernst, M., Lynch, N.S., et al. (1991) Factors related to haloperidol response and dyskinesias in autistic children. Psychopharmacology Bulletin, 27, 119–126.

Lochman, J.E., Coie, J.D., Underwood, M.K., and Terry, R. (1993) Effectiveness of a social relations intervention program for aggressive and nonaggressive, rejected children. Journal of Consulting and Clinical Psychology, 61, 1053–1058.

Long, P., Forehand, R., Wierson, M., and Morgan, A. (1994) Moving into adulthood: Does parent training with young noncompliant children have long-term effects? Behavior Research and Therapy, 32, 101–107.

Lovaas, O.L. (1987) Behavioral treatment and normal educational and intellectual functioning in young autistic children. Journal of Consulting and Clinical Psychology, 55, 3–9.

Lutzker, J.R. (1996) Timeout from emotion, time for science: a response to Kemp. Child Fam Behav Ther, 18, 29–34.

Lyon, G.R., and Cutting, L.E. (1998) Learning disabilities. In E.J. Mash and R.A. Barkley (Eds.), Treatment of Childhood Disorders (pp. 468–498). New York: Guilford.

Manassis, K., Mendlowitz, S.L., Scapillato, D., Avery, D., Fiksenbaum, L., Freire, M., et al. (2002) Group and individual cognitive-behavioral therapy for childhood anxiety disorders:a randomized trial. Journal of the American Academy Child and Adolescent Psychiatry, 41, 1423–1430.

March, J.S. (1995) Cognitive-behavioral psychotherapy for children and adolescents with OCD: a review and recommendations for treatment. Journal of the American Academy Child and Adolescent Psychiatry, 34, 7–18.

March, J.S., and Mulle, K. (1995) Behavioral psychotherapy for obsessive-compulsive disorder: A preliminary single-case study. Journal of Anxiety Disorders, 9, 175–184.

March, J.S., and Leonard, H.L. (1996) Obsessive-compulsive disorder in children and adolescents: a review of the past 10 years. Journal of the American Academy of Child and Adolescent Psychiatry, 35, 1265–1273.

March, J.S., Mulle, K., and Herbel, B. (1994) Behavioral psychotherapy for children and adolescents with obsessive-compulsive disorder: An open trial of a new protocol-driven treatment package. Journal of the American Academy of Child and Adolescent Psychiatry, 33, 333–341.

March, J.S., Amaya-Jackson, L., Murray, M.C., and Schulte, A. (1998) Cognitive-behavioral psychotherapy for children and adolescents with posttraumatic stress disorder after a single-incident stressor. J Am Acad Child Adolesc Psychiatry, 37(6), 585–593.

March, J.S., Swanson, J.M., Arnold, L.E., Hoza, B., Conners, C.K., Hinshaw, S.P., et al. (2000) Anxiety as a predictor and outcome variable in the multimodal treatment study of children with ADHD (MTA). J Abnorm Child Psychol, 28(6), 527–541.

March, J.S., Franklin, M., Nelson, A., and Foa, E. (2001) Cognitive-behavioral psychotherapy for pediatric obsessive-compulsive disorder. J Clin Child Psychol, 30(1), 8–18.

Matson, J.L., and Swiezy, N. (1994) Social skills training with autistic children. In J.L. Matson (Ed.), Autism in children and adults: Etiology assessment and intervention. (pp. 241–260). Pacific grove, CA: Brooks/Cole.

McClellan, J., and Werry, J.S. (1997) Practice parameters for the assessment and treatment of children and adolescents with schizophrenia. Journal of the American Academy of Child and Adolescent Psychiatry, 36 (Supplement 10), 177S-193S.

McEachin, J.J., Smith, T., and Lovaas, O.I. (1993) Long-term outcome for children with autism who received early intensive behavioral treatment. American Journal on Mental Retardation, 97, 359–372.

McMahon, R.J., Forehand, R., Griest, D.L., and Wells, K.C. (1981) Who drops out of treatment during parent behavioral training? Behavioral Counselling Quarterly, 1, 79–95.

Miklowitz, D.J., Goldstein, M.J., Neuchterlein, K.H., Snyder, K.S., and Mintz, J. (1988) Family factors and the course of bipolar affective disorder. Archives of General Psychiatry, 45, 225–231.

Miller, G.E., and Prinz, R.J. (1990) Enhancement of social learning family interventions for childhood Conduct Disorder. Psychological Bulletin, 108, 291–307.

Miller, H.L., Coombs, D.W., Leeper, J.D., and Barton, S.N. (1984) An analysis of the effects of suicide prevention facilities on suicide rates in the United States. American Journal of Public Health, 74, 340–343.

Moffitt, T.E., Caspi, A., Dickson, N., Silva, P., and Stanton, W. (1996) Childhood-onset versus adolescent-onset antisocial problems in males: natural history from ages 3 to 18 years. Developmental Psychopathology, 9, 399–424.

Moreau, D., Mufson, L., Weissman, M.M., and Klerman, G.L. (1991) Interpersonal psychotherapy for adolescent depression: Description of modification and preliminary application. Journal of the American Academy of Child and Adolescent Psychiatry, 30, 642–651.

MTA (1999) A 14-month randomized clinical trial of treatment strategies for attention-deficit/hyperactivity disorder. The MTA Cooperative Group. Multimodal Treatment Study of Children with ADHD. Arch Gen Psychiatry, 56(12), 1073–1086.

Mufson, L., Moreau, D., Weissman, M.M., Wickramaratne, P., Martin, J., and Samoilov, A. (1994) Modification of interpersonal psychotherapy with depressed adolescents (IPT-A): Phase I and II studies. Journal of the American Academy of Child and Adolescent Psychiatry, 33, 695–705.

Mufson, L., Weissman, M.M., Moreau, D., and Garfinkel, R. (1999) Efficacy of interpersonal psychotherapy for depressed adolescents. Archives of General Psychiatry, 56, 573–579.

Muris, P., Meesters, C., Merckelbach, H., Sermon, A., and Zwakhalen, S. (1998) Worry in normal children. Journal of the American Academy of Child and Adolescent Psychiatry, 37, 703–710.

NHS Executive (1996) NHS Psychotherapy services in England: Review of Strategic Policy. London: NHSE.

Nixon, R.D., Sweeney, L., Erickson, D.B., and Touyz, S.W. (2003) Parent-child interaction therapy: a comparison of standard and abbreviated treatments for oppositional defiant preschoolers. J Consult Clin Psychol, 71(2), 251–260.

Nugent, W.R., Carpenter, D., and Parks, J. (1993) A statewide evaluation of family preservation and family reunification services. Research on Social Work Practice, 3, 40–65.

Nye, C.L., Zucker, R.A., and Fitzgerald, H.E. (1995) Early intervention in the path to alcohol problems through conduct problems: Treatment involvement and child behavior change. Journal of Consulting and Clinical Psychology, 63, 831–840.

Ollendick, T.H., and King, N.J. (1998) Empirically supported treatments for children with phobic and anxiety disorders. Journal of Clinical Child Psychology, 27, 156–167.

Owens, E.B., Hinshaw, S.P., Kraemer, H.C., Arnold, L.E., Abikoff, H.B., Cantwell, D.P., et al. (2003) Which treatment for whom for ADHD? Moderators of treatment response in the MTA. J Consult Clin Psychol, 71(3), 540–552.

Patterson, G. (1982) Coercive family processes. Aegean, OR: Castilia Publishing Co.

Patterson, G.R., and Chamberlain, P. (1988) Treatment process: A problem at three levels. In L.C. Wynne (Ed.), The state of the art in family therapy research: Controversies and recommendations (pp. 189–223). New York: Family Process Press.

Pelham, W.E., and Hoza, B. (1996) Comprehensive treatment for ADHD: A proposal for intensive summer treatment programs and outpatient followup. In E. Hibbs and P. Jensen (Eds.), Psychosocial treatment research of child and adolescent disorders. Washington, DC: American Psychiatric Assocation.

Piacentini, J., Rotheram-Borus, M.J., and Cantwell, C. (1995) Brief cognitive-behavioral family therapy for suicidal adolescents. In L. VandeCreek, S. Knapp and T. Jackson (Eds.), Innovations in Clinical Practice: A Source Book (Vol. 14, pp. 151–168) Sarasota, FL: Professional Resource Press.

Pisterman, S., McGrath, P., Firestone, P., Goodman, J.T., Webster, I., and Mallory, R. (1989) Outcome of parent-mediated treatment of preschoolers with attention deficit disorder with hyperactivity. Journal of Consulting and Clinical Psychology, 57, 628–635.

Pisterman, S., Firestone, P., McGrath, P., Goodman, J.T., Webster, I., Mallory, R., et al. (1992) The role of parent training in treatment of preschoolers with ADDH. American Journal of Orthopsychiatry, 62, 397–408.

Pollack, M.H., Otto, M.W., Sabatino, S., Majcher, D., Worthington, J.J., McArdle, E.T., et al. (1996) Relationship of childhood anxiety to adult panic disorder: Correlates and influence on course. American Journal of Psychiatry, 153, 376–381.

Quay, H.C., and LaGreca, A.M. (1986) Disorders of anxiety, withdrawal, and dysphoria. In H.C. Quay and J.S. Werry (Eds.), Psychopathological Disorders of Childhood (3rd ed., pp. 111–155) New York: Wiley.

Quinn, M.M., Kavale, K.A., Mathur, S.R., Rutherford, R.B., and Forness, S.R. (1999) A meta-analysis of social skill interventions for students with emotional or behavioral disorders. Journal of Emotional and Behavioral Disorders, 7, 54–64.

Raue, J., and Spence, S.H. (1985) Group versus individual applications of reciprocity training for parent-youth conflict. Behav Res Ther, 23(2), 177–186.

Reinecke, M.A., Ryan, N.E., and DuBois, D.L. (1998) Cognitive-behavioral therapy of depression and depressive symptoms during adolescence: A review and meta-analysis. Journal of the American Academy of Child and Adolescent Psychiatry, 37, 26–34.

Richters, J.E., Arnold, L.E., Jensen, P.S., Abikoff, H., Conners, K., Greenhill, L.L., et al. (1995) NIMH collaborative multisite multimodal treatment study of children with ADHD: I. Background and rationale. Journal of the American Academy of Child and Adolescent Psychiatry, 34, 987–1000.

Rieppi, R., Greenhill, L.L., Ford, R.E., Chuang, S., Wu, M., Davies, M., et al. (2002) Socioeconomic status as a moderator of ADHD treatment outcomes. J Am Acad Child Adolesc Psychiatry, 41(3), 269–277.

Robin, A.L., Siegel, P.T., Koepke, T., Moye, A., and Tice, S. (1994) Family therapy versus individual therapy for adolescent females with anorexia nervosa. Journal of Developmental and Behavioral Pediatrics, 15, 111–116.

Robin, A.L., Siegel, P.T., and Moye, A. (1995) Family versus individual therapy for anorexia: Impact on family conflict. International Journal of Eating Disorders, 17, 313–322.

Robin, A.L., Siegel, P.T., Moye, A.W., Gilroy, M., Baker-Dennis, A., and Sikard, A. (1999) A controlled comparison of family versus individual therapy for adolescents with anorexia nervosa. Journal of the American Academy of Child and Adolescent Psychiatry, 38, 1482–1489.

Rohde, P., Clarke, G.N., Lewinsohn, P.M., Seeley, J.R., and Kaufman, N.K. (2001) Impact of comorbidity on a cognitive-behavioral group treatment for adolescent depression. Journal of the American Academy Child and Adolescent Psychiatry, 40, 795–802.

Roth, A., and Fonagy, P. (1996) What works for whom? A critical review of psychotherapy research. New York: Guilford.

Roth, A., and Fonagy, P. (in press) What works for whom? A critical review of psychotherapy research. Second edition. New York: Guilford.

Roth, A., and Parry, G. (1997) The implications of psychotherapy research for clinical practice and service development: lessons and limitations. Journal of Mental Health, 6, 367–380.

Rotheram-Borus, M.J., Piacentini, J., Van Rossem, R., Graae, F., Cantwell, C., Castro-Blanco, D., et al. (1999) Treatment adherence among Latina female adolescent suicide attempters. Suicide and Life-Threatening Behavior, 29(4), 319–331.

Rotheram-Borus, M.J., Piacentini, J., Van Rossem, R., Graae, F., Cantwell, C., Castro-Blanco, D., et al. (1996) Enhancing treatment adherence with a specialized emergency room program for adolescent suicide attempters. Journal of the American Academy of Child and Adolescent Psychiatry, 35, 654–663.

Routh, C.P., Hill, J.W., Steele, H., Elliott, C.E., and Dewey, M.E. (1995) Maternal attachment status, psychosocial stressor and problem behavior: Followup after parent training course for Conduct Disorder. Journal of Child Psychology and Psychiatry, 36, 1179–1198.

Rubin, A., Bischofshausen, S., Conroy Moore, K., Dennis, B., Hastie, M., Melnick, L., et al. (2001) The effectiveness of EMDR in a child guidance center. Research on Social Work Practice, 11(4), 435–457.

Ruma, P.R., Burke, R.V., and Thompson, R.W. (1996) Group parent training: Is it effective for children of all ages? Behavior Therapy, 27, 159–169.

Russell, G.F.M., Szmukler, G., Dare, C., and Eisler, I. (1987) An evaluation of family therapy in anorexia nervosa and bulimia nervosa. Archives of General Psychiatry, 44, 1047–1056.

Salloum, A., Avery, L., and McClain, R.P. (2001) Group psychotherapy for adolescent survivors of homicide victims: a pilot study. J Am Acad Child Adolesc Psychiatry, 40(11), 1261–1267.

Saltzman, W.R., Pynoos, R.S., Layne, C.M., Steinberg, A.M., and Aisenberg, E. (2001) Trauma- and grief-focused intervention for adolescents exposed to community violence: Results of a school-based screening and group treatment protocol. Group Dynamics, 5(4), 291–303.

Santiseban, D.A., Perez-Vidal, A., Coatsworth, J.D., Kurtines, W.M., Schwartz, S., LaPierre, A., et al. (2003) The efficacy of brief strategic family therapy in modifying Hispanic adolescent behavior problems and substnce use. Journal of Family Psychology, 17, 121–133.

Satterfield, J.H., Satterfield, B.T., and Cantwell, D.P. (1981) Three-year multimodality treatment study of 100 hyperactive boys. Journal of Paediatrics, 98, 650–655.

Satterfield, J.H., Satterfield, B.T., and Schell, A.M. (1987) Therapeutic interventions to prevent delinquency in hyperactive boys. Journal of the American Academy of Child and Adolescent Psychiatry, 26, 56–64.

Schachar, R., Jadad, A.R., Gauld, M., Boyle, M., Booker, L., Snider, A., et al. (2002) Attention-deficit hyperactivity disorder: critical appraisal of extended treatment studies. Can J Psychiatry, 47(4), 337–348.

Schmidt, U., Hodes, M., and Treasure, J. (1992) Early onset bulimia nervosa – who is at risk? Psychological Medicine, 22, 623–628.

Schuhmann, E.M., Foote, R.C., Eyberg, S.M., Boggs, S.R., and Algina, J. (1998) Efficacy of parent-child interaction therapy: Interim report of a randomized trial with short-term maintenance. Journal of Clinical Child Psychology, 27, 34–45.

Scott, S., Spender, Q., Doolan, M., Jacobs, B., and Aspland, H. (2001) Multicentre controlled trial of parenting groups for childhood antisocial behavior in clinical practice. Bmj, 323(7306), 194–198.

Silver, M., and Oakes, P. (2001) Evaluation of a new computer intervention to teach people with autism or Asperger syndrome to recognize and predict emotions in others. Autism, 5(3), 299–316.

Silverman, W.K., Kurtines, W.M., Ginsburg, G.S., Weems, C.F., Rabian, B., and Serafini, L.T. (1999) Contingency management, self-control, and education support in the treatment of childhood phobic disorders: a randomized clinical trial. Journal of Consulting and Clinical Psychology, 67(5), 675–687.

Soberman, G.B., Greenwald, R., and Rule, D.L. (2002) A controlled study of eye movement desensitization and reprocessing (EMDR) for boys with conduct problems. Journal of Aggression, Maltreatment and Trauma, 6(1), 217–236.

Sonuga-Barke, E.J., Daley, D., Thompson, M., Laver-Bradbury, C., and Weeks, A. (2001) Parent-based therapies for preschool attention-deficit/hyperactivity disorder: a randomized, controlled trial with a community sample. J Am Acad Child Adolesc Psychiatry, 40(4), 402–408.

Sonuga-Barke, E.J., Daley, D., and Thompson, M. (2002) Does maternal ADHD reduce the effectiveness of parent training for preschool children's ADHD? J Am Acad Child Adolesc Psychiatry, 41(6), 696–702.

Southam-Gerow, M., Kendall, P.C., and Weersing, V.R. (2001) Examining outcome variability: correlates of treatment response in a child and adolescent anxiety clinic. J Consult Clin Psychol, 30, 422–436.

Stark, K.D., Reynolds, W.M., and Kaslow, N.J. (1987) A comparison of the relative efficacy of self-control therapy and a behavioral problem-solving therapy for depression in children. Journal of Abnormal Child Psychology, 15, 91–113.

Steinhausen, H.C. (1995) Treatment and outcome of adolescent anorexia nervosa. Hormone Research, 43(4), 168–170.

Strauss, C.C., and Last, C.G. (1993) Social and simple phobias in children. Journal of Anxiety Disorders, 7, 141–152.

Target, M., and Fonagy, P. (1994a) The efficacy of psychoanalysis for children with emotional disorders. Journal of the American Academy of Child and Adolescent Psychiatry, 33, 361–371.

Target, M., and Fonagy, P. (1994b) The efficacy of psychoanalysis for children: Developmental considerations. Journal of the American Academy of Child and Adolescent Psychiatry, 33, 1134–1144.

Target, M., and Fonagy, P. (in press) The psychological treatment of child and adolescent psychiatric disorders. In A. Roth and P. Fonagy (Eds.), What works for whom? A critical review of psychotherapy research. New York: Guilford.

The MTA Cooperative Group. (1999) Moderators and mediators of treatment response for children with Attention-Deficit/Hyperactivity Disorder. Archives of General Psychiatry, 56, 1088–1096.

Toren, P., Wolmer, L., Rosental, B., Eldar, S., Koren, S., Lask, M., et al. (2000) Case series: brief parent-child group therapy for childhood anxiety disorders using a manual-based cognitive-behavioral technique. J Am Acad Child Adolesc Psychiatry, 39(10), 1309–1312.

Tracey, S.A., Patterson, M., Mattis, S.G., Chorpita, B.F., Albano, A.M., Heimberg, R.G., et al. (1999) Cognitive behavioral group treatment of social phobia in adolescents: Preliminary examination of the contribution of parental involvement. Paper presented at the Annual meeting of the Anxiety Disorders Association of America, San Diego, CA.

Trowell, J., Ugarte, B., Kolvin, I., Berelowitz, M., Sadowski, H., and Le Couteur, A. (1999) Behavioral psychopathology of child sexual abuse in schoolgirls referred to a tertiary centre: a North London study. Eur Child Adolesc Psychiatry, 8(2), 107–116.

Trowell, J., Kolvin, I., Weeramanthri, T., Sadowski, H., Berelowitz, M., Glaser, D., et al. (2002) Psychotherapy for sexually abused girls: psychopathological outcome findings and patterns of change. Br J Psychiatry, 180, 234–247.

Turk, J. (1993) Cognitive approaches. In B. Lask and R. Bryant-Waugh (Eds.), Childhood Onset Anorexia and Related Eating Disorders. Hillsdale, NJ: Lawrence Erlbaum Associates, Inc.

van der Ham, T., van Strien, D.C., and van Engeland, H. (1994) A four-year prospective followup study of 49 eating-disordered adolescents: Differences in course of illness. Acta Psychiatrica Scandinavica, 90, 229–235.

Vitiello, B., Severe, J.B., Greenhill, L.L., Arnold, L.E., Abikoff, H.B., Bukstein, O.G., et al. (2001) Methylphenidate dosage for children with ADHD over time under controlled conditions: lessons from the MTA. J Am Acad Child Adolesc Psychiatry, 40(2), 188–196.

Walker, H.M., Hops, H., and Greenwood, C.R. (1984) The COR-BEH research and development model: Programmatic issues and strategies. In S.C. Paine, G.T. Bellamy and B. Wilcox (Eds.), Human services that work: From innovation to clinical practice (pp. 57–77). Baltimore: Paul H. Brookes.

Webster-Stratton, C. (1996) Early-onset conduct problems: Does gender make a difference? Journal of Consulting and Clinical Psychology, 64, 540–551.

Webster-Stratton, C., and Hammond, M. (1997) Treating children with early-onset conduct problems: A comparison of child and parent training interventions. Journal of Consulting and Clinical Psychology, 65, 93–109.

Webster-Stratton, C., and Reid, M.J. (2003) The incredible years parents, teachers and children training series. In A.E. Kazdin and J.R. Weisz (Eds.), Evidence-based psychotherapies for children and adolescents (pp. 224–240). New York: Guilford.

Weisz, J.R., Weiss, B., Morton, T., Granger, D., and Han, S. (1992) Meta-analysis of psychotherapy outcome research with children and adolescents. Los Angeles: University of California.

Weisz, J.R., Weiss, B., Han, S.S., Granger, D.A., and Morton, T. (1995) Effects of psychotherapy with children and adolescents revisited: A meta-analysis of treatment outcome studies. Psychological Bulletin, 117, 450–468.

Wells, K.C., Epstein, J.N., Hinshaw, S.P., Conners, C.K., Klaric, J., Abikoff, H.B., et al. (2000) Parenting and family stress treatment outcomes in attention deficit hyperactivity disorder (ADHD): an empirical analysis in the MTA study. J Abnorm Child Psychol, 28(6), 543–553.

Whalen, C., and Schreibman, L. (2003) Joint attention training for children with autism using behavior modification procedures. J Child Psychol Psychiatry, 44(3), 456–468.

Wolchik, S.A., Weiss, L., and Katzman, M.A. (1986) An empirically validated, short term psychoeducational group treatment program for bulimia. International Journal of Eating Disorders, 5, 21–34.

Wood, A., Trainor, G., Rothwell, J., Moore, A., and Harrington, R. (2001) Randomized trial of group therapy for repeated deliberate self-harm in adolescents. J Am Acad Child Adolesc Psychiatry, 40(11), 1246–1253.

Wood, A.J., Harrington, R.C., and Moore, A. (1996) Controlled trial of a brief cognitive-behavioral intervention in adolescent patients with depressive disorders. Journal of Child Psychology and Psychiatry, 37, 737–746.

Individual and Group Psychotherapies for Children and Adolescents

John R. Weisz, Eunie Jung

12.1 Psychotherapy: Definition and Historical Background – 141

12.2 Problems Addressed in Psychotherapy with Children and Adolescents – 142

12.3 Identifying Evidence-Based Treatments – 142

12.4 Therapies for Fears and Anxiety Disorders – 143
12.4.1 Background – 143
12.4.2 Indications and Significance – 143
12.4.3 Overview of Beneficial Treatments – 144
12.4.4 Techniques of Treatment and Management – 144
12.4.4.1 Modeling Treatments: Conceptual Basis and Procedural Overview – 144
12.4.4.2 Multicomponent Cognitive-Behavioral Treatments: Conceptual Basis and Procedural Overview of the Coping Cat and Family Anxiety Management Programs – 145

12.5 Therapies for Depressive Symptoms and Disorders – 147
12.5.1 Background – 147
12.5.2 Indications and Significance – 147
12.5.3 Overview of Beneficial Treatments – 148
12.5.4 Techniques of Treatment and Management – 148
12.5.4.1 The Coping with Depression Course for Adolescents: Conceptual Basis and Procedural Overview of a CBT Program – 148
12.5.4.2 Interpersonal Therapy for Adolescents: Conceptual Basis and Procedural Overview – 149

12.6 Therapies for Attention Deficit/Hyperactivity Disorder – 150
12.6.1 Background – 150
12.6.2 Indications and Significance – 150
12.6.3 Overview of Beneficial Treatments – 150
12.6.4 Techniques of Treatment and Management – 151
12.6.4.1 Behavioral Parent Training: Conceptual Basis and Procedural Overview – 151
12.6.4.2 Behavioral Intervention in Classroom and Camp Settings: Conceptual Basis and Procedural Overview – 152

12.7 Therapies for Conduct Problems, Oppositional Defiant Disorder, and Conduct Disorder – 153

12.7.1 Background – 153
12.7.2 Indications and Significance – 154
12.7.3 Overview of Beneficial Treatments – 154
12.7.4 Techniques of Treatment and Management – 154
12.7.4.1 Youth Anger Management Training: Conceptual Basis and Procedural Overview – 154
12.7.4.2 Problem Solving Skills Training: Conceptual Basis and Procedural Overview – 155
12.7.4.3 Parent-Child Interaction Treatments: Conceptual Basis and Procedural Overview – 156
12.7.4.4 Video-Guided Group Behavioral Parent Training: Conceptual Basis and Procedural Overview – 157
12.7.4.5 Multisystemic Therapy: Conceptual Basis and Procedural Overview – 158

12.8 Treatment Results: Efficacy, Effectiveness, and Issues for Attention in Future Research – 160

References – 161

Nine-year-old Ellie has been a worrier since early childhood. In the preschool years, she was afraid to be alone in her room, and terrified when her parents left her with a babysitter. Now in primary school, Ellie is afraid to speak in class, and she is so shy during lunch that she looks for empty classrooms, where she can eat hidden from view. Melanie, age 13, has long tended to see dark clouds rather than silver linings, but she has seemed genuinely depressed since members of her social group began to exclude her. She has lost confidence in herself, can't sleep, has no appetite, cries behind her locked bedroom door, and recently told her mother, »No one likes me. I'm an outcast.« Eleven-year-old Max speeds through his house leaving a path of destruction in his wake. He means no harm, but he is so impulsive and distractible that each day is a series of collisions, spills, scars on the wall, and broken objects. At school he is unable to attend to his teacher or a class discussion for more than a few minutes, he sometimes blurts out inappropriate comments, and some of his peers joke that Kevin is »from outer space«. Aaron, age 12, gets in trouble at school almost every week, sometimes for defying teachers, sometimes for fighting with other students. He has been suspended from school three times this year, once for stealing, once for starting a fistfight with another child, and once for swearing at a teacher. At home, too, Aaron is disobedient and disrespectful, and his single parent mother cannot control him.

Young people like Ellie, Melanie, Max, and Aaron can be found in homes and schools all around the world. For most such troubled youngsters there are concerned parents and teachers, seeking help. In this chapter, we focus on one form of help: psychotherapy. We consider both individual and group psychotherapies for youths in the four categories illustrated by the four case examples.

12.1 Psychotherapy: Definition and Historical Background

The term psychotherapy refers to an array of non-medical interventions designed to relieve psychological distress, reduce maladaptive behavior, or enhance adaptive functioning through counseling, structured or unstructured interactions, training programs, or specific environmental changes. Tracing the history of psychotherapy is difficult, but the tradition of helping by listening and discussing is certainly older than recorded history. It is unclear when psychotherapy began to be a profession, but a case could be made for the era of the classical Greek philosophers, who used discourse to probe the life of the mind. Socrates (469–399 BCE) developed both a method and a thesis that arguably set a pattern for some modern forms of psychotherapy (see Plato's Apology). His philosophical dialectic, later called the »Socratic method«, involved questioning others in ways designed to prompt examination of their beliefs and bring them closer to truth. His »midwife thesis«, the notion that the philosopher's role was to deliver the truth that is already within others, much like the midwife delivers the baby that is within a mother, is not far from the view many modern therapists have of their own professional roles. By asking others to tell him what they thought, rather than telling them what to think, Socrates sought to reach the rational soul or psyche of those he talked with. The term psyche denoted the mind, inner nature, and capacity for feeling, desire, and reasoning, and was precursor to the word psychology. Finally, Socrates maintained that thought

and outward behavior are closely connected, presaging a tenet of many modern therapies.

Formal designation of psychotherapy as a type of professional intervention and an area of study can be traced back about a hundred years (Freedheim 1992). Arguably, contemporary psychotherapy grew out of the work of Sigmund Freud (1856–1939) and his intellectual heirs. Early markers in the application to children were Freud's (1909) treatment of a boy (»Little Hans«) who was afraid of horses by consulting with the boy's father, and Freud's psychoanalysis of his own daughter, Anna (1895–1982), who became a prominent child analyst in her own right beginning in the 1920s. The acceleration of child psychotherapy through the century was propelled by other models and methods, as well, including a radically different behavioral approach. Mary Cover Jones (1924), for example, used modeling and »direct conditioning« to help a two-year-old, Peter, overcome fear of a white rabbit. This work helped to launch a remarkable burgeoning of behavioral psychotherapies for young people, complementing psychoanalysis and humanistic treatments. By the late twentieth century, child and adolescent psychotherapy had expanded remarkably in the variety of its forms and the extent of its reach.

The growth of psychotherapy soon prompted a growing curiosity about its effects. Although psychotherapy research developed later and more slowly than psychotherapy practice, studies began to accumulate. Eysenck (1952) reviewed studies of adult psychotherapy and concluded that the evidence did not show it to be effective. Levitt (1957, 1963) reviewed studies that included children or adolescents and concluded that rates of improvement among children (67–73%) were about the same with or without treatment. This conclusion was reinforced by Eysenck (1960, 1966) in later reviews encompassing youth and adult therapy.

These early reviews were highly influential, but many of the studies they relied on were methodologically weak by today's standards. Subsequent research has grown stronger, and much more plentiful. Indeed, by the year 2000, well over a thousand treatment outcome studies of child and adolescent psychotherapy had been completed (Durlak et al. 1995; Kazdin 2000). The studies are increasingly sophisticated, with many meeting the standards of randomized clinical trials. Another important development is that research has shifted, more and more, from tests of unspecified »treatment« or generic »psychotherapy« to tests of well-articulated therapies with specific treatment procedures described in manuals. Of course, tests of therapy that are not manualized but rather done as a part of usual clinical care, with therapists free to choose the methods they prefer, are potentially very useful in helping us understand whether usual care is beneficial (see Weisz 2004). However, the upsurge of studies in which treatment procedures are specified in advance and therapists follow those procedures make it possible to know, when results are published, which specific intervention methods worked or did not. This is a major strength, bolstering prospects for both understanding and disseminating what works. So, thanks to several historical developments, we are now in a position to profit from a large and increasingly rigorous body of evidence on youth psychotherapies and their effects.

12.2   Problems Addressed in Psychotherapy with Children and Adolescents

Psychotherapy is used to address diverse problems and disorders that cause emotional distress, interfere with daily living, undermine the development of adaptive skills, or threaten the well-being of others. Many of the youth problems addressed fit within the broad syndromes known as internalizing (e.g., sadness, fears, shyness) and externalizing (e.g., disobedience, fighting, stealing; Achenbach 1991). Problems within both syndromes are common reasons for referral to clinics. Problems that undermine school performance also generate many treatment referrals (see Burns et al. 1995; Bussing et al. 1998; Leaf et al. 1996). Another way to describe the targets of treatment is to focus on categorical diagnoses within the formal Diagnostic and Statistical Manual of Mental Disorders tradition (e.g., American Psychiatric Association 1994). Recent evidence from North American clinics (e.g., Jensen and Weisz 2002) suggests that four clusters of disorders account for a very high percentage of youth referrals:

1. Fears and anxiety disorders (e.g., social phobia, generalized anxiety disorder)
2. Depressive symptoms and disorders (e.g., dysthymic disorder, major depressive disorder)
3. Attentional problems and attention deficit/hyperactivity disorder (ADHD)
4. Conduct problems and disorders (e.g., oppositional defiant disorder, conduct disorder)

These four clusters match the four case examples that began this chapter. In the rest of the chapter, we con-

centrate on treatments for disorders and related referral problems associated with these four clusters.

12.3   Identifying Evidence-Based Treatments

To identify psychotherapies relevant to the four clusters, we draw information from three sources. First, we look to four published meta-analyses of the youth treatment outcome literature that have been particularly broad in their inclusion criteria, encompassing studies of diverse problems and disorders and diverse treatments (Casey and Berman 1985; Kazdin et al. 1990; Weisz et al. 1987, 1995). Across these four meta-analyses, mean unweighted effect sizes were all .71 or higher, indicating that the average treated youth scored better than more than 3/4 of control group youths on a variety of outcome measures at the end of treatment. Effect sizes are more modest, but still positive and substantial, when weighting is introduced (e.g., adjusting for sample size; Weisz et al. 1995) and when one focuses on studies not subject to publication bias (e.g., doctoral dissertations; McLeod and Weisz, in press). Meta-analytic findings also suggest that treatment effects show specificity – i.e., effects are larger on measures of the problems actually targeted in treatment than on measures of other mental health outcomes not targeted (Weisz et al. 1995).

As a second source of evidence-based treatments, we look to a report by a task force on empirically supported treatments for children and adolescents (Lonigan et al. 1998). This group applied a published set of review criteria to the outcome research evidence base to identify treatments satisfying one of two levels of support: well-established or probably efficacious. Well-established treatments were those supported by either group comparison studies or within-group studies. In group comparison studies, there had to be two such studies demonstrating that the treatment was superior to medication, a psychological placebo condition, or an alternate treatment, or by showing that the treatment was equivalent to an already established treatment. Treatments could also be classified as well-established based on at least nine well-designed within-group experiments comparing the target treatment to an alternative treatment. Treatments were also required to (a) use a manual, (b) clearly specify the sample used, and (c) garner support from at least two independent investigators or research teams. To qualify as probably efficacious, a treatment had to be supported by either (a) two group comparison studies showing the treatment to be more effective than a waitlist control group, (b) at least one experiment meeting most of the »well-established treatment« criteria, or (c) at least three within-group or single case design experiments; this category also required treatment manuals and clear description of client samples, but it did not require independent replication by different investigators. It also did not require that the target treatment be shown to be superior to an alternative treatment or even an active control condition; superiority to waitlist was sufficient if demonstrated in at least two studies. The task force identified well-established and probably efficacious treatments for the four broad clusters of problems and diagnoses that will be addressed in this chapter: fears and anxiety (Ollendick and King 1998), depression (Kaslow and Thompson 1998), ADHD (Pelham et al. 1998b), and conduct-related problems and disorders (Brestan and Eyberg 1998).

A third source we used to identify evidence-based youth treatments is a current review of the published evidence, which is being carried out by our research team at this writing. We are using a variety of sources. First, we search standard computerized databases housing publications beginning in 1965 and continuing through December, 2002. For psychotherapy, we use the PsychInfo database, employing 21 psychotherapy-related key terms (e.g., »psychother-«, »counseling«, »treatment«) derived from previous youth psychotherapy meta-analyses (Weisz et al. 1987, 1995). In addition, we survey published reviews and meta-analyses of the youth psychotherapy literature to identify studies not found in PsychInfo. We also follow reference trails of reviewed studies and screen studies suggested by investigators in the field. To be included, studies must focus on youths averaging between 3.5 and 18.4 years old who have been selected for having psychological problems or maladaptive behavior. Youths who have been self-referred, teacher-referred, parent-referred, or selected based on pretest scores are all acceptable. Several methodological criteria are applied (e.g., random assignment to treatment and control conditions). Although the first step of our search led to a pool of more than 3,000 published articles, applying our screening and review procedures (e.g., ruling out studies that lack random assignment) has reduced the pool to about 400 studies. For the present chapter, we reviewed these studies to identify treatment programs that have replicated support (i.e., two or more studies) in the published evidence base.

Throughout the chapter, treatments are named and described as generically as the evidence warrants. Thus, we describe one »brand name« treatment with one specific manual if the evidence is that specific; but we describe generic approaches (e.g., cognitive behavioral therapy for child depression) if multiple manuals or versions have been tested and found to be beneficial. Finally, we should note that the space available within this chapter precludes comprehensive coverage of all evidence-based treatments and all treatments that may have merit. So, we have tried to simply illustrate the literature on beneficial treatments by focusing briefly on some of the most thoroughly studied approaches. A much more detailed examination of multiple treatments can be found in the recent Cambridge Press book, Psychotherapy for Children and Adolescents: Evidence-Based Treatments and Case Examples (Weisz 2004).

12.4   Therapies for Fears and Anxiety Disorders

12.4.1   Background

Maladaptive fears in young people have been a focus of study and treatment since the beginning of psychological theory and intervention. Sigmund Freud's (1909/1955) case of »Little Hans«, Watson and Rayner's (1920) famous experiment with Little Albert, and Mary Cover Jones' (1924) treatment of two-year-old Peter, all concerned anxiety in children. In the eight or nine decades since Freud and the behaviorists did their early work, an enormous number of theorists, investigators, and therapists have addressed fears and anxieties in young people. The result is a massive literature on the nature and treatment of anxiety in youth, probably outpacing the literature on any other childhood condition.

12.4.2   Indications and Significance

The conditions for which anxiety-related treatments are indicated span a broad range from uncomplicated (e.g., fear of being in the dark alone) to more complex (such as generalized anxiety disorder) with diverse forms and manifestations. Taken together, anxiety-related conditions are the most common class of behavioral and emotional dysfunction among children and adolescents (see Albano et al.

1996). Silverman and Ginsburg's (1995) review of ten epidemiologic studies led them to estimate the prevalence of »any anxiety disorder« at 6–18% among youths in the general population. In addition to its high prevalence, severe anxiety can be highly debilitating, undermining a youngster's adaptation and development in numerous ways. Development of peer relationships can be hampered, school performance may suffer, efforts to learn new skills may be thwarted, and normative challenges (e.g., presenting an oral report, meeting a new person) may become major life crises.

12.4.3   Overview of Beneficial Treatments

The adverse impact of anxiety on social relationships, learning, and development establishes a clear need for beneficial treatments. Treatment developers have responded with diverse interventions. Freud's (1909/1955) psychoanalytic approach evolved over time into a variety of psychodynamic treatments, some involving play. However, most of the literature bearing on the outcome of such treatments involves case reports. In keeping with our emphasis here on strong empirical support, we will focus, in this chapter, on only those treatment procedures supported in experimental tests (see review by Ollendick and King 1998). Those tests have been focused on treatments that have grown out of the more behavioral tradition, traceable to the early work of Watson and Rayner (1920) and Jones (1924), as discussed above. For example, Jones' procedure of gradually bringing Peter into increasing proximity to the rabbit (while Peter ate food that he liked) is a sort of template for a cluster of exposure procedures that are now a common part of behavioral treatment for fear and anxiety. Similarly, Jones' efforts to have Peter observe other children interacting happily with the rabbit form a basic foundation for anxiety treatments that involve modeling, or observational learning.

Exposure and modeling have become mainstays of most empirically supported treatments for youth anxiety. For relatively uncomplicated fears and anxiety disorders, such as simple phobia, four relatively simple clusters of intervention approaches have proven helpful. In modeling or observational learning, nonanxious responses are modeled for the fearful youth by others; in systematic desensitization, youngsters are exposed to fear-producing objects or situations while they are very relaxed (or in some other fear-incompatible state); in reinforced exposure, youngsters are rewarded for showing nonfearful behavior; and in simple cognitive-behavioral treatment, self-talk and other ways of linking thoughts and behavior are brought to bear on the object of the child's fear. For more complex anxiety disorders, such as separation anxiety disorder, social phobia, and generalized anxiety disorder, more complex multicomponent cognitive-behavioral treatment programs have been shown to be beneficial.

12.4.4   Techniques of Treatment and Management

12.4.4.1   Modeling Treatments: Conceptual Basis and Procedural Overview

For fearful boys and girls, the sequence of feared object, anxious thoughts, aversive arousal, avoidance, relief, can be quite powerful and self-sustaining. Altering the sequence is not an easy task, as many parents and many therapists have learned. One way the sequence can be broken is by exposing fearful youths to a model who violates the assumptions underlying the fear. Having the model engage in the feared behavior shows that it can be done, illustrates how, and illustrates that the consequences the child has feared do not actually occur. When the treatment works, the child who observes emulates the behavior of the model and learns that it can be done without harmful repercussions. Multiple treatment studies have shown beneficial effects of modeling interventions in the treatment of children's fears. A common practice is to start the child at a modest level of intensity (e.g., sitting at a distance from the feared object) and add increments (e.g., moving closer, touching the object, picking it up) following each successful exposure. Optionally, the therapist may praise or reward the child for successes. Three general forms of modeling have been supported in outcome studies thus far:

1. Live modeling involves in-person observation of the models' nonfearful behavior.
2. Symbolic modeling employs video or other representations of models showing nonfearful behavior.
3. Participant modeling pairs the fearful youngster with a model who encourages shared involvement in the feared activity.

All three forms of modeling have been used and tested most often with preschool through primary school children, although some applications to adolescent fears have also been found helpful. Sessions tend to be brief (8–35 min) and limited in number (e.g., 1–8 sessions total). For reasons that are not clear, the current zeitgeist in youth anxiety treatment does not emphasize modeling approaches, even though the evidence suggests that such treatments can be quite helpful and the focus and brevity of the treatments is consistent with current pressures for efficiency and cost-effectiveness. Because so much of the evidence supporting the modeling approaches was generated through studies published in the 1960s and 1970s, some of the trappings of successful treatments from the 1990s are missing. For example, detailed treatment manuals and related materials, common in the current treatment literature, are hard to find for modeling treatments. However, the relative simplicity of these treatments means that the descriptions provided in the original published articles may provide sufficient guidance for clinical use.

Modeling treatments: in brief*

Designed for	Specific fears (e.g., dogs, swimming) in children aged 3–12
Number of sessions	Range: 1–8
Session length	Range: 8–35 min
Session participants	Therapist, live or video model, children (individually or in small groups)
Theoretical orientation	Observational learning

Treatment steps:
1. Assess fear levels in children who are to be treated
2. Arrange for children to observe live or video model performing feared activity, with level or intensity increasing over time (e.g., observing dog, then approaching, then petting)
3. Invite children to engage in the activity, initially at low level, then increasing intensity
4. (optional) Arrange positive consequence for successful imitation of the model
* In Brief section reprinted from JR Weisz (2004) Psychotherapy for children and adolescents: Evidence-based treatments and case examples. Cambridge University Press, Cambridge, UK.

12.4.4.2 Multicomponent Cognitive-Behavioral Treatments: Conceptual Basis and Procedural Overview of the Coping Cat and Family Anxiety Management Programs

Such complex conditions as separation anxiety disorder, social phobia, and generalized anxiety disorder may require a multicomponent cognitive behavioral therapy (CBT) program. The most thoroughly studied of such programs is Coping Cat, developed by Philip Kendall and colleagues (Kendall et al. 2003). Coping Cat is designed to address the interplay of biological arousal, anxious thoughts, and behavioral avoidance that are thought to converge in creating and sustaining anxiety disorders. Biological arousal can be a problem in part because children often do not recognize it (they only know that they feel scared) and in part because they don't know how to cope with arousal even when they do notice it. Anxious thoughts are another problem; young people often lack skills in identifying their thoughts and in modifying the ones that are maladaptive. Avoidance of feared situations is also an issue in that avoiding prevents youngsters from learning that the situations are not actually so bad. Moreover, avoidance can be quite entrenched because it is self-reinforcing (i.e., avoiding feared situations reduces arousal, which in turn rewards the avoidance).

To tackle this trio of presumed causal factors – arousal, cognition, and avoidance – Coping Cat therapists teach their young clients a cluster of related skills. These include (a) recognizing how the body signals anxious arousal, (b) making one's body relax when anxious feelings arise, (c) identifying and altering fearful cognitions, (d) planning and carrying out exposures to feared situations, and (e) evaluating one's effort and rewarding oneself for trying hard. Roughly the first half of the treatment is devoted to educating the child about the somatic, cognitive, and behavioral components of anxiety, with particular emphasis on the individual child's distinctive pattern. The second half involves real-world application of what has been learned, through a series of personally tailored in vivo exercises involving direct exposure to feared situations. Over time, the situations progress from those that are mildly upsetting to those that evoke major fears. The goal is that by the end of therapy, treated youngsters will be able to design and carry out their own exposures, and thus be their own therapists.

12

The Coping Cat Program: in brief*

Designed for	Youth aged 8–13, diagnosed with Generalized Anxiety Disorder, Separation Anxiety Disorder, and Social Phobia
Number of sessions	16–20
Session length	50–60 min
Session participants	Therapist and child
Theoretical orientation	Cognitive behavioral

Treatment steps:
1. Youth identifies situations that make him/her feel anxious, and describes his/her response to those situations
2. Youth makes a hierarchy of anxiety-provoking situations, ranked from least to most feared
3. Therapist and youth identify cues (e.g., pounding heart, dry mouth) that signal the onset of anxiety
4. Therapist trains child to relax and provides a relaxation audiotape for home use
5. Therapist and youth identify anxious self-talk – i.e., cognitions that can make situations anxiety-provoking (e.g., the thought »If I flunk this test, my teacher will think I'm stupid«)
6. Therapist helps youth to identify coping self-talk and other strategies for confronting fears
7. Youth practices self-evaluation (e.g., of coping efforts) and self-reward
8. In a series of imaginal, role-play, and in vivo experiences, the youth is exposed to various feared situations, starting low in the hierarchy (see #2, above) and progressing upward
9. Throughout these exposures, the youth practices the »FEAR steps« – i.e., identifying physical sensations that signal anxiety (»Feeling frightened«) and cognitions that exacerbate the anxiety (»Expecting bad things to happen«), altering the cognitions and making themselves try the feared activity (»Attitudes and actions that can help«), and evaluating and rewarding their own coping efforts (»Rate and reward«)

* In Brief section reprinted from JR Weisz (2004) Psychotherapy for children and adolescents: Evidence-based treatments and case examples. Cambridge University Press, Cambridge, UK.

Given parents' potential impact on anxious children, it is sometimes important to bring parents into the treatment process. Doing so may help curb parents' tendencies to instigate, nurture, or magnify their children's worries, and tolerate or reward fearful avoidance. Moreover, in cases where the parents' own anxiety creates displays of fear and avoidance for their children to see, including parents in treatment may help reduce harmful parental modeling. This is part of the rationale for the Family Anxiety Management (FAM) Program, developed in Australia by Barrett and colleagues (see Barrett and Shortt 2003).

The program entails 12 sessions, most of which include child, parents, and therapist (sometimes meeting in family groups) and focus on conveying information and skills to help both child and parent cope with anxiety. The last few sessions involve only the parents and therapist; these sessions emphasize three broad themes. First, parents are taught basic behavioral principles to use in creating a home environment in which the child's displays of anxiety are not rewarded and displays of courage are. Second, parents are helped to identify the anxious responses they are displaying for their children and to replace them with coping responses. Third, training in communication and problem-solving skills is used to help the parents work as a team; they learn ways to reduce their own conflict, particularly over child-rearing issues and how to respond to child displays of anxiety, and they are encouraged to have regular problem-solving discussions, to help them reach consensus solutions and present a unified front at home.

The Family Anxiety Management (FAM) Program: in brief*

Designed for	Families of 7–14 year-old youth diagnosed with Generalized Anxiety Disorder, Separation Anxiety Disorder, and Social Phobia
Number of sessions	12
Session length	40 min to 1.5 h

Session participants	Primarily therapist with child and family, sometimes in multifamily groups; but last few sessions with parents and therapist only
Theoretical orienta-tion	Cognitive behavioral

Treatment steps:

1. Talk about how to recognize different feelings (e.g., sadness, happiness, anger), the situations that produce the feelings, and how thoughts are connected to feelings

2. Develop a hierarchy for the child, rank-ordering situations from least to most feared; begin trying low-level exposures to situations low in the hierarchy

3. Learn how bodies give off hints of fear or worry (e.g., muscle tension), and learn procedures for relaxing the body

4. Learn how thoughts or »self-talk« relate to feelings; for example, thinking about bad things that can happen in a situation may cause worried feelings

5. Practice changing negative, worried self-talk into positive self-talk, or expecting good things to happen

6. Learn how to praise and reward self for trying to do hard things; extend this concept to self-praise and self-reward for coping with feared situations

7. Review the F-E-A-R plan children have learned for coping with worries; F is for »Feeling Good« (by relaxing, and by doing positive activities), E is for »Expecting Good Things to Happen« (using positive self-talk), A is for »Action« (doing things to make a situation less frightening, so as to enter it), R is for »Reward« (praising and rewarding oneself for self-exposure to frightening situations, and for trying to cope)

8. Practice via homework using the F-E-A-R plan on real-life frightening situations, celebrate with a party

9. »Partner Support« sessions with parents and therapist only. Parents learn how to react when a problem occurs with the child (e.g., keep voice calm, back up your partner, debrief afterward), how to arrange »casual discussions« about family matters, and how to have systematic problem solving discussions to generate well thought-out solutions.

* In Brief section reprinted from JR Weisz (2004) Psychotherapy for children and adolescents: Evidence-based treatments and case examples. Cambridge University Press, Cambridge, UK.

12.5 Therapies for Depressive Symptoms and Disorders

12.5.1 Background

Depression is a relative newcomer to the literature on child and adolescent psychopathology, and particularly to the treatment literature. Hammen and Rudolph (1996) suggest attention to youth depression was delayed by several historical myths – i.e., the notions that depression did not or could not exist in children, that it was merely a transitory or developmentally normal state, or that it was most often »masked« by »depressive equivalents« such as disruptive behavior or somatic complaints. Over the past three decades, however, youth depression has come to be viewed as genuine and as an appropriate target for descriptive psychopathology and intervention research.

12.5.2 Indications and Significance

About 2% of preadolescents in the general population meet diagnostic criteria for either major depressive disorder or dysthymic disorder, and prevalence increases to about 6% in adolescence (Angold et al. 1999; Weisz and Hawley 2002). Of course, rates of these disorders are much higher in clinics and other treatment settings for youths than in the general population. Moreover, many youths suffer from symptoms that fall just short of major depressive disorder or dysthymic disorder but are nonetheless significantly distressed and appropriate targets for treatment.

The symptoms of depression can be painful and serious in their impact, not only for depressed youngsters but for their family and friends as well. Depression may undermine social development, learning in school, and other kinds of growth and skill-building (e.g., sports and music) that are important to maturation and self-esteem. Moreover, depression increases the risk of suicide. Between 6% and 13% of adolescents, across surveys, report that they have attempted suicide at least once, and suicide is the third most common cause of death among USA 15–19-year-olds (Garland and Zigler 1993). For many reasons, then, there is a clear need to develop effective treatments.

12.5.3   Overview of Beneficial Treatments

A hallmark of depression is sad mood, sometimes expressed by children and teens as irritability or anger. Beyond this emotional state, depressed youths often show characteristic styles of thinking and behaving. On the thinking front, they may interpret events in unduly negative ways. Compared to their peers, depressed youngsters may see themselves as less able or worthy, and their situations as more hopeless. On the behavioral front, depressed youths may be more passive than their peers in situations that need to be changed, and they may show skill deficits that undermine school performance and interfere with peer relationships. Depression, then, can involve problems in mood and emotion, problems in cognitive style, problems in behavior and skill development, and problems with peer relationships. Difficulties of each type are targeted in the two forms of treatment that we review in this section.

In CBT, for example, therapists work with depressed children to deal with problems of sadness and irritability, partly by focusing on how the children think, and partly by addressing deficits in behavioral skills. One of the best-known CBT approaches for children is the Coping with Depression Course for Adolescents (CWD-A; Clarke et al. 2003). Although CBT is the most thoroughly tested approach to youth depression treatment, a second approach, Interpersonal Therapy (ITP), has shown encouraging effects in recent trials. As the name implies, ITP focuses special attention on social relationships in the youth's life. Here we consider both CBT and ITP.

12.5.4   Techniques of Treatment and Management

12.5.4.1   The Coping with Depression Course for Adolescents: Conceptual Basis and Procedural Overview of a CBT Program

The CWD-A course, in keeping with its cognitive-behavioral pedigree, construes depression primarily as a matter of skill deficits – cognitive (e.g., pessimistic or irrational thought patterns), behavioral (e.g., poor social skills, insufficient engagement in pleasurable activities), and affective (e.g., unawareness of one's mood). In addressing these deficits, the treatment developers drew on a number of related cognitive and behavioral treatment methods. These methods all share a key assumption: the depressed youth has acquired maladaptive patterns of behavior that can be unlearned. Thus, the symptoms of depression (e.g. dysphoric mood, fatigue, suicidal thoughts) are viewed as the proper targets of treatment, as opposed to underlying conflicts or general personality dysfunction.

The CWD-A program is called a »course« and presented in the format of an interactive seminar. The participants are called »students«, and the therapist is called a »group leader«. The course thus has a »classroom« rather than a »clinical« tone; the goal is to provide a nonstigmatizing, psychoeducational experience. Teaching methods include lecture, discussion, role play, and homework assignments. The topics covered include improving social skills, decreasing anxiety, changing unpleasant cognitions, resolving conflicts, and planning for the future. Topics covered in the early sessions (e.g., social skills, mood monitoring, pleasant activities) are tied together as a foundation for more challenging material later in the course (e.g., constructive thinking, negotiation and problem solving, and maintaining gains). To keep early lessons fresh in the students' minds, key points are reviewed repeatedly and incorporated into new material. To make the program user-friendly to teens, homework is kept to five or ten min and involves no reading; instead, it stresses practicing the skills learned in the course. Humorous cartoons are used to illustrate maladaptive behaviors. A protocol for booster sessions has also been developed, as has a component for parents, aimed at (a) familiarizing parents with what their children are learning, so they can buttress the adolescents' new skills; and (b) teaching the parents themselves the same skills.

The Coping with Depression Course for Adolescents: in brief*	
Designed for	Depression (or elevated depressive symptoms) in adolescents aged 14–18
Number of sessions	16 with adolescents, optional 7 with parents
Session length	2 h (for adolescents and for parents)

Session participants	Therapist with groups of teens, therapist with parent groups
Theoretical orientation	Cognitive-behavioral

1. Learn how emotions are related to thoughts and actions, practice monitoring own mood
2. Learn social skills, such as how to start a conversation, listen actively, show understanding
3. Identify pleasant activities and arrange schedule to increase their frequency
4. Develop and carry out a personal plan for change – setting goals and working toward them
5. Identify negative thoughts and their cause; learn to use realistic, positive counter-thoughts
6. Learn to deal with stress by using two relaxation methods (deep muscle, quiet breathing)
7. Learn ways to interrupt negative thoughts (thought-stopping, rubber band, worry time)
8. Learn problem-solving and negotiation skills for dealing with interpersonal conflict
9. Discuss how to maintain gains by overcoming fears and obstacles; advance planning for coping with future stressors

* In Brief section reprinted from JR Weisz (2004) Psychotherapy for children and adolescents: Evidence-based treatments and case examples. Cambridge University Press, Cambridge, UK.

12.5.4.2 Interpersonal Therapy for Adolescents: Conceptual Basis and Procedural Overview

Although CBT for depression has the most extensive evidence base with children and adolescents, recent evidence suggests that interpersonal psychotherapy for adolescents (IPT-A) may also be beneficial (see Mufson and Dorta 2003; Rossello and Bernal 1999). IPT-A is designed to reduce depressive symptoms by focusing on common adolescent developmental issues. Examples include separation from parents, authority in relationships, development of dyadic relationships with peers, grief over the death of relatives or friends, dealing with peer pressure, and (where relevant) functioning within single-parent families, an issue that has been shown to be problematic for many depressed adolescents.

The program has three phases. In the initial phase, the therapist works with parents and adolescent to assess familial and other social relationships, decide which interpersonal problem areas to focus on, and develop a treatment contract. In the middle phase, therapist and adolescent work directly on the designated problem areas, as the adolescent is encouraged to monitor the depressive symptoms, express affect, link affect with events, examine conflicts and styles of communication, and use various strategies (e.g., role play) to try out various forms of behavior change. In the termination phase, the adolescent works toward giving up the relationship with the therapist and establishing a sense of competence to deal with future problems. Therapists may add booster sessions to the standardized protocol as needed.

Interpersonal Therapy for Adolescents: in brief	
Designed for	Youths aged 12–18, diagnosed with a non-bipolar, nonpsychotic, major depressive disorder
Number of sessions	12–15
Session length	30–60 min
Session participants	Therapist and adolescent
Theoretical orientation	Interpersonal

Treatment steps:
Initial Phase (sessions 1–4)
1. Gather information about the adolescent's depression and explain the disorder
2. Assess the adolescent's familial relationships
3. Identify the problem areas
4. Explain the treatment
5. Establish a treatment plan
6. Explain what is expected of the patient
Middle Phase (sessions 5–8)
1. Work on one or two of the selected problem areas
2. Implement intervention strategies
3. Monitor depressive feelings
4. Establish a positive therapeutic relationship
5. Involve family members in treatment
Termination Phase (sessions 9–12)
1. Discuss ending treatment
2. Acknowledge feelings related to separation with therapist
3. Review progress, and establish the adolescent's future competence to deal with problems

12.6   Therapies for Attention Deficit/Hyperactivity Disorder

12.6.1   Background

Problems involving overactivity and attentional difficulties have certainly existed for centuries but probably came into sharper focus with the advent of compulsory schooling, which requires sustained self-control in group settings (see Hinshaw 1994). Self-control is a critical skill for school-aged youngsters, and deficits in this skill pose major problems. In the late 1950s, professional and research attention was focused mainly on unusual levels of physical activity in youths, and terms such as hyperkinesis and the hyperactive child syndrome were used to label the problems. By the 1970s, Douglas (e.g., 1972) and others argued that the difficulties in attention and impulse control were at least as important as problems in motor activity. This notion – that there is a syndrome that includes hyperactivity, impulsivity, and poor attentional control – is reflected in the current diagnostic term, Attention-Deficit/Hyperactivity Disorder (ADHD), used in DSM-IV (American Psychiatric Association 1994).

In the typical developmental course of ADHD, hyperactivity and impulsivity appear earliest, often by age three or four, with attentional problems identified in the early school years, about ages five to seven. While the hyperactivity and impulsivity may fade somewhat during the primary school years, the poor attention control remains relatively stable up to adolescence. All three clusters of symptoms decline somewhat in adolescence, and 25–50% will lose the ADHD diagnosis by adolescence or young adulthood, but most children diagnosed with ADHD will have some related problems throughout their lives, even as adults.

12.6.2   Indications and Significance

Current estimates suggest that 3–5% of all school-aged youths meet diagnostic criteria for ADHD; this translates into an average of about one child per classroom of 20–40 youngsters (Mash and Wolfe 2002). The diagnosis is about three times as common in boys as in girls. A third to a half of all clinic-referred children show ADHD characteristics, either alone or together with other disorders (Barkley 1997).

The behavioral patterns associated with ADHD result in diverse problems, across multiple settings. Life at home can be difficult for the child, and perhaps even more difficult for others in the family, who must cope with the chaos, clutter, forgetfulness, unfinished jobs, spills, property destruction, and sleeplessness. At school, poor attending and impulsivity can be a potent combination, jeopardizing the child's relationship with the teacher, undermining academic performance, and leading to conduct problems borne not so much of ill will as of impulses the child's will cannot curb. Among peers, the child with ADHD may well be a misfit, as poor attention control makes conversations awkward, play activities frustrating, and performance in sports erratic. Given this scope of impact, it is clear that attentional problems, overactivity, and ADHD warrant treatment, but what forms of treatment?

12.6.3   Overview of Beneficial Treatments

Treatment decisions in the ADHD area are enriched, but complicated, by the existence of empirically supported interventions in both psychological and pharmacologic forms. Numerous studies document the benefits of stimulant medication in reducing the intensity of ADHD symptoms. However, some 20–30% of ADHD youngsters show either no response or an adverse response to stimulant medication (Swanson et al. 1995) and thus need some alternative treatment. Even those who benefit from stimulants may experience unwanted side-effects, especially sleep and appetite problems, as well as possible growth suppression, and this may make nonmedical alternatives appealing to some youths and parents. Beyond these matters, some parents may not want to see their children depend on drugs for acceptable social and school behavior. Thus, the search for effective psychological interventions has continued for many years.

That search has led to tests of a number of psychological-behavioral treatments. Because diagnostic categories and criteria have changed over the years, much of the research did not employ samples selected to fit DSM-IV criteria. However, for at least two decades, intervention research has tested treatments aimed at the prevailing diagnostic counterparts of DSM-IV ADHD. Additionally, for more than 30 years now, treatments have been tested that address core symptoms now associated with the ADHD diagnosis (e.g., disruptive behavior, overactivity, impulsivity, poor attentional control). So, for simplicity of presentation, we will use the term »ADHD« to refer to the problems addressed by these treatments.

According to one widely accepted view, ADHD is a disorder of performance (Barkley 1997). That is, people with ADHD may know what they should do but often find it difficult to do these things when they should. From this perspective, the treatments most likely to help will be those that support appropriate behavior at points of performance – i.e., at those times and in those situations where success depends on overcoming the deficits, by paying attention and managing behavior, for example. By this logic, the best psychosocial treatments for ADHD children may be those emphasizing environmental intervention – i.e., specific adjustments in the contingencies within children's settings. The two broad classes of environmental interventions that have particularly strong empirical support are behavioral parent training and behavioral interventions in classroom and camp settings.

12.6.4 Techniques of Treatment and Management

12.6.4.1 Behavioral Parent Training: Conceptual Basis and Procedural Overview

A number of experts (e.g., Barkley 1997) believe that ADHD youngsters' biological abnormalities generate specific deficits in rule-governed behavior – i.e., reduced capacity to adjust behavior in response to commands, rules, and self-directed speech. Behavioral parent training programs address this reduced child responsiveness by training parents to (a) use explicit, systematic, and salient methods to convey rules and instructions, and (b) ensure clear, consistent, and powerful consequences for compliance and noncompliance with the rules and instructions. The idea is that a parentally-organized environment rich in appropriate cues and contingencies can help children stay on track for appropriate behavior (e.g., attending, thinking before acting, persisting at tasks) and avoid inappropriate behavior (e.g., carelessness, impulsivity, hyperactivity) in spite of their relatively enduring biological deficits. A second part of the rationale for parent training is the well-documented fact that ADHD is often accompanied by serious conduct problems, and that children who show this combination tend to have particularly poor adoles-

cent and adult outcomes. Thus, it seems important to address oppositional behavior and other conduct problems in any treatment for ADHD youths.

The most thoroughly tested and well-supported approach for addressing this combination of problems is behavioral parent training. A typical format for such training includes assigned readings on the use of behavioral principles with children and a series of 820 weekly sessions, focused on applying the principles with the individual children involved. Coverage usually includes such core behavioral concepts as maximizing parental attention (and praise) in response to appropriate child behavior, withholding attention (and praise) when behavior is inappropriate, developing reward and incentive systems (e.g., charts, points, tokens) to encourage desired behavior, and effective use of time-out for noncompliance. So, therapists first teach parents about the nature and causes of ADHD, disobedience, and defiance, next teach and supervise practice in the use of behavioral principles at home, and then work on applying the principles at school and other out-of-home settings. Here we illustrate the components of a representative parent training program by focusing on Barkley's (1997) Defiant Children Program.

Behavioral Parent Training for Defiant Children (Barkley 1997): in brief*	
Designed for	Defiant and ADHD children, aged 2–12
Number of sessions	10, plus booster session and follow-up meetings
Session length	1 h for individual families, 2 h for groups of families
Session participants	Therapist with parents, child included for parts of individual family sessions
Theoretical orientation	Behavioral

Treatment steps:
1. Therapist leads parents through a review of information on nature, etiologies, developmental course, and prognosis of ADHD; may include video illustrations and reading material

2. Therapist and parents discuss and practice procedures for, attending to appropriate child behavior; procedures include close visual attending, narrative descriptions, and praise. Procedures implemented in daily »special time« at home
3. Parents learn how to give effective commands to child, and how to respond immediately with positive attention when the child complies
4. Parents learn how to make reinforcement concrete and external, by establishing a token economy at home
5. Parents learn to use consequences for noncompliant and inappropriate behavior. Such consequences include loss of points or chips in the token economy, and time-out
6. Parents and therapist fine-tune the time-out procedure, discussing problems in implementation at home, and new applications that can be tried
7. Parents learn procedures for managing noncompliance and inappropriate behavior in public places
8. Parents learn procedures for improving the child's school behavior – coordinating communication with school personnel via the daily school behavior report card
9. Parents and therapist discuss future problems that may arise, and how the skills learned may be applied
10. Booster session, one month after end of Step 9, to review the main ideas of Steps 1–9, and to plan solutions to problems that have arisen during the month

* In Brief section reprinted from JR Weisz (2004) Psychotherapy for children and adolescents: Evidence-based treatments and case examples. Cambridge University Press, Cambridge, UK.

12.6.4.2 Behavioral Intervention in Classroom and Camp Settings: Conceptual Basis and Procedural Overview

The conceptual basis for classroom and camp intervention with ADHD is closely linked to the notion that youngsters with ADHD suffer from performance deficits more than comprehension deficits – i.e., they know what they should do, but their biological deficits hamper their ability to do it (see Barkley 1997). Addressing such deficits may require putting interventions into the contexts where problems arise for the child. Prominent among such contexts are group learning situations, including classrooms, camps, and other contexts where the goal is to convey information and skills in the company of peers. Behavioral classroom and camp programs aim for such goals as (a) improving attention to assigned tasks, (b) reducing overactive and impulsive behavior, (c) reducing disobedience and conduct problems, and (d) improving learning. In these programs, typically, specific behavioral goals and objectives are identified for the child, a procedure is set up to monitor target behaviors, rewards are made contingent on the desired behaviors, and unattractive consequences are attached to unwanted behaviors such as disobeying, drifting off-task, or disrupting class. These consequences may be loss of points or chips in a token economy, loss of privileges (e.g., no outdoor time during recess), or brief time outs.

Making adaptive and appropriate behavior possible on a regular basis may require both reminders and rewards. The classroom or camp environment can be altered to include salient cues for appropriate behavior, and to insure that rewarding consequences follow such behavior. In addition, there may be adverse consequences for failing to show the appropriate behavior. Evidence suggests that such consequences, called response cost, improve child behavior beyond the effects of reward alone. Each of these features – i.e., salience, reward, and response cost – can be incorporated into classroom and camp settings and coordinated by teachers, counselors, or staff. In addition, a regular report to parents (e.g., a simple daily report card) may be used to link the child's behavior in the group situation to consequences at home, thus bolstering the strength of the intervention by arranging for continuity across settings. To illustrate this form of intervention, we focus on a very comprehensive program that has been used and refined over a period of two decades, and described in what is very likely the most thorough and detailed treatment manual available for behavioral intervention in group settings: The Children's Summer Treatment Program (STP), developed by William Pelham and his colleagues (Pelham et al. 1998a). STP camps are staffed by undergraduate and graduate students, supervised by permanent staff, some at the doctoral level. In addition, developmental and educational specialists teach academic subjects, and medical specialists consult on stimulant medication. Elements of the STP are shown in the In Brief box.

Pelham's Summer Treatment Program for ADHD: in brief*

Designed for	ADHD children, aged 5–15
Duration of the program	360 h over 8 weeks of summer; parent training, Saturday treatment, and/or school follow-up may be added
Session length	8:00 AM to 5:00 PM, every weekday, for 8 weeks
Participants	Children in age-matched groups of 12, each group has 5 clinical staff
Theoretical orientation	Social Learning Theory, Operant, Cognitive-Behavioral

Treatment components:
1. Daily schedule for children that includes training in social skills, cooperative projects, academic subjects, arts and crafts, sports, and computer use
2. Token economy with points/chips awarded for appropriate behavior and withdrawn for inappropriate behavior throughout the day, to be exchanged for privileges (e.g., field trips)
3. Use of appropriate commands (e.g., brief, specific) with generous reinforcement for compliance – i.e., points/chips, liberal praise by staff, public recognition, parental rewards
4. Use of time out and loss of privileges as consequences for specific prohibited behaviors
5. One h per day in a school-like classroom learning academic subjects, with token economy and consequences to support appropriate behavior and learning
6. Peer relationship training, with daily group sessions to learn specific skills, daily cooperative group task, group problem solving training, and buddy system to learn dyadic/friend skills
7. Sports training, 3 h/day, to learn rule-following, improve motor coordination, skill in the sport, thus to improve self-esteem and self-efficacy and reduce risk of rejection by peers
8. Parent involvement: Weekly behavioral training sessions, near-daily parent contact with camp staff, daily report cards, with home token economy, praise, and privileges as reward
9. Trials to assess whether stimulant medication improves child behavior beyond effects of other camp components
10. Follow-up treatment options including Saturday treatment program, intervention in schools to which children return, and parent booster sessions

* In Brief section reprinted from JR Weisz (2004) Psychotherapy for children and adolescents: Evidence-based treatments and case examples. Cambridge University Press, Cambridge, UK.

12.7 Therapies for Conduct Problems, Oppositional Defiant Disorder, and Conduct Disorder

12.7.1 Background

Conduct problems – aggression toward peers, disobedience and disruptive behavior, and defiance of authority – are sources of great concern in most societies, and the prevalence of oppositional and defiant behavior may have increased over the past two decades, at least in the USA (Achenbach et al. 2003). Such shocks as the murders of students and teachers by armed youths in schools have served as wakeup calls, a reminder of the extremes to which aggressive tendencies can be taken if not curbed in childhood. One of the most consistent findings of research is that aggression and conduct problems are persistent across developmental periods. Children as young as 2–3 years old who show high levels of conduct problems across different settings are at risk of continued behavior problems for years. Further, conduct problems that are stable at the time of school entry are apt to persist into adolescence. The fact that conduct problems in early life predict subsequent delinquency and criminal behavior underscores the need for treatments that work with children.

The challenge of understanding and treating conduct problems is complicated by the heterogeneity of such problems and the youth who display them, and by the fact that multiple causes (biological, cognitive, interpersonal, sociological) interact to produce them. A particularly worrisome trend is the developmental progression of conduct problems from childhood through adolescence, with early oppositional behavior presaging later more violent forms, including fighting and vandalism at the intermediate level, and stealing and mugging at the more extreme end. Many experts agree that any search for a simple causal explanation is doomed from the outset. Similarly, any search for a single treatment to address all forms of disruptive and deviant conduct, may be fruitless; different treatments may differ in their impact on different subsets of youth, depending in part on which factors converge to maintain the various youngsters' conduct problems. Thus, it may be quite apropos that the treatments developed and tested thus far are so variegated, focus on a range of target problems, and address various hypothesized causal and maintaining factors.

12.7.2 Indications and Significance

Conduct problems are the most common reason for child clinical referrals in North America (Hinshaw et al. 1996). Of course, this is partly due to the high prevalence of such problems. Formal diagnoses of conduct disorder are found in 2–6% of school-aged youth in community samples (see Hinshaw and Anderson 1996); rates of oppositional defiant disorder are found to be uniformly higher, with estimates ranging from 10–22% in the general population (Nottelman and Jensen 1995). But other evidence (Weisz 2004) indicates that even when problem prevalence in the general population is controlled, conduct problems are much more likely than other problems to be the reason children are taken to clinics for treatment, at least in North America. This fact, coupled with the obviously high stakes for society, may help account for the high activity level among researchers in developing treatments for conduct problems.

12.7.3 Overview of Beneficial Treatments

These treatments range from very focused techniques for teaching young people self-control to broader methods of restructuring family and social environments. One set of approaches (Feindler et al. 1984; Lochman et al. 2003) emphasizes teaching youngsters to manage their anger. Another youth-focused approach emphasizes the value of prob-

lem-solving skills (Kazdin 2003). Several approaches employ behavioral parent training principles and procedures reflecting the early work of Patterson and Gulion (1968) and Hanf (1969). Another method, designed for particularly difficult antisocial youths, intervenes within multiple systems that touch the errant youth's life. Treatments for conduct problems and conduct disorder include a rich array of evidence-based options, addressing multiple possible causal factors and spanning a broad developmental range.

12.7.4 Techniques of Treatment and Management

12.7.4.1 Youth Anger Management Training: Conceptual Basis and Procedural Overview

Anger management programs (e.g., Feindler et al. 1984; Lochman et al. 2003) emphasize teaching self-control and problem solving skills. These treatments have grown out of social-cognitive models of anger arousal and aggressive behavior. In the Lochman et al. model, for example, the youth encounters a potentially anger-arousing event, but the youth's physiological and emotional response is due to the youth's perception of the event, not the event itself. The perception is derived from such sources as the youth's learning history and selective attention to specific aspects of the event. The way such factors converge sets the stage for the youth's response. That response is followed by some consequence for the aggressive youth (e.g., school suspension). The model posits multiple deficits that make aggressive youth prone to maladaptive behavioral responses. The deficits include, for example, (a) attributional biases toward perceiving hostile intentions by others when their intentions are unclear, (b) a tendency to underestimate the youth's own role in conflict and overestimate others' responsibility, and (c) a belief that problems cannot be resolved through nonaggressive means.

Lochman and colleagues developed their Anger Coping Program to confront such deficits. Youngsters meet in groups for exercises designed to counter their reflexive responses to perceived threat. The following three steps are considered critical. Therapists teach the children (a) to inhibit their initial angry and aggressive reactions, (b) to cognitively relabel stimuli perceived as threatening, and (c) to solve problems by generating alternative coping responses and choosing adaptive, nonaggressive alternatives. An overall aim is to enhance children's cognitive processing of their stressful encounters, and strengthen their ability to plan effective and adaptive responses. In addition, as the program has evolved, an emphasis on learning to set and achieve specific behavioral goals has become quite central, as well.

Anger Coping Program: in brief*	
Designed for	Aggressive school children aged 9–13
Number of sessions	1218
Session length	40–60 min
Session participants	Therapist with youth in small groups
Theoretical orientation	Cognitive behavioral

Treatment steps:

1. Discuss group goal of learning about members' similarities and differences; take pictures of each group member with instant camera; use visual exercises (e.g., face/vase) to illustrate how different people can have different perceptions of the same thing
2. Exercises and discussion to explore children's reactions to cooperating with, being controlled by, and being distracted by peers. For example, build domino towers while peers try to verbally distract
3. Use stories and role plays to practice identifying the problem – i.e., which specific aspect(s) of an interpersonal situation create a problem and lead to anger
4. Use cartoon sequences and role plays to practice generating alternative solutions to problems
5. Use cartoon sequences and role plays to practice evaluating pros and cons of various alternative solutions to problems
6. Use modeling videotape to learn to identify bodily cues that signal angry arousal, and to identify negative and positive thoughts (or »self-statements«) that can increase or diminish angry arousal
7. Use other modeling videotapes to practice integrating (a) physiological awareness of angry arousal, (b) self-talk (e.g., »Stop! Think! What should I do?), and (c) social problem solving, to resolve interpersonal problems without aggression

8. Use role plays to continue practicing physiological awareness + self talk + interpersonal problem solving. Videotape the role plays and discuss them. Plan for extending anger control skills to future situations at school and home
9. Practice setting specific behavioral goals – e.g., no arguments with teacher – achieving them, and being rewarded for doing so; this component may be introduced at any point in treatment, and may operate concurrently with other treatment components

* In Brief section reprinted from JR Weisz (2004) Psychotherapy for children and adolescents: Evidence-based treatments and case examples. Cambridge University Press, Cambridge, UK.

12.7.4.2 Problem Solving Skills Training: Conceptual Basis and Procedural Overview

A second intervention approach aimed at creating change within the individual youth is Problem Solving Skills Training (PSST; Kazdin 2003), a program designed to teach aggressive youngsters to use their heads before using their fists. PSST grows out of a particular model of how antisocial behavior and conduct disorder develop and are maintained (see Kazdin 2003). The model focuses on »packages« of risk factors (biological, social-environmental, and cognitive) that may combine to produce behaviorally toxic outcomes, and on the »snowballing« of these factors over time. For example, children with difficult temperaments who are exposed to poor parenting may fail to develop adequate self-control. Disciplinary problems may follow, along with deficient school performance and impulsively aggressive behavior. Aggression, together with other social and academic problems, may lead to social rejection, and then by default to affiliation with deviant peer groups, in which antisocial behavior is modeled and rewarded.

The challenge for a treatment developer is to identify a process which, if properly addressed, can interrupt the developmental progression toward increasingly serious conduct problems and antisocial behavior. One component quite central to PSST is youth cognition. PSST aims to help youngsters (a) identify the specific interpersonal problems they confront, (b) generate alternative solutions they might use to address the problems, (c) think through the steps needed to carry out these solutions, and (d) anticipate the likely consequences of various solutions for others and for themselves. Two central goals of PSST warrant attention here. One is to improve the process by which children reason as they confront various interpersonal problems – e.g., to make the process more systematic and less impulsive, and to bring a broader range of solutions into focus for consideration. Another goal is to increase the number of prosocial solutions children consider and ultimately employ.

In PSST, children aged 7–13 take part in about 20 weekly sessions with a therapist. Each session lasts about 40–50 min. During these sessions, children are taught five steps they can apply to problems of many different types. The steps range from simply identifying the problem to laying out potential solutions and selecting the most promising of these to try. These problem solving steps are first practiced in the context of simple games, and then gradually applied to the kinds of real-life social problems that have caused difficulties for the youngsters in the past. Parents are also taught the skills, so they can help their children outside the sessions. PSST is sometimes paired with behavioral parent training in child management, based in part on the valuable work of Patterson and colleagues (e.g., Patterson and Gullion 1968), and called Parent Management Training (PMT) by Kazdin and colleagues. PMT involves about 16 weekly one-hour sessions, most of which include some explanation of behavioral concepts and procedures, some teaching of the relevant skills, some planning of how to apply the skills at home with the child, and some role-playing and rehearsal with the therapist. Parents try the skills with the child at home and use therapy sessions, in part, to help trouble-shoot and refine their application of PMT skills.

Problem Solving Skills Training: in brief*	
Designed for	Aggressive and antisocial children aged 7–13
Number of sessions	20 (range: 20–25)
Session length	40–50 min
Session participants	Therapist with child, plus parent contact
Theoretical orientation	Behavioral

Treatment steps:
1. Therapist teaches child five problem-solving steps (identify the problem, list possible solutions, evaluate them, choose one, try it and evaluate the outcome)
2. Child practices the steps on various games (e.g., Checkers, Connect Four)
3. Child practices applying the steps to real-life, everyday problems (e.g., peer conflict)
4. Parent learns the steps; learns to prompt and praise child's use of steps with real-life problems (called »supersolvers«), including problems that originally led to referral
5. Child continues to practice applying steps to real-life situations (e.g., peer taunting, social exclusion, peers encouraging antisocial behavior); solutions re-enacted with therapist
6. Wrap-up, review of what has been learned, role-reversal in which child teaches the skills to the therapist

* In Brief section reprinted from JR Weisz (2004) Psychotherapy for children and adolescents: Evidence-based treatments and case examples. Cambridge University Press, Cambridge, UK.

12.7.4.3 Parent-Child Interaction Treatments: Conceptual Basis and Procedural Overview

While anger management training and PSST focus primarily on the individual youth, another approach targets the parent and child together and addresses their style of interaction. Parent-child interaction treatments (Brinkmeyer and Eyberg 2003; McMahon and Forehand 2003) are built partly on the notion that noncompliance is a foundation on which other conduct problems are built (see McMahon and Forehand 2003), and that it thus warrants focused and early attention. Accordingly, parent-child interaction treatments are generally used to address noncompliance and conduct problems in the preschool through mid-primary school years.

The treatment procedures used in the most prominent parent-child interaction programs were derived in part from a model developed by Hanf (1969). In this paradigm, the therapist works directly with the parent, serving as both teacher and coach, while the parent engages in a series of play-like interactions with the child. In the first phase of the process, the child chooses the play activities. As the child takes the lead, the parent learns to attend closely, comment descriptively, and praise the child liberally. In a second phase, the parent takes the lead in play activities, and the coaching and training focus on evoking child compliance, dealing with noncompliance (e.g., via ignoring or time-out procedures), and generally establishing effective management of child behavior. In this therapeutic two-step, the goals and methods of behavioral parent training are combined with some of the relationship-building goals and methods used in play therapy. Several treatment programs have been built on the basic Hanf model. Here we provide an »In Brief« description of one exemplar, Parent-Child Interaction Therapy (Brinkmeyer and Eyberg 2003).

Parent-Child Interaction Therapy: in brief*	
Designed for	Oppositional children aged 2–6 (but clinical trials have included 8 yr olds)
Number of sessions	13 (range: 9–16)
Session length	60 min
Session participants	Parent-child dyads, therapist
Theoretical orientation	Behavioral, psycho-dynamic, attachment

Treatment steps:
1. Therapist observes parent-child interactions, identifies problems, sets goals
2. Child-Directed Interaction sessions: child leads play activity, parent follows child's lead, using praise, reflection, imitation, description, and enthusiasm (PRIDE)
3. Parent-Directed Interaction sessions: parent leads play activity, gives directives, sets limits, learns to use time-out for noncompliance, learns to reward compliance and appropriate behavior
4. Therapist observes parent-child interactions to assess parent learning, child disruptive behavior
5. Treatment continues until key skills have been mastered and interactions meet pre-determined criteria

*In Brief section reprinted from JR Weisz (2004) Psychotherapy for children and adolescents: Evidence-based treatments and case examples. Cambridge University Press, Cambridge, UK.

12.7.4.4 Video-Guided Group Behavioral Parent Training: Conceptual Basis and Procedural Overview

Another approach to early intervention that is based partly on the Hanf model adds the element of video guidance to the treatment regimen. This approach, called The Incredible years (Webster-Stratton and Reid 2003), is especially notable due to its unusually extensive evidence base (see Weisz 2004). In the parent component of their Incredible years BASIC program, a therapist shows brief videos of parent-child interactions to groups of parents and leads discussions on themes illustrated in the videos. Why train parents using videotapes? One important reason is that theory and research on modeling suggest that it is a highly efficient form of learning. It is also more engaging for many parents than didactic learning in a classroom format, or being tested on readings. Another strength is that the video material is the same at every presentation, which supports consistency across therapists and settings. Such standardization may help limit the impact of variations in therapist training, orientation, and skill. Finally, and notably in an era of fiscal concern, video modeling is cost-effective; it limits expensive therapist training time, and therapist intervention time, in ways that cost-conscious mental health administrators can appreciate.

Although the Hanf model and observational learning form part of the conceptual basis for the treatment, other theoretical perspectives have been influential as well. Building on Bandura's (1977) self-efficacy theory, Webster-Stratton and her colleagues train therapists to work as collaborators with parents, rather than as dispensers of advice; the purpose is to enhance parents' »efficacy expectations« – i.e., the conviction that they can successfully change their own and their child's behavior. CBT theory is also highly relevant, as therapists work with parents to identify and modify unproductive cognitions (e.g., »I'll never be an effective parent« or »My child is impossible to control«) or to reframe distressing events (e.g., a difficult child's demands can be construed as »testing limits« or »moving toward independence«).

In Webster-Stratton's Incredible years BASIC parent training program, groups of 10–14 parents meet with a therapist or »group leader« for 13–14 weekly 2-h sessions. Parents view a series of 1–2-min video vignettes showing parents dealing with their children in a variety of situations, sometimes successfully, sometimes not. These videos are used to stimulate discussion of behavioral principles and how they might be used by parents in the group. Parents practice these principles in homework assignments, some of which include tracking their children's behavior to look for changes after the new parenting methods are implemented. Over the series of sessions, four themes are addressed: constructive use of play, using praise and reward effectively, setting and enforcing limits, and handling misbehavior. Other elements of the BASIC procedure are shown in the In Brief box. Evidence on the beneficial effects of this program, for parents and children, is unusually strong and well-replicated.

The Incredible years BASIC Parent Training Program: in brief*

Designed for	Parents of children aged 3–8 who have conduct problems
Number of sessions	12–14
Session length	2 h
Session participants	Therapist with groups of 10–14 parents
Theoretical orientation	Observational learning, operant, cognitive-behavioral, relationship, group support

Treatment steps:
1. Constructive use of child-directed play. Therapist uses video vignettes and role plays to focus parent discussion on constructive use of child-directed play skills to help build children's self-esteem and self-confidence, help children handle boredom, avoid power struggles with peers, improve language skills (including emotion language) and problem solving, and cope with frustration
2. Effective use of praise and reward. Using other videos, role plays, and guided discussion therapist teaches parents ways to use praise and tangible rewards to increase the frequency of specific, desirable child behaviors. Parents are helped to generalize principles of praise to other relationships such as partners and teachers

3. Limit-setting. With videos, role plays, and discussion, therapist helps parents learn basic rules for effective limit-setting – e.g., limit commands to the ones that really matter, make them clear and concise, fit them to child's maturity level, don't insert a barb, and use distraction to enhance compliance
4. Handling misbehavior. Videos, role plays, and discussion focus on dealing with child misbehavior through preventing it, strategic ignoring, time-out, logical and natural consequences, and problem-solving
Other features, present throughout the steps. Intervention individualized through parent goal-setting and self-monitoring, solution-focused assignments with identification of personal barriers, notes to/from therapist in parent folders, home assignments, and therapist phone calls to parents at home; peer support comes through a support group and through »buddy« calls at home.
* In Brief section reprinted from JR Weisz (2004) Psychotherapy for children and adolescents: Evidence-based treatments and case examples. Cambridge University Press, Cambridge, UK.

12.7.4.5   Multisystemic Therapy: Conceptual Basis and Procedural Overview

Our final example of evidence-based treatments for conduct problems is a program designed for especially difficult youth: adolescents who have histories of serious antisocial behavior, often with arrest records to match. A core idea underlying Multisystemic Therapy (MST; Henggeler and Lee 2003) is the notion that such youth antisocial behavior is multidetermined – i.e., shaped and maintained by multiple elements of the youth's social world – and that the influence is reciprocal, in that the youth both receives and exerts influence. These elements of the social world include immediate and extended family members, teachers and other school personnel, neighbors, peers, religious leaders, various professional agencies, and even law enforcement officers. Of course, the various individuals and systems to which the youth and family are connected interact with one another as well. Antisocial behavior can result from this interplay of youth, key individuals, and social systems, but figuring out how is part of the detective work of MST. Once the therapist has an understanding of how the individuals and systems have converged to produce undesirable behavior, the task is to reconstruct the environment, changing individuals and systems at points where there is some given and where change can have a desirable impact on the youth.

Conceptually, MST is built on general systems theory (von Bertalanffy 1968) and Bronfenbrenner's (1979) theory of social ecology. A major contribution of systems theory is its rich conceptualization of causality. Unlike more mechanistic and linear notions, systems theory describes causality in terms of the reciprocal influence of multiple interacting forces. Instead of arguing that A causes B, which in turn causes C, the systems theorist argues that A, B, and C all influence one another and that any specific behavior may have multiple causes, some reflecting the interplay of A, B, and C. Applying this notion to a delinquent youth, a therapist might consider not only how parental practices influence the youth, but also how the youth's behavior influences the parents, and what function the youth's behavior may serve in the family system, including the extended family. Bronfenbrenner's (1979) theory of social ecology also contributed importantly to the development of MST. In this view, the individual's ecosystem is »a set of nested structures, each inside the next, like a set of Russian dolls« (p. 3). The innermost doll is the developing individual, who is influenced by and who in turn influences other elements or layers of the ecosystem. Thus, an individual's behavior can only be fully understood in relation to its context.

Following these theoretical principles, the ideal MST therapist enters multiple settings in which troubled and troubling youths live their lives, gets acquainted with multiple individuals and entities with whom the youths interact regularly, and works with those individuals and entities to shape changes in the youths' environment that will support desirable behavior and discourage undesirable behavior. Treatment is tailored and adapted to fit each individual case, but several core principles and procedures are intended to lend conceptual consistency to the interventions carried out. Some of the core elements of the MST intervention process are summarized in the In Brief box.

Multisystemic Therapy: in brief*

Designed for	Seriously antisocial, delinquent youths, at high risk of out-of-home placement (e.g., in a corrections facility), often with prior arrests; ages 12–18
Number of sessions	Highly variable; sessions are combined with various brief contacts (some by phone) and diverse environmental interventions; typical treatment duration is about 60 h (plus phone contact and collateral meetings) spanning 4–5 months
Session length	Highly variable; range is about 10 min to several hours, with mean >1 h
Session participants	Therapist with parents, with youth and parents, with youth and family, with family members and extra-family systems (e.g., teachers, neighbors)
Theoretical orientation	Emphasizes empirically-tested procedures that are mainly behavioral (operant), cognitive-behavioral, and pragmatic family therapies

Treatment elements:
1. Therapist carries out assessment, to map (a) youth, family, and system strengths, and (b) the connection between the youth's identified problems and his or her social systems (family, school, neighborhood, peer group, etc.)
2. Therapist together with parents, youth, and others in the social systems, designs interventions to help the social systems support responsible youth behavior and discourage irresponsible behavior

3. Therapist has sessions with family members, to coordinate implementation of the planned interventions, evaluate their progress, adjust them as needed
4. Therapist has multiple weekly contacts with family, in person or by phone, and is available to family through cell phone/pager at all times, for consultation on problems, crises
5. Weekly supervision with an MST expert, and on-call supervision available to therapist at all times, through cell phone/pager
6. Establish family connections to community support systems, and introduce other changes to support staying power and generalization of treatment effects

* In Brief section reprinted from JR Weisz (2004) Psychotherapy for children and adolescents: Evidence-based treatments and case examples. Cambridge University Press, Cambridge, UK.

12.8   Treatment Results: Efficacy, Effectiveness, Issues for Attention in Future Research

The treatments reviewed here are examples of a broader array of evidence-based interventions that have been developed for children and adolescents. Taken together, the literature on the full array of treatments reveals a number of strengths. Meta-analytic reviews cited previously point to mean effects of tested treatments that (a) fall within the »medium« to »large« range (as per Cohen 1988), (b) are relatively specific to the problems and disorders targeted in treatment, not just general improvements in overall adjustment, and (c) show substantial holding power, at least over the 5–6 month periods characteristic of most follow-up assessments. Another strength is the creative array of treatment delivery models employed across the various interventions. The traditional weekly office visit model still predominates in the research base, but alternative approaches have also been developed. Some are geared to school breaks and summer camp programs, some employ parent group discussions guided by videotaped vignettes, others include treatment supplements in the form of posttherapy booster sessions, and at least one employs a peripatetic therapist intervening within multiple layers of the youth's social environment.

On the other hand, there are significant gaps in the evidence base, suggesting directions in which future research might be directed. First, for some problem areas in which risk is great and need for interventions is pronounced we have relatively little in the way of evidence-based, beneficial programs. Anorexia, substance abuse, and suicidal behavior, for example, need increased research attention, and we lack strong nonmedication interventions for ADHD in adolescence. The problem of limited coverage is even more pronounced if we consider covariation and comorbidity. Most treatment research with children and teens has focused on single problems or disorders. Extensive evidence (e.g., Angold et al. 1999) indicates that co-occurrence of disorders and problems is quite characteristic of the youngsters seen in everyday clinical care. Rates of comorbidity, striking even in community samples, are markedly higher in clinical samples (Angold et al. 1999). We need to understand the extent to which comorbidities of various kinds moderate the effects of treatments, and we may well need more treatments designed to encompass multiple problems and disorders.

A second area in need of attention concerns theoretical models of treatment. Meta-analyses that encompass both children and adolescents (Kazdin et al. 1990; Weisz et al. 1987, 1995) have found a heavy emphasis on tests of behavioral and cognitive-behavioral treatments, with nonbehavioral approaches (e.g., psychodynamic, client-centered, psychoanalytic, existential-humanistic) constituting 18–26% of the studies sampled. Yet, these nonbehavioral approaches are actually much more representative of the treatment models used in most everyday clinical practice. It seems appropriate for researchers to broaden the array of models tested, working to include more of the approaches service providers use and trust.

A third concern is that many of our treatments are omnibus in style – packing a variety of procedures and training a variety of skills, but without a clear or coherent picture of which ones really matter. Researchers have barely begun to dismantle most treatment packages to identify the specific components that are actually necessary for good outcomes. As a result, many of our treatments may be a rather poor fit to the current emphasis in real-world clinical care on session limits and maximum efficiency. Making treatment programs more streamlined and efficient could enhance their attractiveness to practitioners, render the procedures more teachable, increase treatment viability in the marketplace of clinical care, and thus perhaps reach more of the children who need their benefits.

A fourth topic for future research is treatment outcome moderation. For each treatment in the armamentarium, we need to understand the range of youth clinical and demographic characteristics within which the treatments produce the greatest benefit and outside of which benefit diminishes. Even the best-supported programs are good for some conditions but not others, with benefit potentially constrained by comorbid conditions, age, SES, ethnicity, family configuration, or other clinical and demographic factors. Although many researchers have begun the process of testing for moderation of treatment effects, we remain poorly informed about the boundary conditions surrounding most of the evidence-based treatments. As an example, racial, ethnic, and cultural factors are embedded but unexamined in most of our treatment outcome research (Weisz 2004), and this makes it difficult to know how robust most treatment effects are across various population groups. At this early stage in youth treatment development research, it is understandable that most tested treatments have not been designed to take into account broad variations in language, values, customs, child-rearing traditions, beliefs and expectancies about child and parent behavior, and distinctive stressors and resources associated with different cultural traditions. But this theme certainly warrants attention in the next generation of research.

A fifth goal for the future is to expand our grasp of the change processes in treatment that account for observed outcomes. At present, we know much more about what outcomes our treatments produce than about what actually causes the outcomes (Kazdin 2000). If we fail to identify core causal processes, we risk a proliferation of treatments administered rather superstitiously because studies show they work, but without an understanding of the change processes therapists actually need to set in motion to produce results. To understand how the treatments work, we need a generation of research testing hypothesized mediators of outcome, using procedures outlined by several leaders in the field (e.g., Baron and Kenney 1986; Kraemer et al. 2002).

A sixth area in need of attention is the therapeutic relationship. The current array of evidence-based treatments is strong in describing principles and procedures to apply in treatment, but weak in helping therapists build a warm, empathic relationship and a strong working alliance with children and families. This gap is striking in light of the widespread belief that the quality of the therapeutic relationship or alliance is important to success in most treatment encounters. Indeed, many child therapists rate the therapeutic relationship as more important than the specific techniques used in treatment. What we lack thus far is a strong body of evidence (a) clearly defining what a positive therapeutic relationship is, (b) establishing how best to measure it, (c) identifying therapist characteristics and behaviors that foster it, and (c) testing the extent to which it actually predicts outcome when evidence-based treatments are used.

A final topic for future research is the relation between evidence-based practices and everyday clinical care. Given the nature of the research conducted to date, we know a good deal about the efficacy of our EBTs, i.e., their effects under experimentally contrived conditions. However, we know little about their effectiveness, i.e., their effects in representative clinical practice conditions. This is a problem in its own right, but it also contributes to a number of other problems, including the very limited dissemination the tested treatments have enjoyed to date. If we want these treatments to reach the youths and families who need them, we may need a body of evidence on how the treatments fare with precisely those youths and families in the clinical practice settings where they typically receive care. Moreover, if this evidence suggests that treatments that fare well in efficacy trials produce less impressive outcomes in everyday clinical practice, we may need models of treatment development and testing designed to bridge the gap between research and practice, e.g., the Deployment-Focused Model described by Weisz (2004), and we may need a generation of research built on such models.

References

Achenbach TM (1991) Manual for the Child Behavior Checklist/ 4–18 and 1991 profile. University of Vermont Department of Psychiatry, Burlington, VT.

Achenbach TM, Dumenci L, Rescorla LA (2003) Are American children's problems still getting worse? A 23-year comparison. Journal of Abnormal Child Psychology 31:1–11.

Albano AM, Chorpita B, Barlow DH (1996) Childhood anxiety disorders. In: Mash EJ, Barkley RA (eds) Child psychopathology. Guilford, New York, pp. 196–241.

American Psychiatric Association (1994) Diagnostic and statistical manual of mental disorders, fourth edition. American Psychiatric Association, Washington, DC.

Angold A, Costello EJ, Erkanli A (1999) Comorbidity. Journal of Child Psychology and Psychiatry 40:57–87.

Bandura A (1977) Self-efficacy: Toward a unifying theory of behavioral change. Psychological Review 84:191–215.

Barkley RA (1997) Defiant children: A clinician's manual for assessment and parent training. Guilford, New York.

Baron RM, Kenny DA (1986) The moderator-mediator variable distinction in social psychological research: Conceptual, strategic, and statistical considerations. Journal of Personality and Social Psychology 51:1173–1182.

Barrett PM, Shortt AL (2003) Parental involvement in the treatment of anxious children. In: Kazdin AE, Weisz JR (eds) Evidence-based psychotherapies for children and adolescents. Guilford, New York, pp. 204–223.

Brestan EV, Eyberg SM (1998) Effective psychosocial treatments of conduct-disordered children and adolescents: 29 years, 82 studies, and 5,272 kids. Journal of Clinical Child Psychology 27:180–189.

Brinkmeyer MY, Eyberg SM (2003) Parent-Child Interaction Therapy for oppositional children. In: Kazdin AE, Weisz JR (eds) Evidence-based psychotherapies for children and adolescents. Guilford, New York, pp. 204–223.

Bronfenbrenner U (1979) The ecology of human development. Harvard University Press, Cambridge, MA.

Burns BJ, Costello EJ, Angold A, Tweed D, Stangl D, Farmer EMZ, Erkanli A (1995) Children's mental health service use across service sectors. Health Affairs 14:147–159.

Bussing R, Zima BT, Perwien AR, Belin TR, Widawski M (1998) Children in special education programs: Attention deficit, hyperactivity disorder, use of services, and unmet needs. American Journal of Public Health 88:880–886.

Casey RJ, Berman JS (1985) The outcome of psychotherapy with children. Psychological Bulletin 98:388–400.

Clarke GN, DeBar LL, Lewinsohn PM (2003) Cognitive-behavioral therapy for adolescent depression: Comparative efficacy, mediation, moderation, and effectiveness. In: Kazdin AE, Weisz JR (eds) Evidence-based psychotherapies for children and adolescents. Guilford, New York, pp. 120–134.

Cohen J (1988) Statistical power analysis for the behavioral sciences (2nd ed.). Erlbaum, Hillsdale, NJ.

Douglas VI (1972) Stop, look, and listen: The problem of sustained attention and impulse control in hyperactive and normal children. Canadian Journal of Behavioral Science 4:259–282.

Durlak JA, Wells AM, Cotton JK, Johnson S (1995) Analysis of selected methodological issues in child psychotherapy research. Journal of Clinical Child Psychology 24:141–148.

Eysenck HJ (1952) The effects of psychotherapy: An evaluation. Journal of Consulting Psychology 16:319–324.

Eysenck HJ (1960) The effects of psychotherapy. In: Eysenck HJ (ed) Handbook of abnormal psychology: An experimental approach. Pitman Medical Publishing, London.

Eysenck HJ (1966) The effects of psychotherapy. International Science Press, New York.

Feindler EL, Marriott SA, Iwata M (1984) Group anger control training for junior high school delinquents. Cognitive Therapy and Research 8:299–311.

Freedheim DK (ed) (1992) History of psychotherapy: A century of change. American Psychological Association, Washington, DC.

Freud S (1955) Analysis of a phobia in a five-year-old boy (1909). In: Standard Editions of the complete psychological works of Sigmund Freud. Hogarth Press, London.

Garland AF, Zigler E (1993) Adolescent suicide prevention: Current research and social policy implications. American Psychologist 48:169–182.

Hammen C, Rudolph KD (1996) Childhood depression. In: Mash EJ, Barkley RA (eds) Child psychopathology. Guilford, New York, pp. 153–195.

Hanf C (1969) A two-stage program for modifying maternal controlling during mother-child interaction. Paper presented at the Western Psychological Association meeting, Vancouver, BC, Canada.

Henggeler SW, Lee T (2003) Multisystemic treatment of serious clinical problems. In: Kazdin AE, Weisz JR (eds) Evidence-based psychotherapies for children and adolescents. Guilford, New York, pp. 301–322.

Hinshaw SP (1994) Attention deficits and hyperactivity in children. Sage, Thousand Oaks, CA.

Hinshaw SP, Anderson CA (1996) Conduct and oppositional defiant disorders. In: Mash EJ, Barkley RA (eds) Child psychopathology. Guilford, New York.

Jensen AL, Weisz JR (2002) Assessing match and mismatch between practitioner-generated and standardized interview-generated diagnoses for clinic-referred children and adolescents. Journal of Consulting and Clinical Psychology 70:158–168.

Jones MC (1924) A laboratory study of fear: The case of Peter. Pedagogical Seminary 31:308–315.

Kaslow NJ, Thompson MP (1998) Applying the criteria for empirically supported treatments to studies of psychosocial interventions for child and adolescent depression. Journal of Clinical Child Psychology 27:146–155.

Kazdin AE (2000) Psychotherapy for children and adolescents: Directions for research and practice. Oxford University Press, New York.

Kazdin AE (2003) Problem-Solving Skills Training and Parent Management Training for conduct disorder. In: Kazdin AE, Weisz JR (eds) Evidence-based psychotherapies for children and adolescents. Guilford, New York, pp. 241–262.

Kazdin AE, Bass D, Ayers WA, Rodgers A (1990) Empirical and clinical focus of child and adolescent psychotherapy research. Journal of Consulting and Clinical Psychology 58:729–740.

Kendall PC, Aschenbrand SG, Hudson JL (2003) Child-focused treatment of anxiety. In: Kazdin AE, Weisz JR (eds) Evidence-based psychotherapies for children and adolescents. Guilford, New York, pp. 81–100.

Kraemer HC, Wilson T, Fairburn CG, Agras WS (2002) Mediators and moderators of treatment effects in randomized clinical trials. Archives of General Psychiatry 59:877–883.

Leaf PJ, Alegria M, Cohen P, Goodman SH, Horwitz SM, Hoven CW, Narrow WE, Vadem-Kierman M, Reiger DA (1996) Mental health service use in the community and schools: Results from the four-community MECA Study. (Methods for the Epidemiology of Child and Adolescent Mental Disorders Study) Journal of the American Academy of Child and Adolescent Psychiatry 35:889–897.

Levitt EE (1957) The results of psychotherapy with children: An evaluation. Journal of Consulting Psychology 21:189–196.

Levitt EE (1963) Psychotherapy with children: A further evaluation. Behaviour Research and Therapy 60:326–329.

Lochman JE, Barry TD, Pardini DA (2003) Anger control training for aggressive youth. In: Kazdin AE, Weisz JR (eds) Evidence-based psychotherapies for children and adolescents. Guilford, New York, pp. 263–281.

Lonigan C J, Elbert JC, Bennett-Johnson S (1998) Empirically supported psychosocial interventions for children: An overview. Journal of Clinical Child Psychology 27:138–145.

McLeod BD, Weisz JR (in press) Increasing the accuracy of treatment effect estimates in youth therapy trials: Using dissertations to assess and address publication and file drawer bias. Journal of Consulting and Clinical Psychology.

McMahon RJ, Forehand R (2003) Helping the noncompliant child: Family based treatment for oppositional behavior (2nd ed.). Guilford Press, New York.

Mash EJ, Wolfe DA (2002) Abnormal child psychology, 2nd ed. Wadsworth, Belmont, CA.

Mufson L, Dorta KP (2003) Interpersonal psychotherapy for depressed adolescents. In: Kazdin AE, Weisz JR (eds) Evidence-based psychotherapies for children and adolescents. Guilford, New York, pp. 148–164.

Nottelman ED, Jensen PS (1995) Comorbidity of disorders in children and adolescents: Developmental perspectives. In: Ollendick TH, Prinz RJ (eds) Advances in clinical child psychology. Plenum, New York, pp. 109–155.

Ollendick TH, King NJ (1998) Empirically supported treatments for children with phobic and anxiety disorders: Current status. Journal of Clinical Child Psychology 27:156–167.

Patterson GR, Gullion ME (1968) Living with children: New methods for parents and teachers. Research Press, Champaign, IL.

Pelham WE, Greiner AR, Gnagy EM (1998 a) Children's Summer Treatment Program manual. State University of New York at Buffalo, New York.

Pelham WE, Wheeler T, Chronis A (1998 b) Empirically supported psychosocial treatments for attention deficit hyperactivity disorder. Journal of Clinical Child Psychology 27:190–205.

Rossello J, Bernal G (1999) The efficacy of cognitive-behavioral and interpersonal treatments for depression in Puerto Rican adolescents. Journal of Consulting and Clinical Psychology 67:734–745.

Silverman WK, Ginsburg CS (1995) Specific phobias and generalized anxiety disorder. In: March JS (ed) Anxiety disorders in children and adolescents. Guilford Press, New York, pp. 151–180.

Swanson, JM, McBurnett K, Christian DL, Wigal T (1995) Stimulant medication and treatment of children with ADHD. In: Ollendick TH, Prinz RJ (eds) Advances in Clinical Child Psychology (Vol. 17). Plenum, New York, pp. 265–322.

von Bertalanffy L (1968) General systems theory. Braziller, New York.

Watson JB, Rayner R (1920) Conditioned emotional reactions. Journal of Experimental Psychology 3:1–14.

Webster-Stratton C, Reid MJ (2003) The Incredible years Parent, Teachers, and Children Training Series: A multifaceted treatment approach for young children with conduct problems. In: Kazdin AE, Weisz JR (eds) Evidence-based psychotherapies for children and adolescents. Guilford, New York, pp. 224–240.

Weisz JR (2004) Psychotherapy for children and adolescents: Evidence-based treatments and case examples. Cambridge University Press, Cambridge, UK.

Weisz JR, Jensen PS (1999) Efficacy and effectiveness of child and adolescent psychotherapy and pharmacotherapy. Mental Health Services Research 1:125–157.

Weisz JR, Hawley KM (2002) Developmental factors in the treatment of adolescents. Journal of Consulting and Clinical Psychology 70:21–43.

Weisz JR, Weiss B, Alicke MD, Klotz ML (1987) Effectiveness of psychotherapy with children and adolescents: A meta-analysis for clinicians. Journal of Consulting and Clinical Psychology 55:542–549.

Weisz JR, Weiss B, Donenberg GR (1992) The lab versus the clinic: Effects of child and adolescent psychotherapy. American Psychologist 47:1578–1585.

Weisz JR, Weiss B, Han SS, Granger DA, Morton T (1995) Effects of psychotherapy with children and adolescents revisited: A meta-analysis of treatment outcome studies. Psychological Bulletin 117:450–468.

Family Therapy

David Cottrell, Paula Boston, Dawn Walker

13.1   Introduction   – 164

13.2   The Early Development of Family Therapy, Different Schools of Family Therapy and the Techniques Associated with Them   – 165
13.2.1   Development of Systemic Family Therapy   – 165
13.2.2   Early Systemic Therapy   – 166
13.2.3   Second-Order Cybernetics and Constructivism   – 166
13.2.4   Social Constructionism   – 166
13.2.5   Contemporary Systemic Family Therapy Models   – 167
13.2.5.1 Minuchin's Structural Family Therapy   – 167
13.2.5.2 Post-Milan Therapy   – 167
13.2.5.3 Brief Solution-Focused Therapy   – 168
13.2.5.4 White and Epston's Narrative Therapy   – 169
13.2.5.5 Anderson, Goolishan and Andersen's Post-modern Collaborative Approach   – 170
13.2.5.6 Cognitive Behavioral Family Therapy   – 171

13.3   Assessment and Indications for Family Therapy   – 171
13.3.1   Introduction   – 171
13.3.2   The Context of Assessment   – 172
13.3.3   Family Typologies   – 173
13.3.4   Conducting an Evaluation or Assessment   – 173
13.3.5   Post-modern Assessment   – 176
13.3.6   Conclusion   – 178

13.4   The Effectiveness of Family Therapy Approaches   – 178
13.4.1   Introduction   – 178
13.4.2   Outcome Trials of Family Therapy   – 178
13.4.2.1 Conduct Disorders, Delinquency and Substance Misuse   – 178
13.4.2.2 Eating Disorders   – 179
13.4.2.3 Other Presenting Problems   – 179
13.4.3   Service-User Perspectives on Family Therapy   – 180
13.4.4   Conclusions   – 180

13.5   Service-User Involvement in Family Therapy   – 180

13.6   Conclusions   – 182

        References   – 182

13

13.1   Introduction

Family therapy was initially defined as any psychotherapeutic endeavor that explicitly focused on altering the interactions between or among family members, and sought to improve the functioning of the family as a unit, or its subsystems, and/or the functioning of the individual members of the family (Gurman et al. 1986). With time, the working definition of »family« has changed substantially. Family therapy (or, more appropriately, systemic therapy) usually refers to the inclusion in treatment of people who have a significant relationship to the individual concerned, not necessarily bounded by biological, legal, or household designations. The »system« of treatment is now seen as including those who have a part in the concern about the problems and those who could provide resources and support for change, i.e., the system includes the therapy team.

The boundaries between different therapeutic modalities are becoming increasingly blurred. Parent training programs, and cognitive behavior therapy for individual children that also involves parents as cotherapists, might also seem to fit the definitions above. What distinguishes therapists who may be observed to be acting in similar ways in the therapy session is their therapeutic intention in intervening, the theoretical rationale for the interventions they make. An observational and interview study of family therapists in the UK suggested eleven guiding principles that characterize systemic family therapists: a systems focus; seeing relationships in terms of connections and patterns; circularity; an emphasis on strengths and solutions; meaning seen as relating to context; coconstructed practice; reflexivity; use of narrative; interest in language; attention to power; and constructivism (Pote et al. 2003).

Within this chapter, we will focus on therapies that draw on these systemic, cybernetic, narrative, constructivist, or constructionist theories. We will discuss the development of family therapy over time and the schools of family therapy most commonly practiced today, giving a brief account of the underlying theory and the techniques most commonly associated with each school. We will consider the question of assessment and the relative indications for family therapy alongside the evidence for the effectiveness of family therapies. Family therapists have always been concerned with the imbalances of power in the therapeutic relationship and latterly have been at pains to make more transparent the therapeutic process and to empower clients to be as involved with the process of therapy as the therapist. We will therefore conclude with some discussion of child users' views of therapy and how service users can be included in the development of family therapy services.

13.2 The Early Development of Family Therapy, Different Schools of Family Therapy and the Techniques Associated with Them

13.2.1 Development of Systemic Family Therapy

Systemic family therapy traces its origins from the 1950s and currently encompasses several models. There are numerous differences in the practice and use of theory and the definitions of different schools of systemic practice are varied. This section will review the development of the most prominent contemporary strands of family therapy, and briefly describe the theory and techniques associated with each. Early systems family therapy was not the offspring of any individual person or theory but rather a product of several key players and significant meetings. In the UK some of the ground was laid by Bowlby's work on mother-child attachment and his research on children separated from parents during the war (Bowlby 1961). RD Laing's radical perspective on schizophrenia and its creation by family and society (Laing and Esterson 1964), and later, Robin Skynner's application of psychodynamic ideas to families (Skynner 1976) were also influential.

Developers of family therapy in the USA were typically psychoanalysts who had become disen-

chanted with the limitations of a psychotherapy that excluded consideration of current relationships other than that between therapist and client (Ackerman 1958; Bowen 1966; Whitaker 1975). These analysts saw pathology as a function of family dynamics, and treatment as having to do with seeing the whole family rather than the individual and their internalized »family experiences«. They were frustrated with the failure of classical psychoanalytic methods to reach difficult-to-treat patients, for example, people with schizophrenia and adolescents with behavioral problems, but at this point they lacked a common theoretical position.

In the 1950s, a group was established in Palo Alto, later known as the Mental Research Institute, to investigate patterns of communication. They produced numerous seminal papers (see for example Bateson et al. 1956; Weakland and Jackson 1958). The concept of homeostasis, originally suggested by Jackson, became a prominent explanation of family resistance to treatment (Jackson 1957). This interest in patterns of communication between people, initially dyads, led to the search for a theory that would account for interpersonal, rather than intrapsychic exchange and general systems therapy (von Bertalanffy 1969) became an important influence.

General systems theory purports that living organisms can be seen as a group of elements in interaction with one another, forming stability over time, with boundaries and subparts within itself and between itself and the environment. The system has properties such as wholeness and nonsummativity (the whole is greater than the sum of its parts), feedback incorporated to maintain the function of the system, and equifinality (the same end points can be reached by different stimuli (the organization of the system is more significant in determining reactions). Bateson contributed an elaborate vocabulary to describe these patterns of interactions: complementarity and symmetry, for example. He later employed the theory of logical types (Whitehead and Russell 1910) to give a more detailed explanation of the confusion around »schizophrenic« communication. The double bind theory of schizophrenia was developed which looked at paradox in communication (Bateson et al. 1956; Jackson 1957). In conjunction with Norbert Wiener, who was discussing the new field of cybernetics, Bateson linked general systems theory and cybernetics, thus starting the mechanistic metaphor which would have such a major impact in the field for decades (Wiener 1948).

Given the application of general systems therapy to families and the notion of family homeostasis, the question remained »what is the specific mechanism that kept families from changing?« Cybernetics seemed to provide a more specific metaphor for thinking of the internal processes that might be at work to maintain equilibrium. The principal conceptual leap was the recognition that a host of physically different situations involving regulation of behavior in mechanical, electrical, biological, and even social systems could be understood as manifestations of one basic phenomena: the return of information to form a closed control loop. This return of information to form a closed control loop was »feedback«.

13.2.2   Early Systemic Therapy

From these disparate sources a consensus emerged of what was held in common for systemic therapists, the main points being as follows: the family is a system with boundaries/subsystems/and wider systems; patterns of interaction connect the different parts of the system; these patterns are rule governed and recursive; a system contains processes for both change and stability; problems can be functional as a way to maintain the stability of the system; certain behavior patterns can be categorized as symmetrical or complementary; change can be minor or more significant in terms of levels of abstraction; and patterns at one level may be seen at a higher level (Carr 2000 a). Problems, in this view, become social phenomena whose development, persistence and elimination take place within the interactional arena (Anderson 1997).

There was a split within the original members of the Mental Research Institute, ostensibly around irreconcilable ideas on the nature of power in human relationships. One group, led by Jay Haley, developed an orientation that placed emphasis not on the homeostatic function of the problem in the management of feedback loops, but rather on the system's responses to difficulties and problems maintaining behavior. They developed the use of paradoxes into a pragmatic brief therapy, called strategic therapy. This was the precursor to what is now known as brief, solution-focused therapy, which will be described in a following section.

In the same period, another psychoanalyst, Salvador Minuchin, was also breaking away from individual treatment. His client population comprised deprived inner city families with children with be-

havioral difficulties and conduct disorder (Minuchin et al. 1964, 1967). He developed the view that healthy families had clear interpersonal boundaries, drawing from organizational theory. Minuchin's model became known as structural family therapy and has remained true to its early roots. This model will be discussed in greater detail in later sections.

13.2.3   Second-Order Cybernetics and Constructivism

Second-order family therapy was marked by the inclusion of the concept of constructivism. Inherent in this body of thought is the notion that what is »known« in the external world is determined by our innate mental and sensory structures (Maturana and Varela 1984; Kelly 1955). This was a change from the former position that external reality was »knowable«. Systems were no longer »out there« to be observed in isolation, the mental constructions of the observer needed to be included. In terms of family therapy, this now meant that therapists were called upon to include their own personal or theoretical bias as part of the systemic formulation.

13.2.4   Social Constructionism

Another profoundly different way of considering »reality« came from the body of work known as social constructionism. This suggests that reality is created through language in an ongoing interactional and relational process. Discourse about the world is not a reflection or map of the world but an artifact of communal interchanges (Gergen 1985). Family therapists now became interested in an active process of meaning making, a greater variation of possible realities and in the inherent assumptions in particular discourses and ideas that had been excluded.

13.2.5   Contemporary Systemic Family Therapy Models

The primary schools of family therapy are most accurately referenced by their major developers rather than by their theory or even techniques as they continue to be redefined and do not always maintain clear distinctions. The major schools of systemic family therapy currently are as follows: Minuchin's

Structural Therapy, Boscolo and Cecchin's Post-Milan Therapy, De Shazer's Brief Solution Focused Therapy, White and Epston's Narrative Therapy and Anderson, Goolishan and Andersen's Postmodern Collaborative Approach.

13.2.5.1 Minuchin's Structural Family Therapy

Here the underpinning theory of change is that problems result from inappropriate family structure and organization (Minuchin et al. 1967; Minuchin 1974, 1978). The symptom arises from a dysfunctional organization and will disappear when the family organization alters. The therapist is concerned with the boundaries between the parental subsystem, the child subsystem and the extended family and sees the family in terms of spatial relationships, extremes being enmeshed or disengaged. There is a normative map of the family life cycle and the design for the best support of individuals within the family according to their developmental needs. The aim of therapy is to redesign the family to a form that is closer to the ideal. Probably the most characteristic feature of structural family therapy is the intentional use of commands, directions, and suggestions, as the therapist takes responsibility for the direction in which she or he is pushing the family (Camp 1973). The therapist attends to verbal and behavioral indications of the structure, for example, who speaks with authority, where people sit and the nature of small interactional sequences. The therapist develops a very active style, moving in and out of relationships with the family members. Interventions are also very active, a family may be directed to demonstrate the pattern of the difficulty or be instructed to talk directly to each other in the room instead of being side-tracked by a third person.

Techniques associated with structural family therapy include:

1. Joining (making connections and rapport with family members to get »into« the system)
2. Accommodation (the therapist's adjustment in order to maintain alliance)
3. Life cycle stages (a key concept in therapist formulation in terms of family capacity to meet the developmental needs of individuals)
4. Family mapping (the construction of genograms that indicate interactional patterns, alliances, and the quality of emotional connections)
5. Creating a »workable« reality and reframing (changing description of problems or activity to make change more possible or to offer a different explanation for phenomena in order to increase the possibility for change)
6. Enactment (getting the family to demonstrate the problem pattern in the therapy room)
7. Intensification (the therapist acts in a way to increase emotional reactions and encourage interactions, for example disagreements to continue beyond the point at which they would normally stop)
8. Unbalancing (the therapist uses his/her power to side with a less powerful member to change homeostasis)
9. Boundary making and restructuring (intervening to make distinctions between subsystems in the family, acting to alter the family dysfunctional structure)
10. Task setting (the therapist sets specific tasks for the family to enact between sessions that build on one or more of the above techniques)

13.2.5.2 Post-Milan Therapy

Milan Therapy arose out of the Palo Alto-based work on systems theory and cybernetics. Four Italian therapists developed these concepts into a school of family therapy that was to be highly influential for decades and continues to have a major impact in the field (Palazzoli et al. 1978). The original Milan version, referred to as their strategic phase, was based on the idea that the family system »needed« the problem to maintain its equilibrium. Their theory of change suggested that pathology was a result of hidden loyalties and family games, and if these were declared as understandable responses to various pressures, then the family would be free to develop in a healthier way. The double bind theory and paradox played a key role in the thinking. A circular hypothesis was developed that linked family members' positions to the presented problems and then the paradoxical (in the sense that psychotherapists are usually on the side of change) instruction was given to stay the same. The method was further outlined in a seminal paper by Palazzoli et al. (1980).

Post-Milan therapy refers to the more contemporary manifestation of the Milan Method. The strategic emphasis was replaced by Bateson's work on communication and learning, and the stance of working against resistance was replaced with an emphasis on curiosity about the relationships between beliefs and behaviors in the family (Cecchin 1987). Family difficulties were understood to arise not out of some systemic need for a problem but were more to do with a limitation in terms of alternatives, an unhelpful linking of explanations and/or behaviors. The therapy was more about the process of posing questions that would facilitate different connections and the intervention became the questions themselves (Tomm 1987 a, b, 1988). Post-Milan ideas encompass second-order cybernetics: an incorporation of the beliefs and behaviors of the therapist as part of the therapy system of family and therapist (Boscolo et al. 1987; Campbell and Draper 1985).

Techniques associated with Milan therapy include:

1. Circular questions: aimed at looking at difference and therefore a way of introducing new information into the system. They are effective at illuminating the interconnectedness of the family subsystems and ideas and are based on the notion of feedback and building on the preceding answer or a connection to a hypothesis. Circular questions may relate to comparison of time, beliefs, and behaviors.

2. Neutrality: the position taken by the therapist to ensure that all points of view are attended to without bias. The therapist is trying not only to hear everyone's views but also to establish their interest in different perspectives that may be held within the system. At this point unless serious concerns arise regarding safety/confidentiality the therapist should remain neutral to the difficulties and issues that the family are presenting and their views about them.

3. Hypothesizing: the development of ideas about interactional patterns in relation to beliefs and behaviors of family members that are connected to the presenting problems. A systemic hypothesis is a more fully developed notion that includes all members in the system and may be linked to the notion that the problem has served a function for the family, akin to a defense mechanism.

4. Positive connotation: the therapist conveys the message that the family actually needs the problem based on greater fears of what would happen if the problem were not there.

5. End of session message: This includes the sharing of the circular hypothesis with the family and is structured in such a way that the protective function of the problem is placed in a broader family context.

6. Post-Milan practice placed emphasis on the therapeutic value of the questions themselves. Interventive interviewing is the practice of therapists asking questions with the intention of the questions having therapeutic impact. Examples include: embedded suggestions questions, questions that point to difference, questions that recontextualize answers, questions that ask one person to comment on the relationship of two others, agreement/disagreement questions that contrast periods of time, explanations, responses, etc. Reflexive questions include the assumptions of the therapists, thus making those assumptions more explicit but less imposing, while asking the family member to reflect on its own patterns.

13.2.5.3   Brief Solution-Focused Therapy

Brief solution-focused therapy arose from work on cybernetic patterns of information. The focus was on problem-perpetuating behavior, rather than the underlying need for the problem in terms of maintaining homeostasis. Milton Erikson's work on hypnosis and indirect methods of working with »resistance« played a key role in the development of the model (Haley 1973) as did the work of the MRI group (see for example Watzlawick et al. 1974; Weakland et al. 1974). The theory is that problems are maintained by the way difficulties are viewed and by the repetitive behavioral sequences surrounding attempts to solve them. Inherent is also the belief that clients already have solutions to their difficulties and that their own particular resources are most likely to bring results, if these can be brought to bear on the problem. The therapist is very goal orientated, seeking to track problem-perpetuating ideas or behavior and interrupting it. Methods employed might include a reframing of a client's explanation, an instruction to do something else, or a paradoxical suggestion that prescribes the symptom, for example, telling the depressed client to have a »practice« depression session daily.

A significant shift in the model arose with the change in emphasis from problem maintaining behavior to the search for solutions. Steve de Shazer developed the notion that interventions need not be specific to each family, but that formula interventions can be used in any number of cases (de Shazer 1985). For example, if a client presents with a phobic reaction in a particular location, suggest that the site of the reaction be moved, thus beginning the change of pattern around the reaction and the embedded assumption about the lack of control of the symptom. The task for the therapist is to develop knowledge of the client's strengths and solutions to other problems and then to set about the process of applying these to the particular problem at hand. Social constructionism and the thinking of Wittgenstein have both influenced Brief Solution-Focused Therapy. It has responded to these influences by placing emphasis on the part played by language in creating reality. Thus the therapy, in search of more solutions, will place emphasis on the therapist's linguistic selections of the positive, and techniques to facilitate the family's ability to imagine and speak of a problem-free alternative. As clients talk more and more with the therapist about the solution they want to construct together, they come to believe in the truth or reality of what they are talking about. It is argued that this builds on the way that language works naturally (Berg and de Shazer 1993).

Techniques associated with the Solution Focused Therapy include:

1. Goal setting: the development of small and achievable aims for therapy
2. The »miracle question«: helps the clients to imagine life without problems
3. Ranking questions: used to obtain numerical representation of the severity of difficulties and to chart their reduction
4. Determining factors that contribute to the reduction of the problem
5. Exceptions: the capacity to notice and accentuate the positives or exceptions to problems is seen as a major therapeutic skill
6. Task development: clients are ask to carry out tasks related to noticing the circumstances around exceptions.

13.2.5.4 White and Epston's Narrative Therapy

The early systemic narrative model owes much to the work on learning of Gregory Bateson (1972). The major idea incorporated into narrative work is the importance of the process of comparison for learning, »the difference that makes the difference«. Australian Michael White noticed that people failed to be able to make comparisons between the problem and other areas of their life in which the problem was absent. He developed a technique, externalization, which acted to separate the problem from the person, such that there could be distinctions between times when the problem was an influence and

those times when it was not. Circular questions derived from the Milan method were employed to consider the relationship of the problem to people and their identities and lives. The beginning of the distinction of this model was by virtue of incorporation of the work of Bruner (1986) who used a story metaphor to explain how people make sense of their lives and how these stories include and inevitably exclude various data.

Latterly, narrative therapy has drawn more directly on the French poststructuralists. Derrida's (1976) concept of deconstruction and Foucault's (1975) ideas about dominant and subjugated discourses are central notions. Moving from the importance of narrative structure in meaning making for individuals, White has linked societal discourses to these individual narratives (White and Epston 1990), such that people can be offered more choice about the ideas that they employ to define themselves. The main ideas in this model include: individual identity is in the form of a personal narrative that includes different versions of the self; clients come to therapy with a »problem-saturated narrative« which has become internalized; and problem stories/identities are created, lived, and kept alive by their connection to important others. The therapist looks for »unique outcomes« and positive exceptions to the problematic story, and amplifies change by use of letter writing, specific audiences (others who have successfully conquered the same issue) and personal enthusiasm. The problem recedes into relative insignificance as a more positive account of the individual emerges.

Techniques associated with narrative therapy include:

1. Externalization: a linguistic construction that signifies that the person has a problem rather than is the problem, thus removing the problem description from the identity of the individual.
2. Naming the problem whether it is about an action, emotional state, or interaction.
3. Deconstruction: questions aimed to explore various dimensions of the situation, reveal unstated cultural assumptions and what is not said. Helps to move the problem from an individual to a societal level.
4. Mapping the influence of the problem: therapist and client determine the degree to which the problem inhibits the possibility of more desirable descriptions of self, relationships with others, etc. Provides information to both about desired outcomes.

5. Externalizing conversations: questions that place the problem in language of something other than the person identity, the problem is spoken about as something that interferes with a better life story. This conversation places client/family and therapist in a position to work together to defeat problem.

6. Search for an alternative story: the therapist listens for unique outcomes or sparkling moments where the problem story was not around, picking up threads of a different character description to build and amplify. »How« questions invite people to make sense or meaning about these times of protest against the problem.

7. Unique Re-description Questions: invite people to make meaning of the significance/influence/impact of the unique account. These questions focus on how people think and feel about their relationships in a new/different way from the descriptions of the past.

8. Constructing a history of the preferred story: looking for a more positive self-definition and connecting it to traits and abilities that showed themselves in earlier development. Re-storying the client with abilities and events that were discovered to have existed all along in order to enhance their strength in relation to problem story. This alternative story has always been there but has been oppressed by the problem story.

9. Unique possibility questions (future developments/the forthcoming chapters) invite people to speculate/wonder about the future relations that may be possible in the alternative story.

10. Experience of experience questions (bringing in the co-author) invite people to re-experience themselves and their own story during the session by reflecting on the therapist's experience.

13.2.5.5 Anderson, Goolishan and Andersen's Post-modern Collaborative Approach

Anderson and Goolishan (1988, 1992) define their practice as postmodern collaborative therapy. Social constructionism, as defined by Gergen (1991), has played a large part in the development of this model. The other important cornerstone is the philosophical theory of hermeneutics, the science of interpretation and explanation. The main components of the model are that language rather than interactional pattern is seen as the system, difficulties are constructed in the language system and can be »dis-

solved« through language, and change occurs through development of new language. The therapist is the participant manager of the conversation, not »the expert« and takes a »not knowing« stance, asking questions to develop expanded or alternative understandings. The structure of therapy is less about beginning, middle, and end points, more about creating space for a specific kind of conversation among participants. Advice or research evidence in relation to a particular problem might be offered as one of many potential new ideas. The therapist would appreciate that »information« might not fit with the client's experience and be genuinely respectful and interested in different thoughts and reactions of the client. The therapist's primary contribution to the process of change is in the construction of a particular style of conversation. »Reflecting team conversations« are used; these are conversations in which team members speak to one another in front of the family (Andersen 1987). The team elaborates and embellishes themes from the session, introduce their own ideas that have emerged as they have been listening, and actively respond to the emergent meanings within the conversation. The family and therapist are then free to ignore, negate, or develop ideas in more detail.

The collaborative therapist would be less inclined to speak about techniques and would prefer to consider therapy as a philosophical activity and a particular way of being. However, there are elements of practice that could be seen as techniques and these include:

1. Taking a nonexpert stance involves moving away from the traditional hierarchical therapeutic relationship. Emphasis is placed on the client's own knowledge and the therapist's collaborative stance.

2. Creating a context for dialogue: the therapist behaves with a slow pace, patience, and a respectful approach to understanding of difference. There is a skill that is aimed at creating a particular kind of conversation in which meanings are the problem and can unfold and evolve.

3. Attending to conversational space: the therapist pays attention to the linguistic constructions of the client/family and considers the implications of what has been said and what has been left out.

4. Questions are gently aimed at the expansion and uncovering of meanings for individuals in the system.

5. Reflecting team discussion: although this technique is used in narrative and other models, it originated with this model. Ideas developed in

the session by the clients are considered in conversation by observing therapy team members, with some developments in the meanings or potential directions in aid of offering difference. The family and therapist are then free to ignore, negate, or develop the reflecting team's ideas in more detail.

13.2.5.6 Cognitive Behavioral Family Therapy

This model was derived from behavioral parent training developed by Patterson (1971) and cognitive behavioral marital therapy by Stuart (1969). The model places emphasis on the identification of problematic interactional sequences and the cognitive schema that supports them. A behavioral analysis will determine the contingencies that support the perpetuation of the problematic behavior. These sequences are mapped and the family members are taught to alter their behavior. Negative reinforcements and assumptions are replaced with rewards and alternative explanations. Epstein added more detail in terms of a cognitive approach in work with couples with five types of cognitions that are applicable to intimate relationships: assumptions about relationships, standards about how relationships should be, selective attention – systemic bias, attributions – inferences about the partner's behavior, expectations – about future behavior in the partner (Epstein 1997).

Techniques associated with cognitive behavioral family therapy include:
1. Observation: watching the problem in action
2. Identification of problematic interactions: mapping the behavioral sequence
3. Behavioral reward systems: developing specific rewards/reinforcers for particular behaviors
4. Cognitive restructuring: reframing or developing alternative explanations
5. Contracting agreements: parties agree on consequences for behavior
6. Problem solving skills: identification of smaller and more manageable components in issue
7. Communication skills: defining the problem in a nonblaming way, empathetic listening, reformulating »I want« statements, generating solutions, deciding on a solution and implementation
8. Task setting: agreement between therapist and client about activities between sessions.

13.3 Assessment and Indications for Family Therapy

13.3.1 Introduction

Assessment and diagnosis have well-established traditions in individual psychotherapy. Symptoms cluster in a particular way end to a diagnosis based on agreed operational definitions within the medical and psychological disciplines (DSM IV, etc.). L'Abate (1994) makes the point that assessment, evaluation, and diagnosis are sometimes used interchangeably. He defines assessment as a formal process of interview and administration of objective and projective instruments. Evaluation includes the interviewer's subjective judgment, based on knowledge, experience, and biases. Usually, this includes the question of »treatability«. Will this particular family benefit from family therapy? Diagnosis means labeling, in the case of the family, using the characterization of the most salient qualities of the family. This rather tidy distinction is not reflected in most family therapy practice and some therapists would challenge the notion of »objectivity« and the relevance of projective tools. Therefore, the terms assessment and evaluation will be used interchangeably, to reflect the common usage in the field and including the elements of subjectivity and experience, etc.

Mental health difficulties usually present to professionals as an individual phenomenon rather than a family or systemic one. The naming of the phenomena by the professional often has significant implications for the individual concerned and the treatment they receive. Family therapy often proceeds from an »individual« diagnosis although in practice, most »assessments« for family therapy are based on a combination of less explicit variables: the skills and theoretical orientation of the clinicians, the family's enthusiasm for meeting as a group, and the institutional and cultural context. Although it sometimes happens, it is unusual for a therapist to find themselves telling a family that their worries are disproportionate to the problems and that they do not require treatment. The norm is that the therapist appreciates the logistical and emotional efforts involved in getting a family to attend assessment meetings and rather than look for factors that argue against treatment, the emphasis is on how to support it. The following part of this chapter will address the question of assessment, the past and current issues in relation to family therapy and assessment, and provide a very basic guide to conducting an assessment interview.

13.3.2   The Context of Assessment

The degree to which the diagnosis and assessment is a prerequisite to treatment is highly dependent on the mental health context of the country. Family therapy as described above grew from work in the USA and Europe, and thus reflects a bias towards European and North American culture in its history, theories, research, and practices (Barratt et al. 1999; McDowell et al. 2003). This has led family therapists to consider the importance of culture, for both families and the therapists working with them. Two approaches have been prominent: the etic, suggesting that psychotherapy is generalizable across cultures (Ma 2000) and the emic, suggesting that psychotherapy needs to be culture specific (Tamura and Lau 1992; Adeksou 2003). Rivett and Street (2003) advocate the concept of cultural competency as a means of resolving the etic and emic debate. A culturally competent therapist would have an understanding of the way their own culture influences the way they perceive things, and be open to learning specific, local knowledge from families. Several therapists describe the successful combination of family therapy practices with local knowledge throughout the world (Ng 2003; Prabhu 2003; Varga 2003; Lavee 2003; Haug 2003; Bakker and Snyders 1999; Ma 2000). Family therapy training programs in the USA and Europe include multicultural course elements, and these appear to have increasing prominence (McDowell et al. 2003; Guanapina 2003; Khan 2003).

Although family therapy is practiced in much of the world, it has differing levels of state legitimacy, being a licensed activity in, for example, the USA, UK, Australia, Italy, and Austria. In other countries such as India, Malaysia, France, and Ecuador, it is largely practiced as part of a wider service within, for example, child guidance, schools counseling, general psychotherapy and family support (Prabhu 2003; Ng 2003; le Goff 2003; Haug 2003). In some countries family therapy is practiced largely in health settings, in Japan for eating disorders, school phobia, and behavioral problems (Tamura 2003); in Italy and the UK within child mental health settings (Rivett and Street 2003; Bertrando 2003). In Singapore it has emerged within social services and fits with government policy on strengthening families (Tan 2003). In Central and South America family

therapy sits alongside family and community support offered by religious groups and elders. The focus may be on behavior such as juvenile delinquency, drug use, and family violence (Bucher and da Costa 2003; Haug 2003).

Training courses that include clinical supervision are offered in the USA, Australia, and much of Europe; these are accredited by the Associations for Family Therapy in those sites. The European Family Therapy Association has published minimum criteria for approved training (Periera et al. 2002). Asia has fewer training programs; formal training was set up in Singapore in the 1990s and there are programs in Japan that have a clinical supervision element. Tel Aviv University saw Israel's first family therapy training program in 1984, several now exist in social work and psychology departments throughout the country. In Ecuador, the first formalized training was in structural family therapy and lay people recruited to work with indigenous populations made up 30% of the trainees. Argentina has systemic institutes offering both undergraduate and graduate courses, as does South Africa (where many are developing multicultural programs; Marchetti et al. 1999). Thus family therapy training is at different stages in different parts of the world.

Two contrasting examples of the way in which context influences assessment are provided by the UK and the USA. In the former, the National Health Service provides most mental health treatment. The General Practitioner (family physician) usually determines which specialist services are offered to the client. Whether the individual is referred for family therapy or individual treatment will be governed by the particular specialist seen, the service availability, family preference, degree of concern, etc. Diagnosis and assessment has remained more flexible as funding is not linked specifically to diagnosis. However, government is putting increasing pressure on services to demonstrate value for money and to use only interventions that are supported by evidence. In this context, for family therapy to be seen as a valid form of treatment in the future, it must enhance its evidence base. This argument moves the field closer to considerations of standardization of treatment and the establishment of baselines of family functioning or recognized categorizations of family pathology.

In the USA, a very high percentage of treatment is funded by private insurance, which is dependent on an individual diagnosis. Families get treatment on the »back« of a named member, depending on the treatment inclinations of the initial service.

There currently exists a secondary diagnosis of parent-child difficulties, but nothing more specific about family dynamics. The lack of a »family diagnosis« undermined the professional status and funding for family therapy in the private sector. Strong (1993) writes of family therapists in the USA having to straddle two languages, that of the medical/insurance profession and that of the family. Efforts have been made to include a diagnostic category that would reflect the notion that systems have disorders. The notion of a relational diagnosis was offered in the early 1990s and continues to be a lively issue (Kaslow 1993; Sholevar 2003). Karl Tomm (1991) has developed a diagnostic system based on pathological interactions (PIPS) which are constructed by the client and therapists. Reciprocal behaviors are named and are seen to reside »between« people rather than within individuals.

According to Sholevar (2003), a diagnosis has three main purposes: a common language for the professionals involved; facilitation of understanding of etiology and prognosis; and an aid to selection of treatment approaches in conjunction with particular family presentations. He argues for the relational diagnosis as shifting blame from the individual to the group but warns of several problems inherent in the concept. There are difficulties in defining boundaries when working with groups; families are ever flexible in the redrawing of their boundaries and definitions of membership. There continues to be a lack of adequate evidence which connects the individual diagnosis to family patterns or makes the case for a causal relationship. Finally, there is the problem of potential misuse of the diagnostic system in terms of the potential for it to be applied in a way that is not sensitive to cultural diversity (Cuellar 1996). The term »diagnosis« is based in the medical discourse, which creates a very lively debate amongst family therapists. This debate will be discussed in more detail in a subsequent section.

13.3.3 Family Typologies

Another significant approach to the work of describing family functioning has come from the field of family research. People who worked with families began to consider whether the system could demonstrate salient characteristics consistent over time and whether there was a relationship between certain family types and particular individual symptoms. Although this might be construed as a family diagnosis, little of the work has been tied to an individual pathology paradigm. Most of the work drew from structural family therapy and theories of group behavior. Four examples will be discussed in brief.

The McMaster Model of family function describes families with respect to six aspects of functioning: problem solving, communication, roles, affective responsiveness, affective involvement and behavior control (Epstein 1978; Olson 1986). The Beavers/Timberlawn places families on two intersecting dimensions: the centripetal (family turning inward) and centrifugal (family turning outward) dimension and the health competence dimension.

The work of David Reiss (1981, 1987) on Family Paradigm has focused on the family's relationship to the outside world. It incorporates three dimensions: the capacity of the family to see patterns or coherence in a confusing situation, the family's belief in facing difficulties in a cohesive and coordinated manner, and the capacity to change in response to new information. The Global Assessment of Relational Functioning, currently under development, focuses on three areas of family functioning: problem solving, family organization, and emotional climate. It is designed to be used in conjunction with an intake meeting and does not require a sophisticated clinician to administer it. It is currently being field tested in the USA and Europe and has been included in the DSM-IV Appendix (Sholevar 2003).

These typologies are still largely research tools and are not widely used in clinical practice. The following is a description of some of the elements that are included in the early, assessment stages of a systemic interview(s).

13.3.4 Conducting an Evaluation or Assessment

Often there will have been some preliminary assessment of the individual child prior to referral for family therapy, but if this is not the case consideration must be given to whether this is necessary. The probability is that, to some degree, another professional has discussed the idea of a family approach prior to the initial meeting. This assumption does not always hold true, so it is an important element to clarify in the first meeting. Some of the factors that inform the »starting position« of the assessment will be dependent on what has gone on before: the degree to which the referring professionals have discussed the referral to family therapy, the degree to which the family feels it has a choice and is interested in the idea of working as a family, and the degree of complexity and urgency around clinical issues. In Lambert's (1992) meta-analysis of psychotherapy outcome research, 40% of improvements in clients in psychotherapy are attributed to client and extra therapeutic factors (client characteristics, inner strengths, religious faith, goal directedness, personal agency and motivation, and things outside the control of the client, social support, etc.). For family therapy, the »client« is the constellation of people with whom the therapy takes place and the therapist should therefore facilitate a consideration of the resources available to support treatment.

Assessments are often seen as containing three elements; engagement in the assessment process itself, development of a formulation, and finally, building a therapeutic alliance (Carr 2000 a). Some practices would include a clear and rigid distinction between the evaluation and treatment phase, while others would see the process in a more recursive way. The former position might have the benefit of making a contract for therapy more explicit and avoid the possibility that families are seduced into family therapy. The latter might place more emphasis on attempts to build a therapeutic alliance in the initial session as part of addressing the question of treatability and motivation. This orientation would place more emphasis on the evaluation experience being mutual, so that the family considers whether they want to participate in family therapy while the clinician is forming an idea about the suitability of family therapy. It would be important for the family to have an experience in the assessment process itself, which is closer to what would actually happen in treatment, so as to be able to make informed decisions about participation.

Whether there are distinct dichotomies between evaluation and treatment or not, there are general topics of inquiry in initial meetings that are part of the development of an agreement for treatment. These ingredients include consideration of the family's:

1. Hopes and expectations of treatment
2. Presenting problems
3. Explanations held by family members for these difficulties
4. Expressive style
5. Capacity to become interested in the relational aspect of the problem
6. Capacity to engage in treatment and potential for forming an alliance
7. Response to the initial formulation(s)

The assessment often includes questions about the family's hopes and expectations of treatment and their history in relation to seeking help. Some families want a better understanding of how the difficulties developed in the first place and are already interested in family work. Individual members may have different agendas for therapy. Families as a whole vary in their expectations of treatment, some expect the professionals to »fix« the individual with presenting problems and feel completely confused about the notion of meeting as a family. Others simply want advice or medication, as opposed to therapy. Coercion by education or child protection services or other professionals making it a requirement as part of the package of obtaining individual treatment of the child may be a significant issue to address. None of these positions immediately negate a family approach, but the more problematic ones do require skilled responses by the therapist to determine whether there might be some movement within the early interview(s) toward a more therapeutically amenable perspective on the part of the family. The »story« of the family's previous treatment history gives invaluable information to the therapist about their problem solving responses and their actual experiences with other professionals. It is particularly important to listen to what has been helpful in the past as a way to inform future work.

A very specific question from the brief solution focused model, referred to as the miracle question, asks clients to imagine what life would look like if the problem had disappeared. It is useful in helping clients formulate more specific treatment goals (O'Hanlon 1989; George 1990). Implied in the general question about hopes for treatment are queries about the elements of fear and »resistance«. The model of therapy will, to a large degree, shape the extent to which these issues will be taken up directly or be left for more indirect consideration. Most current systemic models will place more emphasis on identification of the potential for positive change and note exceptions to the problem pattern. The constraints or ambivalence toward change may be explored but the therapist would be most interested in learning about the client's preferences for the future.

The assessment interviews include discussion of the presenting problems from different members in the family or may include the perspectives of other professionals or representatives from institutions, for example, schools and social services. Although theoretical models will affect the degree to which therapists becomes engaged in a detailed account of the problems, it is important for the therapist to hear about the problems directly from the clients. Clients may be concerned about something other than that described in the initial referral. Clients cite feeling heard by the therapist as a key feature in successful treatment and this sense of being heard is most critical in the early work or assessment stage. The therapist will try to attend to every participant's perspective, while also respecting the family structure and the degree to which people wish to share their thoughts. Understanding the child's perspective in the family context is particularly important. Developmentally appropriate methods need to be employed to encourage full consideration of their point of view, whilst respecting their sense of timing and the constraints they might feel in the situation.

In addition to the discussion of the problems, it is important to obtain information about the explanation held by family members for the difficulties encountered. Sometimes there is a shared view, more often this is a source of difference between members. The systemic therapist is interested in the different views and the impact of these differences on the relationships. Family therapists may have quite a wide field of inquiry, including extended family members, friends, or other significant people who are seen as relevant to the difficulties.

Often, a genogram is constructed which maps at least three generations of family membership and the transmission of particular themes. The purpose of the genogram is to develop an historical view of the family as a system of relationships and patterns over time. Males are indicated by squares and females as circles and there are drawing conventions that show marriages, divorces, births and deaths, and sibling relationships. Dates marking significant transitional events are included. There may be markers reflecting alliances and conflictual relationships and themes. These themes are usually based to some degree on the presenting problems. For example, if the presenting issue was behavioral problems and aggressiveness, possible ADHD, then there would be a particular interest in the accounts of behavioral problems, school difficulties in other family members, and also in connected issues: anxiety, parenting problems, aggressiveness, and »medicalization« in other parts of the family system. The genogram should not be used in a static manner, with the therapist rigidly sticking to preconceived interview questions. The information that is offered spontaneously by the family is seen as valuable and what may appear to be tangential may place the present-

ing problems in a context that the therapist has not previously considered. The construction of a genogram is often used as a method of engaging younger children in the family interview, as they often enjoy drawing the boxes and circles and naming the people they represent.

The family's expressive style will often be a significant aspect of the assessment process. Therapists will pay attention to the overall affective component and to the differential communication between individuals. The degree of frustration, antagonism, hopelessness and withdrawal will be considered, along with more positive attributes, attachment, positive regard, and resilience. Some therapists will take a position of nonintervention in order to let patterns emerge without influencing them. The child may be left to run around the room and climb on the furniture to observe the manner and threshold for the institution of parental boundaries. Other therapists will place a greater weight on the engagement aspect of the assessment process, and actively intervene or structure the session to assure the family that the therapy room is a safe place and that their interactions will be contained. The therapist notes the child's activity and offers a puzzle or to take a short break. The therapist will inevitably be forming an idea of the degree to which he/she will need to actively structure the session, and the duration and frequency of meetings. Families that present as highly chaotic and emotionally reactive may benefit from a higher degree of therapist containment and structure (Weitzman 1985).

A significant element of the assessment process involves questions that are derived from the relational aspect of the systemic model. The particular construction of these questions will depend on the family therapy model. The family's capacity to engage with questions that open up the possibility that the presenting difficulties of an individual child have some connection to their interactions, beliefs, and feelings with each other will also be a central issue in considering a family approach. Although it is not expected that family members will have a bird's eye view of their familial interactional pattern, it is hoped that they show at least a minimal degree of curiosity about their mutual influence. The systemic therapist will hope that family members, through the initial interviews, will see each other as resources in the treatment rather than subjects of blame or criticism.

The greatest challenge to the family therapist is when a family presents with a rigid and all-inclusive negative account of the child's character that fails to shift in its potency despite the therapist's efforts to draw out any evidence of a more positive view. This task is quite demanding for the therapist. If he/she asks questions that invite positive remarks about the child prematurely, before the parents feel that their frustration has been heard, the potential for a therapeutic alliance is greatly diminished. The therapist will also be concerned to develop a relationship with the child or young person and create a therapeutic environment that derails the »scapegoating« and negative interactions. This is a delicate balance to be achieved in the assessment period.

Part of the assessment is developing an idea of who needs to participate in family therapy in order for change to occur. Family therapy has moved on from requiring all household members to attend every session. The treatment group may be organized around those who have seemed most involved in the concern: the »problem« determined systems, rather than the system creating the problem (Anderson and Goolishan 1988; Anderson 1997). The child may be asked to invite particular friends, relatives or a school counselor to the sessions who may be seen as providing support for change. Therapists may include important absent members metaphorically, by use of an empty chair, asking people what the absent person would think or say if they were there or by writing a summary of the session in a letter to them. Family therapists will also think about risk factors related to meeting as a family. In some situations, meeting as a group may be contraindicated as it might actually increase the potential of domestic violence or harm to a child or adult individual. Meetings with a high degree of threat or emotionally abusive material may be stopped or reconfigured into separate meetings with family members.

The therapeutic alliance has three components: consensus between the therapist and client on the goals of therapy; an agreement and collaboration on the relevance and implementation of various therapy tasks (how the therapy is conducted, including such things as the frequency of meetings, topics of conversation, interview procedures, and specific techniques), and a strong, positive affective bond between therapist and client (Bordin 1982). If the assessment process has given the clients a fair preview of the general conduct of therapy and the differences between the client and therapists in the elements listed above have been explored and worked through, then treatment is more likely to be effective.

An initial formulation is generated over a brief period, usually one to three sessions. This formulation includes both notions about the etiology and ideas about the family's suitability for treatment. The task of the formulation is to create an explanation that both fits with the family's experience and also offers additional clarity, coherence, and enough difference to add to the family's original explanations. Increasingly, formulations include explicit attention to the strengths and resources found within the material generated as part of the history taking and assessment interviews (Walsh 1995; Allison 2003). This is fed back to the family and a decision about engaging in treatment is made. The formulation may be presented directly to the family or may come in the form of the reflecting team discussion (Anderson 1995).

13.3.5   Post-modern Assessment

As described in a previous part of this chapter, family therapy has been influenced to a large degree by two theories, constructivism and social constructionism. It is important to consider how these ideas relate to the concept of assessment. From a constructivist frame of reference, the assessment process is heavily influenced by the internal schema or constructs of the observer. What is »seen« and »understood« in the process depends to a large degree on the internal framework of the person doing the interviewing. These filters will include a large range of elements, from personal, gender, life experiences, and institutional and professional assumptions. The range of models in the field of family therapy will also play a large part in the assessment outcome (Carlson 1997). The structural therapist would be most »at home« with the notion of an assessment and formulation in which pathological patterns were described by the therapist. For example, the structural family therapist (Minuchin 1981) will be looking for the degree of closeness or distance between family members (enmeshment/disengagement on either end of the spectrum), inappropriate generational boundaries (father/son alliances against mother), and unhelpful patterns of dealing with conflict (triangulation). They may assign tasks for the family in order to determine the degree of commitment and motivation, and attend to the family's emotional reactivity by actively intensifying or reducing the tension in the session.

Brief solution-focused therapists dismiss the traditional notion of delving deeply to discover the hidden causes for family pathology. They place an emphasis on solution building, believing it is more important to understand what the clients deem to be the criteria for successful completion of therapy. When have the family been able to circumvent problems in ways that have surprised them? Brief solution-focused therapists would happily engage with the notion of assessment in terms of working with very specific and attainable goals for therapy (de Shazer 1985; Klar 1999). They would attend to the degree to which this goal setting seemed possible in the initial stage of therapy and perhaps aim for a small degree of change. The other element in which they would fit happily with the more traditional approach to assessment is that of noting the issue of motivation for treatment. They are distinct in the field by virtue of naming the level of motivation in terms of whether a client is a visitor, complainant, or customer. The visitor is there by virtue of pressure from an external source, the complainant has a problem but it resides in someone else, and the customer is presenting an investment in personal change. They tailor their therapeutic responses to the position of the client. One family member may be a customer and receive therapist questions related to change while another may be more of a visitor, who would receive appreciative responses about his/her support from the therapist.

The original Milan group placed a great deal of emphasis on the development of systemic hypotheses about the nature of the family interaction and the perpetuation of problems. Latterly, the Post-Milan orientation leads its practitioners to think carefully about the fit or misfit between beliefs held by individuals and their consequent actions. Therapists are not really interested in the development of a formulation or »professional« diagnosis but focus on asking circular questions designed to help the family generate more useful ways of thinking about difficulties (Campbell 1989; Jones 1993). For example, the therapist may ask the father about his idea that, for example, ADHD is the problem and consider how this idea affects his response to his son's oppositional behavior. The father may elaborate by saying that it is a medical condition and that the doctors should medicate him. When asked, the mother says that her son's oppositional behavior is a result of the highly distant father and that they argue about this issue. The son says that he gets into trouble because of being fed up with his sister being so good and clever at school. The Post-Milan therapist would consider the family members' capacity to open up their own thinking and to genuinely consider the position of the other family members.

The Narrative therapist would listen for the client's problem-saturated story and develop an understanding of the client's preferred way of being in relation to this story. What would the family call the difficulties that have come into their life, what would the child call this thing that people were concerned about and to what degree is it a concern of his? The child might name this thing the »rumble« in his head that gets him angry and distracts him. The influence of this story would be mapped in terms of how it affects the sense of self, significant relationships, and aspirations for life. The »rumble« makes him feel stupid, causes him to fight and be disobedient. Further exploration would take place in terms of the various elements that sustain the problem and negate other positive attributes and alternative descriptions of the individual. Narrative therapists are highly attuned to the power of the mental health professional to promote a pathological description of an individual, therefore they would be disinclined to participate in a traditional diagnostic process, although they would consider the diagnosis as another story to be understood (White 1990; Madigan 1998). The label of ADHD would be considered in terms of the influences it had on the child's identity, relationship with school, etc.

The very notion of assessment and diagnosis has come under intense criticism from followers of more contemporary models of family therapy (narrative and collaborative models). Diagnosis has been situated in the modern discourse of scientific certainty and expertise, a position that was challenged by the inclusion of postmodern thinking in current practice. It has been referred to as »psychiatric hate speech« (Gergen 1996). From a social constructionist frame, diagnostic labels are not seen to reflect a reality but rather to create one and are more an expression of the culture that creates distinctions between people in terms of pathology and deviancy (Gaines 1992). This theory places emphasis on the constitutive nature of conversation and language. The nature of »languaging« together is what contributes to the present construction of the self, and is always »in process«. Therefore, an initial assessment interview will be informing all participants in the interview (including the therapist) of the »selves« that will be experienced and created together in that context. The meanings associated with assessment and treatment will be more relevant. The therapist brings an expertise, but one that is introduced »lightly«. The therapist may have notions about families who present in similar ways and information derived from their training, research, and past experience but these are not certainties or prescriptions. The uniqueness of each encounter is emphasized rather than the capacity to categorize and standardize.

13.3.6   Conclusion

The concept of assessment in systemic family therapy is best seen as a work in progress. While there are many indications for the effectiveness of family therapy in conjunction with specific presenting problems, the research base is still in its early days. The major indicator of successful treatment other than factors that reside in the clients themselves is that of the therapeutic alliance (Lambert 1992). While there is a significant gap between the work of family diagnosis or typology and clinical use, it seems most helpful to consider the assessment approach that is most likely to attend to alliance building.

13.4   The Effectiveness of Family Therapy Approaches

13.4.1   Introduction

Traditionally, although with some notable exceptions, family therapy practitioners have not favored quantitative research techniques. More recently, despite theoretical models that dispute the notion of an objective, measurable reality, a number of well-designed controlled trials have been reported. Family therapy outcome research is complicated by the inclusion of more than one person in therapy. As suggested in the section on assessment, the development of generally agreed methods of measuring family interaction is still in its infancy. The measurement of individual outcomes is complicated by difficulties in agreeing whose outcome should be measured (the identified patient, other family members, or patterns of family interaction) and whose perspective on outcome should be privileged. It is recognized that agreement between parents for ratings of behavior in their children is not always good (Achenbach 1995; Bird et al. 1992). In this section we will describe two domains of evidence about outcome: controlled trials of interventions, and user perspectives on family therapy.

13.4.2   Outcome Trials of Family Therapy

Meta-analyses of family therapy (Hazelrigg et al. 1987; Markus et al. 1990; Shadish et al. 1993) and descriptive but systematic reviews (Estrada and Pinsof 1995; Carr 2000b; Cottrell and Boston 2002) consistently report positive effects for family therapy. However, these reports are tempered by the usual methodological problems found in much of the outcome research literature in children and young people. Thus, there are concerns about the size and age range of samples, generalizability from nonrepresentative samples, inadequate descriptions of interventions and lack of measures of treatment integrity, problems with measurement of outcome, and lack of follow-up. Nevertheless, there is sufficient evidence from well-conducted studies to suggest that family therapy may be the treatment of choice in conduct disorders in older children, substance misuse, and in eating disorders. It may also have something to offer in depression and for children with physical illness.

13.4.2.1   Conduct Disorders, Delinquency and Substance Misuse

Two research programs have demonstrated the effectiveness of family therapy-based interventions for teenagers with conduct problems and delinquency. Functional family therapy has been shown to be effective in controlled trials (not always randomized) at reducing offending behavior (Alexander and Parsons 1973; Parsons and Alexander 1973; Barton et al. 1985; Gordon et al. 1995). Functional family therapy sees problems as having a function for the family. It includes elements of behavioral management such as positive reinforcement and contingency management, but focuses on improving communication and changing maladaptive, repetitive patterns family interaction (Alexander and Parsons 1982). Multisystemic treatment (MST; Henggeler and Borduin 1990) delivers an intensive, tailor-made package of interventions designed to reduce an adolescent's offending behavior. MST is systemic in the broadest sense as it attends to the family's relationships with local education and welfare services, but also includes formal family therapy interventions drawn from the structural and strategic schools of therapy alongside other psychological interventions for family members. A number of randomized, controlled trials of

MST have demonstrated significant reductions in behavior problems and offending behaviors that have been maintained at 30-month follow-up. Economic analyses suggest that despite its intensity, MST is not more expensive than treatment as usual control groups (Borduin 1999).

In addition, structural family therapy has been shown in one randomized, controlled trial of conduct problems in 6- to 12-year-old boys to produce equivalent change to individual therapy and significantly greater improvement than in a no-treatment control group (Szapocznik et al. 1989). Improvements in child function were maintained at 12-month follow-up when family functioning had deteriorated in the individual treatment group but improved in the group that had received family therapy.

A systematic review of random allocation trials for substance abuse has concluded that family-couples therapy is superior to individual counseling-therapy, peer group therapy, and to family psychoeducation for both adults and adolescents (Stanton and Shadish 1997). Reported drop-out rates were also lower for those in receipt of family therapy interventions, a finding supported in a study specifically designed to evaluate the effectiveness of family therapy in engaging families of substance abusers in therapy (Szapocznik et al. 1988). Multisystemic therapy (described above) has also been shown to be effective in reducing substance misuse (Borduin 1999).

13.4.2.2 Eating Disorders

There is good evidence to support the use of family therapy for the treatment of anorexia nervosa in younger people. Family therapy was found to be more effective than individual therapy for non-chronic patients with onset before the age of 19 years in a randomized, controlled trial of individuals with anorexia nervosa (Russell et al. 1987). Improvements were maintained at 5-year follow-up (Eisler et al. 1997). Out-patient family therapy was also found to be as effective as in-patient treatment or out-patient individual therapy and more effective than no treatment in a separate random allocation trial with patients with anorexia nervosa (Crisp et al. 1991). Improvements in this evaluation were maintained at 2-year follow-up (Gowers et al. 1994). Robin et al. (1994, 1999) have also compared a family therapy with an individual therapy in a random allocation trial for anorexia nervosa. Although both groups made equal improvement on some measures (including family functioning), the family

therapy group made greater weight gains and had higher rates of resumption of menstruation post-treatment and at 1-year follow-up. All of these studies used different forms of family therapy but had in common structural techniques that attended to boundaries and alliances, especially cross-generational alliances, problem solving strategies, and communication patterns.

13.4.2.3 Other Presenting Problems

There are three unrelated studies that investigate the use of family therapies in depression and/or bereavement. Family therapy was included as one of the treatment options in a random allocation trial of cognitive behavioral therapy, family therapy, and nondirective supportive therapy for adolescents with depression (Brent et al. 1997; Birmaher et al. 2000). The family therapy intervention was another structurally based model and the main finding was that although cognitive behavioral therapy was more effective in reducing depression at the end of treatment, at 2-year follow-up there were no differential effects of the three treatments. However, further analysis of the results has indicated the possibility that family therapy may be more effective in the presence of maternal depression or where the mother was more controlling (Brent et al. 1998). At 2-year follow-up, family therapy may also have produced some positive differential effects on family functioning (Kolko et al. 2000). Harrington et al. (1998) used a random allocation model to evaluate the effectiveness of a brief (four sessions), structured, home-based family intervention for young people who had deliberately self-poisoned. There were no significant differences in primary outcome measures of suicidal ideation and hopelessness, but compliance with family treatment was better than for routine care and parents were significantly more satisfied with treatment at 2-months follow-up. An interesting incidental finding was that at 6-month follow-up the control group had made significantly more use of foster care and residential care. Black and Urbanowicz (1987) randomly allocated bereaved families to either family-based guided mourning or no treatment. There was a trend for better outcomes at 1-year follow-up for the family therapy but few differences at 2-year follow-up.

There have been a number of random allocation trials evaluating family therapy for children with chronic physical illness – often the outcomes investigated have related to the physical symptoms not to family functioning or the psychological status of the child. Thus family therapy has been shown to significantly improve lung function in children with severe asthma when compared with routine pediatric care in two random allocation trials, albeit both with small numbers (Lask and Matthew 1979; Gustaffson et al. 1986). Evaluation of family therapy interventions in diabetes show promise but results are inconclusive as yet (Ryden et al. 1994; Wysocki et al. 2000).

13.4.3 Service-User Perspectives on Family Therapy

Several studies could be described as service-user satisfaction surveys using questionnaires sent to families (Frude and Dowling 1980; Bowen 2000; Fee and Hendra 2000; Seligman 2002). Some satisfaction studies begin to address specific areas, for example, reflecting teams (Baldwin and Jones 2000). These indicate a general level of satisfaction with family therapy although the questions asked were conceived by the services rather than in conjunction with service-users. It is acknowledged that service-user satisfaction and outcome share a complex relationship (Woodward et al. 1978; Reimers 2001).

Some qualitative research studies of service-user experience have attempted to address the potential differences between carers and children by focusing specifically on children's views (McNab et al. 2000; Stith 1996; Strickland-Clark 2000; Lobatto 2002). These small studies found that children had different views about aspects of the process of therapy, for example, whereas some preferred activities to talking as part of the therapeutic process (McNab et al. 2000; Stith 1996), some used activities as a way of taking time out of the process (Lobatto 2002). Some children found exploration of the technical aspects of family therapy helpful (Stith 1996; McNab et al. 2000).

Children generally expressed a wish to be included though not to be the sole focus of attention. They wanted to be involved in generating solutions and not to be blamed. Time and a greater understanding of the purpose of therapy increased their willingness to be involved, but even younger children seemed to understand the purpose of therapy and found talking about problems helpful (Stith 1996). In a study of younger children (aged 8–12 years) interviewed in the presence of their parents, children reported difficulties in knowing how or when to move in and out of the therapeutic circle and uncertainty about the rules of therapy. The use of toys and play materials were highlighted as important in helping children to feel secure within the therapeutic setting (Lobatto 2002).

13.4.4 Conclusions

Despite some impressive evidence to support the effectiveness of family therapies for some conditions, there is still a marked lack of formal evaluation of family therapy interventions. Current approaches to family therapy could be seen as relying too heavily on language and verbal communication and therefore potentially excluding children. However, studies of children's perceptions of therapy suggest that it is possible to include even quite young children in the therapeutic process and that they want to be included. Children were also aware of the potential negative consequences of talking about family life in front of their carers.

It is striking that all of the family therapies evaluated tend to be of older structural/behavioral type therapies and that there have been no formal evaluations of the postmodern therapies that are found most commonly in clinics today. The evidence also suggests that family therapies may reduce drop-out and increase engagement of families in the therapeutic process. This is perhaps already being recognized with the blurring of boundaries and sharing of techniques between different therapeutic modalities. Therapeutic interventions for children have to take into account the child's developmental level and position within the family and cannot be delivered in isolation. Practitioners intending to deliver cognitive behavioral or individual psychodynamic interventions often make use of family therapy techniques to engage families in therapy and ensure the ongoing support of families for the therapeutic process. There is also a suggestion that family therapy interventions may have a beneficial impact that is maintained and might even increase with time. The lack of studies that follow-up participants after cessation of treatment has made it hard to draw conclusions about this and more research is needed.

13.5 Service-User Involvement in Family Therapy

Service-user involvement refers to the active participation of children, young people and their carers

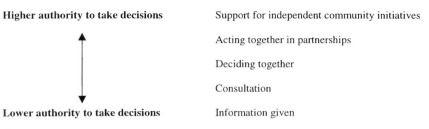

Higher authority to take decisions

Support for independent community initiatives

Acting together in partnerships

Deciding together

Consultation

Lower authority to take decisions

Information given

◘ **Fig. 13.1.** Ladder of empowerment (Willcox 1995)

(and sometimes potential service-users and the public) in the planning, development, and delivery of health services.[1] For family therapy, it tends not to refer to the process of therapy with individual families, rather to the broad range of activities outside of this that aim to increase the involvement of these groups. This is a complex area for all children's mental health services since there are three potential groups of service users to consider: parents and carers (and the gender implications thereof), young people, and children. Their needs and wishes may differ and, at times, be opposed.

One framework for conceptualizing these activities is the ladder of empowerment (Arnstein 1969; Willcox 1995; Hart 1997). Different rungs of the ladder offer service-users different levels of power in decision-making processes. The original model suggested all services should aspire to having service-users involved at the highest levels of decision-making (Arnstein 1969). Current thinking would suggest that the level of participation should be appropriate to the task, for example, a service might consult service-users about preferred appointment times if it was considering starting an evening clinic but not if appointment times were rigidly fixed (◘ Fig. 13.1).

Most of the examples of family therapy offering high authority to service-users are to be found in community-based approaches by workers sometimes referred to as Community Family Therapists (Doherty 2003). In these approaches family therapists are actively engaged in communities and are participating in projects to develop sustainable communities. Much of this work takes place outside of clinic settings and is longstanding in duration. Members of the communities are encouraged to take leadership positions. Whilst ideas from family therapy are used, it is in the context of community development and often explicitly includes aspects of

social justice (Waldegrave and Tamasese 1993; Kennedy 1994). Public services having service-users in paid positions where they are able to influence decision-making would offer this level of authority. Searches have not revealed examples of this in family therapy literature, nor of family therapists and service-users forming equal partnerships from which to plan, develop, and deliver services.

Policy on healthcare is increasingly including the preference for service-users to participate in decision-making (Council of Europe 2000; Department of Health 2001). Suggested methods for this include service-user and public members of advisory boards, service-user fora, and workshops or seminars. These methods constitute examples of deciding together within the ladder of empowerment framework. None of the national associations for family therapy appear to have included service-users in this way although some licensing boards in the USA have lay members. One creative example of bringing together a group of young people using family therapy services in the UK seemed to begin as an information-sharing exercise (McNab et al. 2000). It then clearly developed into a forum for sharing ideas between the young people and the group facilitators, with the young people involved in role-playing therapy sessions, quizzes, and games. These activities enabled young people to become comfortable in giving feedback about their experiences.

It is in the area of consultation with service-users that most of the examples of service-user involvement in family therapy are to be found. The service-user experiences described in the previous section are examples of consultation with service-users, although they are presented as research rather than explicit attempts to consult with service-users about specific issues. None of them include any detail of feedback to the service-users taking part in the studies (an integral aspect of service-user involvement processes). In the UK, Reimers and Treacher (1995) have worked on integrating their find-

[1] Sometimes also called patient participation or consumer involvement.

ings from research on families' experience of therapy into their practice. They have also been guided in their focus by information given by families in previous research/practice cycles.

The first rung of the ladder of empowerment relates to giving information about services. Many family therapy services produce literature for service-users. Some services use information designed by young service-users themselves, for example, leaflets, videos, and posters. Reimers and Treacher (1995) found that families preferred to have an introduction to the process and technology of family therapy prior to commencing. This practice appears to have been adopted within the UK (McNab et al. 2000; Reimers 2001).

13.6   Conclusions

Systemic family therapy has traveled a long way from its roots in the 1950s and has been influenced along the way by psychoanalysis, anthropology, cybernetics, general systems theory, and social constructionism. The central importance of considering the child in the family context and the family in a wider social context is now accepted as standard practice. Whilst this has not come about solely because of the influence of family therapists, they have played a major part in determining every day clinical practice with children and families across the world.

As with other therapeutic developments, the growth of family therapy has proceeded in advance of a quantitative evidence base to support it. The growth of mixed methods research and the integration of qualitative and quantitative approaches to evaluation is appealing to systemic therapists and should lead to increased outcome research—this is much needed. However, good quality evidence for its effectiveness has starting to emerge and in some problem areas (anorexia nervosa and substance misuse) family therapy is probably the treatment of choice, whilst in others there are indications that family therapy, or elements of family therapy practice may have an important contribution to make to integrated treatment packages.

More recently family therapists, driven by constructionist theoretical models, have become concerned with involving clients more in the process of therapy. This has led to changes in practice that seek to acknowledge and minimize the power imbalance inherent within the therapeutic relationship, and attempt to involve the client more in decisions

about the therapeutic process and where possible about the wider development of therapeutic services.

Family therapy remains a broad church, including many different schools of practice. If we look to the future, family therapists are also seeking to make links not just within systemic practice but also with other therapeutic modalities. There is a movement away from approaches that create treatment dichotomies (psychopharmacological versus therapy, individual therapy versus family, qualitative versus quantitative research) and towards the integration of multiple approaches in the best interests of the child and family.

References

Achenbach, T. M. (1995) Diagnosis, assessment, and comorbidity in psychosocial treatment research. Journal of Abnormal Child Psychology, 23, 45–64.

Ackerman, N. (1958) The psychodynamics of family life: Diagnosis and treatment of family relationships. New York: Basic Books.

Adeksu, M. (2003) Indigenous family work in Nigeria: the Yoruba experience. In (Ed. Ng, K.S.) Global Perspectives in Family Therapy: Development, Practice, Trends. New York: Brunner-Routledge.

Alexander, J. F., & Parsons, B. V. (1973) Short-term behavioral intervention with delinquent families: Impact on family process and recidivism. Journal of Abnormal Psychology, 81, 219–225.

Alexander, J. F., & Parsons, B. V. (1982) Functional Family Therapy. Monterey, CA: Brooks/Cole.

Allison, S., Stacey, K., Dadds, V., Roeger, L., Wood, A. & Martin, G. (2003) What the family brings: gathering evidence for strengths-based work. Journal of Family Therapy, 25, 263–284.

Andersen, T. (1987). The reflecting team: dialog and meta dialog in clinical work. Family Process, 26, 415–481.

Andersen, T. (1995) Reflecting processes; acts of informing and forming; you can borrow my eyes, but you must not take them away from me! In Friedman, S. (Ed.) The reflecting team in action: collaborative practice in family therapy. New York: Guilford.

Anderson, H. (1997) Conversation, language, and possibilities – a post modern approach to therapy. New York: Basic Books.

Anderson, H. & Goolishan, H. (1988) Human systems as linguistic systems. Family Process, 27, 371–393.

Anderson, H. & Goolishan, H. (1992) The client as the expert: a not knowing approach to therapy. In McNee, S. & Gergen, K. (Eds.) Therapy as a social construction. London: Sage Publications.

Arnstein, S. (1969) A ladder of citizen participation. Journal of the American Planning Association, 35, 216–224.

Bakker, T. M. & Snyders, F. J. A. (1999) The (HI)Stories we live by: power/knowledge and family therapy in Africa. Contemporary Family Therapy, 21, 133–154.

Baldwin, L. & Jones, A. (2000) The reflecting team: client perspectives Context: the Magazine for Family Therapy and Systemic Practice 50, 31–33.

Barratt, S., Burck, C., Dwivedi, K., Stedman, M., & Raval, H. (1999) Theoretical bases in relation to race, ethnicity and culture in family therapy training. Context: the Magazine for Family Therapy and Systemic Practice 44, 4–12.

Barton, C., Alexander, J. F., Waldron, H., Turner, C. W., & Warburton, J. (1985) Generalising treatment effects of Functional Family Therapy: Three replications. American Journal of Family Therapy, 13, 16–26.

Bateson, G. (1972) Steps to an ecology of mind. Chicago: University of Chicago Press.

Bateson, G., Jackson, D. D., Haley, J. & Weakland, J. (1956) Toward a theory of schizophrenia. Behavioral Science, 1, 251–264.

Berg, I. K. & de Shazer, S. (1993) Making numbers talk: Language in therapy. In Friedman, S. (Ed.) The new language of change: Constructive collaboration in psychotherapy. New York: Guilford Press.

Bertrando, P. (2003) The effects of family therapy in Italy. In (Ed. Ng, K.S.) Global Perspectives in Family Therapy: Development, Practice, Trends. New York: Brunner-Routledge.

Bird, H. R., Gould, M. S. & Staghezza, B. (1992) Aggregating data from multiple informants in child psychiatry epidemiological research. Journal of the American Academy of Child & Adolescent Psychiatry, 31, 78–85.

Birmaher, B., Brent, D. A., & Kolko, D. (2000) Clinical outcome after short-term psychotherapy for adolescents with major depressive disorder. Archives of General Psychiatry, 57, 29–36.

Black, D. & Urbanowicz, M. (1987) Family intervention with bereaved children. Journal of Child Psychology & Psychiatry. 28, 467–476

Bordin, E. S. (1982) A working alliance based model of supervision. The Counseling Psychologist, 11, 35–42.

Borduin, C. M. (1999). Multisystemic treatment of criminality and violence in adolescents. Journal of the American Academy for Child and Adolescent Psychiatry, 38, 242–249.

Boscolo, L., Cecchin, G., Hoffman, L. & Penn, P. (1987) Milan systemic family therapy: Conversations in theory and practice. New York, Basic Books.

Bowen, B. (2000) »The Jersey Family Therapy Service: feedback from families. Context: the Magazine for Family Therapy and Systemic Practice. 50, 27–28.

Bowen, M. (1966) The use of family theory in clinical practice. Clinical Psychiatry, 7, 345–374.

Bowlby, J. (1961) Childhood Mourning and its Implications for Psychiatry. American Journal of Psychiatry, 118, 481–498.

Brent, D. A., Holder, D., Kolko, D., Birmaher, B., Baugher, M., Roth, C., Iyengar, S. & Johnson, B. A. (1997) A clinical psychotherapy trial for adolescent depression comparing cognitive, family and supportive treatment. Archives of General Psychiatry, 54, 877–885.

Brent, D. A., Kolko, D., Birmaher B., Baugher, M., Bridge, J., Roth, C., & Holder D. (1998) Predictors of treatment efficacy in a clinical trial of three psychosocial treatments for adolescent depression. Journal of the American Academy of Child and Adolescent Psychiatry, 37, 906–914.

Bruner, E.M. (1986) Ethnography as narrative. In Turner, V.W. & Bruner, E.M. (Eds.) The anthropology of experience. Chicago: University of Illinois Press.

Bucher, J. & da Costa, I. (2003) Family therapy in Brazil: memoir and development. In (Ed. Ng, K.S.) Global Perspectives in Family Therapy: Development, Practice, Trends. New York: Brunner-Routledge.

Camp, H. (1973) Structural family therapy: An outsider's perspective. Family Process, 12, 269–277.

Campbell, D. & Draper, R. (1985) Applications of systemic thinking: the Milan approach. London: Grune and Stratton.

Campbell, D., Draper, R. & Huffington, C. (1989) Second Thoughts on the Theory and practice of the Milan Approach to Family Therapy. London: DC Publishing.

Carlson, J., Sperry, L. & Lewis, J. (1997) Family Therapy: Ensuring Treatment Efficacy. Pacific Grove: Brooks/Cole Publishing.

Carr, A. (2000 a) Family Therapy: Concepts, process, and practice. Chichester: Wiley.

Carr, A. (2000 b) Evidence based practice in family therapy and systemic consultation. I Child-focused problems. Journal of Family Therapy, 22, 29–60.

Cecchin, G. (1987) Hypothesizing, circularity, and neutrality revisited: an invitation to curiosity. Family Process, 26, 405–413.

Cottrell, D. & Boston, P. (2002) The effectiveness of systemic family therapy for children and adolescents. Journal of Child Psychology & Psychiatry, 43, 573–586.

Council of Europe (2000) Recommendation Rec. (2000)5 on the development of structures for citizen and patient participation in decision-making processes affecting health care. Strasbourg: Council of Europe.

Crisp, A. H., Norton, K. R. W., Gowers, S. G., Halek, C., Levett, G., Yeldham, D., Bowyer, C., & Bhat, A. (1991). A controlled study of the effect of therapies aimed at adolescent and family psychopathology in anorexia nervosa. British Journal of Psychiatry, 159, 325–333.

Cuéllar, I. & Glazer, M. (1996). The impact of culture on the family. In Harway, M. (Ed.) Treating the changing family. New York: Wiley.

Department of Health (2001) Involving patients and the public in healthcare. London: HMSO

Derrida, J. (1976) Of grammatology. Baltimore: Johns Hopkins University Press.

De Shazer, S. (1985) Keys to solutions in brief therapy. New York: Norton.

Doherty, W. (2002) The families and democracy project. Family Process. 42, 579–589.

Eisler, I., Dare, C., Russell, G. F. M., Szmukler, G., le Grange, D. & Dodge, E. (1997) Family and individual therapy in anorexia nervosa: A 5-year follow-up. Archives of General Psychiatry, 54, 1025–1030.

Epstein, N.B., Baucom, D. & Daiton, A. (1997) Cognitive Behavioral Couples Therapy. In Halford, W.K. (Ed.) Clinical Handbook of Marriage and Couples interventions. New York: Wiley.

Epstein, N.B., Bishop, D.S. & Levine, S. (1978) The McMaster model of family functioning. Journal of Marriage and Family Counseling, 4, 19–31

Estrada, A.U. & Pinsof, W.M. (1995) The effectiveness of family therapies for selected behavioral disorders of childhood. Journal of Marital & Family Therapy, 21, 403–440.

Fee, J., Hendra, T. (2000) Survey of family therapy feedback in Hampshire. Context: the Magazine for Family Therapy and Systemic Practice. 50, 29–30.

Foucault, M. (1975). The archaeology of knowledge. London: Tavistock.

Frude, N., Dowling, E. (1980) A follow-up analysis of family therapy clients. Journal of Family Therapy, 2, 149–162.

Gaines, A. (1992) From DSM-I to III-R; voices of self, mastery and the other: A cultural constructivist reading of US psychiatric classification. Social Science & Medicine, 35, 3–24.

George, E., Iveson, C. & Ratner, H. (1990) Problem to solution: Brief therapy with individuals and families. London: Brief Therapy Press.

Gergen, K.J. (1985) The social constructionist movement in modern psychology. American Psychologist, 40, 266–275.

Gergen, K.J. (1991). The saturated self. New York: Basic Books.

Gergen, K.J. Hoffman, L. and Anderson, H. (1996) Is diagnosis a disaster?: A constructionist dialogue. In Kaslow, F. (Ed.) Handbook for Relational Diagnosis. New York: Wiley.

Jones, E. (1993) Family Systems Therapy: Developments in the Milan Systemic Therapy. Chichester: Wiley.

Gordon, D. A., Graves, K., & Arbuthnot, J. (1995) The effect of Functional Family Therapy for delinquents on adut criminal behavior. Criminal Justice and Behavior, 22, 60–73.

Gowers, S., Norton, K., Halek, C., & Crisp, A.H. (1994) Outcome of outpatient psychotherapy in a random allocation treatment study of anorexia nervosa. International Journal of Eating Disorders, 15, 165–177.

Guanapina, C. (2003) Sharing a multicultural course design for a marriage and family therapy program: one perspective. Journal of Family Therapy, 25, 86–106.

Gurman, A.S., Kniskern, D.P. & Pinsof, W.M. (1986) Research on marital and family therapies. In S.L. Garfield & A.E. Bergin (Eds.) Handbook of psychotherapy and behavior change. (3rd ed.). New York: Wiley.

Gustafsson, P. A., Kjellman, N.-I. M., & Cederblad, M. (1986). Family therapy in the treatment of severe childhood asthma. Journal of Psychosomatic Research, 30, 369–374.

Haley, J. (1973) Uncommon Therapy. New York: Norton

Harrington, R., Kerfoot, M., Dyer, E., McNiven, F., Gill, J., Harrington, V., Woodham, A., & Byford, S. (1998). Randomized trial of a home-based family intervention for children who have deliberately poisoned themselves. Journal of the American Academy of Child and Adolescent Psychiatry, 37, 512–518.

Hart, R. (1997) Children's participation: the theory and practice of involving young citizens in community Development and Environmental Care. London: Earthscan Publications and New York: UNICEF

Haug, I.E. (2003) Observing the growth and development of family therapy in Ecuador. In (Ed. Ng, K.S.) Global Perspectives in Family Therapy: Development, Practice, Trends. New York: Brunner-Routledge.

Hazelrigg, M.D., Cooper, H.M. & Borduin C.M. (1987) Evaluating the effectiveness of family therapies: An Integrative Review and Analysis. Psychological Bulletin, 101, 428-442.

Henggeler, S.W. & Borduin, C.M. (1990) Family Therapy and beyond: A multisystemic approach to teaching the behavior problems of children and adolscents. Pacific Grove, CA: Brooks/Cole.

Jackson, D. (1957)The question of family homeostasis. Psychiatric Quarterly, 3, 79–90.

Kaslow, F.W. (1993) Relational diagnosis: An idea whose time has come? Family Process. 32, 255–259.

Kelly, G. (1955) A theory of personality: The psychology of personal constructs. New York: Norton.

Kennedy, J. (1994) Living and working in a poor community: an evolving conversation. Human Systems: the Journal of Systemic Consultation and Management, 5, 209–218.

Khan, S. (2003) Editorial: changing contexts, changing minds. Context: the Magazine for Family Therapy and Systemic Practice, 67, 1–3.

Klar, H. & Berg, I.K. (1999) Solution Focused Therapy. In Lawson, D. & Prevatt, F. (Eds.) Casebook in Family Therapy. Belmont: Wadsworth Publishing Company.

Kolko, D. J., Brent, D.A., Baugher, M., Bridge J. & Birmaher B. (2000) Cognitive and family therapies for adolescent depression: treatment specificity, mediation, and moderation. Journal of Consulting & Clinical Psychology, 68, 603–14.

L'Abate, L. (1994) Family Evaluation: A psychological approach. Thousand Oaks: Sage.

Laing, R.D. & Esterson, A. (1964) Sanity madness and the family. Vol. 1. The families of schizphrenics. London: Tavistock Publications

Lambert, M.J. (1992) Psychotherapy Outcome Research: Implications for integrative and eclectic therapists. In Norcross, N.J. & Goldfried, M.R. (Eds.).Handbook of psychotherapy integration. New York: Basic.

Lask, B. & Matthew, D. (1979) Childhood asthma: A controlled trial of family psychotherapy. Archives of Disease in Childhood, 54, 116–119.

Lavee, Y. (2003) Family therapy in a multicultural society: the case of Israel. In (Ed. Ng, K.S.) Global Perspectives in Family Therapy: Development, Practice, Trends. New York: Brunner-Routledge.

le Goff, J.F. (2003) Family therapy in France: a brief overview. In (Ed. Ng, K.S.) Global Perspectives in Family Therapy: Development, Practice, Trends. New York: Brunner-Routledge.

Lobatto, W. (2002) Talking to children about family therapy: a qualitative study. Journal of Family Therapy, 24, 330–343.

Ma, J.L.C. (2000) Treatment expectations and treatment experiences of Chinese families towards family therapy:

appraisal of a common belief. Journal of Family Therapy. 22, 296–307.

McDowell, T., Ruei Feing, S., Gomez-Young, C., Khanna, A., Sherman, B. & Brownlee, K. (2003) Making space for racial dialogue: our experience in a Masters in Family Therapy training program. Journal of Marital and Family Therapy, 29, 179–183.

McNab, S., Wagstaff, S., Smith, A. (2000) Everything you wanted to know about family therapy but were afraid to ask! Context: the Magazine for Family Therapy and Systemic Practice, 50, 2–5.

Madigan, S. (1998) Praxis. Vancouver: The Cardigan Press.

Marchetti Mercer, M.C., Beyers, D. & Dews, L. (1999) Training family therapists in a multicultural setting. Contemporary Family Therapy, 21, 187–202.

Markus, E., Lange, A. & Pettigrew, T.F. (1990) Effectiveness of family therapy: a meta-analysis. Journal of Family Therapy 12, 205–221.

Maturana, H. & Varela, F. (1984) The tree of knowledge: Biological roots of human understanding. London: Shambhala

Miller, S.D., Duncan, B.L. & Hubble, M.A. (1997) Escape from Babel: toward a unifying language for psychotherapy practice. New York: Wiley.

Minuchin, S. (1974) Families and family therapy. Cambridge, Mass: Harvard University Press.

Minuchin, S. (1981) Family Therapy Techniques. Cambridge: Harvard University Press.

Minuchin, S., Auerswald, E., King, C. Rabinowitz, C. (1964) The study and treatment of families that produce multiple acting-out boys. American Journal of Orthopsychiatry. 34, 125–134.

Minuchin, S., Montalvo, B., Guerney, B., Rosman, B. & Schumer, F. (1967) Families of the slums. New York: Basic Books.

Minuchin, S., Rosman, B.L., & Baker, L. (1978) Psychosomatic Families. Cambridge, Mass: Harvard University Press.

Ng, K.S. (2003) Family therapy in Malaysia: an update. In (Ed. Ng, K.S.) Global Perspectives in Family Therapy: Development, Practice, Trends. New York: Brunner-Routledge.

O'Hanlon, W. (1989) In search of solutions. New York: W.W. Norton.

Olson, D.H. (1986) Circumplex Model VII: Validation studies and FACES III. Family Process. 25, 337–351.

Palazzoli, S., Boscolo, L., Cecchin, G. & Prata, G. (1978) Paradox and counterparadox. New York: Aronson.

Palazzoli, S., Boscolo, L., Cecchin, G. & Prata, G. (1980) Hypothesizing, circularity & neutrality: Three guidelines for the conductor of the session. Family Process, 19, 3–12.

Parsons, B. & Alexander, J. (1973) Short term family intervention: a therapy outcome study. Journal of Consulting and Clinical Psychology, 41, 195–201.

Patterson, G (1976) The Aggressive Child: victim or architect of a coercive system. In Leitenberg, H. (Ed.) Behavior Modification and Behavior Therapy. Prentice Hall: New Jersey.

Periera, R., Kurimay, T., Onnis, L., Eisler, I., Goldbetter, E. & Stratton, P. (2002) Minimum criteria for training in Family Therapy. European Family Therapy Association/www.efta-europeanfamilytherapy.com

Pote, H., Stratton, P., Cottrell, D., Shapiro, D. & Boston, P. (2003) Systemic family therapy can be manualized: research process and findings. Journal of Family Therapy, 25, 236–262.

Prabhu, R. (2003) The beginning of family therapy in India. In (Ed. Ng, K.S.) Global Perspectives in Family Therapy: Development, Practice, Trends. New York: Brunner-Routledge.

Reimers, S., (2001) Understanding alliances. How can research inform user-friendly practice. Journal of Family Therapy. 23, 46–62.

Reimers, S. & Treacher, A. (1995) Introducing user-friendly family therapy. London: Routledge

Reiss, D. (1981) The Family's Construction of Reality. Cambridge: Harvard University Press.

Reiss, D., & Klein, D. (1987) Paradigm and pathogenesis: a family centered approach to problems of etiology and treatment of psychiatric disorders. In Jacob, T. (Ed) Family Interaction and Psychopathology: Theories, Methods, Findings. New York: Plenum.

Rivett, M. & Street, E (2003) Family Therapy in Focus. London: Sage.

Robin, A.L., Siegel, P.T., Koepke, T., Moye, A., & Tice, S. (1994) Family therapy versus individual therapy for adolescent females with anorexia nervosa. Journal of Developmental and Behavioral Pediatrics, 15, 111–116.

Robin, A.L., Siegel, P.T., Moye, A.W., Gilroy, M., Baker-Dennis, A., & Sikard, A. (1999) A controlled comparison of family versus individual therapy for adolescents with anorexia nervosa. Journal of the American Academy of Child and Adolescent Psychiatry, 38, 1482–1489.

Russell, G. F. M., Szmukler, G., Dare, C., & Eisler, I. (1987). An evaluation of family therapy in anorexia nervosa and bulimia nervosa. Archives of General Psychiatry, 44, 1047–1056.

Ryden, O., Nevander, L., Johnsson, P., Hansson, K., Kronvall, P., Sjoblad, S. & Westbom, L. (1994) Family therapy in poorly controlled juvenile IDDM: effects on diabetic control, self evaluation and behavioral symptoms. Acta Paediatrica, 83, 285–291.

Seligman, P. (2002) Clients views of systemic psychotherapy. Context: the Magazine for Family Therapy and Systemic Practice, 50, 19–23.

Shadish, W.R., Montgomery, L.M., Wilson, P., Wilson, M.R., Bright, I. & Okwumabua, T. (1993) Effects of family and marital psychotherapies: A meta-analysis. Journal of Consulting and Clinical Psychology, 61, 992–1002.

Sholevar, G. & Schwoeri, L. (2003) Textbook of Family and Couples Therapy: Clinical Applications. Washington: American Psychiatric Publishing Inc.

Skynner, A.C.R. (1976) Systems of family and marital psychotherapy. New York, Brunner/Mazel.

Stanton, M.D., & Shadish, W.R. (1997) Outcome, attrition and family/couples treatment for drug abuse: A meta-analysis and review of the controlled and comparative studies. Psychological Bulletin, 122, 170–191.

Strong, T. (1993) DSM IV and describing problems in family therapy. Family Process, 32, 249–253.

Stuart, R. B. (1969) Operant–interpersonal treatment for marital discord. Journal of Consulting and Clinical Psychology, 33, 675–682.

Szapocznik, J., Perez-Vidal, A., Brickman, A. L., Foote, F. H., Santisteban, D., Hervis, O., & Kurtines, W. M. (1988) Engaging adolescent drug abusers and their families in treatment: A strategic structural systems approach. Journal of Consulting and Clinical Psychology, 56, 552–557.

Szapocznik, J., Rio, A., Murray, E., Cohen, R., Scopetta, M., Rivas-Valquez, A., Hervis, O., V., P., & Kurtines, W. (1989). Structural family versus psychodynamic child therapy for problematic Hispanic boys. Journal of Consulting and Clinical Psychology, 57, 571–578.

Tamura, T. (2003) The development of family therapy and experience of fatherhood in a Japanese context. In (Ed. Ng, K.S.) Global Perspectives in Family Therapy: Development, Practice, Trends. New York: Brunner-Routledge.

Tamura, T. & Lau, A. (1992) Connectedness vs. separateness: the applicability of family therapy to Japanese families. Family Process, 31, 319–340.

Tan, A. (2003) The emergence of family therapy in post-modern Singapore. In (Ed. Ng, K.S.) Global Perspectives in Family Therapy: Development, Practice, Trends. New York: Brunner-Routledge.

Tomm, K. (1987 a) Interventive interviewing: Part I. Strategizing as a fourth guideline for the therapist. Family Process. 26, 3–13.

Tomm, K. (1987 b) Interventive interviewing: Part II. Reflexive questioning as a means to enable self-healing. Family Process, 26, 167–83.

Tomm, K. (1988) Interventive interviewing: Part III. Intending to ask lineal, circular, strategic, or reflexive questions? Family Process, 27, 1–15.

Tomm, K. (1991) Beginnings of 'HIPs and PIPs' approach to psychiatric assessment. The Calgary Participator. Spring, 21–24.

Varga, A (2003) Family therapy and family life cycle in Russia. In (Ed. Ng, K.S.) Global Perspectives in Family Therapy: Development, Practice, Trends. New York: Brunner-Routledge.

von Bertalanffy, L. (1968) General systems theory: Foundations, developments, applications. New York: Braziller.

Waldegrave, C. (1995) Some central ideas in the 'Just Therapy' Approach. Australian and New Zealand Journal of Family Therapy, 14, 1–8.

Walsh, F. (1995) From family damage to family challenge. In Mikesell, R., Lusterman, D. & McDaniels, H. (Eds.) Integrating family therapy: Handbook of family psychology and systems theory. Washington: American Psychological Association.

Watzlawick, P., Weakland, J. & Fisch, R. (1974) Change: Principles of problem formation and problem resolution. New York: Norton.

Weakland, J., & Jackson, D. (1958) Patient and therapists observation on the circumstances of a schizophrenic episode. Archives of Neurolog, 79, 554–574.

Weakland, J., Fisch, R., Watzlawick, P. & Bodin, A. (1974) Brief therapy: Focused problem resolution. Family Process. 13, 141–168.

Weitzman, L. C. S. W. (1985) Engaging the Severely Dysfunctional Family in Treatment: Basic Considerations. Family Process, 24, 473–485.

Whitaker, C. (1975) Psychotherapy of the absurd. Family Process, 14, 1–16.

White, M. & Epston, D. (1990) Narrative means to therapeutic ends. New York: Norton.

Whitehead, A.N. & Russell, B. (1910) Principia Mathematica, Cambridge: Cambridge University Press.

Wiener, N. (1948) Cybernetics or Control and Communication in the Animal and the Machine. New York: Wiley.

Willcox, D. (1995) A guide to effective participation York: Rowntree.

Woodward, C.A., Santa-Barbara, J., Levin, S. & Epstein, N. (1978) Aspects of consumer satisfaction with brief family therapy. Family Process, 17, 399–407.

Wysocki, T., Harris, M.A., Greco, P., Bubb, J., Danda, C.E., Harvey, L.M., McDonell, K., Taylor, A. & White, N.H. (2000) Randomized, controlled trial of behavior therapy for families of adolescents with insulin-dependent diabetes mellitus. Journal of Pediatric Psychology, 25, 23–33.

13

Innovative Interventions in the Community

Ernesto Caffo, Barbara Forresi, Carlotta Belaise, Giampaolo Nicolais, Nathaniel Laor,
Leo Wolmer, Helmut Remschmidt

14.1   **Telefono Azzurro: A Multiprogram Approach to**
Problems of Child Abuse – 188
Ernesto Caffo, Barbara Forresi, Carlotta Belaise,
Giampaolo Nicolais

14.1.1   Introduction   – 188
14.1.2   Telefono Azzurro: Theoretical Framework   – 188
14.1.2.1 Developmental Psychopathology Model   – 188
14.1.2.2 Multiagency Approach   – 189
14.1.3   Program Elements   – 189
14.1.3.1 National Call Center: Helplines   – 189
14.1.3.2 Tetto Azzurro: Clinical Intervention   – 193
14.1.3.3 Emergency Team   – 194
14.1.4   The Future   – 196
14.1.5   Conclusions   – 196

14.2   **Implementing Relief Programs in Communities**
Affected by Disaster: Theory, Principles,
and a Case Study – 196
Nathaniel Laor, Leo Wolmer

14.2.1   Introduction   – 196
14.2.2   Principles for Disaster Interventions   – 197
14.2.3   Disaster Intervention Teams:
Task and Leadership   – 197
14.2.4   A Disaster Preparedness and Intervention Program:
The Tel-Aviv Model   – 198
14.2.5   A Teacher-Mediated School-Based Intervention
Program   – 199
14.2.6   Conclusion   – 200

14.3   **A Mobile Mental Health Service for Children and**
Adolescents in Germany – 200
Helmut Remschmidt

14.3.1   Historical Background   – 200
14.3.2   General Guidelines for Child and Adolescent
Mental Health Services   – 201
14.3.3   The Mobile Mental Health Service for Children
and Adolescents as Part of a Comprehensive
Service System   – 201
14.3.3.1 Conception of the Mobile Service   – 201
14.3.3.2 Utilization of the Mobile Service   – 202
14.3.4   Conclusions   – 204

References   – 204

This chapter describes three different services in three different countries that have two things in common:

1. They are directly addressed to and based in a community.
2. They are innovative in terms of the addressed population, in terms of methodology and also in terms of funding.

The first part (Ernesto Caffo et al.) focuses on three different Italian services for children who are abused or neglected, and also children with other problems: Telefono Azzurro's helpline, Tetto Azzurro and Emergency Team. The second part (Nathaniel Laor and Leo Wolmer) describes a program for communities affected by disaster in Tel Aviv, and the third part (Helmut Remschmidt) presents a Mobile Service for psychiatrically disturbed children and families in a rural district in Germany.

The experiences with the three different services are promising. All of them, however, have problems with regard to appropriate financing and to getting integrated into the systems of care in the respective country. Nevertheless, they demonstrate that both private and NGO initiatives play an important role in the development of mental health services for children and adolescents and their families.

14.1 Telefono Azzurro: A Multiprogram Approach to Problems of Child Abuse

Ernesto Caffo, Barbara Forresi, Carlotta Belaise, Giampaolo Nicolais

14.1.1 Introduction

Telefono Azzurro is a nonprofit organization, dedicated to enhancing child and adolescent well-being and health, especially for those living situations of developmental difficulty, trauma and emergency. The mission of Telefono Azzurro is to promote child and adolescent rights and develop good practices for care.

Telefono Azzurro is composed of several different structures (Call Center, Emergency Team, Tetto Azzurro, Training and Study Center) and is involved in primary prevention, emergency intervention, treatment, research and training. Centers are currently located in Milan (National Call Center), Rome (Tetto Azzurro and Study Center) and Treviso (Emergency Team), Italy.

Launched in 1987, Telefono Azzurro Helpline is a confidential service that enables young children to talk to professional counselors, toll free, 24 hours a day. All Telefono Azzurro telephone counselors are trained professionals. The service provides assessment, emotional support, information, and referrals to local agencies. For emergency and life-threatening situations, Telefono Azzurro offers crisis intervention and the mobilization of emergency response services.

Begun in 1999, Tetto Azzurro is the Province of Rome's clinical center for diagnosis, treatment, and residential care of abused and neglected children. Children are referred by the juvenile court, social services, and national health system child care units, for second-level, focused clinical intervention. Tetto Azzurro also provides a psychosocial help-desk for parents, teachers, or children who may have experienced abuse or maltreatment. In the first years of activity, the center has trained professionals working in social services as well as the national health system's clinical units on the management of child abuse, and the promotion of a multiagency and interdisciplinary network approach to child maltreatment.

Telefono Azzurro Emergency Team is a project developed in 1997, in collaboration with the Yale Child Study Center and the New Haven Police Department (Child Development and Community Policy Program). The Team is composed of psychologists trained to immediately intervene in emergency situations where children and adolescents are victims or witnesses of traumatic events (abuse, antisocial behaviors, natural disasters, domestic violence, juvenile prostitution, delinquency, runaway, and psychiatric emergencies). Telefono Azzurro Emergency Team is engaged in promoting the development of a multiagency and multidisciplinary intervention network for child and adolescent care.

This chapter focuses on the issues and difficulties involved in building an interagency response and adopting a developmental psychopathology model as a framework for intervention.

14.1.2 Telefono Azzurro: Theoretical Framework

The Telefono Azzurro intervention approach is based on an ecological and developmental psychopathology model (Cicchetti 2002; Pine and Cohen 2002; Cummings et al. 2000; Pynoos et al. 1999) and a »multidisciplinary and multiagency approach« (Henggeler et al. 2002; U.S. Department of Health and Human Services 1999).

14.1.2.1 Developmental Psychopathology Model

Organizational theorists believe that each stage of development confronts children with new challenges. An individual who has adaptively met the developmental tasks of a particular stage will be better equipped to meet successive new challenges in development. In contrast, incompetence in development leads to difficulties or maladaptive efforts to resolve the challenges of a developmental period. However, the progression is probabilistic, not inevitable. Changes in the environment may lead to improvements in the ability to deal with developmental challenges, resulting in a redirection in the developmental course (Cicchetti 2002; Cummings et al. 2000; Cicchetti and Cohen 1995).

Even before the emergence of psychopathology, certain pathways signify adaptational failures in normal development that probabilistically lead to pathology (Cummings et al. 2000). Thus, knowledge derived from research in the field of developmental psychopathology bears considerable relevance for the prevention and treatment of high risk and maladaptive conditions. »By thoroughly understanding factors that pull subjects toward or away from increased risk at various age periods, one not only acquires a deeper understanding of development but one also gains valuable information for primary prevention« (Sroufe and Rutter 1984).

According to a developmental psychopathology model, a mental health professional needs to do an accurate analysis of individual/environmental risk and protective factors. The U.S. Surgeon General's Report on Children and Mental Health (1999) stated that »psychopathology in childhood arises from the complex, multilayered interactions of specific characteristics of the child (including biological, psychological and genetic factors), his or her environment (including parent, sibling, family relations, peer and neighborhood factors, school and community factors, and the larger social-cultural context) and the specific manner in which these factors interact with and shape each other over the course of development.«

14.1.2.2 Multiagency Approach

The multidetermined nature of problems such as child abuse and neglect has been explicated by decades of research. To a large extent, Telefono Azzurro's intervention strategy is based on the findings in this literature. Children at greatest risk of sexual abuse, for example, appear to come from families characterized by multiple sources of difficulties and dysfunction, including marital conflict, parental separation, step-parenthood, parental psychopathology, and impaired parent-child relationship (Forresi 2003; Purtois 2000; Fergusson and Mullen 1999).

If a problem is multidetermined, in order to optimize the probability of favorable outcomes, intervention should address the complex array of factors that are related to the problem (Henggeler et al. 2002; Cohen and Caffo 1998). This is the reason why, in many cases, a single mental health professional cannot be expected to effectively address the broad range of challenging problems presented by children and families. Managing a case of childhood maladjustment or abuse, for example, is a complex process, demanding collaboration between different and specific agencies (school, social services, court, law enforcement) and different professionals, such as doctors, psychologists, social workers, lawyers, judges, and policemen. This is clearly

evident in emergency situations in which the child/adolescent is acutely and imminently in danger or is at high risk for trauma (e.g., runaway, suicide, sexual or physical abuse). Safe and effective interventions can be best developed understanding individual, family, peer, and community factors sustaining or diminishing the crisis. Parents and other caregivers play essential roles in the child's socioemotional development. Cognizant of this fact, Telefono Azzurro promotes healthy caregiving and enhancing the role of family and school (Forresi 2003).

A multiagency intervention can be implemented in ways that prioritize youth, that are developmentally appropriate, and fit the developmental needs of the youth. The aim of the interagency approach is to bring together all relevant statutory and voluntary sector agencies in order to build joint responses in child protection matters. The ability to collaborate within a national network of services and sharing common language, methodologies, and goals represents the real challenge for the successful care of children. Meaningful and effective multiagency work requires constructive sharing of policies, procedures, and practices on a wider interagency basis. It is required that there be operating protocols within a network to promote an ongoing exchange of information, to define roles, to set limits, and delineate areas of expertise for each agency or professional involved.

14.1.3 Program Elements

To foster prevention, Telefono Azzurro enhances coordination among community agencies and professionals. Over the past decade, Telefono Azzurro has developed partnerships and collaborative ways of working with health and nonhealth sectors, such as police, schools, community services, and courts.

In the following paragraphs, we will focus on intervention programs developed by Telefono Azzurro: Telefono Azzurro helpline, Tetto Azzurro and Emergency Team.

14.1.3.1 National Call Center: Helplines

Clinical and research literature produced in the United States, United Kingdom, and Canada suggest that telephone counseling can be used to provide help and support for those individuals whose access to services is limited by geographical/physical and emotional barriers. Positive features include anonymity and accessibility. The recent explosion in the use of mobile phones among adolescents and children (Caffo 2003a, Rosenfield 1997) adds to the potential use of the telephone for telephone counseling.

The Telefono Azzurro National Call Center, located in Milan, provides two different helplines. The 19696 line is dedicated to children and adolescents 4–14 years of age who wish to report abuse and maltreatment or discuss problems that they might be experiencing. The 199.15.15.15 line is for adolescents 15–18 years of age, parents, teachers, and adults who need to report child and adolescent difficulties, to get information, or to be supervised. Both lines are available 24 hours a day, 7 days a week. Children and adolescents determine what, how much, and the manner in which they are going to state their problems. All their problems are »legitimated« through the interaction.

According to a developmental psychopathology model, the primary purpose of a childline is »prevention«, identification of children at risk, and improvement of factors that affect well-being by enhancing coping capacities as well as support systems (e.g., extended family, school, neighbors, friends; Caffo 2003a; Alperstein and Raman 2003). The emphasis is on the positive, using family and community strengths as levers for change. For example, the child calling 19696 may be asked to phone again together with a family member, a teacher, or an adult. This way a counselor can promote responsible behavior and decrease irresponsible behavior among family members. Thus, a childline can improve the quality of family-school linkage, and engage school professionals.

Even though each call is different from the next, there are clear phases in the childline use process. These phases are: (1) making the contact with the caller, (2) engaging the caller, (3) clarifying the presenting problem, (4) developing solutions, and (5) terminating the call (Caffo 2003a). In the initial phase the caller needs to be welcomed and listened to. In order to establish an effective helping relationship, the initial contact with the caller is very important. A calm, open, accepting, and supporting approach is required to facilitate communication. In case of an emergency, the operator should try to get information about what happened, but only if the emotional turmoil subsides is the person likely to be reflective.

Using counseling skills, a telephone operator has to explore the situation (in order to establish if the child may be at immediate risk). It is essential to take time to get to the real problem and trying to learn as much as he/she can about the caller, his/her feelings, family's internal and external resources, and possibilities for change. Exploration is an ongoing process that occurs throughout the counseling. Active listening and carefully responding to the child or adolescent are useful to avoid being sidetracked by superficial concerns. It is possible, in fact, that the caller does not present their primary concern and may cover up more pervasive problems.

Telephone counseling may have different outcomes. Once the problem has been identified, the counselor can decide if he/she is able to provide help. If not, can the counselor help the caller in obtaining support and help elsewhere by means of a referral to community resources? Sometimes one consultation is enough to set up a helpful relationship with the caller, to help him/her be empowered, to develop his/her own awareness of what may have happened, or improve his/her relationships and interactions.

In other cases, the caller is requested to call again, alone or together with an adult (parents, teachers), who may be helpful to him/her. In this case, the operator and the caller can develop more specific goals for the next call or plan strategies to be adopted in order to overcome a difficulty. Sometimes a referral to local social services, mental health services, courts or police may be necessary. According to January–June 2003 data, in 93% of cases, children and adolescents who called the National Call Center received telephone counseling by a professional (psychologist or pedagogist). In the other 7% of cases, a referral to another agency (e.g., mental health service, social service, court, police) was made.

In any of the previous cases, a telephone operator is requested to:

1. Identify individual and community resources to be mobilized as well as to try to locate a possible support for the future;
2. Explore different solutions and propose an intervention;
3. Try to establish a final agreement with the caller, who is supposed to be the subject and not the object of the intervention.

The last phase of a telephone consultation is the follow-up. When external agencies are mobilized (e.g., social and mental health services, court), counselors are also asked to make a follow-up call to them, within two weeks of the original call. Unfortunately, in some cases the follow-up cannot be realized. The latter happens when the caller asks for anonymity or when the agency is not collaborative and does not give a feedback on intervention outcomes.

14.1.3.1.1 Data

A computer-assisted form concerning each case is usually filled out by the telephone operator. The form is structured in order to gather the most complete information and details provided by the child or adult during the telephone call. The main topics are: demographic information for the child; information about the caller; information about child/ adolescent's problem or distress; information about the abuse and the alleged offender; professionals/institutions who already know the case; information about the family; agreement and case referral.

From January to June 2003, Telefono Azzurro received a total of 194,000 phone calls, on both its lines. The calls on relevant problems were 1,909. Most callers were females (57.8% females and 42.2% males). As regards the age groups, children who call Telefono Azzurro are mainly 11–14 years

of age (43%), followed by children under 10 years (41.3%) and teenagers (15.7%).

◘ Table 14.1 shows some data on presenting problems. Almost 50% of reasons for a call concern family difficulties: relational difficulties between children and parents or parental conflicts after a divorce. In the first 6 months of 2003, Telefono Azzurro received 608 calls (31.8% of the total calls) for physical abuse (38.4%), sexual abuse (17.4%), psychological abuse (22.8%) and neglect (21.4%). Considering these four major causes for children calling Telefono Azzurro, we notice a predominance of female children and adolescents experiencing abuse (55.8% vs. 44.2% of males; see ◘ Table 14.2).

For the last three years, it has been noted that there are an increasing number of foreign children and adolescents' calls, raising multicultural issues. In 2001, foreign children and adolescents calls were 6% of the total, in 2002 they were 8.8%, while in the first 6 months of 2003 they reached 9.8%. The main reasons for calls by foreign children and adolescents are problems in relationships with parents (29.8%); physical abuse (25.1% vs. 13.6% of the national sam-

◘ **Table 14.1.** National Call Center presenting problems

Presenting problems	Sex		Total
	Male (%)	Female (%)	(%)
Relational problems with parents	32.8	35.1	34.1
Problems related to parental divorce	18.1	15.3	16.3
Physical abuse	16.3	14.1	14.8
Need to talk	11.6	15.9	14.0
Relational problems	14.0	12.9	13.3
Psychological abuse	10.8	7.1	8.8
Relational problems with peers	8.0	8.5	8.4
Neglect	10.3	6.6	8.3
Sexual abuse	4.3	8.7	6.7
Fears	5.6	6.8	6.3
Loneliness	6.1	6.3	6.1
Academic difficulties	8.3	4.0	5.8
Sentimental reasons	1.1	5.5	3.8
Sexual difficulties	2.3	4.2	3.6
Relational problems with strangers	2.8	2.5	2.6
Parents with alcohol problems	2.8	2.5	2.6
Grief	2.1	1.1	1.5
Drugs use	1.3	1.5	1.4
Learning difficulties	1.9	1.2	1.4
Runaway	1.3	1.4	1.3
Problems related to adoption	1.1	1.0	1.0
Suicidal intention	1.3	0.7	1.0
Pregnancy	0.1	1.1	0.8
Child labor	0.8	0.6	0.7
Separation anxiety	0.7	0.5	0.6
Prostitution	0.5	0.2	0.3%

❏ **Table 14.2.** Characteristics of telephone calls

Type of abuse	Sex		Total
	Male	Female	
Physical	46.0%	54.0%	270
Sexual	26.7%	73.3%	122
Psychological	52.9%	47.1%	160
Neglect	53.5%	46.5%	151
TOTAL	44.2%	55.8%	608

ple); and neglect (19.3% vs. 18.3% of the entire national sample). Some cases are specifically linked to the child's family culture, such as female genital mutilation, children in the international illegal trade, serious labor exploitation, and precocious marriage. Many children also report situations that have to do with integration difficulties, both social and educational, as well as home problems usually linked to parents' and children's conflicting expectations of living in a new country.

14.1.3.1.2 Effectiveness and Quality

In order to guarantee that all European children receive an effective answer and professional service, both public and private organizations sponsoring hotlines are requested to offer a service according to basic quality requirements. But how to define the »effectiveness« of a helpline? Does it deal with the number of case referrals or with a reduction of risk factors for maladjustment or psychopathology? During its 16 years experience, Telefono Azzurro made many efforts to develop a quality service for children and adolescents. Two major steps are relevant to this point (Caffo 2003 a).

The Daphne project has been an opportunity for European Helplines (Telefono Azzurro, Italy; SNATEM, France; NSPCC, England; ANAR, Spain; RAF, Austria; and BAG, Germany) to discuss best practices, procedures, telephone operators' competencies and training. »Quality« has been defined as »the observance of fundamental principles«, defined in two main documents: the European Chart of Telephone Helpline and the European Helpline Operators Competencies: Value base requirements for good practice.

The Telefono Azzurro quality system aims to identify common guidelines for the consultation process. They can be described according to ISO9000 norms and total quality management organization principles. Process rationalization and on-

going monitoring permit a constant control over the telephone consultation process, to evaluate internal and external satisfaction, to identify critical aspects of the service according to quantitative (questionnaires, performance indicators, number of calls, waiting time, etc.) and qualitative (according to quality principles defined by main European helplines) parameters.

14.1.3.1.3 Competencies

»Conditio sine qua non« for the effectiveness of a telephone consultation is represented by counselor's competencies (Caffo 2003 a). Competencies include: (a) being able to communicate with children of different ages by creating a trusting relationship with the caller and by reassuring him/her about the real possibility to be helped and protected; (b) understanding and evaluating the caller situation, especially if it represents an emergency, after having gathered detailed information in respect of the caller's confidentiality and point of view; and (c) planning a way to empower the caller by involving him/her directly and by using child, family and environmental resources.

Professional counselors need to be competent in psychological, psychiatric, and sociological matters. They also need to know about normal and pathological development, psychological assessment, personality, and gender development. Telephone operators working in Telefono Azzurro are specifically trained to deal with children, adolescents, and adults from different cultures, races and religions. The operators pay special attention to the study of different cultural habits, cultural influences on children and adolescents' development, relationships between family members, and specific, culturally relevant interventions.

In addition to communication skills and knowledge required for specific problems (child abuse, suicide, domestic violence, etc.), telephone counselors also need to be trained in role, organization, and interagency relations. Counselors involved in intervention need to become familiar with resources available in the community. Such knowledge is also useful in making good referrals to social services and mental health services (to police and court if necessary). In the document »European helpline operators' competencies: Value base requirements for good practice«', competencies for the development of training courses include performance indicators, guidelines for the helpline service evaluation and guidance for the development of specific assessment instruments (checklist, questionnaires, etc.). Training efforts are addressed to volunteers that manage the first phase of the call, as well as telephone operators and coordinators (Caffo 2003 a).

14.1.3.2 Tetto Azzurro: Clinical Intervention

Tetto Azzurro, the diagnostic and treatment unit (Unit), provides a clinical intervention in cases of child abuse using a child and family diagnostic assessment and psychotherapeutic treatment.

So far, the Unit has provided interventions for more than 100 abused children, ranging from 18 months to 18 years of age. While the number of children referred to the Unit for sexual and physical abuse has slightly decreased within 4 years of activity (from 41% in the first 2 years to 34% in the last two), domestic violence and neglect have increased especially during the last year, and now represent 48% of intakes. Whatever kind of abuse, nearly 90% of intakes are because of intrafamilial abuse.

14.1.3.2.1 Theoretical Orientation

The Unit clinical activity fits a transactional-ecological model of intervention (Belsky 1993), where child abuse is understood as the result of a balance between risk and protective factors operating at different levels of the child's context. Specific to the Unit's clinical approach and methodology is the focus, derived from attachment theory (Bowlby 1973, 1980), on child-primary caregivers' vicissitudes. The way infant-parent attachments develop in the context of child abuse is considered of primary relevance in terms of assessment, in the light of the intergenerational transmission of maladaptive parenting patterns (Belsky 1984).

As a consequence of the main theoretical assumptions, the aims of the diagnostic intervention may be outlined as follows:
1. To have a clear picture of the child's developmental status, both in terms of actual clinical assessment and retrospectively as a balance between developmental risk and protective factors
2. To assess the quality of the child's attachment to the primary caregivers
3. To assess the personality of the parents and other significant adults (foster parents, relatives, etc.).

14.1.3.2.2 Clinical Assessment

Child observation (free, structured, and interactional) is the core of the assessment procedure. The Strange Situation (Ainsworth et al. 1978) is usually administered to children of 1–2 years of age, in order to obtain a child's attachment profile. With children 2–7 years of age, the Crowell Procedure (Crowell and Feldman 1988) is usually administered to the mother-child and/or father-child dyad, as a measure of dyadic regulation. Children of 3–7 years of age are administered the structured play procedure of the MacArthur Story Stem Battery (MSSB; Bretherton et al. 1990), for evaluating the attachment representational level. Children 10–18 years of age are interviewed with the Modified Adult Attachment Interview (AAI) for early adolescence (Ammaniti et al. 1991). Finally, the Child Behavior Checklist (CBCL; Achenbach 1978) is administered to parents to assess the child's developmental and symptomatological profile.

Adults are involved in clinical sessions to the evaluate their personality traits and to the identify criteria for a possible Axis I or II diagnosis. The Symptom Checklist-90-R (SCL-90-R; Derogatis 1983) for the assessment of symptoms and the Adult Attachment Interview (AAI; Main and Goldwyn 1985–1994) for the evaluation of the attachment representational status are also administered. As previously underlined, great emphasis is placed on the analysis of the intergenerational level.

14.1.3.2.3 Data

Preliminary data on samples of abusing and nonabusing parents (Nicolais et al. 2002, Speranza and Nicolais 2002; Speranza et al. 2002) have shed an interesting light on what appears to be the long-neglected issue, in the field of child maltreatment, the role of the so-called nonabusing parent in child intrafamilial abuse. These data, that are currently being verified in a control-group study, seem to quite clearly indicate that in child intrafamilial abuse there is often a constellation of »insensitive parenting« (Lyons-Ruth 1999) that also involves the nonabusing parent, and that therefore worsens the effects of the actual abuse leading to more psychopathological outcomes for the »at risk« child.

14.1.3.2.4 Treatment

In terms of treatment, it is clear that Tetto Azzurro has to provide treatment for individuals (children, parents) and for »relationships«, as relationship trauma is believed to be the core mechanism of child intrafamilial abuse. Consequently, different treatment models are devised for the child as victim; the parent as abuser; the nonabusing parent and the dyadic-relationship. An accurate diagnosis of the context allows the therapist to understand the relationship(s) trauma within the family and leads to focused and effective treatments.

Methodologically speaking, it does not make much sense to distinguish, a priori, between expressive versus supportive treatment with the child. Rather, treatment modalities are offered in relation to specific characteristics of the age range of the child as follows:

1. 1–3 years old: dyadic therapy
2. 3–6 years old: play therapy, with a recommended focus on narratives
3. 6 (or more) years old: play therapy and a focus on narratives.

In the program, treatment lasts approximately 1 year. The therapy is carried on until all following conditions are fully satisfied:

1. Symptoms are over or at least dramatically reduced
2. Criteria are no longer fulfilled for a DSM/ICD disorder
3. The child is able to symbolize the trauma.

Adult treatment inevitably confronts a major challenge, i.e., the promotion and establishment of a therapeutic alliance in absence of a spontaneous request for treatment. This challenge can be engaged only through a preliminary phase where diagnostic data are shared with the parent. In this sense, the Unit's procedure defines a strong continuity between the diagnostic and the treatment phases. For all treatment intakes the diagnostic phase is the first step, both to verify crucial aspects of the individual's presentation, and prepare him/her for psychotherapeutic treatment. The diagnostic phase obviously gathers data which will be used as the basis for treatment. For parents' treatment, this procedure is of particular importance. In fact, after a diagnostic evaluation, the therapist will explain to the parent his/her diagnostic profile, highlighting the dysfunctions and/or psychopathologies, and letting him/her undergo an appraisal of personal psychological difficulties, often for the first time. The intergenerational transmission construct is shared at this same time, so that the parent will have the chance to see the abuse (either actively perpetrated or not recognized) as a relationship trauma across generations (data from the Adult Attachment Interview).

In methodological terms, this introductory phase of treatment, if successful, makes it possible for the therapist to place personal dysfunction/psychopathology within a meaningful family context, actively nurturing the therapeutic work. Sometimes at this stage, high levels of symptomatology and/or psychopathology require an associated pharmacological intervention. In these cases, the therapeutic emphasis will be specifically put on the »working through« of dysfunctional representational expectations. In other words, a perspective of change will now not only be shared, but actively sought, moving towards the establishment of new procedural models of relationship(s).

Finally, a distinguishing feature of the Tetto Azzurro unit's clinical approach has to be stressed: the previously mentioned close continuity between the diagnostic and treatment phases to make possible sound monitoring of treatment efficacy. Every diagnostic instrument has in fact a twofold aim, not only serving in the here and now of the diagnostic assessment, but also representing a possible repeated measure that can be administered at different moments of the therapeutic intervention in order to have an evidence-based evaluation process.

14.1.3.3 Emergency Team

Another project supported by Telefono Azzurro may exemplify how the insights derived from psychotraumatology research may be translated into health care systems (Caffo 2003 b). The »Emergency Team« Project was launched in Treviso (Italy) in 1998 as an experimental partnership between Telefono Azzurro and the community agency responsible for safeguarding children and adolescents. The project has been carried out in partnership with the Yale Child Study Center (USA), which has been running the »Child Development and Community Policing« Program (CD-CP) since 1991 (Marans et al. 1995). Their common goals are: (a) better understanding of the relationship between a child's or adolescent's involvement with or exposure to a crisis situation and the following traumatic stress symptoms; (b) creating a multiagency and interdisciplinary network able to face emergencies; (c) arranging a care strategy on a clinical, legal, and social level with a child perspective; (d) promoting community activities aimed at increasing public and professional awareness of the effects of crisis situations on children and adolescents; (e) giving useful advice in order to prevent emergencies; and (f) organizing training courses.

The Emergency Team is composed of trained psychologists available 24 hours a day, 365 days per year. These psychologists deal daily with emergency cases such as abused or neglected children/ adolescents, self-destructive or dangerous behaviors, victims of catastrophic situations, and new social emergencies.

The abuse and neglect cases include sexual abuse, physical abuse, severe neglect, psychological abuse, and violence exposure. Self-destructive or dangerous behaviors refer to suicide attempts, self-harm, runaways, drug and alcohol abuse, sensation seeking, and medical-psychiatric emergencies. Harmful or destructive behaviors towards other people encompass aggressiveness (threatening to kill or seriously harm someone; going beyond the control of significant adults; serious antisocial behaviors including sexual assault); destructiveness (violent, destructive behaviors against things; fire setting; sensation seeking); and violent psychotic behaviors (acute psychotic episodes and other severe forms of psychotic confusion).

Catastrophic/stressful situations refer to accidents (personal or external involvement in: car accidents, train or plane disasters, domestic accidents); natural disasters (earthquake, flood, fire, volcanic eruption); kidnapping or robbery (both involvement and witnessing) and war traumas (migrant children from war-torn countries). New social emergencies include juvenile prostitution involving trafficked adolescents and children; pedo-pornography (often by Internet) and young immigrants without parents.

14.1.3.3.1 Interventions

The Emergency Team intervention in case of an emergency is based on the following steps (Caffo and Belaise 2003; Caffo 2003 b): (1) identify the emergency; (2) contact other specific agencies and professionals; (3) evaluate resources, limits, and role of each agency; (4) evaluate the child's or adolescent's personal and environmental coping abilities; (5) plan and conduct an intervention on a clinical and/or legal and/or social level; (6) provide joint follow-up.

14.1.3.3.1.1 Community Reactivation Program

A multidisciplinary and multiagency approach is also evident in the Community Reactivation Program (see Sect. 14.2) run by Telefono Azzurro's Emergency Team in Molise, Italy, where on October

31st (2002) an earthquake caused the death of 29 citizens, most of them children from the first-grade class in an elementary school, in the village of San Giuliano di Puglia (Caffo 2003 b; Caffo et al. 2003). A joint Italian–Israeli team (consisting of professionals of Telefono Azzurro and of the Cohen-Harris Center for Trauma and Disaster Intervention) worked together in order to map the affected area in terms of type and amount of the community's psychosocial needs and to apply a model of Community Revitalization and Reactivation, adapted to the specific characteristics of the Molise community.

The Community Reactivation Program is based on the premise that not only individuals and families, but the whole community is affected by a catastrophe like an earthquake. Therefore, the program addresses the special needs of the community in terms of empowerment, revitalization, and rehabilitation of the community's main institutions, roles, and values. These institutions include formal and informal leadership, school system (kindergarten, elementary, and high school), community centers, primary care clinics, mental health services, etc.

The program is also based on the assumption that local professionals (leaders, mental health professionals, community workers, and volunteers) need to be empowered and trained to take the responsibility for and lead the implementation of the process, supervised by expert professionals who stay committed throughout the process. This is necessary because most affected communities have large-scale needs that are unable to be met by the existing professional forces. Programs need to be implemented through mediators within the local community (e.g., teachers) who, also, have a deep knowledge of the community, its residents, culture, and historical background.

Specific contents of the program (still under study) included:
1. Development of the community's formal and informal leadership.
2. Screening of the population in order to identify individuals at risk for the development of long-term psychological responses.
3. School reactivation – the provision of mental health relief to administrators and teachers, and role adaptation and empowerment of the educators as social mediators – is implemented through a Class Activation Program. This Program is a consumer-friendly process consisting of 8 sessions lasting 90 min each, led by the teachers and focused on the psychological relief of the students in parallel with the implementa-

tion of the normal teaching curriculum. The program integrates cognitive, behavioral, educational, and dynamic concepts and techniques that follow teachers and students not only during the program but throughout the school year.

4. Training of local mental health professionals to offer group, family and individual psychological relief for children and adults who continue to suffer from posttraumatic or grief symptoms after the implementation of the above-mentioned projects.

14.1.4 The Future

For the future, Telefono Azzurro is making efforts to promote an Internet counseling service and developing new emergency procedures for helplines. Since March 2003, in fact, Telefono Azzurro has been given by the Italian government the task of developing a 114 line, an emergency line dedicated to children and adolescents. Emergency intervention through telephone counseling is actually different from the counseling model usually adopted by helplines. The same communication skills are required, but emergency intervention is something more active, brief, and direct: telephone calls are time-limited and focused on caller's immediate needs. While the operator is trying to communicate support to the caller, he also has to intervene promptly in order to seek medical help, to arrange for some kind of immediate placement, to involve the police, etc., according to the presenting problem.

14.1.5 Conclusions

If a problem is multidetermined, intervention should address the complex array of factors that are related to it, in order to optimize the probability of favorable outcomes (Henggeler et al. 2002; Cohen and Caffo 1998). Managing a case of childhood maladjustment or abuse is therefore a complex process, demanding collaboration between different and specific agencies (school, social services, court, law enforcement) and different professionals (doctors, psychologists, social workers, lawyers, judges, and policemen). To this end, Telefono Azzurro has developed, over the past decade, partnerships and collaborative ways of working with health and nonhealth sectors, such as police, schools, community services, and courts. Incorporating approaches based on an

understanding of developmental psychopathology and the usefulness of a multiagency approach will remain a challenge worth pursuing.

14.2 Implementing Relief Programs in Communities Affected by Disaster: Theory, Principles, and a Case Study

Nathaniel Laor, Leo Wolmer

14.2.1 Introduction

Disasters, whether natural or instigated by human beings, occur unexpectedly and result in physical loss and massive harm. Such emergencies inflict acute and extensive damage on property and lives, and their impact can persist for years, disrupting the livelihood and the basic daily routines of individuals and communities.

Mental health interventions for relief, revitalization, and reactivation can have a contributory impact upon diverse social institutions (families, schools, local leadership) (Galante and Foa 1986; Goenjian et al. 1997). Nevertheless, experience has shown that professionals in charge need to endorse a systemic, socially oriented perspective (Pynoos et al. 1998). The difficulties are more pronounced in the field of children's mental health, because professionals must work across various public and private systems, among them medical, educational, and communal. Yet most position papers and guidelines for organizing emergency mental health services remain almost entirely oblivious to disaster preparedness as well as to the specific local and municipal systemic context within which emergency mental health services for children ought to be implemented (DeWolfe 2000; Young et al. 1998).

In this section, we put forth a philosophy of disaster intervention based on ecological-systems theory (Laor 2002) and on principles borrowed from public health, preventive medicine, communal welfare, education, and urban planning. We then propose two models: a disaster intervention model oriented to children living in urban areas and a model for teacher-mediated, school-based intervention.

14.2.2 Principles for Disaster Interventions

The complexities of working with communities affected by mass disaster require the implementation of a number of basic principles (Laor and Wolmer 2002; Laor et al. 2003):

Principle 1: Conduct risk assessment early and reach as many people as possible. Professionals need to employ rapid, easy-to-use, reliable and sensitive screening tools (Cochrans and Holland 1969; Ohan et al. 2002) to assess the numerous potential clinical disorders (posttraumatic stress, anxiety, dissociation, depression, grief) as well as the risk and vulnerability factors (e.g., past functioning, disaster-related events).

Principle 2: Implement systematic, broad-scale outreach programs. Bear in mind that survivors of disasters are often reluctant to seek professional help (Norwood et al. 2000; Schwarz and Kowalski 1992). Outreach programs should be followed by clinical triage protocols to match risk groups with intervention programs (Austin and Godleski 1999; Lindy et al. 1981; Saltzman et al. 2003; Pfefferbaum et al. 1999).

Principle 3: Be sensitive to the environment in which you work. Subordinate clinical evaluations to social considerations, and collaborate with the regular care system to achieve good results. Provide guidance to government and social institutions, school communities, and intervention teams in adapting to newly emerging needs; use data derived from population screening to direct allocation of institutional responsibilities and resources.

Principle 4: Manage regressive and progressive shifts in professional groups. Disasters initially result in a regressive loss of boundaries (dedifferentiation) among the traditional roles (psychiatrists, psychologists, social workers, child caretakers, educators) caring for survivors' basic needs. This process needs to be monitored by taking into account the unique contribution of these groups in later stages (redifferentiation).

Principle 5: Integrate mediators who work adjacent to the mental health system. A systemic perspective facilitates integration of information from various fields. Still, it lacks an ecological perspective that views the need to rehabilitate survivors within their most natural environment, while remaining sensitive to their culture. Social agents (educators, nurses, community workers) are properly suited to serve as mediators for such interventions as they occupy central positions in the community institutions that constitute the normal social matrix (Laor et al. 2003). Rehabilitated institutions (schools, primary care clinics, community centers) could serve as social reactivation centers within which large-scale interventions are implemented.

14.2.3 Disaster Intervention Teams: Task and Leadership

A fundamental task of mental health leaders is to facilitate a series of transitions that disaster survivors must undergo in order to recover normal functioning: from a freeze on past experience to a creative future orientation; from fixation on death and loss to involvement with life and revitalization; from passive submission to grief, shame, and anger to engagement of personal strengths; from withdrawal and alienation to involvement with nature, family, society, and technology; and from a mythological world view to a revised socio-cultural identity (Laor 2001).

Professionals need to coordinate their efforts with local authorities as well as to empower other professionals who have trustful relationships with children and parents (teachers, nurses, community workers) to serve educational-therapeutic roles (Laor and Wolmer 2002). These local mediators may themselves require relief of their symptoms, training in disaster-related interventions, and an opportunity to reclaim their original functions. Empowerment is the process by which individuals and communities recover their dignity and self-esteem by expanding their critical self-awareness, their control over resources and objectives, and their sense of personal and collective responsibility (Rappaport 1987). In displaced populations, this process of identifying specific needs, discovering leadership qualities, and gaining a greater sense of interdependence, cohesion, and cooperation allows newly formed communities to achieve greater control over their natural and social environment.

Collaboration between professionals in the field of children's mental health and agents in various systems could generate a child and adolescent emergency care team focused on the well-being of children and families. The task of such a team would be to integrate the various dimensions of reality decimated by the disaster (Laor et al. 2003) and to delegate professional authority to each of its members.

14.2.4   A Disaster Preparedness and Intervention Program: The Tel-Aviv Model

Mass disasters call for large-scale interventions that are accessible to everyone affected, without regard for socio-economic class. A system capable of properly functioning in unstable times must be established in advance. The Tel-Aviv Model lays the foundation for an urban framework for preparedness, resilience, and intervention. The model relies on a municipal headquarters for mental health that is accountable for integrating, training, and operating all services within its area of responsibility by bringing together municipal, governmental, military, and HMO systems under one operational structure (Laor et al. 2003). The uniqueness of the model stems from its ability to use its programs not only for disaster preparedness but also to resolve the sense of alienation that characterizes communities affected by privatization and urbanization. All this is accomplished while focusing specifically on the welfare of children. In the following discussion, we describe the model in action.

In an emergency, once rescue teams have completed their task, municipal immediate **intervention teams** carry out screening in the disaster vicinity and refer identified victims to Regional Trauma Centers. These multidisciplinary intervention teams provide immediate physical and mental health assistance at the disaster site, and/or at the evacuation centers.

Victims evacuated to hospitals are monitored by the Emergency Headquarters **Liaison Unit**, which, upon discharge, follows up with a home visit and refers victims to Regional Trauma Centers if needed. Information about casualties is transferred from the hospital and from the Victim Identification Facility to the **Family Notification Unit**. This unit is comprised of a member of the city council, a clergyman, a physician/paramedic, a social worker, and a police officer, whose job it is to notify the families of the deceased and assist in funeral arrangements.

At the **Victim Identification Facility**, the intervention teams work with families who are waiting for information, and special mental health teams work closely with the pathologist and the families in helping to identify the remains of their loved ones.

The **Regional Trauma Centers** integrate primary care, well-baby care, education, and welfare services. Each center is comprised of multidisciplinary professional units responsible for screening, treatment (individual, group, family and community), and fol-low-up of all victims in the community. The Regional Trauma Centers are also involved in community preparedness and resilience. In this, their goal is to design and develop programs for community preparedness, intervention, and rehabilitation, in particular through special programs geared towards infants, children and teens, the elderly, the disabled and sick, and special population groups such as new immigrants, foreigners, and minorities. These programs are run through community institutions, including schools, kindergartens, well-baby clinics, primary care clinics, mental health clinics, old-age homes, and community centers.

The community intervention team of the Trauma Center, in coordination with the Mental Health Headquarters and the primary care system, trains representatives from the fields of primary care, nursing care, education, and mental health in providing mental health services during emergencies and major disasters. This preparedness and resilience program supports the existing mental health system by means of planned and organized use of volunteers and activists, who work to enhance community resilience and restore community functioning.

The **Mental Health Headquarters** is responsible for pooling resources, integrating systems (beyond the local government level), and training and providing continuing education to professionals, paraprofessionals, and support teams. It is also responsible for conducting assessment and research programs, forecasting different scenarios and preparing accordingly, providing support and guidance to the teams and operating a hotline service. Furthermore, intervention protocols where military and civilian professionals work together in the community are applied to facilitate the smooth transition from traumatic military service into normal social routines.

The **Municipal Headquarters**, of which the Mental Health headquarters is a part, sets down strategic organizational and professional emergency principles by integrating representatives of organizations within the local government (e.g., welfare services, education, public health, tourism, security, and emergency services) as well as outside the local government (the Mental Health Command, HMOs, the army's Home Front Command and the Mental Health Department of the Medical Corps, the Ministries of Health, Education and Welfare, the National Insurance Institute and volunteer organizations).

This dynamic system, if properly created and securely established during routine times, can integrate institutions and professionals from diverse fields to create a comprehensive matrix within which a community can be adequately equipped to prepare for and handle the chaos, stress, and severe mental consequences of large-scale disaster. The model is child-oriented, integrating services from infancy (well-baby clinics) to young adulthood (army), and providing programs sensitive to the culture of this population group. Following is one example.

14.2.5 A Teacher-Mediated School-Based Intervention Program

Schools are the second most important natural environment for children. Thus, rehabilitating this environment, preferably based on the schools' own resources, ought to receive priority in any postdisaster relief program. For the program to be successful, mental health professionals specializing in schoolchildren need to provide teachers with clinical knowledge formulated as effective didactics for class activation (Wolmer et al. 2003) as well as with social theory that is practically formulated and converted to school activities to be applied to school revitalization (Laor and Wolmer 2002).

Postdisaster support at school is one of the significant predictors of posttraumatic stress disorder after disasters (Udwin et al. 2000), and school-based screening allows clinicians to identify and treat children exhibiting the most severe posttraumatic symptoms (Chemtob et al. 2002). School-based intervention models include single-session debriefings, small group programs for high-risk children or agitated children who need closer attention (Goenjian et al. 1997; Gillis 1993), and class activation programs with or without the presence of the teacher (Klingman 1993; Eth 1992; Pynoos and Nader 1988), intended to minimize stigma, teach normal reactions to stress, and reinforce the expectation that the children will soon resume their roles as students (Klingman 1993; Vernberg and Vogel 1993; Pfefferbaum 1997).

To implement teacher-mediated interventions where teachers become true partners, mental health consultants need to genuinely address three issues: **Why to intervene?**; **Why to intervene in the school?**; and **Why to intervene through the teacher?** Teacher-mediated intervention, which encompasses teacher relief, role enhancement, and empowerment, is comprised of three phases (Wolmer et al. 2003).

The first phase addresses the symptomatic responses of the teachers to the disaster. Most exposed teachers benefit from participating in interventions that allow them to process and restructure personal experiences as well as to clarify those of their students. In the **second phase**, teachers are empowered and instructed to assume their role as »educators« who prepare students for living in society under extreme circumstances they have never before encountered and for which they have not been didactically equipped. The **third phase** addresses teachers' needs to simultaneously manage the regular curriculum while implementing intervention programs for traumatized students. This effort requires continuous support and supervision from the staff, who provide a much needed holding environment by analyzing previous meetings, sharing experiences and doubts, and collaboratively preparing the contents of subsequent meetings.

A teacher-mediated intervention based on the model described above was implemented in a prefabricated village adjacent to Adapazari, Turkey following the 1999 earthquake (Wolmer 2001; Wolmer et al. 2003). First, a group intervention among teachers was implemented, with the objective of processing and restructuring their traumatic experiences, normalizing their responses, and enabling their trauma-related affects to be expressed and worked through. Although teachers reported an improvement in their feelings, they were still reluctant to take responsibility for the intervention. Thereafter, teachers were helped to redefine their role as »educators« and »leaders« vis-à-vis the students, in addition to focusing on the regular curricula. In their transformed role as educators, a team of local professionals taught teachers about children's responses to trauma and trained them in implementing the disaster-related school reactivation program. The local professionals were also responsible for ongoing weekly training, supervision, and support. In addition to the class work, the professional team consulted with the principal and facilitated revitalization in the school at large (e.g., parent involvement, celebrations, sport activities, memorials).

The teachers took charge of class activation, and all the children in the class participated. Parents were also engaged in the process, receiving information about the program and the children's expected reactions to the disaster. The program consisted of eight two-hour meetings, which combined psychoeducational modules, cognitive-behavioral techniques, play activities, and ongoing documentation in personal diaries, and covered various aspects of trauma and recovery.

Following the intervention, children reported a significant decrease in posttraumatic symptoms (50% reduction in severe symptoms) and dissociation, whereas grief symptoms increased for a few weeks, indicating that normal grieving had been set in motion once dissociative symptoms had been alleviated. For many of these children, this was the first opportunity they had to cope openly with their suffering, after having been granted legitimacy by caring adults ready to contain their emotions.

Our results, supported by feedback from both teachers and students, suggest that the program facilitated availability and containment of traumatic material, as well as initiation of adaptive grieving. The teachers, who were initially unwilling to take responsibility for implementing the program, reported significant accomplishments: an increased capacity among the students to concentrate in class and study the regular curriculum; a significant improvement in classroom climate; and increased motivation among teachers, who were able to control their teaching and feel closer to their students as well. Furthermore, a follow-up conducted 3 years later (Wolmer 2003) showed that compared to a control group matched for age and exposure, children who participated in the program were described by their teachers as functioning more adaptively in terms of academic performance, social behavior and general discipline.

14.2.6   Conclusion

Our global village enjoys rapid communication that brings the entire world community closer. As a consequence, however, we are also affected by remote disasters in real time. Our reactions may range from disconnection to caring to fear. Most countries tend to offer help to other nations affected by massive emergencies, but rarely do we invest in our own preparedness and resilience. Even though it is hard to envision massive damage and remain engaged in our daily routine, pretending a calamity will not happen does not eliminate it as a possibility. The responsible solution to this problem is to make preparedness and resilience part of our daily routine. It is not enough, however, to design a plan, not even if its implementation is supported by manuals. Building preparedness and resilience ought to penetrate all systems of community care and become integrated in their operation. For both professional

and systemic reasons, childcare offers an excellent heuristic for such a program.

Children may be vulnerable, but with proper support for their matrix, and sensitivity to their capacity to assume responsible roles even in times of disaster, they may serve as active reminders, recipients, and mediators of systemic integration. The model described here incorporates this perspective in order to fill the communal fissures created by disasters and to facilitate resilience and rehabilitation. We envisage the model as also applicable during ordinary times for coping with ongoing strains such as massive immigration, economic constraints, and the challenges of privatization, urban alienation, and violence, as well as today's constant threat of terrorism. Leaders who endorse the viewpoint at the foundation of this model may be better able to transmit hope to their communities, and, in particular, to the next generation.

14.3   A Mobile Mental Health Service for Children and Adolescents in Germany

Helmut Remschmidt

14.3.1   Historical Background

With regard to progress in child and adolescent mental health in Germany, five developments during the last 25 years have been decisive:
1. The Psychiatry Enquête of the Federal Government of Germany (Report 1975)
2. The Model Program »Psychiatry« of the Federal Government of Germany (1980–1985)
3. The Psychiatry Personnel Equipment Act (stepwise introduction between 1991 and 1995)
4. The inclusion of psychotherapy in the training curriculum and in the name of the specialty since 1992 »child and adolescent psychiatry and psychotherapy«
5. The law on psychological psychotherapists that allows psychologists to perform psychotherapeutic treatment with children and adolescents, but also with adults independently (1998).

These five developments have influenced current mental health services in a remarkable way.
1. The Psychiatry Enquête opened the possibility for a broad inquiry about the situation of psychiatry and child and adolescent psychiatry all

over what was then West Germany. After the report of the commission (1975), a Model Program »Psychiatry« was created which was carried out in 14 regions of the Federal Republic of Germany and which evaluated different types of services and created new ones. One region (Marburg) was devoted exclusively to the evaluation and establishment of child and adolescent mental health services. Many of these newly created services were continued.

2. The Psychiatry Personnel Equipment Act was responsible for more satisfactory staffing of psychiatric hospitals and services, which led to a remarkable improvement in everyday work.

3. The inclusion of psychotherapy in the curriculum for child and adolescent psychiatrists and the permission for psychologists to perform psychotherapy independently have also substantially contributed to the improvement of mental health services for children and adolescents.

14.3.2 General Guidelines for Child and Adolescent Mental Health Services

The Expert Commission for the Model Program »Psychiatry« of the Federal Government of Germany proposed guidelines for services based on the following general principles (Report of the Expert Commission, 1988, pp. 383–385):

1. Mental health services for children and adolescents should be equalized with services for children with other disorders or diseases.

2. This equality requires an integration of the relevant services into the field of medicine, though there is a broad overlap with other nonmedical services.

3. The services should be community-based, avoiding too long distances and too high thresholds for consultation. It was proposed to define a region of approximately 250,000 inhabitants for outpatient services and a region of between 500,000 and 750,000 inhabitants for inpatient and complementary services. It should be the aim of service planning to treat most of the children and adolescents within their home region.

4. The services should be qualified to value age and developmental stage, the individuality of each child and his or her family, and to consider risk factors and protective factors in the patient and his or her environment.

14.3.3 The Mobile Mental Health Service for Children and Adolescents as Part of a Comprehensive Service System

14.3.3.1 Conception of the Mobile Service

The Mobile Service was conceptualized in order to fill the gap between clinical outpatient, inpatient, and day treatment services delivered in institutional settings, in the community, and in the homes of the patients. The Mobile Service concentrated on three major aims:

1. Provide aftercare for former inpatients following discharge
   - This group of patients comprised those with severe psychiatric disorders such as psychotic states, obsessive-compulsive disorders, eating disorders, affective disorders, etc. The patients had been treated either as inpatients, outpatients, or day patients and were contacted by the Mobile Service at their homes and with the permission of their parents and also in the kindergarten, at school, or at work.

2. Provide consultations in the countryside
   - The members of the Mobile Service were located in Marburg. They had a vehicle at their disposal and held consultation hours in five communities within two rural counties in the Marburg region with a total population of 400,000 inhabitants.
   - As far as the activities of the Mobile Service were concerned, all kinds of assessment and treatment were possible, except by means of medical device. If these were required, the patients had to be referred to the outpatient, inpatient, or day patient unit of the university department for child and adolescent psychiatry of the Philipps University in Marburg.
   - The times for the consultation hours were published in the press or announced by broadcasting services..

3. Provide expert consultation in institutions
   - The third aim of the Mobile Service was to provide consulting services for institutions working with children, adolescents, and their parents that might not have suitable expertise. Included were community agencies such as the youth support system and the social support system as well as kinder-

garten, clinical institutions, and homes for children. These consulting services were offered upon request to all institutions working with children. The consulting service was strictly confined to the individual case and special case conferences were offered to the respective institution. In addition, patient-centered supervision was offered to the different institutions.

– Furthermore, when the Mobile Service was implemented, intensive public relations activities were conducted in the press in the Model Region. Press conferences were held to inform the population about the mode of operation of the Mobile Service. The local broadcasting services reported several times on the Mobile Service and announced the consultation hours. Different newspapers in the region published articles about the Mobile Service.

– The region that was served by this service comprised two rural counties (County I: Marburg-Biedenkopf and County II: Waldeck-Frankenberg) with a population of 400,000 inhabitants and a distance of 100 km from north to south and 55 km from east to west. The population as 1/14 of the total population of the federal state of Hesse. The region has a predominantly rural character with rather poor public transport facilities and an equally poor infrastructure. Whereas the city of Marburg as a university location is characterized by a very good inpatient and outpatient service structure, this is not at all true for the rural counties around Marburg. The Model Program covered three counties, but only two of them (Counties I and II) accepted the Mobile Service as a major part of the mental health services structure.

14.3.3.2 Utilization of the Mobile Service

◻ Table 14.3 gives an overview of the population of children and adolescents up to 17 years and the number of patients of that age group who attended all inpatient, outpatient, and day patient facilities during a one-year period.

◻ Table 14.4 gives data from a survey of all patients attending the different services (nine) which were subdivided into primary consultation services (PC) and secondary consultation services (SC). The inpatient services are not included in the table.

As ◻ Table 14.4 demonstrates, the Mobile Service served 11.4% of all outpatients and ranked 4th for all outpatient visits, while outpatient units in hospitals ranked 1, child guidance clinics ranked 2, and early intervention centers ranked 3. Thus, the Mobile Service was a remarkable contribution to overall service capacity.

The staff for the Mobile Service was subdivided into two teams, each of them serving one county. Every team included a child psychiatrist, a clinical psychologist, and a social worker. As already mentioned, the teams of the Mobile Service performed diagnostic and therapeutic services and were very important for fostering interdisciplinary cooperation in all mental health services in the region. The team members of the Mobile Service were all trained in the university department of child and adolescent psychiatry in Marburg and were supervised by experienced child psychiatrists and psychologists in this department.

One of the main aims of our evaluation study was to find out how the different services (not only the Mobile Service) were utilized by children and their families. We analyzed the proportion of patients from the respective three counties who utilized the in- and outpatient services within the whole Model Region. As ◻ Table 14.3 demonstrates, the proportion of the service users is very different in the three counties:

◻ **Table 14.3.** Utilization of mental health services by children and adolescents (0–17 years) in the three counties (Model Region) during the period of 1 year in percent of the total population of that age group

Counties	Population (0–17 years)	Number of patients (clients) utilizing inside and outside of model region	Percentage of the population of minors (0–17 yrs)
County I (Marburg-Biedenkopf)	50,393	1,859	3.7
County II (Waldeck-Frankenberg)	33,566	785	2.3
County III (Schwalm-Eder)	40,029	630	1.6
Total	123,988	3,274	2.6

▢ **Table 14.4.** Survey of all patients attending the following outpatient mental health services during the period of 1 year

Primary consultation services	Number of users	Percent of users
1. Early intervention centers	490	15.3
2. Child guidance clinics	634	19.8
3. Adolescent services and public health agencies	50	1.6
4. Psychological practices	115	3.6
5. Other psychological services	72	2.3
Primary consultation services	1,361	42.6
Secondary consultation services		
6. Public consultation centers	58	1.8
7. Outpatient units in hospitals	1,105	34.5
8. Child psychiatric private practices	307	9.6
9. Mobile Service	366	11.4
Secondary consultation services	1,836	57.4
Total	3,197	100.0

▢ **Table 14.5.** Mean value of consultation rates per patient and month in the Mobile Service in comparison with other primary and secondary consultation services

Primary consultation services	Mean relative consultation rate			N	No data available
	In the institution	Home visits	Total		
1. Early intervention centers	0.75	0.13	0.88	488	2
2. Child guidance clinics	1.54	0.02	1.56	629	5
3. Adolescent services and public health agencies	0.66	0.02	0.68	50	–
4. Psychological practices	2.96	0.07	3.03	111	4
5. Other psychological services	3.78	0.27	4.05	69	3
Secondary consultation services					
6. Public consultation centers	0.90	0.15	1.06	58	–
7. Outpatient units in hospitals	0.94	0.01	0.95	1,100	5
8. Child psychiatric private practices	2.37	0.00	2.37	57	–
9. Mobile Service	2.36	0.35	2.72	354	12

1. The most advanced county with the best equipped services (County I) shows the highest rate of service attenders (3.7%; $n = 1,859$) among children and adolescents below the age of 18. County III with the lowest density of services shows also the lowest attendance (1.6%; $n = 630$).
2. Nevertheless, in the relatively well-equipped County I (Marburg-Biedenkopf), the total rate of attenders does not reach the level of 5%, which is postulated as a minimal estimate of patients in need of treatment (Castell et al. 1980; Weyerer et al. 1988).

As far as inpatient treatment is concerned (which is not the focus of this chapter), three results seem to be interesting:

1. With increasing distance between the place of residence and the place of inpatient units, there was a decrease in the utilization rate of inpatient treatment.
2. Regions with a better array of outpatient services had a higher rate of referral for inpatient treatments, but a significantly shorter duration of inpatient treatment.
3. Patients from regions with fewer in- and outpatient facilities differed from those where more in- and outpatient facilities were available on three variables: On average, they were one year older (15.1 vs. 14.2 years), had a more severe psychiatric diagnosis, and their treatment duration was significantly longer (median: 65.0 vs. 32.0 days).

As far as social class is concerned, the Mobile Service reached – next to the outpatient units at hospitals – the highest rate of patients from the lower social classes (21.1% vs. 31.5%).

❏ Table 14.5 gives an overview of the intensity of treatment of the Mobile Service as compared to other primary and secondary consultation services.

The table shows the mean value of the consultation rates per patient and month, including home visits. As the table demonstrates, every patient gets 2.72 consultations with the Mobile Service, which is the third rank after the other psychological services and psychological practices. The consultation rates are similar to those of patients in child psychiatric private practices. With regard to home visits, the Mobile Service holds rank 1: home visits are carried out with every third patient.

With regard to the diagnoses of the patients that were served by the Mobile Service, there is no remarkable difference between this service and a child psychiatric private practice. The clientele is also similar to outpatient units at hospitals. Approximately one third of the patients suffer from emotional disorders, one quarter from special symptoms and syndromes (according to ICD-9), 17% from conduct disorders and ADHD, 3.4% from psychotic disorders, 9.1% from neurotic disorders, 4.7% from adjustment disorders, and less than 1% from brain damage. These are only the diagnoses on the 1st axis (psychiatric syndrome), according to the multiaxial classification system of psychiatric disorders in children and adolescents (Remschmidt and Schmidt 1986). Of course, there were many patients suffering from developmental disorders. The numbers are not described in this context.

Within the study described here, we did not investigate the efficacy of treatment; we could, however, demonstrate that, during an interval of 42 months, hospital admissions (in relation to the number of inhabitants) decreased in those counties where outpatient services for children and adolescents had been improved. The establishment of the Mobile Service contributed to this major improvement.

14.3.4   Conclusions

Within the Model Program »Psychiatry« of the Federal Government of Germany, we had the unique opportunity to study a complete child and adolescent psychiatric in- and outpatient user population in three German counties comprising a total of 574,000 inhabitants out of whom 123,988 were under 18 years of age. The total user rate for in- and outpatient services differed between the three counties and was for the outpatient service 3.7% for the most advanced county I (Marburg) and 1.6% for County III, which had the lowest density of all types of services. In all counties, the proportion of users was below the rate of 5% of the total population under 18 years, which was postulated as a realistic figure for psychiatrically disturbed children and adolescents in need of some kind of treatment. As the distance between the place of residence and the place of services played an important role in service utilization, the conclusion could be drawn that more community-based services were necessary. In response to this conclusion, we developed a Mobile Service for psychiatrically disturbed children and adolescents for two of the three counties of the Model Region. This Mobile Service existed for more than 10 years in County I (Marburg) and worked successfully (Remschmidt and Walter 1989; Remschmidt et al. 1986). In spite of this successful work and its acceptance by the population, the service had to be shut down for financial reasons.

References

Achenbach T (1978) The Child Behavior Profile: I. Boys aged 6–11. Journal of Consulting and Clinical Psychology 46: 478–488

Ainsworth MDS, Blehar MC, Waters E, Wall S (1978) Patterns of attachment: A psychological study of the Strange Situation. Hillsdale, NJ: Erlbaum.

Alperstein G, Raman S (2003) Promoting mental health and emotional well-being among children and youth: a role for community child health? Child: Care, Health and Development 29(4):269

Ammaniti M, Candelori C, Dazzi N, De Coro A, Muscetta S, Ortu F, Pola M, Speranza AM, Tambelli R, Zampino F (1990) I.A.L.: Intervista sull'attaccamento nella latenza (A.I.C.A., Attachment Interview for Childhood and Adolescence). Manoscritto non pubblicato, Università di Roma »La Sapienza«.

Austin LS, Godleski LS (1999) Therapeutic approaches for survivors of disaster. Psychiatric Clinics of North America 22:897–910

Belsky J (1984) The determinants of parenting: A process model. Child Development 55:83–96

Belsky J (1993) Etiology of child maltreatment: A developmental-ecological analysis. Psychological Bulletin, 114: 413–434

Bowlby J (1973) Attachment and loss: Vol. 2. Separation. New York, Basic Books

Bowlby J (1980) Attachment and loss: Vol. 3. Loss: Sadness and depression. New York, Basic Books.

Bretherton I, Ridgeway D, Cassidy J (1990) Assessing internal working models of the attachment relationship: an attachment story completion task for 3-year-olds. In MT Greenberg, D Cicchetti, EM Cummings (a cura di), Attachment in the preschool years: Theory, research, and intervention. Chicago: The University of Chicago Press.

Buie J (1989) Therapy by telephone does it help or hurt? APA Monitor 20:14–15

Bundesministerium für Jugend, Familie, Frauen und Gesundheit (ed) (1988) Empfehlungen der Expertenkommission der Bundesregierung zur Reform der Versorgung im psychiatrischen und psychotherapeutisch/psychosomatischen Bereich. Aktion Psychisch Kranke, Bonn

Burns JM, Patton GC (2000) Preventive intervention for youth suicide: a risk factor-based approach. Australian and New Zealand Journal of Psychiatry 34:388–407

Caffo E (2003a) Consulenza telefonica e relazione di aiuto. La qualità dell'ascolto e dell'intervento con i bambini e gli adolescenti. Milano: McGraw-Hill.

Caffo E (2003b) Emergenza nell'infanzia e nell'adolescenza. Interventi psicoterapeutici e di comunità. Milano: McGraw-Hill.

Caffo E, Belaise C (2003) Psychological aspects of traumatic injury in children and adolescents. Child Adolesc Psychiatric Clin N Am 12:493–535.

Caffo E, Forresi B, Lopez G, Nicolais G, Rossi M. (2003) Emergenza, rischio e trauma. Gestione dell'emergenza in Molise e confronto con altre realtà internazionali. In: Telefono Azzurro, Eurispes 2003, IV Rapporto Nazionale sulla Condizione dell'Infanzia e dell' Adolescenza.

Castell R, Biener A, Artner K (1980) Häufigkeit psychischer Störungen bei Kindern und Jugendlichen. Münchner Medizinische Wochenschrift 122: 591–592

Chemtob CM, Nakashima JP, Hamada RS (2002) Psychosocial intervention for postdisaster trauma symptoms in elementary school children. Archives of Pediatric and Adolescent Medicine 156:211–216

Cicchetti D (1984) The emergence of developmental psychopathology, Child Development 55:1–7

Cicchetti D (2002) The impact of social experience on neurobiological systems: illustration from a costructivist view of child maltreatment, Cognitive Development 17:1407–1428.

Cicchetti D, Cohen DJ (1995) Perspectives on developmental psychopathology. In: D Cicchetti, DJ Cohen (Eds) Developmental psychopathology (Vol. 1, Theory and Methods), Wiley, New York, pp 3–20

Cicchetti D, Toth S (1995), A developmental psychopathology perspective in child abuse and neglect. Journal of the American Academy of Child and Adoelscent Psychiatry 34:541–564

Cochrane A, Holland W (1969) Validation of screening procedures. British Medical Journal 27:3–8

Cohen DJ, Caffo E (1998) Developmental Psychopathology: a framework for planning child mental health, Epidemiologia e Psichiatria Sociale 7:156–160

Crowell JA, Feldman SS (1988) Mothers' internal models of relationships and children's behavioral and developmental status: A study of mother-child interaction. Child Development 59:1273–1285

Cummings EN, Davies PT, Campbell SB (2000) Developmental Psychopathology and family process. Theory, research and clinical implications. The Guilford Press, New York.

Derogatis LR (1983) SCL-90R Administration, Scoring and Procedure Manual. Towson, MD: Clinical Psychometric Research.

DeWolfe DJ Field Manual for mental Health and Human Service workers in major disasters. Center for Mental Health Services; Washington, DC. Available at: http://www.mentalhealth.org/publications/allpubs/ADM 90-537/Default.asp Accessed January 5, 2004

Eth S (1992) Clinical response to traumatized children. In: Austin LS (ed) Responding to disaster. A guide for mental health professionals. American Psychiatric Press, Washington, DC, pp 101–123

Forresi B (2003) Un nuovo approccio alla relazione di aiuto: la psicopatologia dello sviluppo. In: E Caffo (2003a). Consulenza telefonica e relazione di aiuto. La qualità dell'ascolto e dell'intervento con i bambini e gli adolescenti. Milano: McGraw-Hill.

Galante R, Foa D (1986) An epidemiological study of psychic trauma and treatment effectiveness after a natural disaster. Journal of the American Academy of Child and Adolescent Psychiatry 25:357–363

Gillis HM (1993) Individual and small group psychotherapy for children involved in trauma and disaster. In: Saylor CF (ed) Children and disasters. Plenum Press, New York, pp 165–186

Goenjian AK, Karayan I, Pynoos RS, Steinberg A, Najarian L, Asarnow J, et al (1997) Outcome of psychotherapy among early adolescents after trauma. American Journal of Psychiatry 154:536–542

Henggeler SW, Schoenwald SK, Rowland MD, Cunningham PB, (2002) Serious emotional disturbance in children and adolescents. Multisystemic Therapy. Guilford Press, London.

Kazdin AE, Kraemer HC, Kessler RC, Kupfer DJ, Offord DR, (1997) Contributions of risk factor research to developmental psychopathology. Clinical Psychological Review 17:375–406

Klingman A (1993) School-based interventions following a disaster. In: Saylor CF (ed) Children and Disaster. Plenum Press, New York, pp 187–210

Laor N (2001) The role of mental health professionals after mass disasters. Presented at the Promised Childhood Congress, Tel Aviv

Laor N (2002) The open and closed society from the perspective of disaster situations. The Centennial Popper's Conference, Vienna

Laor N, Wolmer L (2002) Children exposed to disaster: The role of the mental health professional In: Lewis M (ed) Textbook of Child and Adolescent Psychiatry, 3rd ed. Williams and Wilkins, Baltimore, pp 925–937

Laor N, Wolmer L, Spirman S, Wiener Z (2003) Facing war, terrorism, and disaster: Toward a child-oriented comprehensive emergency care system. Child and Adolescent Psychiatric Clinics of North America 12:343–361

Lindy JD, Grace MC, Green BL (1981) Survivors: Outreach to a reluctant population. American Journal of Orthopsychiatry 51:468–478

Lyons-Ruth K, Jacobvitz D (1999) Attachment disorganization: In Cassidy J, Shaver PhR, Handbook of attachment, The Guilford Press, New York

Main M., Goldwyn R. (1985–1994) Adult attachment scoring and classification systems, Unpublished manuscript, University of California at Berkeley

Marans S, in collaboration with Adnopoz J, Berkman M, Esserman D, MacDonald D, Nagler S, Randall R, Schaefer M, Wearing M, (1995) The Police-Mental Health Partnership. A Community-Based Response to Urban Violence. New Heaven, Yale University Press.

Nicolais G, Ricceri F, Pandolfo MC, Ferrero E (2002) Memoria, attaccamento e resilience nell'abuso all'infanzia: un percorso di integrazione. Infanzia e Adolescenza, 1:81–95.

Norwood AE, Ursano RJ, Fullerton CS (2000) Disaster psychiatry: Principles and practice. Psychiatry Quarterly 71:207–266

Ohan JL, Myers K, Collett BR (2002) Ten-year review of rating scales. IV: Scales assessing trauma and its effects. Journal of the American Academy of Child and Adolescent Psychiatry 41:1401–1422

Okun FB (2002) Effective Helping: interviewing and counseling techniques. Pacific Grove CA, USA, Brooks Cole

Pennebaker JW (1997) Opening up: The healing power of expressing emotions. New York: Guilford Press

Pfefferbaum B (1997) Posttraumatic stress disorder in children: A review of the past 10 years. Journal of the American Academy of Child and Adolescent Psychiatry 36:1503–1511

Pfefferbaum B, Nixon SJ, Tucker PM, Tivis RD, Moore VL, Gurwitch RH, et al (1999) Posttraumatic stress responses in bereaved children after the Oklahoma City bombing. Journal of the American Academy of Child and Adolescent Psychiatry 38:1372–1379

Pine DS, Cohen JA, (2002) Trauma in children and adolescents: risk and treatment of psychiatric sequelae. Biological Psychiatry 51:519–531

Pynoos RS, Nader K (1988) Psychological first aid and treatment approach to children exposed to community violence: Research implications. Journal of Traumatic Stress 1:445–473

Pynoos RS, Goenjian AK, Steinberg AM (1998) A public mental health approach to the postdisaster treatment of children and adolescents. Child and Adolescent Psychiatric Clinics of North America 7:195–210

Pynoos RS, Steinberg AM, Piacentini JC (1999) A Developmental psychopathology model of childhood traumatic stress and intersection with anxiety disorder. Society of Biological Psychiatry 46:1542–1554.

Ranan W, & Blodgett A (1983) Using telephone therapy for »unreachable« clients. Social Casework: The Journal of contemporary Social Work 64:39–44.

Rappaport J (1987) Terms of empowerment/exemplars of prevention. Toward a theory for community psychology. American Journal of Community Psychology 15:121–145

Reese RJ, Conoley CW, Brossart DF, (2002) Effectiveness of telephone counseling a field based investigation. Journal of Consulting Psychology 49:233–242

Remschmidt H (1998) Structure and organization of services for children and adolescents with psychiatric disorders in Germany. In: Young JG, Ferrari P (eds) Designing mental health services and systems for children and adolescents, A shrewd instrument. Brunner/Mazel, Philadelphia, pp 269–276

Remschmidt H, Schmidt MH (1986) Multiaxiales Klassifikationsschema für psychiatrische Erkrankungen im Kindes- und Jugendalter nach Rutter, Shaffer und Sturge, 2nd ed. Huber, Bern Stuttgart Toronto

Remschmidt H, Walter R (1980) Evaluation kinder- und jugendpsychiatrischer Versorgung. Analysen und Erhebungen in drei hessischen Landkreisen. Enke, Stuttgart

Remschmidt H, Walter R, Kampert K (1986) Der mobile kinder- und jugendpsychiatrische Dienst: Ein wirksames Versorgungsmodell für ländliche Regionen. Zeitschrift für Kinder- und Jugendpsychiatrie 14:63–80

Remschmidt H, Walter R, Kampert K, Hennighausen K (1990) Evaluation der Versorgung psychisch auffälliger und kranker Kinder und Jugendlicher in drei Landkreisen. Nervenarzt 61: 34–45

Remschmidt H, Schmidt MH, Walter R (1998) Survey of the utilization of psychiatric services for children and adolescents. In: Young JG, Ferrari P (eds) Designing mental health services and systems for children and adolescents, A shrewd instrument. Brunner/Mazel, Philadelphia, pp 83–94

Rosenfield M (1997) Counseling by Telephone, London, Sage.

Rutter M (2000) Psychosocial influences: critique, findings and research needs, Development and Psychopathology 12: 375–405

Saltzman WR, Layne CM, Steinberg AM, Arslanagic B, Pynoos RS (2003) Developing a culturally-ecologically sound intervention program for youth exposed to war and terrorism. Child and Adolescent Psychiatric Clinics of North America 12:319–342

Sameroff A (2000) Developmental system and psychopathology. Development and Psychopathology 12:297–312

Schwarz ED, Kowalski JM (1992) Malignant memories: Reluctance to utilize mental health services after a disaster. Journal of Nervous and Mental Disease 180:767–772

Speranza AM, Nicolais G (2002) Dissociazione e rappresentazione dell'attaccamento in genitori coinvolti in abuso e maltrattamento all'infanzia. Maltrattamento e Abuso all'Infanzia 4:61–84.

Speranza AM, Nicolais G, Ammaniti M (2002) Le rappresentazioni mentali dell'attaccamento nella trasmissione intergenerazionale dell'abuso. Maltrattamento e Abuso all'Infanzia 4:187–201

14

Sroufe LA, Rutter M (1984) The domain of developmental psychopathology. Child Development 55:17–29

U.S. Department of Health and Human Services (1999) Mental health: a report of the Surgeon General. Rockville MD: National Institute of Mental Health, National Institute of Health, US Department of Health and Human Services.

Udwin O, Boyle S, Yule W, Bolton D, O'Ryan D (2000) Risk factors for long-term psychological effects of a disaster experienced in adolescence: Predictors of posttraumatic stress disorder. Journal of Child Psychology and Psychiatry 41:969–979

Vernberg EM, Vogel JM (1993) Interventions with children after disasters. Journal of Clinical Child Psychology 22:485–498

Walter R, Kampert K, Remschmidt H (1988) Evaluation kinder- und jugendpsychiatrischer Versorgung in drei hessischen Landkreisen. Praxis der Kinderpsychologie und Kinderpsychiatrie 37:2–11

Weyerer S, Castell R, Biener A, Artner K, Dilling H (1988) Prevalence in treatment of psychiatric disorders in 3 to 14 year-old children: Results of a representative field study in the small town rural region of Traunstein, Upper Bavaria. Acta Psychiatrica Scandinavica 77:290–296

WHO (2002) The World Health Report. Reducing Risks, Promoting healthy Life. www.who.int

Williams S (2000) How is telehealth incorporated into psychology practice? APA Monitor 31:15

Wolmer L (2001) School reactivation after mass disaster: The case of the Israeli Village. Presented at the 48th Annual Meeting of the American Academy of Child and Adolescent Psychiatry, Honolulu, Hawaii

Wolmer L, Laor N, Yazgan Y (2003) Implementing relief programs in schools after disasters: The teacher as clinical resource. Child and Adolescent Psychiatric Clinics of North America 12:363–381

Young BH, Ford JD, Ruzek JI, Friedman MJ, Gusman FD (2003) Disaster Mental Health Services: A Guidebook for Clinicians and Administrators. Department of Veterans Affairs. The National Center for Post-Traumatic Stress Disorder, Vermont. Available at: http://www.ncptsd.org/publications/disaster/index.html. Accessed January 5, 2004

Zhu S, Stretch V, Balabanis M, Rosbrook B, Sadler G, Pierce JP (1996) Telephone counseling for smoking cessation: effects of single session and multiple-sessions interventions. Journal of Consulting and Clinical Psychology 64:202–211.

Medications

Stan Kutcher

15.1 Introduction – 208

15.2 General Considerations – 209
15.2.1 Baseline Medical and Psychiatric Assessment – 209
15.2.2 Concurrent Nonmedication Treatments – 210
15.2.3 Evaluation Points and Treatment Process – 211

15.3 Medication Approaches to Specific Disorders – 211
15.3.1 Early-Onset Depression – 211
15.3.1.1 Acute Treatment – 212
15.3.1.2 Continuation Treatment – 213
15.3.2 Bipolar Disorder – 213
15.3.2.1 Acute Treatment – 213
15.3.2.2 Continuation Treatment – 214
15.3.3 Schizophrenia – 214
15.3.3.1 Acute Treatment – 215
15.3.3.2 Continuation Treatment – 215
15.3.4 Anxiety Disorders – 216
15.3.4.1 Obsessive-Compulsive Disorder – 216
15.3.4.2 Panic Disorder – 216
15.3.4.3 Social Anxiety Disorder – 217
15.3.5 Attention Deficit Hyperactivity Disorder (Hyperkinetic Disorder) – 217
15.3.5.1 Acute Treatment – 217
15.3.5.2 Continuation Treatment – 217
15.3.6 Mental Retardation and Pervasive Developmental Disorders – 218

15.4 Integrating Psychopharmacology into Routine Care – 218

References – 219

15.1 Introduction

Psychotropics are a necessary, albeit not sufficient part of the therapeutic approach to child and adolescent psychiatric illnesses. Indeed, there are few, if any, psychiatric disorders that have their onset in this age group for which medications should not be considered – either as a primary treatment for the syndrome or as a treatment for specific symptoms associated with the syndrome. In other words, medication treatment may be directed towards ameliorating the disorder itself (as in the case of antidepressant treatment of major depressive disorder) or may be directed towards the improvement of specific symptoms known to be sensitive to medication effects, while not directly treating the psychiatric illness per se (for example, aggressive outbursts in autism).

Research in the domain of child and adolescent psychopharmacology has increased immensely over the last decade stimulated in part by a growing recognition that many child and adolescent psychiatric disorders may be amenable to psychotropic interventions and by a policy decision by the United States government which encouraged the pharmaceutical industry to invest in controlled clinical trials of medications in a variety of child and adolescent psychiatric disorders. Presently, there are significant and growing cadres of sophisticated clinical investigators studying the entire gamut of child and adolescent psychiatric disorders in terms of medication use and a number of journal/newsletter publications specific to this field are now available. In some cases, these researches have been directed primarily at the use of medications themselves, while in other cases, investigators are addressing the complexity of joint therapies (for example, antidepressants plus specific psychotherapies in the treatment of major depressive disorder). Spin off studies have included pharmacokinetic aspects of psychotropics in young people, developmental neurobiology, and developmental pharmacology. To date, the available randomized, placebo-controlled clinical trial evidence for the effectiveness of medication treatments in child and adolescent disorders, when taken as a whole, quite likely exceeds that available for any other single therapeutic intervention in this population.

Along with this new information has been the rapid rise in prescription of psychotropics to young people, in the absence of sufficient scientific information to guide optimal treatment. Thus, it is imperative that the practicing clinician be knowledgeable about the various medications used to treat psychiatric illnesses in this age group and also to be proficient in their clinical application. This chapter provides an overview of the clinical approach to pediatric pharmacotherapy and a brief synopsis of practical issues related to the pharmacotherapies of various psychiatric illnesses in this population. For detailed information about pharmacokinetics and pharmacodynamics the reader is encouraged to consult one of the excellent texts currently available (McClellan et al. 2003; Kutcher 1997, 1999, 2002; Osterheld 1998; Koplewicz and Green 1999; Safer 1997; Zito and Riddle 1995; Carrey 2001; March and Vitiello 2001; Carrey and Kutcher 1998).

15.2 General Considerations

Optimal psychopharmacologic intervention begins with careful evaluation of the psychiatric and medical status of the child or adolescent. Central to this is the conduct of a proper diagnostic interview which utilizes a phenomenologically based approach rather than a theory-driven model. As part of this process, some clinicians will utilize semistructured interviews such as the KIDDIE-SADS to invest in their diagnostic interviewing, but others will find this to be a cumbersome task, and outside specific academic centers or clinical research protocols the use of this tool is perhaps not necessary. However, a comprehensive approach to diagnostic interviewing is needed and the use of diagnostic checklists and careful attention to diagnostic criteria is found by most clinicians to be essential. In most cases, when dealing with young people diagnostic interviewing should include not only the identified patient, but information should be sought from other pertinent sources, in particular, family, other significant caretakers, and school teachers. Final diagnosis is based on a composite picture considering all sources of information. When informants provide contradicting information about a young person, it is the responsibility of the diagnosing clinician to ensure that the differences in information are resolved and that a single »best descriptor« is agreed upon (Carlson 2002; Greenhill et al. 2003; Kutcher 2000; Guerrero 2003).

15.2.1 Baseline Medical and Psychiatric Assessment

It is essential to identify the expected therapeutic outcomes prior to initiating pharmacological treatments. In particular, these outcomes must be directed towards anticipated improvement in either the syndrome or in specific symptoms within the syndrome. In some cases, a combination of both might be expected, particularly where medications may have a differential effect on some symptoms yet act to improve the syndrome concurrently.

Evaluation of syndromal improvement will be determined by defining at a particular point in the future whether the individual continues to meet diagnostic criteria for the syndrome in question. Thus, for example, if the treatment is of obsessive-compulsive disorder, then following the appropriate length of treatment with an SSRI medication, the patient will be reassessed for the presence or absence of obsessive-compulsive disorder using the same diagnostic criteria and checklists as at baseline. In some cases, remission of the syndrome will be identified while in other cases, although the syndrome may be significantly improved, it will not be fully remittent. Thus, in addition to syndromal evaluation in terms of outcome, it is necessary to also identify specific symptom outcomes as well.

As a general rule, the optimal manner in which to do so is to use validated and reliable rating scales to measure severity of syndromes or specific constellations of symptoms within a syndrome. It is important to note that these rating scales are not diagnostic instruments and cannot be used in place of an appropriate clinical diagnosis. They do, however, provide an excellent method of measurement of treatment outcome.

A variety of such scales are available and they generally fall into one of two categories, objective and subjective (clinician applied or self-report). While there are pros and cons to each type of rating scale, in general, the busy clinician should select a scale for each specific disorder which is both parsimonious in use and clinically meaningful. Thus, for example, in the treatment of major depressive disorder of an adolescent, the Hamilton Depression Rating Scale would not be a first choice given that it has not been specifically developed for adolescents, but a rating scale such as the Kutcher Adolescent Depression Rating Scale would be of value. The application of these scales at baseline provides the necessary initial evaluation by which to monitor therapeutic change over time.

Baseline medical assessment should address two areas: (1) the physical examination and systems review and (2) particular laboratory or other investigations as necessary. Prior to starting medications, the patient should be carefully questioned about any physical symptoms that he or she might have and an appropriate physical examination should be carried out. For example, if a medication may be suspected to induce tics or extrapyramidal effects, then a baseline neurological examination pertaining to those areas should be conducted and made part of the patient's record. In addition, a physical symptom checklist is recommended covering such common complaints as headaches, diarrhea, etc. This is necessary at baseline, for when somatic complaints arise during the course of medication treatment, without a baseline evaluation of such symptoms it is not possible to tell whether they are indeed medication induced.

Routine laboratory investigations should be limited to those which are known to be associated with psychotropic use. For example, lithium carbonate treatment should always be initiated only after appropriate renal and thyroid indices are evaluated, while it would be medically unnecessary to evaluate similar indices when initiating treatment with an SSRI. Of course, should the medical history and physical symptoms review identify possible somatic disease, then the appropriate diagnostic medical evaluations and laboratory assessments need to be carried out.

Specific attention should be paid to possible drug interactions and a full listing of medications used to treat ongoing medical or psychiatric disorders should be created. In addition, given the widespread use of herbal remedies, the clinician should specifically inquire as to whether any herbal remedies are being used to treat the condition and also notify the family that should they use such remedies that they do so only after consultation with the treating physician. The intent here is not to deny individuals or families the potential of using herbal treatments, but to ensure that potential drug interactions between prescription medication and herbal over-the-counter remedies can be avoided.

15.2.2   Concurrent Nonmedication Treatments

In cases which concurrent nonmedication treatments are to be utilized (such as family therapy) the relationship between these treatments and med-ication use should be explicitly identified. This is particularly important if another individual is conducting »psychological treatments« and the clinician is providing the »medical treatments«. Miscommunication between treatment providers can create major difficulties for the patient and the family and thus consultation and full discussion with any practitioner who is also involved in the child's care prior to the initiation of medication treatment is important. During this discussion, particular attention should be paid to attitudes and beliefs about the use of medications and beliefs about primacy of therapies. There should be a discussion of expected side effects and how they will be managed. In addition, a modus operandi between treatment providers should be determined with clear-cut guidelines of how issues pertaining to medication use will be discussed. It is not uncommon for families and patients to utilize medications as a »fighting point« about family issues and this needs to be understood by all individuals involved in the care of the patient and the family so as to avoid miscommunications.

Psychoeducation is an essential component of medication treatment. This education must be directed both towards the disorder or symptoms of interest and to the medications being used for treatment. In particular, the patient and family should have a good idea of the various alternative medications to be used in the treatment and should participate actively in the choice of a particular medication. As part of that choice process they should be provided with information pertaining to the various types of medicines and have a reasonable understanding of their potential effectiveness and adverse events. In cases in which adverse events may be significant or severe, it may be prudent to provide a written consent form so that patients and families can document their understanding of treatment to be provided. Additionally, patients and families should be instructed on how to deal with common side effects.

During this psychoeducation process, the clinician must actively address possible myths about the medication use ranging all the way from the medication being a »magic bullet« to the medication being harmful to growth and development or »addictive«. It is important that the clinician raise the issue of addiction, as many patients or families will automatically assume that any psychotropic or psychoactive medication is by definition addictive. In other cases, the meaning of medication use as a possible last alternative to other care will also need to be discussed. These issues need to be identified prior to the initiation of medication treatments and in a clinical setting will most likely require a therapeutic intervention that is focused on psychoeducation alone. The availability of written materials to assist the patients and their families in their research will greatly enhance this process and the physician should be encouraged to keep such information easily available. A number of professional organizations in North America and Europe have such information easily accessible, such as the American Academy of Child and Adolescent Psychiatry, and in those cases the patient and family may be referred to their websites.

15.2.3 Evaluation Points and Treatment Process

From the very onset, it is essential to determine a priori when treatment efficacy and side effects of medications will be measured. To a great degree, this is influenced by the characteristics of the patient, the disorder and the medication combined.

In disorders in which symptomatic improvement is expected to occur soon after the onset of pharmacological treatment (such as attention deficit hyperactivity disorder, anxiety disorders) treatment evaluation points (for both symptom and syndrome) should be scheduled within a few days of commencing the medication intervention. For a disorder in which the treatment outcome is expected to have a longer duration before therapeutic emergence, the time period should be more appropriately set (such as major depressive disorder) for a few weeks. For example, in an acute psychotic episode in which the individual is exceedingly aggressive and behaviorally disinhibited, treatment evaluation (of antipsychotic medications or benzodiazepines) should occur within hours of initiation of the initial intervention. In disorders such as attention deficit disorder or anxiety, the treatment evaluation should occur within 3–5 days of initial intervention. In disorders such as major depressive disorder or obsessive-compulsive disorder treatment evaluation is unlikely to be of any value prior to at least 4 weeks of treatment. Thus, treatment evaluation will range from hours to weeks. It is essential that both the patient and the family understand what will be the expected time course for treatment and not to expect therapeutic outcome to occur prior to the first evaluation point and even more likely, not until a specified point thereafter. Thus, not only should measurement be tailored to the disorder, but patient expectation as to time of improvement must be identified relevant to the disorder as well.

Many medications are apt to create side effects, most often soon after they are administered. Side affects such as nausea, vomiting, diarrhea, etc. can be expected to occur within the first 2–3 days of initiating treatment. The patient should be notified a priori about this possibility and the first evaluation of side effects should take place within 2–3 days after beginning medication treatment. Side effects which are expected to occur later (such as tardive dyskinesia) will not need to be assessed soon after treatment but will need to be reviewed at an appropriate time thereafter. Some laboratory parameters which may be changed after treatment will also need to be evaluated at the appropriate time. For example, thyroid status should be evaluated 2–3 months after initiating lithium therapy and prolactin levels within 1–2 months after initiating therapy with an antipsychotic medication known to elevate prolactin.

Patient characteristics may also influence the point of assessment, particularly of side effects. In exceedingly anxious patients or anxious families it is prudent to evaluate side effects sooner than 2–3 days from the onset of treatment and often a telephone conversation regarding how the patient is tolerating the medication will provide both a good window on the tolerability of the treatment and also serve an anxiolytic function in itself.

Behavioral and cognitive side effects may be found with psychotropic medications. These may include irritability, suicidal ideation, and even frank disinhibition. These should also be evaluated as part of the ongoing evaluation of treatment emergent effects from the medications and the patient and family need to be notified about them. These behavioral or cognitive side effects secondary to medication treatment must be managed much in the same way that physical side effects are managed and they need to be carefully assessed over time.

15.3 Medication Approaches to Specific Disorders

15.3.1 Early-Onset Depression

The prevalence of depression is thought to range from less than 1% in preadolescents to up to 5–8% in late adolescence. This disorder onset in youth is predictive of higher rates of mortality often due to suicide, significant morbidity, and a chronic remitting, relapsing illness with significant functional and vocational impairments. Comorbidity is common, particularly with anxiety disorders, and a careful psychiatric history focusing on potential manic or hypomanic symptoms should constitute part of the diagnostic assessment. A family history of affective disorder creates a greater weighting to the diagnosis.

A variety of psychological therapies have shown putative efficacy in depression in young people, albeit mostly in the adolescent group. These are cognitive behavior therapy and (much less so in terms of clinical trial evidence) interpersonal therapy. Tricyclic antidepressants have not shown greater efficacy than placebo and their use is associated with significant and potentially toxic adverse events and so their utilization in this population is not recommended. Data pertaining to the serotonin-specific reuptake inhibitors shows some positive efficacy, but less so than in adult studies. High placebo response rates make effectiveness analysis problematic in some studies. There may be an age gradient effect, with older youth showing a slightly better response than younger youth, but the data at this point is not clear. The best available efficacy available data are for the SSRI fluoxetine.

If SSRIs are to be used, baseline medical evaluation should include an appropriate medical history and a pregnancy test in sexually active females. Further screening investigation such as laboratory tests are not necessary and should not be performed unless clinically indicated. A number of rating scales can be used to provide a measure of symptom severity such as the Beck Depression Inventory, the Child Depression Inventory or the Kutcher Adolescent Depression Scale. These are all scales with reasonably good psychometric properties and can be used not only at baseline, but at appropriate evaluation points during treatment to determine efficacy of care.

Recently, regulatory authorities in the United Kingdom have advised against the use of some SSRIs in the treatment of depressed children and adolescents due to concerns about efficacy and potential suicidal ideation. Such concerns have not in the main been shared by clinical investigators. The FDA is currently reviewing the data on this issue (Schulz et al. 2001; Kastelic et al. 2000; Martin et al. 2000; Brooks et al. 2003; Nobile et al. 2003; Varley 2003).

15.3.1.1 Acute Treatment

Hospitalization can be considered for the youngster who presents with significant suicidal ideation as well as depression. As noted above, in terms of pharmacological treatments, SSRIs are considered to be first-line choices, but care must be taken to discuss with the family the risks and benefits of this intervention. In particular, recent concerns about possible induction of suicidal ideation or suicidal-type behaviors with the use of SSRIs must be discussed and the results of the decision documented in the patient chart. In all cases, national regulatory body directives must be followed by clinicians when prescribing medications. Insufficient data exists to recommend for the use of other antidepressants such as venlafaxine, nefazodone, or bupropion and due to the risk of hypertensive episodes, significant dietary restrictions, and the lack of demonstrated effectiveness with monoamine oxidase inhibitors, their use is not recommended.

If the depression is accompanied with significant psychotic symptoms, the use of an antipsychotic medication combination with SSRIs should be considered, although there is a dearth of research in this domain. Electroconvulsive therapy has been reported in the literature to be effective in cases of psychotic depression in adolescents which have proven to be refractory to antidepressant and antipsychotic combination therapy.

Significant clinical improvement is unlikely to occur prior to 4 weeks of continuous therapy at an appropriate therapeutic dose. It is recommended, however, that a target date of 8–10 weeks be identified at the beginning of treatment as the point at which decisions about further treatment or treatment changes will be entertained if lack of efficacy or partial efficacy has been demonstrated. Intolerable side effects occurring prior to that time will most likely require a change in antidepressant regime and side effects should be measured on a weekly basis. Should a positive treatment response occur, that same medication continued at the dose which led to remission should be continued for about a period of 1 year and if a discontinuation is determined subsequent to that, it is imperative that the medicine be discontinued gradually, perhaps over a period of 23 months.

In the case of partial or nonresponse, it is necessary to re-evaluate the diagnosis, review compliance, and address the possibility of comorbidities, in particular substance abuse. Reasonable treatment strategies consist of the following:

1. Gradual increase of medication to an optimal dose (titrating against adverse effects)
2. Augmenting the initial medication with either lithium or tri-iodothyronine
3. Substituting another antidepressant medication for the initial compound.

Unfortunately, there is very little data available to guide clinicians in any of these alternative strategy choices. Care must be taken if lithium augmentation is implemented, as the lithium is lethal in overdose, its use is associated with significant side effects including neurological, dermatological and metabolic, and it requires blood monitoring, which may not be easily accepted by youngsters. Combination therapies (the combining of two antidepressants), while popular in treatment refractory adult depression, has not been appropriately evaluated in adolescents and should only be considered and implemented in academic settings in which practitioners have extensive use with these compounds. In addition to the difficulties noted above, serotonin syndrome may be more problematic in young people than in adults. If electroconvulsive therapy (ECT) is considered appropriate, safeguards for the patient must be implemented, including independent second opinion and informed consent signed by the patient and parents or legal guardian. Local jurisdictions may have legal qualifications regarding the use of ECT in young people and physicians need to be aware of those. A practice parameter for the use of extra electroconvulsive therapy with adolescents is available from the American Academy of Child and Adolescent Psychiatry. There is insufficient data to support the use of ECT in children.

15.3.1.2   Continuation Treatment

Continuation treatment will be necessary (as mentioned above) in preventing relapse. In cases where psychotherapy has not been initiated during the acute treatment phase, the continuation phase may provide a good opportunity to introduce cognitive behavior or interpersonal therapy so that when medications are withdrawn, the patient can continue on a psychotherapeutic regime. Those patients who have exhibited two or more depressive episodes or who have had serious suicide attempts during a depressive episode may be considered for longer continuation therapy than 1 year's time if they have demonstrated a good response to antidepressant treatment. In every case, duration of treatment

and decisions pertaining to treatment discontinuation must be made in concert with the patient and the patient's family and whenever possible, periods of high stress (such as school exams) should be avoided when medications are being discontinued.

Dysthymic disorder at this time is considered to be treated pharmacologically much the same as major depressive disorder, although sufficient clinical research data to guide its treatment in both pharmacological or psychotherapeutic modalities is not currently available.

15.3.2   Bipolar Disorder

Currently, there is active academic debate about the presentation, prevalence, and clinical components of pediatric bipolar disorder. In adolescence, clear type I bipolar disorder can be diagnosed and small sample studies have suggested a variety of potentially effective treatments, including lithium carbonate, valproate, and some antipsychotics. In prepubertal children, the diagnostic issues are much more confusing and great care must be taken to ensure that the patient does indeed have a bipolar disorder prior to initiating treatment. A family history of bipolarity may be of assistance in this assessment. From a comorbidity standpoint, it is essential to evaluate the potential effects of a substance abuse problem on symptom presentation and in prepubertal cases, the possible diagnosis of attention deficit disorder will need to be addressed. However, the exceedingly high rates of ADHD reported in some studies may be, in the opinion of this author, an artifact of the evaluation process, as many carefully constructed studies addressing this issue are not able to find evidence of attentional problems amongst adolescent-onset bipolars. Prepubertal-onset bipolars (should the diagnosis prove to be a robust one) may have further attentional problems which may not be classic ADHD but part of cognitive disruption that occurs with a bipolar disorder (Kusumakar et al. 2002; Kutcher 2000; Biederman et al. 2000; Ryan et al. 1999; Licht et al. 2003; Kowatch et al. 2003).

15.3.2.1   Acute Treatment

Amongst the thymoleptics, lithium and valproate may be considered first line pharmacological treatments for bipolar disorder in young people. Clinical experience and some preliminary research evidence suggests that antipsychotic medications such as the new atypicals may be useful by themselves or in combination with thymoleptics. Aggressive or disinhibitive behaviors may be addressed by using low potency, highly sedating antipsychotics such as chlorpromazine or low doses of moderate duration benzodiazepines such as clonazepam. In cases where a response to medication treatment is inadequate, electroconvulsive therapy could be considered. In these cases, ECT should be confined to the adolescent population, should be bilateral in its application, and should occur only following informed consent, independent psychiatric consultation and must conform to local therapeutic and regulatory requirements.

The depressive episodes of the bipolar disorder can be treated with antidepressant medications but caution must be taken to prevent cycling. It is essential that compliance to thymoleptic medication be immediately reviewed if depressive symptoms occur, and should serum levels be less than expected, the thymoleptic adherence will need to be addressed. Some evidence suggests that light therapy at 10,000 lux given twice daily may be beneficial when depressive symptoms occur if it added to ongoing thymoleptic treatment. A small case series of lamotrigine added to thymoleptics provided suggestive evidence that it may be of benefit in the depressed phases of a bipolar disorder in teenagers.

15.3.2.2 Continuation Treatment

Continuation therapy is necessary for adolescents with bipolar illness. In every case of bipolar disorder, psychoeducation about the illness and the medicine is necessary. Family interventions may be directed towards instrumental aspects of functioning, and school interventions will be necessary as well. Some evidence suggests that bipolar patients may have specific mathematics deficits which will require careful education academic planning evaluation and vocational counseling.

The treatment goals of the continuation phase are to prevent reoccurrences and to optimize functioning. If the disorder recurs, early intervention with appropriate pharmacological compounds will often abort the episode or decrease its amplitude or duration. At this point in time, there is disagreement amongst authorities about the optimal duration of continuation therapy following the first manic episode. It is my opinion that if a clear bipolar disorder exists, treatment should be continued for a minimum of 2 years of euthymia prior to any dis-

cussions pertaining to discontinuation of medication treatment. If treatment discontinuation is considered, a very gradual tapering of thymolytic medications is indicated, as rapid tapering may be associated with an increased suicidality or enhanced risk of relapse. The bipolar patient taking no medications should be followed as closely as the one who is taking medications in order that should symptoms arise, treatment can be immediately re-established. Such monitoring does not necessarily need to be through the psychiatrist's office, but can be done collaboratively with a well-informed general practitioner or public health nurse.

15.3.3   Schizophrenia

The prevalence of schizophrenia prepubertally is very low, but the incidence increases over the adolescent and into the young adult years, reaching adult levels by about age 25. Antipsychotic medications are a necessary but not sufficient component of the treatment of the schizophrenic youngster and early identification and appropriate intervention has been shown to improve clinical outcomes. While a number of comorbidities may exist concurrent with schizophrenia, perhaps the most common is substance abuse, which needs to be carefully evaluated, particularly in the adolescent patient. This includes alcohol, tobacco, and »soft« drugs as well as »hard« drugs.

Baseline evaluation of the youngster suffering from schizophrenia begins with a thorough diagnostic evaluation. At times, the diagnosis may not be completely clear, for example, a schizophreniform disorder may be a presenting picture or a bipolar disorder may be considered. In such cases, the diagnosis must be made in a tentative manner and treatment should be initiated based on the most reasonable therapeutic consideration. A comprehensive, multimodal intervention program should be available from the beginning of treatment and often short-term hospitalization may be necessary not only to treat an acute psychotic episode but also to ensure that the appropriate community treatment supports are put into place. These should usually include family or group therapy and vocational or academic interventions, as well as antipsychotic medications and case management, where appropriate.

Baseline symptom assessment should be conducted prior to the initiation of antipsychotic treatments. Ideally, this could include either the Brief Psychiatric Rating Scale or the Positive and Negative

Syndrome Scale. A neurological examination focusing on the motor system and documenting presence or absence of any extrapyramidal or dyskinetic movements should be undertaken, and the use of an instrument such as the Extrapyramidal Rating Scale and the Abnormal Involuntary Movement Scale prior to initiating treatment is highly recommended. Medical investigations may include a variety of neuroimaging studies, but these are unlikely to be of diagnostic benefit and, in my opinion, further neurological or laboratory testing should arise from clinical presentation and not be used as a routine screening approach (Findling et al. 2003; Remschmidt et al. 2000; Gillberg 2000; Bryden et al. 2001).

15.3.3.1 Acute Treatment

An acute psychotic episode is usually treated in a general hospital setting both to provide safety for the patient and to commence medication therapy. During the hospitalization, a psychoeducation program pertaining to schizophrenia and the medications used to treat the disorder should be an essential component of the therapeutic intervention. At this time, planning for a comprehensive multimodal outpatient treatment program should be undertaken, and a variety of academic and vocational assessments should be performed as well.

To date there is insufficient evidence to suggest which antipsychotic medication would be most appropriate for treating children and adolescents with schizophrenia or similar psychoses. The »typical« antipsychotics have been successfully used in the past, but the high potency »typical« medications such as haloperidol have the propensity to increase extrapyramidal symptoms and their use is associated with higher rates of dystonias. The low potency »typical« antipsychotics such as chlorpromazine and thioridazine have the disadvantage of sedation. Flupenthixol, which is available in many countries in both oral and intramuscular form, is a reasonable choice of a »traditional« antipsychotic.

The new atypical antipsychotics are currently under investigation and may be more suitable for young patients due to their relative lack of extrapyramidal side effects. However, some of these have their own difficulties, including olanzapine, which is associated with significant weight gain, and risperidone, which may increase prolactin levels. These compounds may also provide advantages over »typicals« in treating negative symptoms; however, this information is not available on the basis of solid research evidence in young people. Clozapine, the first of the atypical agents, has shown good antipsychotic effect in open label studies, but given its potential for inducing agranulocytosis and the complexities of its monitoring, should at this point be reserved for treatment-resistant cases.

For psychotic youth presenting in an acute agitated state, low potency »typical« medications can be given intramuscularly if necessary. Alternatively, sedating, low potency »typical« antipsychotics such as chlorpromazine may be given in a liquid form. Some clinicians prefer to add low doses of rapid acting benzodiazepines such as lorazepam to atypical antipsychotics in the acute phase, using the benzodiazepine to control agitated behavior. Resolution of acute symptomatology follows a pattern in which sleep and vegetative functioning seem to be restored first, followed by improved socialization and then more gradual resolution of the thought disorder. The anticipated initial time line is 4–6 weeks on appropriate amounts of antipsychotic treatment and evidence available clinically to date and from the few studies reported suggest that low doses of atypical antipsychotic medications such as 3 mg of risperidone daily or its equivalent might be a reasonable initial therapeutic dosing target for young people with schizophrenia.

15.3.3.2 Continuation Treatment

Following the resolution of the acute psychotic episode, it is recommended that the same medication be continued at the same dose for a minimum of 12 months. However, the completion of 12 months is not a signal to discontinue treatment, but rather it is an opportunity to evaluate the most appropriate dose for the patient and review the diagnosis. The main goals of treatment are to prevent relapse and optimize functioning, and these require not only antipsychotic medications but a variety of psychosocial interventions as well. Outpatient treatment must include both components.

A portion of patients can be expected to demonstrate a relatively poor response to antipsychotic medication and clinically it is essential to determine whether or not a less-than-optimal response is due to true treatment resistance or is associated with a lack of adherence to treatment. It is exceedingly common, particularly in the adolescent age group, for patients with schizophrenia to forego taking their medications and to seek other forms of chemical intervention, particularly street drugs. Thus, prior to a clinician concluding that the patient is relatively resistant to antipsychotic treatment, a thorough assessment of treatment adherence and potential substance abuse must be conducted. Following that, optimization strategies such as dose increase to tolerability may be considered, as might switching to another antipsychotic medication. Should the individual not show substantive clinical response to a trial of two different antipsychotics, clozapine could be considered.

15.3.4   Anxiety Disorders

Anxiety disorders are arguably the most common psychiatric disturbance in children and adolescents. They have different age points of onset for different disorders. Obsessive-compulsive disorder onsets in latency-aged children and again with a larger incidence peak in early adolescence. Panic disorder tends to come on more strongly in the late adolescent years, although separation anxiety disorder with »panic-like« episodes may occur in younger children and may foreshadow panic disorder. Social anxiety disorder tends to come on in later childhood and early adolescence, but it may be proceeded by generalized anxiety and excessive behavioral inhibition.

In anxiety disorders, as in mild to moderate depressions, psychotherapeutic intervention may be considered prior to pharmacological interventions. For example, cognitive behavior therapy has been demonstrated to be effective in youth with obsessive-compulsive disorder and may be of help in panic disorder and social anxiety disorder as well. If medications are considered in these disturbances, they should be initiated as part of a comprehensive treatment plan which may entail a variety of individual psychotherapies or group interventions. Short-term, focused family treatments may be of help, particularly in dealing with practical issues pertaining to the management of obsessive-compulsive disorder. In all cases, psychoeducation about the illness and the medications should be provided (Varley et al. 2003; Walkup et al. 2002; Findling 2002; Labellarte et al. 1999).

15.3.4.1   Obsessive-Compulsive Disorder

Baseline assessment of obsessive-compulsive disorder should include a comprehensive symptom review and a checklist such as the Yale-Brown Obsessive-Compulsive Scale or the Children's Yale-Brown Obsessive-Compulsive Scale. Medications with strong serotonin inhibition properties are the treatment of choice for obsessive-compulsive disorder. Fluvoxamine, fluoxetine, clomipramine, citalopram, and sertraline may be all effective in this condition. Initiation of treatment should be done at low doses, with gradual increments designed to reach the putative therapeutic dose occurring over 1–2 weeks. A minimum of 10–12 weeks at this initial therapeutic dose is necessary to fully determine effectiveness of treatment. Ideally, medication treatment should be paired with cognitive behavior therapy, if it is locally available.

The assessment of treatment efficacy at 12 weeks is recommended and alterations in medication use or cognitive therapy administration can be made at that time. Partial responders may require higher doses of selective serotonin reuptake inhibitors or may benefit from a switch to a different SSRI. To this point in time, there is insufficient evidence of the efficacy of augmentation therapies in this age group to make data-based recommendations for that use.

15.3.4.2   Panic Disorder

Panic disorder has been shown to be responsive to both SSRIs and medium duration benzodiazepines such as clonazepam. The relative merits of each of those medications should be discussed with the family, and family and patient preference should guide treatment selection. If there are concerns about substance abuse or addiction, including a family history of alcoholism, benzodiazepines may not be the medications of choice. However, they can be often used judiciously in small amounts for short periods of time and can possibly enhance adherence to cognitive behavior therapy or enhance the initial response to SSRI treatment. Baseline assessment should include a panic attacks diary and evaluation of anticipatory anxiety and phobic avoidance, perhaps using a 10 cm visual analogue scale. Behavior therapy may be indicated if severe avoidance has created an agoraphobic type situation. Continuation treatment of 9–12 months following the last panic episode should be clinically considered and upon a decision to terminate medication treatment, a very gradual tapering of medication with ongoing monitoring for the presence of symptom breakthrough is suggested.

15.3.4.3   Social Anxiety Disorder

Social Anxiety Disorder may be responsive to SSRI medications, and currently available data suggests that young people as well as adults tend to show a good response to this intervention. A recommended assessment tool is the Kutcher Social Anxiety Disorders Scale, which provides a comprehensive assessment of both symptoms and disability. Beta blockers may be of value in specific social anxiety such as difficulties in public speaking, but are not recommended for use with generalized socialized anxiety disorder. Optimal duration of initial treatment is unclear, but as many individuals who have social anxiety disorder show a waxing and waning of their anxiety symptoms over time it may be reasonable to reassess treatment at 6-month intervals. Clinically, behavior therapy should be provided to assist in the resolution of most feared social situations and counseling about alcohol abuse risk should be provided.

15.3.5   Attention Deficit Hyperactivity Disorder (Hyperkinetic Disorder)

AHDH is the most prevalent of prepubertal psychiatric disorders and affects both males and females, with a total population prevalence of about 3–5%. The clinical treatment of ADHD is well established, and primary to successful treatment is the use of a psychostimulant medication. Some individuals may additionally benefit from focused behavior therapy, classroom modifications, or parent training interventions. However, the available data does not support full scale individual psychotherapy interventions as the primary approach in this disorder.

The treatment of the child with ADHD should involve not only the child and family, but also the school, as interventions need to be demonstrated to be successful in the classroom as well as in the home. Current clinical thought suggests that treatment be continuous and cover the entire day and not be directed only at school functioning. Long-term treatment for ADHD may be expected to decrease the incidence of future substance abuse and severity of conduct disorder. Comorbidities include learning disabilities, tic disorders, conduct disorder, and oppositional defiant disorder. Some of these comorbidities may require alternative treatment strategies, but in every case an initial trial of medications

directed towards ameliorating ADHD symptoms should be attempted (Greenhill et al. 2002; Pliszka 2001; Kutcher et al. 2004; Markowicz et al. 2003).

15.3.5.1   Acute Treatment

First line medication treatments for ADHD are the psychostimulants, including methylphenidate, dextra-amphetamine, and adderall. A variety of long-acting stimulant preparations are also now available on the market and should an individual patient show a relatively robust treatment response to a short acting psychostimulant, then consideration should be given to continuing treatment with a long-acting stimulant for ease of delivery and enhanced adherence to treatment.

At baseline, a thorough medical evaluation including height and weight should be conducted and appropriate symptom rating scales such as the Connors or SNAP should be used to monitor treatment response over time.

The introduction of atomoxetine into the market place may provide an alternative to psychostimulant treatments as a first-line treatment for ADHD. Tricyclic antidepressants have been utilized in the past, but are not recommended due to their side effects and potential cardiotoxicity. Pemoline, a medication also used in the past, is not recommended due to the possibility of fatal liver failure. Other medications which have some effect in ADHD include clonidine and bupropion. Bupropion may be considered when depression is comorbid with ADHD. The evidence for the efficacy of clonidine is, in my opinion, relatively limited and the difficulties associated with its use clinically preclude widespread adoption of this intervention. Recently, risperidone has been shown to improve a variety of symptoms, particularly in youngsters with comorbid conduct symptoms and ADHD.

15.3.5.2   Continuation Treatment

Long-term medication treatment of ADHD is recommended; however, the data available for continued efficacy for long-term interventions is limited. This in part is due to the fact that appropriately designed long term studies are few and many of them are characterized by an inability to maintain subjects on continuous psychostimulant treatment. Dose response should be evaluated, at least on a yearly basis, as should growth parameters height and weight. Clinically, a number of individuals with mild ADHD may successfully transition from medications into self-developed coping strategies during the adolescent years. Other individuals may require medication treatment for ADHD into adulthood.

Tics may occur concurrently with ADHD or may be found independent of ADHD. When tics occur with ADHD, current clinical approaches suggest utilizing psychostimulants and monitoring the situation with the tics. Should they worsen on psychostimulants a small amount of antipsychotic medication such as risperidone may be indicated. If Tourette syndrome is present without ADHD, treatment with antipsychotic medications at low dose should be considered. Clonidine has been utilized in individuals with ADHD and concomitant Tourette's; however, the efficacy of this compound in ADHD is to my mind underwhelming and the available evidence for its use in this comorbid presentation does not support its use as a first-line intervention.

15.3.6   Mental Retardation and Pervasive Developmental Disorders

There is no pharmacological treatment for mental retardation or pervasive developmental disorders. In these cases, pharmacotherapy is directed towards specific symptoms which are known to be or thought to be amenable to medication intervention. Care must be used prescribing medications to these youngsters, as behavioral and physical side effects of medications may be more profound in this group – in particular – disinhibition with the use of benzodiazepines and extrapyramidal side effects and tardive dyskinesia with antipsychotics. Medications in these groups should be used with caution and »start low and go slow« is an important adage to follow. Careful documenting of symptoms targeted for pharmacotherapeutic intervention should be conducted prior to treatment and then at appropriate points throughout. As treatment is likely to be long term, structured, comprehensive semiannual reassessment is suggested. As consent cannot be given to treatment from the individual, it must be obtained from the parent, or legal guardian (Pliszka et al. 2003; Spencer et al. 2002; Steiner et al. 2003; Tourbiu 2003; Santosh et al. 1999; McCracken et al. 2002).

15.4   Integrating Psychopharmacology into Routine Care

With the rapid rise in the use of psychotropic agents in psychiatric disorders of children and adolescents, there have been many concerns raised about the appropriateness of this use. Undoubtedly, there are cases in which medications are used inappropriately and undoubtedly there are cases in which medications have not been used at all, though they would be highly recommended and highly valuable. At this point in time it is not beneficial and indeed is unhelpful to engage in discussions about whether or not too many medicines are being used in children and adolescents or whether or not as a general theme children and adolescents are being »drugged« instead of »therapized«. Such discussions do little to advance understanding of the complexities of therapeutic intervention for child and adolescent psychiatric disorders and reflect philosophically based and often prejudicial paradigms pertaining to treatment which do more to describe the holder of the constructs than to elucidate helpful interventions for populations to which treatment is directed.

A number of factors impact on the psychopharmacologic treatment of child and adolescent psychiatric disorders. There still exists a social reluctance to diagnosis psychiatric disturbance in childhood, as if brain illnesses were somehow less deserving of medical attention than other disorders. A great deal of stigma, which in adults is expressed as discrimination against the mentally ill, is more subtly presented in the social reluctance to countenance the severity of mental disorders in children and to deny mentally ill young people medicines of proven benefit. The metaphor of the »tabula rasa« of childhood still resonates within the area of mental health, although it has long been superceded in other chronic conditions of childhood such as cancer and cystic fibrosis. In addition, outdated and unvalidated models of intervention arising from analytically driven psychotherapies and child guidance still create predominant influences in the publics' mind as to how mental disturbances should be primarily addressed in children.

In addition, significant concerns about the effect of psychopharmacologic agents on the developing brain and the expression of behavioral side effects from psychotropics have raised popular concern about the use of medicines in children. Recent discussions about the potential suicidal-inducing effects of SSRIs has been an example in point. In the absence of sufficient scientific data on this topic, regulatory bodies in the United Kingdom have come out with strong prohibitory stances about the use of SSRIs in children and adolescents. Such pronouncements may be driven as much by social ideology as by scientific approaches and illustrate the complexities of psychopharmacologic intervention in children and adolescents in which treatment of severe and chronic illnesses is necessary, while at the same time the health of youth needs to be optimally enhanced. More research, such as the recently published study by Olfson et al. 2003 into the relationship between antidepressant medication and suicide in adolescents, is necessary to inform not only clinical practice but health policy as well.

One positive contribution to this issue would be a significant enhancement in the training of child and adolescent psychiatrists in psychopharmacology. To date, insufficient attention has been paid in many training programs in North America and Europe in ensuring that child and adolescent psychiatrists are highly skilled in all areas of psychopharmacology. Additionally, while research programs have begun to develop in this domain, they are still relatively few and far between and have not yet led to a creation of a sufficiently large body of clinically useful knowledge that is scientifically based on appropriate clinical trials evidence. Thus, both training programs and research programs in this area must be a priority in development for the specialty.

In clinical terms, it is essential that health systems have within them expertise in child and adolescent psychopharmacology. The plethora of well-defined and evidence-based therapeutic interventions with the use of medications in many disorders of children and adolescents means that these disorders should be treated appropriately with medications and it means that expertise in their treatment needs to be available to the general public. As health systems are structured in different ways internationally, it is impossible to provide a simple programmatic suggestion for optimizing such interventions. However, as a guiding policy principle, it is possible to suggest that within every health jurisdiction, expertise in child and adolescent psychopharmacology be part of the service provision model available for children and adolescents. Whether this is located within a mental health system or within a pediatric health system frankly is irrelevant as long as it is available. In addition, a facility in which young people can be therapeutically housed for short periods of time, if necessary, to provide sophisticated medication interventions should

also be available, although the vast majority of cases can be treated on an outpatient basis.

While these problems are significant for Western Europe and North America, they are even more magnified within the developing world in which expertise in this domain is sadly lacking and in which universal access to even the most basic pharmacological interventions is very often not available. Therefore, as part of the development of expertise in this domain, care must be taken to ensure that global inequities in knowledge and treatment availability not be continued or further enhanced by focusing all our training and research efforts within the »Western World«. Indeed, through the use of such international organizations as the Global Forum on Health Research, the World Health Organization, the Pan American Health Organization, and perhaps the World Psychiatric Association, the development of training and research programs designed to meet the needs of the developing world in the domain of child and adolescent psychopharmacology should be brought forward as a priority. This of course can be embedded in the larger need for providing evidence-based child and adolescent mental health services in low- and middle-income countries so that when these services are developed that psychopharmacology is a part of them from the beginning (Vitiello 2001; Rey et al. 2003; Mitka 2003; Glenberg 2003; Olfson et al. 2003).

References

Am Acad Child Adolesc Psychiatry. Practice parameter for the assessment and treatment of children and adolescents with schizohprenia. J Am Acad Child Adolesc Psychiatry. 40:45–235, 2001.

Biederman J, Mick E, Spencer T, et al. Therapeutic dilemmas in the pharmacotherapy of bipolar depression in the young. J Child Adolesc Psychopharmacol. 10:185–192, 2000.

Brooks S, Krulewicz S, Kutcher S. The Kutcher Adolescent Depression Scale: assessment of its evaluative properties over the course of an eight week pediatric pharmacotherapy trial. J Child Adolesc Psychopharmacol. 13:337–349, 2003.

Bryden K, Carrey N, Kutcher S. Update and recommendations for the use of antipsychotics in early-onset psychosis. J Child Adolesc Psychopharmacology. 11:113–130, 2001.

Carlson, G. Clinical aspects of child and adolescent psychopharmacology. In S. Kutcher ed. Practical Child and Adolescent Psychopharmacology. Cambridge University Press, Cambridge, pp 70–90, 2002.

Carrey N. Developmental neurobiology: implications for pediatric psychopharmacology. Can J Psychiatry. 46:810–818, 2001.

Carrey N, Kutcher S. Developmental pharmacodynamics: implications for child and adolescent psychopharmacology. J Psychiatry Neurosci. 23:274:276, 1998.

Findling R. The future of pharmacotherapy for pediatric anxiety. Expert Opin Pharmacother. 3:574–574, 2002.

Findling R, McNamara N, Youngstrom E, et al. A prospective, open-label trial of olanzapine in adolescents with schizophrenia. J Am Acad Child Adolesc Psychiatry. 42:170–175, 2003.

Gillberg C. Typical neuroleptics in child and adolescent psychiatry. Eur Child Adolesc Psychiatr. 9: Suppl. 1:12–18, 2000.

Glenberg A. SSRIs for children. Biological Therapies in Psychiatry. 26:1, 2003.

Greenhill L, Pliszka S, Dulcan M, et al. Practice parameter for the use of stimulant medications in the treatment of children, adolescents and adults. J Am Acad Child Adoles Psychiatry. 41:265–495, 2002.

Greenhill L, Vitiello B, Abikoff H, et al. Developing methodologies for monitoring long-term safety of psychotropic medications in children: apart on the NINH conference, Sept. 25, 2000. J. Am Acad Child Adolesc Psychiatry. 42: 651–655, 2003.

Guerrero A. General medical considerations in child and adolescent patients who present with psychiatric symptoms. Child Adolesc. Psychiatr Clin N Am, 12:613–628, 2003.

Kastelic E, Labellarte M, Ridde M. Selective serotonin reuptake inhibitors for children and adolescents. Curr Psychiatry Rep. 2:117–123, 2000.

Koplewicz H., Green K. eds. J of Child and Adolescent Psychopharmacology. Mary Ann Liebert Inc., New York, 1999.

Kowatch R, Sethuramen G, Hume J, et al. Combination pharmacotherapy in children and adolescents with bipolar disorder. Biol Psychiatry. 53: 978–984, 2003.

Kusumakar V, MacMaster F, Kutcher S, Shulman K. Bipolar disorder in young people, the elderly and pregnant women. In Yatham L, Kusumakar V, Kutcher S eds. Bipolar Disorder: A Clinician's Guide to Biological Treatments. Brunner-Routledge, New York, 2002. pp 85–114.

Kutcher S. ed. Child and Adolescent Psychopharmacology News. Guilford Press, New York, 1999.

Kutcher S. Child and Adolescent Psychopharmacology. W.B. Saunders, New York, 1997.

Kutcher S. Adolescent onset bipolar illness. In A. Marneros and Jules Agnst eds. Bipolar Disorders: 100 Years After Manic-Depressive Insanity. Kulwer Academic Publishers, Dordrecht, Netherlands, 2000, pp 139–152.

Kutcher S. Practical clinical issues regarding child and adolescent psychopharmacology. Child Adolesc Psychiatr Clin N Am. 9:245–260, 2000.

Kutcher S ed.. Practical Child and Adolescent Psychopharmacology, Cambridge U. Press, Cambridge, 2002.

Kutcher S, Aman M, Brooks S, et al. International consensus statement on attention-deficit/hyperactivity disorder ADHD and disruptive behavior disorders DBD's: Clinical implications and treatment practice suggestions. Eur Neuropsychopharmacol. 14:11–28, 2004.

Labellarte M, Ginsburg G, Walkup J, et al. The treatment of anxiety disorders in children and adolescents. Biol Psychiatry. 46:1567–1578, 1999.

Licht R, Vestergaard P, Kessing G, et al. Psychopharmacological treatment with lithium and anti-epileptic drugs: suggested guidelines from the Danish Psychiatric Association and the Child and Adolescent Psychiatric Association in Denmark. Acta Psychiatr Scan Suppl. 419:1–22, 2003.

March J, Vitiello B. Advances in pediatric neuropsychopharmacology: an overview. Int J Neuropsychopharmacol. 4:141–147, 2001.

Markowitz J, Straughn A, Patrick N. Advances in the pharmacotherapy of attention-deficit hyperactivity disorder: focus on methylphenidate formulations. Pharmacotherapy. 23:1281–1299, 2003.

Martin A, Kaufman J, Charney D. Pharmacotherapy of early-onset depression: Update and new directions. Child Adolesc Psychiatr Clin N Am. 9:135–157, 2000.

McClellan J, Werry J. Evidence-based treatments in child and adolescent Psychiatry: an inventory. J. Amer Acad Child and Adolesc Psychiatry. 43:1388–1400, 2003.

McCracken J, McGough J, Shah B, et al. Risperidone in children with autism and serious behavioral problems. N Engl J. Med. 347:314–321, 2002.

Mitka M. FDA alert on anti-depressants for youth. JAMA. 290:2534, 2003.

Nobile M, Cataldo G, Marino C. Diagnosis and treatment of dysthymia in children and adolescents. CNS Drugs. 17: 927–946, 2003.

Olfson M. et al. Relationship between antidepressant medication treatment and suicide in adolescents. Arch Gen Psychiatry. 60:978–982, 2003.

Osterheld J. A review of developmental aspects of cytochrome P450. J of Child and Adolesc Psychopharmacology. 8:161–174, 1998.

Pliszka S. New developments in psychopharmacology of attention-deficit hyperactivity disorder. Expert Opin Investig Drugs. 10:1797–1807, 2001.

Pliszka S, Lopez M, Crismon M, et al. A feasibility study of the children's medication alorithm project CMAP algorithm for the treatment of ADHD. J Am Acad Child Adolesc Psychiatry. 42:279–287, 2003.

Remschmidt H, Hennighausen K, Clement H, et al. Atypical neuroleptics in child and adolescent psychiatry. Eur Child Adolesc Psychiatry 9 Suppl:9–19, 2000.

Rey J, Sawyer M. Are psychostimulant drugs being used appropriately to treat child and adolescent disorders? Br J Psychiatry. 182:284–286, 2003.

Ryan N, Bhatara V, Perel J. Mood stabilizers in children and adolescents. J Am Acad Child Adolesc Psychiatry. 38: 529–536, 1999.

Safer D. Patterns of psychotropic medication prescribed by child psychiatrists in the 1990's. J Child Adolesc. Psychopharmacology. 7:267–274, 1997.

Santosh P, Baird G. Psychopharmacotherapy in children and adults with intellectual disability. Lancet. 345:233–242, 1999.

Schulz F, Remschmidt H. Psychopharmacology of depressive states in childhood and adolescence. In I Goodyear ed. The Depressed Child and Adolescent. 2nd, ed. Cambridge University Press, Cambridge, 2001, pp 292–324.

Spencer T, Biederman J. Wilens T, et al. Novel treatments for attention/deficit/hyperactivity disorder in children. J Clin Psychiatry. 63 Suppl 12:16–22, 2002.

Steiner H, Sexena K. Chang K. Psychopharmacologic strategies for the treatment of aggression in juveniles. CNS Spectr. 8:298–308, 2003.

Tourbiu K. Strategies for pharmacology treatment of high functioning autism and Asperger syndrome. Child Adolesc Psychiatry Clin N Am. 12:23–45, 2003.

Varley C. Psychopharmacological treatment of major depressive disorder in children and adolescents. JAMA. 290: 1091–1093, 2003.

Varley CK, Smith CJ. Anxiety disorders in the child and teen. Pediatr Clin North Am. 50:1107–1138, 2003.

Vitiello B. Psychopharmacology for young children: clinical needs and research opportunities. Pediatrics. 108:983–989, 2001.

Walkup J, Labellarte M, Riddle M et al. Treatment of pediatric anxiety disorders: an open-label extension of the research units on pediatric psychopharmacology anxiety study. J Child Adolesc Psychopharmacol. 12:175–188, 2002.

Zito JM, Riddle MA. Psychiatric pharmacoepidemiology for children. Child Adoles. Psychiatric Clin North Am. 4:77–95, 1995.

Outcomes of Treatment

Stephen Scott

16.1   Does It Work? – 222
16.1.1   Well-Conducted Trials That Failed to Show
         Treatments Worked – 223
16.1.2   The Urge to Show an Effect – 223
16.1.3   How Change Is Measured – 223
16.1.4   What Changed? – 224
16.1.5   How Long Does Change Last? – 224
16.1.6   Social Functioning – 225
16.1.7   Statistical Procedures to Increase Effect Size – 225
16.1.8   Levels of Evidence – 225

16.2   For Whom Does It Work? – 226
16.2.1   The Need for Intention-to-Treat Analyses – 226
16.2.2   Prediction of Outcome, Moderators
         and Mediators – 226
16.2.3   Comorbidity – 227

16.3   How Does It Work? – 227
16.3.1   Amount of Therapy Needed – 228
16.3.2   Whole Program at a Fixed Pace or Varied Until a
         Criterion is Reached? – 229

16.4   Will It Work in Ordinary Clinical Practice? – 229
16.4.1   Effectiveness in Real-Life Conditions – 229
16.4.2   Cost-Effectiveness – 229
16.4.3   Disseminability – 229

16.5   Conclusion – 230

         References – 230

This chapter aims to discuss, with examples, four questions that might arise when considering any treatment. Firstly, does it work? Secondly, for whom does it work? Thirdly, how does it work? And fourthly, will it work in ordinary clinical practice?

16.1 Does It Work?

Children are brought to clinics with a problem, and if the treatment gets rid of the problem, it can be said to have worked. There is a growing array of evi-dence for effectiveness of treatments in several do-mains of childhood psychopathology. This chapter does not review these; the reader is referred to the previous chapters in this book, and to recent excel-lent books such as **What Works with Children and Adolescents** by Carr (Carr 2004); **What Works for Whom, a Critical Review of Treatments for Children and Adolescents** by Fonagy and colleagues (Fonagy et al. 2002); **Evidence-based Psychotherapies for Chil-dren and Adolescents** by Kazdin and Weisz (Kazdin and Weisz 2003); and **Handbook of Interventions That Work with Children and Adolescents** by Barrett and Ollendick (Barrett and Ollendick 2004).

Broadly, these suggest that there is good evi-dence for (a) the effectiveness of cognitive-behavior-al approaches with internalizing disorders such as anxiety, depression, phobias, and posttraumatic stress disorder; (b) for parent-training with opposi-tional-defiant disorder, hyperactivity symptoms/ milder ADHD; (c) for behavioral approaches with a number of behavioral problems from bedwetting to sleeping difficulties; (d) for family therapy with anorexia; (e) for multimodal approaches with severe conduct disorder; and (f) for stimulant medication with ADHD/the hyperkinetic syndrome.

In contrast, there is little good evidence for the effectiveness of (g) psychodynamic psychotherapy for any disorder; (h) residential treatment for any disorder, especially conduct disorder; (i) any inter-vention (psychotherapeutic or medical) for the core features of mental retardation or autism; (j) any spe-cific professional intervention for the broader se-quelae of harmful experiences such as sexual abuse or prolonged neglect; (k) tricyclic or specific seroto-nin reuptake inhibitor antidepressants for adoles-cent depression.

Often this is because of a paucity of research rather than confirmation that it is ineffective; so re-garding effectiveness, »lack of evidence is not evi-dence of lack«. However a number of trials have failed to show SSRIs work with depression in adolescents, leading the UK Department of Health in 2004 to virtually ban their use, with the exception of fluoxetine, for which the evidence of effectiveness is also not strong.

16.1.1 Well-Conducted Trials That Failed to Show Treatments Worked

Some plausible treatments have proven notably ineffective when subjected to proper evaluation, underlining the deceptive potential of subjective ideas and »my clinical experience«. For example, in the Cambridge-Somerville trial for delinquency, 325 matched pairs of delinquent boys under 12 were allocated to the best intervention in light of knowledge at the time, or allocated a no-intervention control. The intervention included home visits for the boys twice a month on average over 5 years, together with parent counseling for problems; academic tutoring where indicated, received by half; psychiatric attention where indicated, received by a third; summer camps for half; constructive local activities such as woodwork, sports training and visits to matches. The results showed **worse** outcomes in the treated group (crime, diagnosed alcoholic, or other major psychiatric disorder; McCord 1992). Further analysis has suggested that the summer camps were the ingredient that led to poorer outcomes, probably because when together the boys encouraged each other to more antisocial acts and got kudos for this (Dishion et al. 2001).

The Fort Bragg project (Bickman et al. 2000) allocated considerable funds for clinicians' treatment of choice for child mental health disorders in a defined population in the United States and compared outcomes with a control population without such resources. No improvement was seen in the group given clinicians' treatment of choice. Here a possible explanation is that the treatments actually given were not evidence-based, and included a lot of general counseling and psychotherapy, and expensive but apparently ineffective residential treatments. One message from the above two trials is that it is not good enough to apply an intervention that sounds plausible and assume it will work– yet many services are organized on this principle.

16.1.2 The Urge to Show an Effect

Investigators may have a strong drive to show that a treatment works. There is evidence that allegiance to a therapy by investigators or therapists increases the probability that the trial will show effectiveness. Likewise, pharmaceutical industry-sponsored trials show larger effect sizes than those conducted by independent researchers (Bekelman 2003; Stelfox et al. 1998; Vandenbroucke 1998). Yet to date editors of psychological journals have been slow to insist on conflict of interest statements by psychosocial researchers. This is surprising in light of the fact that a number of interventions for children have, understandably, been evaluated by developers of the studied programs who have a commercial interest in their success. Even where the investigator hasn't invented the type of therapy being used or have a financial stake, huge amounts of effort usually go into organizing the treatment, and a no-effect result is usually very disappointing and has less exciting publishing consequences. As will be shown in this chapter, many devices may be used to try to increase the impression of effects. Therefore, the reader of reports has to have a modicum of skepticism, and an eagle eye for these devices, whilst remembering the huge effort required to mount such trials, which generally are far harder to carry through than nonintervention trials. Replication of findings by practitioners who are independent of the developer and have no conflict of interest are especially desirable.

16.1.3 How Change Is Measured

There is an increasing movement away from only using tests of statistical significance towards using effect size as the preferred indicator of change. The effect size is the difference in mean score following treatment divided by the standard deviation of the sample prior to treatment. This allows one to compare directly the effectiveness of an intervention on different measures. Cohen (1988) describes an effect size of 0.2 as small, 0.5 as moderate, and 0.8 as large. The largest effect size of any intervention in child and adolescent mental health is that found for methylphenidate on hyperactivity, which in some efficacy trials has an effect size of 1.4 standard deviations on hyperactivity symptoms. At the opposite end of the scale, large trials on the effect of aspirin in cardiovascular medicine gave an effect size of about 0.05 or less than a standard deviation. This means that the effect is much more modest, but in terms of total population lives saved, may still be a treatment worthwhile embarking upon since it is cheap and easily administered. An advantage of the effect size is that it is independent of the size of population measured, and so gives different information from statistical significance, which can be high even when the effect size is small, provided the population is large enough – the aspirin studies required a population of thousands to show a significant difference. The issue of different statistical indices of clinically significant change is discussed more fully by Jacobson and Truax (1991). Where the endpoint is categorical, such as having a disorder or not, then a useful expression of effect size is the Number Needed to Treat (Cook and Sackett 1995; Altman et al. 2000). This expresses how many cases would have to be seen with the new treatment compared to controls before one case extra reaches the criterion. Thus the effect size is large if only, 5 cases need to be treated to gain an extra case of generalized anxiety cured, but small if 30 have to be seen.

16.1.4 What Changed?

It is essential that the main objective of change is determined before the trial, and desirable that one main outcome be given precedence. Otherwise, as in many trials, there may be multiple measures of the same construct and the authors may report the positive one with great prominence, but fail to comment much on the negative ones. Thus, trials for antisocial behavior may say show substantial change on one questionnaire, but fail to show much change at all on direct observation, or on another questionnaire measuring similar constructs (e.g., Conduct Problems Research Group 1999). Outcome measures are far more valid if they are well validated and predict future prognosis; they are less useful if they are in-house and, for example, relate to perceived amount of change (Conduct Problems Prevention Research Group 1999). Using multiple informants and multiple methods increases confidence in change, and may reveal practically useful information. Thus, parent training programs for conduct disorder generally improve antisocial behavior in the home, but not at school. This has led to the development of school-based classroom management programs (Scott 2002).

16.1.5 How Long Does Change Last?

This crucial question has not yet been addressed by sufficient treatment trials – typically most do not follow up beyond a year after treatment. The answer is likely to depend on a wide range of factors. Thus, if the natural history of the phenomenon is to recur, as in depression, a treatment may be effective at the time, and again when depression recurs. Certainly relapse rates are high for both pharmacological and cognitive-behavioral treatments (Harrington 2002). The search is on to identify risk factors that can be modified to prevent relapse. Thus, if thinking style is a major determinant of depression, it ought to be modifiable during the recovery phase to prevent relapse, but evidence so far for relapse prevention cognitive therapy has been disappointing. If, on the other hand, external factors such as having critical parents or carers is central to the etiology in someone vulnerable to depression, then reducing this should lead to better outcomes and less relapse – a notion consistent with the findings in adults of the London depression trial, where couple therapy outperformed individual cognitive therapy (Leff et al. 2004). Likewise, if conduct symptoms are in part driven by lack of ability to articulate emotional states, then programs that teach »emotional literacy« should prevent recurrence of antisocial behavior, a notion supported by the impact of prevention programs such as the Promoting Alternative Thinking Strategies program (Greenberg et al. 2004). High chances of relapse have led Kazdin (2000) to liken treatment to dental care, with episodes of specific treatment followed up by regular checks and further treatment courses as indicated. Other disorders such as ADHD have been likened to a chronic illness or handicap, requiring lifelong intervention (Barkley 1990).

In contrast to trials offering treatment for established clinical conditions, a number of prevention programs have been followed up for several years. The best known is perhaps the Perry/Highscope study, where cognitive enrichment of disadvantaged children 2–4 years of age led to early gains in academic attainment, but these disappeared by late adolescence. However, on studying psychosocial functioning rather than academic ability at age 27, treated individuals had notably better employment, were financially better off, and committed far fewer criminal offences (Schweinhart and Weikart 1988).

16.1.6   Social Functioning

There is increasing interest in measuring social functioning and impact of disorders, rather than just symptoms. Yet so far, few studies have included these, despite there being relatively simple instruments such as the Child Global Assessment Schedule (Shaffer et al. 1983), and more detailed and potentially valid ones such as the SAICA (John 2004). The Strengths and Difficulties Questionnaire is an example of a simple, well-validated general psychopathology instrument that includes measures of impact at home, at school, and with friends (Goodman 1999). A treatment for depression is less useful if, for example, it banishes feelings of sadness and hopelessness but the young person is not returning to seeing her friends or doing school work effectively. This need to affect social functioning raises the consideration that treatments should perhaps explicitly target the building of skills. Some do this, but are often not part of mainstream services offered. Thus, social skills training programs are well proven (Spence 2003) but are seldom offered even for disorders where social skills are typically lacking, such as conduct disorders. An example of a treatment approach that explicitly targets skills is Multidimensional Treatment Foster Care (Chamberlain 2003), where the treatment package specifically includes a skills trainer to coach the young person in social and negotiating skills in real life, community settings. Problem-solving skills can be effective with even quite young children, down to say age 4 years (Kazdin and Weisz 2003; Webster-Stratton and Hammond 1997).

16.1.7   Statistical Procedures to Increase Effect Size

A number of measures can be deployed to increase the chances of showing an effect (Boyle and Pickles 2004). Firstly, taking multiple time point measures of outcome (over at least three time points) enables linear growth curves to be computed, so that models can be fitted for the slope of change. These are usually more sensitive to change than pre-post measures only. Secondly, if several different measures of the same construct are used, a new, single measure, a so-called latent variable, can be constructed from them. Here those aspects or scores of the measures that go and up and down together (covary) across subjects and time are selected, whereas those as-

pects or scores which are unique for that measure and behave differently from the others are dropped, on the assumption they are noise or measurement error. Using latent variables can give larger effect sizes in intervention trials, but should only be published alongside raw scores for each of the variables so readers can interpret the results both ways. Thirdly, when constructing new instruments, increasing the number of items increases reliability. Fourthly, ensuring regular interrater reliability checks for semistructured interviews and observational coding schemes will also reduce variability and so increase effect size.

16.1.8   Levels of Evidence

The American Psychological Association (Task Force on Psychological Intervention Guidelines of the American Psychological Association 1995) formalized the difference between **efficacy** studies, that determine whether treatments work under tightly controlled settings where factors such as characteristics of participants, quality of treatment, and amount of treatment received are relatively optimal, and **effectiveness** studies that determine whether treatments work in the »real world« of clinical practice where comorbidity and disorganized lives are common, quality of treatment is often variable since it is given by a generalist, and the amount of treatment received may be less than ideal. However, most of the APA recommendations about treatment were based on efficacy studies only. Initially, two levels of evidence were delineated, then Chambless and Hollon (1998) proposed three: treatments were deemed »well established« if there were at least two independent randomized controlled trials with active controls, »probably efficacious« if there was one RCT with an active control or two with a waiting list control, and »possibly efficacious« otherwise.

One problem with this approach is that while there are, for example, scores of trials on parent training for antisocial behavior, there are not enough to offer any opinion on treatments for some specific aspects of autism. This fails to consider the considerable number of single case trials showing an effect where after a baseline period without treatment, the same child is given the treatment, then it is withdrawn (Lovaas and Smith 2003; Koegel et al. 2003).

16.2   For Whom Does It Work?

16.2.1   The Need for Intention-to-Treat Analyses

Until recently, trials often only reported on those participants who had been studied. Furthermore, those who had dropped out of the treatment program were often not followed up, and were not allowed for in analyses. Trials reported this way are likely to overestimate the effects of a treatment. It is essential to include an analysis of all cases randomized to receive treatment, irrespective of whether they then went on to receive it. In such an »intention-to-treat« analysis, cases for whom there is no follow-up information are typically assumed to have made no progress since last assessed. This then should give a more accurate picture of what would happen to all cases allocated to treatment using admission criteria and treatment conditions similar to those in the trial. Some participants, despite signing up to the trial, may have decided on reflection that the effort, cost, inconvenience, and other disadvantages of taking the treatment offered are too great to even start; others may drop out before finishing the prescribed course, or only attend part of it intermittently, or take less than prescribed. Because they usually won't improve as much as those who received the intervention, this will then reduce the effect size of the treatment according to what proportion drop out; examples include a reduction of 22% in a trial of interpersonal therapy for adolescent depression (Mufson et al. 1999), and a reduction of 16% in a trial of parent training for child antisocial behavior (Scott et al. 2001). One reason why the nontreated group may do worse is because they didn't receive treatment (although they might have gone away to get another kind of treatment). Another is because they may have characteristics that differ from those who received treatment and which mean they would have been less likely to respond even if they did get it. These could include being less well organized, having more life events and stressors at home that prevent giving time or mental space to take on a new approach and practice it, being depressed or ill, being poorer, not believing children's problems matter that much, and so on. Characteristics such as these have been shown to typify dropouts and nonengagers (Kazdin and Wassell 2000).

It is not being argued here that only intention-to-treat analyses should be published, as this might, as it were, »throw the baby out with the bath water«. For

example, if half the target population decline further treatment and assessment, but all those who received it do well, then the conclusion should not necessarily be that the treatment doesn't work, but rather, ways need to be found to improve its acceptability so that uptake is increased. This may involve rather different skills and procedures from those required during treatment, including good help with accessibility, good engagement skills, and a collaborative approach (Herbert 1995). The trial of a maternal depression intervention plus a parenting program for antisocial child behavior by Verduyn et al. (2003) reported only an intention-to-treat analysis, which found no effect. However, half the sample allocated to the treatment arm dropped out before any therapy was given, so it remains a possibility that the treatment worked for those who received it, and might work for any group who receive it.

Intention-to-treat analyses also protect against the risk of overestimating treatment effects where there is differential dropout between groups. For example, in a trial conducted by Sanders et al. (2000) the treatment group lost 40% of cases whereas the control group only lost 8%. The impressive results of the trial would have been reduced if a no-improvement assumption had been made from study dropouts. Whilst authors often show demographic material to show that differences between drop outs and completers are small or insignificant on the demographic measures taken, these do not usually cover more psychological reasons for not taking up treatment, such as life events. Psychological journals have been slow to insist on these reporting standards, which were tightly defined for medical trials in the CONSORT criteria (Begg et al. 1996), which have since been revised (Moher et al. 2004).

16.2.2   Prediction of Outcome, Moderators and Mediators

How well participants respond to treatment includes the impact of nonspecific predictors, of moderators of the effect, and of mediators through which the treatment works. Nonspecific predictors are those that operate irrespective of treatment, and are part of the natural history of the condition. In a trial, they will have a similar impact on intervention and control groups. For example, several factors predict outcome in antisocial behavior, Farrington (2002) identified 26 factors, each with an independent effect.

Moderators of outcome are factors that are present before the trial begins that determine the degree of response to treatment but do not usually change as a result of the intervention. For example, they may include age, gender, and socioeconomic disadvantage. Equally, there may be clinically very relevant factors which usually, in naturalistic studies, predict a poor outcome, but that are overcome or cease to operate in treatment. For example, Scott et al. (2001) found that several factors that are usually known to lead to a worse outcome did not diminish treatment response, including an early age of onset of symptoms, low maternal education, and being in a lone parent family. Ways to calculate impact of moderators in general are given by Holmbeck (1997), but an elegant exposition specifically for treatment trials is given by Kraemer et al. (2002).

For children offered parent training for antisocial behavior, it is widely believed that older age predicts worse response; however, two studies addressing this issue found no effect of age: older children did just as well (Ruma et al. 1996). This has important implications for service planning, since it is often held that prevention or early intervention is bound to be superior than later treatment. However, if treatment response is as good later, waiting until children are older could have better cost-effectiveness since identification is more precise later. Prevention trials may involve a significant proportion of cases who do not need the intervention as they would never have developed difficulties anyway. In general, in the treatment of childhood mental health problems, there is little evidence that gender moderates outcome – boys usually do as well as girls.

16.2.3 Comorbidity

Typically, the majority of children and adolescents referred to clinics have more that one diagnosis (Caron and Rutter 1991). Yet almost all the evidence of effectiveness in child mental health is based on trials designed for one disorder or set of problems, with comorbid cases often being specifically excluded. So how should the empirically minded clinician proceed? Possibly the same causal factors may be held to be relevant for both conditions, so the treatment is the same, as in say a parenting program for conduct disorder and moderate hyperactivity. However, if there is no convincing pharmacological treatment to give alongside a psychological one, and the evidence suggests that two conditions require a different psychosocial treatment, as for example in a case with both depression and hyperactivity, which should be addressed first, and how? Trials are

needed that compare combined treatments that comprise realistic, pared-down manualized treatments with key elements from each, versus sequential application of the best evidence-based treatment for each component.

16.3 How Does It Work?

The literature about trials in child mental health is becoming more interesting in that there is beginning to be empirical testing of **how** interventions work, not just **whether** they work. A mediator refers to a factor through which treatment exerts its effect – it has to change because of treatment, and in turn change in the outcome depends on this. This can be conceptually relatively simple, for example, it might be hypothesized that for depression to lift during cognitive therapy, self-esteem has to change first. However, much child mental health work has an added layer of complexity where treatment aims mainly or partly to change the family or parent, and secondarily to this, change child symptoms or functioning. It follows that to begin to determine how treatment works, each step, and the main likely mediating mechanisms need to be measured.

Thus, if it is hypothesized by a family therapist that recurrent abdominal pain in childhood is related to an overly close relationship with the child's mother, then a measure of closeness needs to be taken. If the children's pain doesn't get better, this could be (a) because the family therapy didn't change the closeness, or (b) because it did, but the child didn't respond to this. Equally, such a study might show (c) that maternal closeness didn't change, but the child in therapy got better. Or indeed, (d) that maternal closeness lessened, and that the abdominal pain got better, but that the two were unrelated. Either of these last two scenarios would suggest that another mechanism was involved in the child getting better, say, for example, because the child now felt listened to by the mother, or perhaps because since coming to the clinic she had changed his diet to a less constipating one. Unless these alternative mediators were measured during the study (or could validly be measured afterwards), confirming them would require another study where these mechanisms were explicitly changed. Indeed, Kraemer et al. (2002) take the view that mediational analysis can only **generate** hypotheses of how treatment works, not **confirm** them, which requires new interventional studies.

Measuring the possible mediator allows these alternatives to be teased out, and then, for example, if it wasn't doing so before, the therapy can be improved so it does change closeness, or, if it were being changed but wasn't related to child improvement, then the theory would need to be revised. However, so far, most intervention trials, for understandable reasons including the difficulty mounting them and the lack of funds to do so, haven't got beyond measuring child outcomes. Yet if, in the instance above, the treatment hadn't worked, it wouldn't be clear why not.

An exception is the study by Martinez and Forgatch (2001). Here it was hypothesized that the main mechanism through which a parenting program for disruptive children would work would be through improved disciplinary practices. The authors separately measured both positive parenting and disciplinary practices. To their surprise, whilst improved discipline did mediate some of the improvement, considerably more was mediated through positive parenting. This finding could in turn influence the design of future parenting programs to include a stronger element targeting positive parenting practices such as pleasurable joint activity amongst family members. The trial by Scott et al. (2001) of parenting groups led to a reduction in maternal depression, but interestingly, this did not mediate the large reduction in antisocial behavior found, which on a preliminary analysis was due to changes in parenting practices (Scott 2003).

Although mediators were not measured, a pair of elegant trials by Sanders and colleagues addressed the usefulness of adjunctive therapy for factors within parents that might impede ability to make use of a parenting program for disruptive child behavior. The first trial took parents whose children had behavior problems and divided them into those with and without marital discord (Scott 2002). Each group then either received a basic parenting course, or the basic course plus extra sessions dealing with marital discord and adult relationships. The results showed that where there was no discord, the extra treatment did not improve child outcome, whereas where there was, it did. The second trial with depressed mothers had a similar design, and likewise found that additional sessions addressing depression improved child outcome when mothers were indeed depressed, but not if they were not (Scott 2002). In retrospect, these findings »make sense« and offer evidence that where there are not complicating factors, extra treatment addressing them doesn't lead to better outcome. However, alternative results could also have been predicted. Thus, in distressed families, basic counseling theory might hypothesize that having a longer course of treatment allows for a more trusting and supportive relationship to be built, which in turn should impact on the children. A longer duration would allow more nonspecific therapeutic factors to operate. That this was not the case may indicate that at least for parents with behavioral problems, the specific content of the treatment is important in addition to the general quality of the relationship.

16.3.1 Amount of Therapy Needed

This question is sometimes addressed by »dose-response« curves, which plot amount of therapy received against outcome. In programs of fixed duration, the assumption might be that those who received most of the planned therapy would do better than those who only got a little. However, this does not turn out always to be the case, and a number of trials have failed to find a relationship. This may be because dropout is nonrandom. People who leave may be a mixture of those who are not at all in control of their lives and are overwhelmed by the child problems so subsequently do badly, and those who get better fairly quickly so choose to leave early as they no longer see the need for treatment. In support of this possibility, there is increasing evidence that for CBT with adults, much of the improvement occurs in the first four sessions (Wilson et al. 1999; Ilardi and Craighead 1999). However, what is needed to settle this is research on dropouts that uses qualitative methods to ask for reasons for dropout, and combines these with quantitative data on outcome.

The best way to determine how much therapy is needed is to address the question directly by a trial of longer versus shorter therapy. Shapiro and colleagues in Leeds did this for depression, expecting that cutting down their course of 24 weeks of therapy to 16 would not be as effective in reducing depression in adults. To their surprise, it was (Barkham et al. 2002). Moreover, there was no moderating effect of initial severity – it might be thought that the more severe cases required longer, but this was not found.

16.3.2 Whole Program at a Fixed Pace or Varied Until a Criterion is Reached?

With therapy for individual children or families, it is possible to vary the pace of the program according to whether change is occurring. Thus, some parent training packages do not proceed to the next stage until a certain level of skill is attained in the current one, such as being able to give, say, three praises for each criticism (Patterson 1982). This presumes attainment of each step is necessary at the time for progress – a testable hypothesis. Group programs are hampered in that they have to go at a rate that is reasonable for most members.

16.4 Will It Work in Ordinary Clinical Practice?

Even if a treatment is shown in efficacy trials to work, three broad issues may stop uptake: effectiveness in real-life conditions, cost-effectiveness, and disseminability.

16.4.1 Effectiveness in Real-Life Conditions

United States trials reviewed by Weisz and colleagues (Weisz et al. 1995; Weisz and Hawley 1998) suggest that »the good news is that child psychotherapy works, the bad news is not in real life«. They showed that while the mean effect size in university-based efficacy trials was around 0.7, in real-life clinics it was at best 0.2, and often zero. Reasons for this may include comorbidity, lower motivation of families and young people, a high number of other life problems that undo treatment effects or stop it working in the first place, the nature of treatment given (eclectic versus manualized and evidence-based), and the degree of training and ongoing supervision and support of therapists giving the particular treatment. Trials in everyday clinics using regular staff and typical referred cases are beginning to appear, and some recent ones show good effect sizes (Taylor et al. 1998; Scott et al. 2001).

16.4.2 Cost-Effectiveness

Even if a treatment is shown to be effective, it may be too expensive for health care authorities, insurance companies, or parents and young people to afford. Health economics has developed considerably in the last decade, and is being applied to child mental health (Romeo 2004). Residential treatment is very expensive and has virtually no strong evidence to support it, yet is still widely used in some countries where outpatient management might be possible (Bickman et al. 2000). Alternatives to prison such as Multisystemic Therapy are proving to be more cost-effective and to have a cost benefit (Henggeler et al. 1998). The long-term cost of childhood mental health problems is only beginning to be calculated. One study following conduct-disordered children up from age 10 to age 28 years found that they had cost ten times more than control in public service use (Scott et al. 2001).

16.4.3 Disseminability

For a treatment to be successfully disseminated, it needs (a) to be delivered at sufficient levels of treatment fidelity to get an effect under everyday treatment conditions (Moncher and Prinz 2004), (b) availability of sufficient training courses and ongoing supervision to get and keep staff at a good level, and (c) organizational support. Short training courses without ongoing supervision are probably not sufficient to ensure treatment fidelity. For example, Henggeler et al. (1998) failed to replicate the effects of MST where fidelity was not upheld. More research is needed to measure the degree of skill and fidelity required to achieve reasonable results – this may vary according to type of condition and severity of cases. Even when this is achieved, if the organization in which the therapy is occurring is not supportive and well organized, the intervention may not be effective. Kam et al. (2003) found that for the PATHS emotional skills curriculum to work, good school involvement and commitment was needed, otherwise it failed to improve child functioning even when delivered to a sufficient standard.

16.5   Conclusion

Treatment outcome research is taking off, with far more papers being published than years ago. However, much remains to be discovered, and new treatments need to be invented and refined. Then the »final frontier« of universal prevention will need to be addressed – this opens up a whole now vista of land to conquer.

References

Altman DG, Machin D, Bryant TN, Gardner MJ (2000) Statistics with Confidence. Bristol: BMJ Books.

Barkham M, Rees A, Stiles WB, Hardy GE, Shapiro DA (2002) Dose-effect relations for psychotherapy of mild depression: A Quasi-experimental comparison of effects of 2, 8, and 16 sessions. Psychotherapy Research, 12(4), 463–474.

Barkley R (1990) Attention Deficit Hyperactivity Disorder. A Handbook for Diagnosis and Treatment. New York: The Guildford Press.

Barrett P, Ollendick T (2004) Handbook of Interventions That Work with Children and Adolescents: Prevention and Treatment. New York: Wiley.

Begg C, Cho M, Eastwood S, Horton R, Moher D, Olkin I, Pitkin R, Rennie D, Schulz KF, Simel D, Stroup DF (1996) Improving the quality of reporting of randomized controlled trials: The CONSORT statement. Journal of the American Medical Association, 276(637), 639.

Bekelman JE, Li Y, Gross CP (2003) Scope and impact of financial conflicts of interest in biomedical research. Journal of the American Medical Association, 289, 454–465.

Bickman L, Lambert EW, Andrade AR, Penaloza RV (2000) The Fort Bragg continuum of care for children and adolescents: Mental health outcomes over 5 years. Journal of Consulting & Clinical Psychology, 68, 710–716.

Boyle MH, Pickles AR (2004) Strategies to manipulate reliability: Impact on statistical associations. Journal of the American Academy of Child and Adolescent Psychiatry, 37(10), 1077–1084.

Caron C, Rutter M (1991) Comorbidity in child psychopathology: concepts, issues and research strategies. Journal of Child Psychology and Psychiatry, 32(7), 1063–1080.

Carr A (2004) What Works With Children and Adolescents? London: Routledge.

Chamberlain P (2003) Treating Chronic Juvenile Offenders. Advances made through the Oregon multidimensional treatment foster care model. Washington: American Psychological Association.

Cohen J (1998) Statistical Power Analyses for the Behavioral Sciences. Hillsdale NJ: Lawrence Erlbaum Associates.

Conduct Problems Prevention Research Group (1999) Initial Impact of the Fast Track Prevention Trial for Conduct Problems: 1. The High-Risk Sample. Journal of Consulting and Clinical Psychology, 67(5), 631–647.

Cook RJ, Sackett DL (1995) The number needed to treat: A clinically useful measure of treatment effect. British Medical Journal, 310(452), 454

Dishion TJ, Poulin F, Burraston G (2001) Peer group dynamics associated with iatrogenic effects in group interventions with high-risk young adolescents. In E. C. Nangle DW (Ed.), The Role of Friendship in Psychological Adjustment. New directions for Child and Adolescent Development (pp. 79–92)

Farrington DP (2002) Key Results from the First Forty Years of the Cambridge Study in Delinquent Development. In Thornberry TP and Krohn MD (Ed.), Taking Stock of Delinquency: An Overview of Findings from Contemporary Longitudinal Studies (pp. 137–183) New York: Kluwer Academic/Plenum Publishers.

Fonagy ., Target MCD, Phillips J, Kurtz Z (2002) What Works for Whom? A Critical Review of Treatments for Children and Adolescents. New York: The Guilford Press.

Goodman R (1999) The extended version of the Strengths and Difficulties Questionnaire as a guide to child psychiatric caseness and consequence burden. Journal of Child Psychology and Psychiatry, 40, 791–801.

Greenberg MT, Kusche CA, Cook ET, & Quamma JP (2004) Promoting emotional competence in school-aged children: The effects of the PATHS curriculum. Development & Psychopathology, 7(1), 117–136.

Harrington R (2002) Affective Disorders. In Rutter M and Taylor E (Ed.), Child and Adolescent Psychiatry. Oxford: Blackwell Science Ltd.

Henggeler SW, Schoenwald SK, Borduin CM, Rowland MD, Cunningham PB (1998) Multisystemic Treatment of Antisocial Behavior in Children and Adolescents. New York: The Guildford Press.

Herbert M (1995) A collaborative model of training for parents of children with disruptive behavior disorders. British Journal of Clinical Psychology, 34(3), 325–342.

Holmbeck GN (1997) Toward terminological, conceptual and statistical clarity in the study of mediators and moderators: Examples from the child-clinical and pediatric psychology literatures. Journal of Consulting & Clinical Psychology, 65(4), 599–610.

Ilardi SS, Craighead WE (1999) The role of nonspecific factors in cognitive behavior therapy for depression. Clinical Psychology, 6, 289–292.

Jacobson NS, Truax P (1991) Clinical significance: A statistical approach to defining meaningful change in psychotherapy research. Journal of Consulting & Clinical Psychology, 59(1), 12–19.

John K (2004) Measuring children's social functioning. Child Psychology and Psychiatry Review, 6(4), 181–188.

Kam C, Greenberg MT, & Walls CT (2003) Examining the role of implementation quality in school-based prevention using the PATHS curriculum. Prevention Science, 4(1), 55–63.

Kazdin AE, Weisz JR (2003) Evidence-Based Psychotherapies for Children an Adolescents. New York: The Guildford Press.

Kazdin AE, Wassell G (2000) Therapeutic changes in children, parents, and families resulting from treatment of children with conduct problems. Journal of the American Academy of Child & Adolescent Psychiatry, 39, 414–420.

Kazdin AE, Wassell G (2000) Predictors of barriers to treatment and therapeutic change in outpatient therapy for antisocial children and their families. Mental Health Services Research, 2, 27–40.

Koegel RL, Koegel LK, Brookman LI (2003) Empircally Supported Pivotal Response Interventions for Children with Autism. In Kazdin AE and Weisz JR (Ed.), Evidence-Based Psychotherapies for Children and Adolescents (pp. 341–357) New York: The Guildford Press.

Kraemer HC, Wilson T, Fairburn CG, Agras WS (2002) Mediators and moderators of treatment effects in randomized clinical trials. Archives of General Psychiatry, 59, 877–883.

Leff J, Vearnals S, Brewin CR, Wolff G, Alexander B, Asen E, Dayson D, Jones E, Chisolm D, Everitt B (2004) The London Depression Intervention Trial: Randomized controlled trial of antidepressants v. couple therapy in the treatment and maintenance of people with depression living with a partner: Clinical outcome and costs. British Journal of Psychiatry, 177, 95–100.

Lovaas OI, Smith T (2003) Early and Intensive Behavioral Intervention in Autism. In Anonymous, Evidence-Based Psychotherapies for Children and Adolescents (pp. 325–340) New York: The Guildford Press.

Martinez Jr CR, Forgatch MS (2001) Preventing problems with boys' noncompliance: Effects of a parent training intervention for divorcing mothers. Journal of Consulting & Clinical Psychology, 69(3), 416–428.

McCord J (1992) The Cambridge-Somerville Study: A Pioneering Longitudinal-Experimental Study of Delinquency Prevention. In: J McCord, RE Tremblay (Eds.), Preventing Antisocial Behavior: Interventions from Birth through Adolescence. New York: The Guildford Press.

Moher D, Schulz K, Altman DG (2004) The CONSORT Statement: Revised recommendations for improving the quality of reports of parallel-group randomized trials. Lancet, 357, 1191–1194.

Moncher FJ, Prinz RJ (2004) Treatment fidelity in outcome studies. Clinical Psychology Review, 11(3), 247–266.

Mufson L, Weissman MM, Moreau D, Garfinkel R (1999) Efficacy of interpersonal psychotherapy for depressed adolescents. Archives of General Psychiatry, 56(6), 573–579.

Patterson GR (1982) Coercive Family Process. Eugene, Oregon: Castalia Publishing Company.

Romeo R, Byford S, Knapp M (in press) Economic evaluations of child and adolescent mental health interventions: A systematic review. Journal of Child Psychology and Psychiatry.

Ruma PR, Burke RV, Thompson RW (1996) Group Parent Training: Is It Effective for Children of All Ages? Behavior Therapy, 27, 159–169.

Sanders MR, Markie-Dadds C, Tully LA, Bor W (2000) The Triple P-Positive Parenting Program: A comparison of enhanced, standard and self-directed behavioral family intervention for parents of children with early onset conduct problems. Journal of Consulting & Clinical Psychology,

Schweinhart L, Weikart D (1988) The High/Scope Perry preschool program. In: R Price, E Cowen, R Lorion, J Ramos-McKay (Eds.), 14 ounces of prevention: A casebook for practitioners (pp. 53–66) Washington DC: American Psychological Association.

Scott S (2002) Parent Training Programs. In Rutter M and Taylor E (Ed.), Child and Adolescent Psychiatry (pp. 949–982) Oxford: Blackwell Publishing.

Scott S (2003) Developmental science and clinical intervention: Chalk and cheese? Conference Presentation.

Scott S, Knapp M, Henderson J, & Maughan B (2001) Financial cost of social exclusion: Follow up study of antisocial children into adulthood. British Medical Journal, 323, 1–5.

Scott S, Spender Q, Doolan M, Jacobs B, Aspland H (2001) Multicentre controlled trial of parenting groups for child antisocial behavior in clinical practice. British Medical Journal, 323, 1–5.

Shaffer D, Gould MS, Brasic J Ambrosini P, Fisher P, Bird H, Aluwahlia S (1983) A children's global assessment scale (CGAS) Arch Gen Psychiatry, 40(11), 1228–1231.

Spence SH (2003) Social skills training with children and young people: Theory, evidence and practice. Child and Adolescent Mental Health, 8(2), 84–96.

Stelfox HT, Chua G, O'Rourke K, Detsky AS (1998) Conflict of interest in the debate over calcium-channel antagonists. New England Journal of Medicine, 338, 101–106.

Task Force on Psychological Intervention Guidelines of the American Psychological Association (1995) Template for developing guidelines: Inteventions for mental disorders and psychosocial aspects of physical disorders. Washington DC: American Psychological Association.

Taylor TK, Schmidt F, Pepler D, Hodgins H (1998) A comparison of eclectic treatment with Webster-Stratton's parents and children series in a children's mental health center: A randomized controlled trial. Behavior Therapy, 29, 221–240.

Vandenbroucke J (1998) Medical journals and the shaping of medical knoledge. Lancet, 352 2001

Verduyn C, Barrowclough C, Roberts J, Tarrier N, Harrington R (2003) Maternal depression and child behavior problems. British Journal of Psychiatry, 183, 342–348.

Webster-Stratton C, Hammond M (1997) Treating Children With Early-Onset Conduct Problems: A Comparison of Child and Parent Training Interventions. J Consulting and Clinical Psychology, 65(1), 93–109.

Weisz JR, and Hawley KM (1998) Finding, evaluating, refining and applying empirically supported treatments for children and adolescents. Journal of Consulting & Clinical Psychology, 27 206–216.

Weisz JR, Donenberg GR, Han SS (1995) Bridging the Gap Between Laboratory and Clinic in Child and Adolescent Psychotherapy. Journal of Consulting and Clinical Psychology, 63(5), 688–701.

Wilson GT, Loeb KL, Walsh BT, Labouvie E, Petkova E, Liu X, Waternaux C (1999) Psychological versus pharmacological treatment of bulimia nervosa: Predictors and processes of change. Journal of Consulting & Clinical Psychology, 67, 451–459.

Prevention and Early Detection

17 Interventions That Are CURRES: Cost-Effective, Useful, Realistic, Robust, Evolving, and Sustainable 235

Mary Jane Rotheram-Borus, Diane Flannery, Naihua Duan

18 Prevention of Risks for Mental Health Problems: Lessons Learned in Examining the Prevention of Depression in Families 245

William R. Beardslee, Tracy R.G. Gladstone

19 Prevention and Early Detection of Developmental Disorders 256

Sophie Willemsen-Swinkels, Herman van Engeland

20 Prevention and Early Detection of Emotional Disorders 272

Andreas Dick-Niederhauser, Wendy K. Silverman

21 Prevention and Early Detection of Conduct Disorder and Delinquency 287

David P. Farrington, Brandon C. Welsh

22 Early Detection and Prevention of Attention Deficit/Hyperactivity Disorders 301

Eric Taylor

23 Prevention and Intervention in Primary Care 313

Kelly Kelleher

24 Prevention and Intervention in School Settings 326

Amira Seif El Din

Interventions That Are CURRES: Cost-Effective, Useful, Realistic, Robust, Evolving, and Sustainable

Mary Jane Rotheram-Borus, Diane Flannery, Naihua Duan

17.1   Introduction   – 235

17.2   Current Strategies for Preventing Negative
        Outcomes for Children   – 235
17.2.1 Designing the Prevention Program   – 235
17.2.2 Demonstrating a Program Is Evidence-Based   – 236

17.3   Proposed New Criteria: CURRES   – 237
17.3.1 Cost-Effective   – 237
17.3.2 Useful   – 238
17.3.3 Realistic   – 239
17.3.4 Robust   – 239
17.3.5 Evolve over Time   – 240
17.3.6 Sustainable   – 241

17.4   Summary and Conclusion   – 242

        References   – 242

17.1   Introduction

Currently, the United States is the single largest financial contributor to a prevention research portfolio, spending about $4 billion annually on psychosocial research (Kobor et al. 2002). The National Institutes of Health sets criteria for reviewers on which to evaluate newly proposed interventions (NIMH 2002; Public Health Service 2003). The primary criteria are that the intervention is theory-based (usually a social cognitive theory), innovative, has a solid research design with a detailed implementation plan, is led by competent researchers with a track record to implement the project, follows ethical principles, and has a reasonable budget. These criteria and a set of norms operating among review panels, government staff, and the research community structure a research portfolio with a set of characteristics. Our goals are to: (a) review the existing norms regarding »good« interventions, (b) suggest alternative criteria, and (c) examine the implications of the new criteria for the conduct of intervention research.

17.2   Current Strategies for Preventing Negative Outcomes for Children

17.2.1   Designing the Prevention Program

The rhetoric of intervention design is based on a linear process of systematically developing empirical theories. A great deal of the prevention research portfolio is devoted to the first step in the process: identifying risk and protective factors that provide a rationale for theories that underlie any specific intervention. Typically, at least 5 years of research are required to document the existence of deficits that interventions are aimed at improving. For example, when Sandler and colleagues began to address the challenges of children of divorce, a 5-year study of risk and protective factors in families coping effectively with divorce were compared to families who did not appear to be adjusting well (Sandler et al. 1991).

A complementary strategy is adopted by developmental psychopathologists; these researchers often focus on the types of skills that are necessary to effectively navigate predictable developmental challenges. For example, preadolescents are likely to confront challenges regarding their gender roles as males or females as their parents, teachers, and peers shift their culturally-based expectations about the preadolescent's social behaviors. Developmental psychopathologists often focus on building universal skills and normative beliefs that will assist children and families to successfully accomplish their age-specific tasks. However, documentation of the skills needed for successful development (e.g., Communities that Care; Hawkins and Catalano 1992) or the individual deficits or competencies that are linked to specific outcomes (e.g., drug use) provide little insight for how to design interventions for the targeted outcome. The identification of risk and protective factors does not guide how, when, or the context of behavior change programs. It addresses the content of an intervention, but not the delivery process. Little is learned in this linear approach to the strategies about how to change risk and protective factors.

For example, variations in children's interpersonal problem solving skills have been repeatedly linked to poor social outcomes across early and middle childhood, as well as adolescence (Spivack et al. 1976). Across children of different ages, social learning theory (Bandura 1994) is invoked to assist researchers in designing interventions to improve children's social problem solving (e.g., Spivack et al. 1976; Shure 1991). Programs are designed based on the learning principles of successive approximation, shaping, modeling, extinction, and generalization in order to reach specific, behaviorally defined goals. Some social learning programs emphasize identifying emotional states and teaching self-regulation as a skill (e.g., Wolpe 1953); others have a greater focus on cognitive skills (e.g., Meichenbaum 1993); and some shape social and personal identities (e.g., Oyserman 2001). Yet, while there are slight variations in emphasis of the social learning program, almost all successful prevention programs are grounded in a social learning model.

Researchers attempt to maximize the impact of their interventions by including skills in multiple domains (cognitive, emotional, and behavioral skills), linking a broad range of mediators (e.g., problem-solving coping style, self-regulation, self-system, role perceptions), generating as much social support for the change process as possible, both in members of the social network (e.g., typically implemented in small groups such as classrooms or family groups) and in the norms that characterize the group. Activities are generated in potentially four areas: (1) norms, expectations, and beliefs; (2) skills and competencies; (3) reducing environmental barriers to change or promoting environmental protectors; and (4) relationship factors, both those internal to the change process and those that are external (NIMH Intervention Workgroup 2001).

This social engineering is usually attempted around a very narrowly defined behavioral outcome: stopping drug use, stopping bullying, encouraging prosocial playground behavior, or delaying sexual debut. Once an attractive prevention program has been designed, through integration of a large number of strategic principles around a specific

goal, researchers attempt to demonstrate its effectiveness.

17.2.2 Demonstrating a Program Is Evidence-Based

Behavioral and social intervention research has been based on a model parallel to the model of biomedical interventions (Pequegnat and Stover 1994). There are four phases of research development of an intervention: (1) establishing safety; (2) identifying benefits of the innovative intervention; (3) proving efficacy, typically in a randomized controlled trial that is a proof of the concept; and (4) effectiveness trials mounted in real world settings. Each phase focuses on whether the prevention program will achieve change of a targeted behavior. There is little concern whether the prevention program will be utilized by providers, is within the skill repertoire of providers or existing funding streams, whether the intervention is consistent with the ability of targeted participants to attend and adhere to intervention activities or to sustain the behavior change over time.

These criteria have led to a focus on investigator driven, theoretically-based randomized controlled trials of interventions (Rotheram-Borus and Duan 2003). Phase I and II trials are typically accomplished by qualitative research conducted during the first 6 months of an intervention's development phase. After a relatively brief preparatory stage, there is implementation of a randomized controlled design or potentially a comparison and intervention community design. The National Institutes of Health typically funds studies of risk and protective factors, but not examinations of 10–15 strategies for combining various intervention components during extended exploratory phases I and II, in which dramatically different strategies for intervention delivery are tested empirically with relatively small samples. Almost immediately after conceptualizing an intervention need or specifying hypothesized risk and protective factors, pilot data are expected to be generated suggesting that a specific intervention strategy should be pursued.

The investment strategy used in behavioral prevention research is very conservative. In contrast, biomedical researchers in the pharmaceutical industry devote a substantial effort towards phase I and II trials (Heyd and Carlin 1999). Based on the data of DiMasi and colleagues (1991, 1995), 59% of the capitalized cost in clinical testing is devoted to phase I (27%) and phase II (32%) trials; only 41% is devoted to phase III trials. Development of new drugs is a risky business. Among candidate medicines tested in clinical trials, only 23% make it through phases I through III to be approved by the Food and Drug Administration (DiMasi et al. 1991, 1995). Similarly, the Pharmaceutical Research and Manufacturers Association (1999) estimates that approximately one in five potential medicines tested in clinical trials are approved by the FDA.

The pharmaceutical industry accepts the need to test a large number of potential drugs, knowing that the vast majority will end up as failures. The industry devotes substantial resources into those innovations, to give themselves an opportunity to find the next miracle drug like Prozac or Viagra. Miracle drugs do not come from miracles; they come from intensive research efforts and substantial investments. Successful drugs emerge from among a pyramid of experiments, supported by a solid (and costly) foundation of numerous failed innovations.

In social science, both the identification of innovative approaches and the testing of safety and benefits are underemphasized. Nor is there a focus on tailoring an efficacious intervention to a variety of different audiences. Once an effective behavioral intervention is identified, investigators typically want to replicate the program with fidelity (Bauman et al. 1991). Yet, the intervention must be tailored to different market segments (e.g., those motivated to change sexual risk because it limits future options vs. those who change for their partner) with different modalities (individual, small group, telephone, broadcast media) and in different contexts (physician offices, shopping malls, schools). These are typically conceptualized as phase IV questions, but these questions are rarely asked (i.e., effectiveness trials). After an efficacious intervention trial has been completed, review groups should ask: is a replication project with a different modality warranted?

Ultimately, there is an underlying assumption that real science is about creating an innovation. The applicability, accessibility, feasibility, and adoption of the innovation are not concerns of the »scientist«. However, there is no identified group, other than some government agencies (e.g., Center for Disease Control), who are responsible for taking science to the world. In contrast, application of innovations in the basic sciences has been further refined, modified, and marketed by private industry. Congress has established funding streams to facilitate the transfer of technologies from the basic laboratory sciences to profitable business enterprises

(NIH, Office of Extramural Research 2003). While this funding mechanism also is available for social and preventive sciences, it is used far less often in the behavioral sciences than in the biomedical sciences. A parallel process has been lacking for the social sciences to prepare prevention programs aimed at social outcomes to be taken to scale. If we focused on different criteria in the initial design of interventions, we might generate innovations in interventions, which make for broader adoptions of evidence-based programs.

17.3 Proposed New Criteria: CURRES

We propose that new interventions routinely be evaluated as to their cost-effectiveness (C), usefulness (U), ability to be realistically implemented in community settings (R), utilize robust components (R), have mechanisms to evolve over time (E), and are sustainable (S). Adopting a consumer focus is at the heart of these criteria (Duan et al. 2002). We must define consumers as not only the clients who may receive the intervention, but also the providers who must mount our interventions and the funders and policy makers whose ongoing support is necessary in order for the intervention to be sustainable.

17.3.1 Cost-Effective

In a climate of increasing fiscal responsibility for both private, nonprofit, and governmental sectors (Office of State Attorney General Eliot Spitzer 2003; Bradley et al. 2003; Riedl 2003), the cost-effectiveness of all potentially new interventions is going to be a key criterion used by policy makers to determine if funding streams should or can be designated for a new intervention or innovation. However, fiscal funding streams are not typically considered by prevention researchers when designing interventions. For example, in the world of HIV prevention, there have been 102 efficacious interventions identified in phase III efficacy trials (Rotheram-Borus et al. 2000). Yet, at best, only 17 of these interventions have cost-effectiveness evaluations that accompany the original efficacy trial. To increase the visibility and potential adoptability of interventions, economists must routinely be included on all intervention trials, and the costs of delivery should be considered throughout the development and evaluation phases of each new intervention. For example, our team designed an efficacious intervention for families living with HIV delivered in a small group format (Rotheram-Borus et al. 2001 a, b). It cost a $55 taxi ride and child care costs to deliver the intervention for each participant. It is unlikely that policy makers will ever authorize a fee of $55 to disenfranchised families to attend small groups. If an economist had been part of the initial design team, it is likely that other strategies would have been used to build social support for families with HIV other than a small group meeting in central Manhattan, New York that required an expensive cab ride. Internet, telephone, or peer visits may have accomplished the same goal with a less expensive price tag. Expanding research teams to routinely include economists at the beginning of designing interventions will lead to very different strategies for implementing an intervention.

Not only may cost-effectiveness assist in designing new interventions, but it may also guide which strategies should be pursued for interventions. In HIV prevention, increased HIV detection among those who are seropositive is one of the most cost-effective interventions available; yet, the international momentum is not for early HIV detection, but for funding antiretroviral therapies for persons living with HIV at a cost of US$125 to $14,000 annually (Shapiro et al. 1999). Postexposure prophylaxis with antiretroviral therapies is an expensive strategy that is not very viable for HIV prevention (Holtgrave 2002). In addition, it appears to be a strategy only used by highly educated white men in the United States, rather than by those who are members of the exploding epidemic among African-American and Latino men. If an economist was guiding the decisions on which preventive interventions should be pursued, the HIV intervention portfolio would look very different from that currently held by the National Institutes of Health in the United States. Over the past 20 years, substantial investment has demonstrated that psychosocial prevention programs can and do reduce risk among those routinely engaging in unprotected sexual and substance use acts. Again, an economic perspective is critical for each stage of the design, selection, tailoring, and implementation of preventive interventions.

17.3.2   Useful

Useful refers to the outcome of an intervention, as being relevant to the goals of society, policy makers, funders, providers, and consumers. Typically, an intervention is considered important on the basis of the significance of the problem that it seeks to impact and its ability to shed light on the utility of its theoretical underpinnings. An intervention is useful only if it is feasibly relevant and has benefits for each segment of consumers.

There are at least two components of consumer input that are important. First, is the intervention acceptable to the consumers? The example below demonstrates that the use of recreational vehicles as the intervention was not acceptable to the policy makers. Second, are the outcomes used in assessing the intervention relevant to the consumers? Many clinical interventions are focused on outcomes that are not that relevant to patients or their families.

The key is to have market research a formal procedure to establish the potential usefulness of the intervention before it is even designed. Yet, there are many examples in which the intervention's utility to a key audience is not considered during the design process. In the 1970s, one of the most innovative and effective preventive interventions was developed to reduce gang violence: providing gangs with recreational vehicles from which to engage in positive community activities (Schwitzgebel and Schwitzgebel 1980). While efficacious, no policy maker was willing to »reward« gang members with recreational vehicles in order to divert youth away from gang violence. Similarly, prevention researchers often care about children's problem solving ability and design school-based programs to improve problem solving skills. Yet, parents and teachers care less about problem solving and more about their ability to control children's behavior. Even though problem solving skills are highly related to children's social behaviors, the direct link may often not be relevant to teachers and administrators who must support implementation of the program. There are parallel examples in clinical interventions. For example, interventions may be targeted at reducing depressed or anxious feelings. Yet depressed clients and their families may care more about functional outcomes, such as the ability to hold a job.

Any intervention that is to be designed or delivered must gain the acceptance and endorsement of the stakeholders at every level: policy makers, funders, community leaders, providers, and consumers (i.e., perspective clients). Interventionists who design successful preventive interventions usually recognize the need to secure the endorsements and ownership of these stakeholders, even though this process is often not acknowledged within journal articles summarizing the research. Furthermore, market research may be needed to give interventionists the tools needed for the intervention to be useful to its consumers. In order for interventions to be acceptable and salient to stakeholders, it is often necessary to market to these populations or, at a minimum, to identify the potential gains for each stakeholder in the community whose operation may be impacted by the intervention. Again, this is often an implicit process, not well documented or considered a component of an evidence-based program.

17.3.3   Realistic

Interventionists are not typically guided by the feasibility of disseminating their intervention when in the design process. Demonstrating a »proof of concept«, that a particular intervention approach can be efficacious, is the typical standard. Yet, in many cases it is not feasible that the providers could implement a designed intervention. In the 1980s, most social workers and psychologists in New York City were trained in psychodynamic approaches to interventions (Feldman 1998). Yet, behavioral and cognitive-behavioral programs were proliferating. It is not feasible to implement behavioral programs with providers trained in psychodynamic approaches. Substantial commitment must be made to overcome the limitations and accommodate the capacities of providers to implement an intervention.

Currently, »capacity building« is a theme of much of the funding of organizations such as the Centers for Disease Control [e.g., CDC, Division of HIV/AIDS Prevention (DHAP), 2004]. Staff at community-based organizations can benefit substantially from technical assistance and skill-building activities (e.g., Cheadle et al. 2002; US Department of Health and Human Services 2002). In most social service agencies, however, the average length of employment is less than 2 years (US GAO 2003) and personnel turnover is high (Tebb 2002). Despite the efforts for capacity building, constant staff turnover will make sustained intervention very difficult. Rather than design programs that are beyond the abilities of the current staff, researchers should devote their efforts to designing programs that existing staff members can implement, by making the implementation procedures explicit and identifying the key stakeholder audiences.

17.3.4   Robust

The current emphasis on replication with fidelity has meant that many efficacious interventions contain multiple components and intervention strategies, with multiple persons in the environment involved (NIMH Intervention Workgroup 2001). For example, the Fast Track Project combines a number of family, peer, and school-focused intervention components for youth at high risk for significant conduct problems later in life (Bierman et al. 2002). When positive outcomes are observed, it is often unclear which components, strategies, or change agents were responsible for the benefits. For example, in the highly efficacious and cost-effective nurse home-visit program for infants (Olds et al. 1994, 2002), it is not clear why nurses are necessary in the intervention. Is it the training of nurses, society's attributions towards nurses, personality types, or some other characteristic that makes nurses desirable as the implementers of the program?

In order to answer fundamental questions about the robust ingredients in an intervention, it is critical to shift our research paradigms from phase I to a phase IV biomedical model of intervention development. Prior to efficacy (phase III) and effectiveness trials (phase IV), it is critical to consider that the »whole is greater than the sum of the parts« in preventive intervention programs. After a program has been shown to be efficacious, it would be desirable to conduct a series of small trials that identify the intervention's robust components, not a large effectiveness trial that answers whether a program will remain efficacious when mounted by typical clinicians in typical settings. Questions must be answered about the process of research: is the main intervention effect associated with the intervention facilitators, the social support provided, the skills imparted, the social norms that are changed, shifts in self-perceptions, or the social pressure generated by peers committed to behavior change? Few interventions have been examined in enough detail to begin to disentangle these effects and the synergistic impact of the combination of factors is not currently addressed in our theories or methodologies. For example, many interventionists have believed that a match is needed between the characteristics of the intervention and the deficits of the consumer targeted (e.g., COMMIT trial). Yet, there has been little empirical support for such a relationship and a failure to find effects in large trials.

In addition, issues associated with the delivery process such as consumer adherence to the intervention or provider fidelity to the program's manuals are defined by researchers as »problems« of consumers or providers. Consumers are often labeled uncooperative or nonadherent and blamed for not attending the intervention. If researchers used the considerable data amassed by private industry, they would attend much more closely to »market conditions« both in initial design of interventions and in tailoring the intervention to specific market segments once it has been developed.

For example, there are few psychosocial interventions offered in multiple modalities. Yet, some people prefer telephone contact, others the Internet, others need the support of a small group, and others prefer one-on-one contact. There are few studies that tailor a single intervention to delivery in multiple modalities. Yet, if we wanted to diffuse interventions broadly, we must recognize that this diversity is needed in dissemination strategies for a single intervention. Does the intervention increase or decrease its potency when delivered in alternative formats? There has been little research on these questions.

However, for most of society's major health problems, there are a range of treatment options. For smokers, there are programs based on self-help models (Smokefree.gov; QuitNet.org), biomedical interventions such as nicotine patches (Jolicoeur et al. 2003), a range of psychotherapeutic approaches (Abbot et al. 2000; Haustein 2003; Marlow and Stoller 2003), social marketing campaigns (e.g., TheTruth.com; National Library of Medicine 2003), and structural interventions (e.g., increase taxes; Leverett et al. 2002). Similarly, weight control is approached by a variety of for-profit companies that specialize in providing behavioral management strategies, drugs, food preparations, social support, and self-help strategies. Once a problem enters the private sector, experimentation in the range of options available for different market segments is widely conducted. When social problems are not perceived as having a market in the private sector, little experimentation occurs after a main effect has been demonstrated.

Duan and Rotheram-Borus (1999) have pointed to quality engineering as a model for researchers to improve their interventions on an ongoing basis (Demmings 1986). Once a positive intervention effect has been observed, product developers in private enterprise companies experiment to streamline the intervention program and eliminate or de-emphasize nonessential ingredients. Quality engineers make efforts to build quality into the product design, so that the product will perform satisfactorily without demanding the consumer to read and follow detailed instructions. They recognize consumers' preferences on issues such as color, size, and taste, and design the products to accommodate such preferences. They also build in safeguards to ensure that the product can tolerate a reasonable level of consumer abuse and misuse, such as not following the recipes exactly. Product developers, product disseminators, and marketers collaborate seamlessly in private enterprise models that broadly impact the culture and create new markets. Psychosocial researchers could benefit from such perspectives and by introducing experts in these areas in the initial design of psychosocial interventions.

Entrepreneurs typically perceive an opportunity to satisfy or to create a need among consumers. In social science preventive programs, the need to mount a trial or to offer a service arises from the consumer or perceived consumer need. Social science researchers often perceive a need that the consumer may not want to change. Smoking is a pleasurable habit to most smokers and it is only social pressure, fear of negative consequences, payment of high personal costs to maintain the habit, and a desire to be socially responsible that may motivate many people to shift this highly addictive habit. Marketers and product developers could assist researchers in considering these issues for solving serious public health problems, rather than selling video recorders, soap, or deodorant.

17.3.5   Evolve over Time

The conditions that elicit the need for an intervention shift over time. Stopping smoking in the year 2004 has many different characteristics from stopping smoking in 1970.

Environmental shifts occur: in 1970, approximately 33% of women and 43% of men 18 or older in the US population smoked (MMWR 1999); there were no bans in public places against smoking, and there was controversy about the validity of data demonstrating that smoking caused cancer. Advertisements that may have been effective in 1970 are unlikely to be effective in the present. Most psychosocial interventions are designed with the perspective that adaptation and evolution are not useful: replication with fidelity is a holy grail.

In addition to the environmental shifts that demand reexamination of efficacious programs, there are two other forces that demand that programs evolve over time. First, the definition of a problem shifts dramatically as the perception of issues evolves from the fringe to becoming mainstream. When an issue has reached the »tipping point«, it will become mainstream and the strategies used to shift the behavior must also change. Different populations must be addressed when a problem is only among »fringe« persons in contrast to when the mainstream has adopted a behavior or a perspective. When dealing with children and families, developmental shifts lead to changes in the individual's capacities to understand and/or exert control over the circumstances maintaining the problem.

The benefits of the evolution of an intervention program over time were most evident for our research team on a project implemented in Calcutta, India (Basu et al. in press; Jana et al. in press). The Sonagachi Project (Dugger 1999) is an intervention with sex workers that has been slated for replication and dissemination by the Gates Foundation to reduce the risk of HIV among sex workers. In its initial implementation, a high-status Brahmin medical doctor bartered employment conditions of sex workers with the pimps, police, and political officials that controlled the lives of sex workers. It was not in the financial best interests of these stakeholder groups if sex workers became infected with HIV; therefore, there were economic incentives that allowed the doctor in charge of occupational health to mount the program. The program involved establishing a clinic to treat sexually transmitted diseases and visits by peer educators (i.e., other sex workers) to encourage protection of one's sexual health. Over time this program grew, evolved, and expanded. It now is a social enterprise that sells condoms, loans money, runs group homes, teaches reading to children of sex workers, and has become a social movement as an international trade union with about 60,000 workers. The process by which this intervention was transformed from an occupational health intervention to a social movement would not have been allowed if this was an evidence-based intervention.

It is critical that researchers begin to recognize the need for evolution of interventions over time and to design strategies that collect and analyze the evolutions over time so that improvements can be noted, emphasized, and replicated. Simultaneously, innovations that detract from robust outcomes must not be maintained. Researchers are needed throughout the dissemination process.

The concept of sustained involvement of researchers as programs evolve is typically perceived as an undesirable role. Researchers want to be innovators and not the people who take the intervention to scale or maintain its relevance over time. Researchers often assume that the identification of a program effect is the accomplishment of science and solving the technological glitches involved in mounting and implementing a program is the role of social workers, technocrats, or program evaluators. It is such attitudes that keep efficacious psychosocial interventions unused and not broadly disseminated.

17.3.6   Sustainable

Some of the most vexing behavioral problems are associated with chronic conditions. For example, weight control, smoking, alcohol abuse, and sexual risk reduction are behaviors whose risk emerges over time as new developmental challenges are encountered. Yet, our intervention programs are designed to work on models that are more similar to immunizations; a single dose is delivered and expected to shift risk for a sustained period of time. Relapse prevention is an entire field in psychosocial intervention and not routinely designed into the initial prevention programs. Changing a behavior is influenced by factors quite different from those that will sustain the change over time (NIMH Intervention Workgroup 2001). It is critical to plan for feasible methods to maintain positive outcomes over time. In addition, physical and mental health symptoms are likely to rise and fall repeatedly over this period, having a concurrent positive and negative impact on children. Children's developmentally linked needs will also shift; for example, as children become old enough to drive an automobile, the types of risk situations that they encounter are dramatically different and require their own type of intervention (Paikoff et al. 1995). A strategy for providing ongoing support and skill training for newly emerging challenges is routinely needed. Again, this calls for innovations by the researchers. First, we must emphasize to consumers and providers that change is slow, must be maintained, and needs intermittent reinforcement over time. Second, researchers must select delivery sites that are accessible on an ongoing basis in order to sustain behavior change over time. In general, this recommendation calls for shifting the basis of most advertising in the United States from a »quick fix« to a »long-term quality life«.

17.4   Summary and Conclusion

The field of preventive psychosocial interventions has grown dramatically over the last 30 years, demonstrating that programs can and do change people's behavior, especially the behaviors of children and families. There are many opportunities, however, for improvement in the existing norms and strategies used by researchers to exact this behavior change. In particular, the members of research teams designing and evaluating must be expanded to include economists, marketers, product developers, quality engineers, and delivery experts. The norms regarding the field of research must be shifted in order to encourage an emphasis on intervention delivery, the consumers of our research (i.e., clients, policy makers, providers), providing diversity in delivery formats, and identification of robust components of the research. Efficacious intervention programs must be made »consumer proof«, not able to be easily derailed by a failure to implement with fidelity or to provide intensive training and feedback. Finally, programs must be allowed and encouraged to evolve over time and to be designed initially to anticipate the need for sustained interventions over time. By re-examining our intervention models, we may be able to design programs that substantially increase their applicability to real-world challenges faced by children and families on a daily basis.

Acknowledgements. This work was completed with the support of National Institute of Mental Health grants #1ROI MH49958-04 and P30 MH58107.

References

Abbot NC, Stead LF, White AR, Barnes J, Ernst E (2000) Hypnotherapy for smoking cessation. Cochrane Database Syst Rev 2:CD001008

Bandura A (1994) Social Cognitive Theory and Exercise of Control over HIV infection. In: DiClemente R, Peterson, JL, eds. Preventing AIDS: Theories and Methods of behavioral Interventions. New York, NY: Plenum Press, pp. 25–59

Basu I, Jana S, Rotheram-Borus MJ, Swendeman D, Lee S-J, Newman P, Weiss R (In press) HIV Prevention Among Sex Workers in India. JAIDS

Bauman LJ, Stein RE, Ireys HT (1991) Reinventing fidelity: the transfer of social technology among settings. Am J Community Psychol 19:619–639

Bierman KL, Coie JD, Dodge KA, Greenberg MT, Lochman JE, McMahon RJ, Pinderhughes EE (2002) Conduct Problems Prevention Research Group. Using the Fast Track randomized prevention trial to test the early-starter model of the development of serious conduct problems. Dev Psychopathol 14(4):925–943

Box GEP, Draper NR (1987) Empirical Model-Building and Response Surfaces. New York: John Wiley & Sons Publishing.

Bradley B, Jansen P, Silverman L (2003, May) The Nonprofit Sector's $100 Billion Opportunity. Harvard Business Review.

Centers for Disease Control, Division of HIV/AIDS Prevention (DHAP) (2004) Capacity Building Assistance Announcement # 04019 Application Kit. Available at: http://www.cdcnpin.org/scripts/pa04019/. Accessed on January 6, 2004

Cheadle A, Sullivan M, Krieger J, Ciske S, Shaw M, Schier JK, Eisinger A (2002) Using a participatory approach to provide assistance to community-based organizations: the Seattle Partners Community Research Center. Health Educ Behav 29(3):383–394

Demmings WE (1986) Out of the Crisis. Massachusetts: MIT Press.

DiMasi JA, Hansen RW, Grabowski HG, Lasagna L (1991) Cost of innovation in the pharmaceutical industry. J Health Econ 10:107–142

DiMasi JA, Hansen RW, Grabowski HG, Lasagna L (1995) Research and Development Costs for New Drugs by Therapeutic Category: A Study of the US Pharmaceutical Industry. PharmacoEconomics 7(2):152–169

Duan, N, Rotheram-Borus MJ (1999) Development and dissemination of successful behavioral prevention interventions: Safety, innovation, essential ingredients, robustness, and marketability. In: Translating prevention research into social work practice [Monograph]. University of Washington School of Social Work Prevention Research Center

Duan N, Gonzales J, Braslow J, Chambers D, Kravitz R (2002) Evidence in mental health services research: what types, how much, and then what? Opening remarks presented at NIMH Conference, Washington, DC, April 1.

Dugger CW. »Dead Zones: Fighting Back in India: Calcutta's Prostitutes Lead the Fight on AIDS.« New York Times, January 4, 1999, sec. A, p. 2

Feldman HA, McKinlay JB, Potter DA, Freund KM, Burns RB, Moskowitz MA, Kasten LE (1997) Nonmedical Influences on a Medical Decision Making: An Experimental Technique Using Videotapes, Factorial Design, and Survey Sampling. Health Services Research 32:3

Feldman RA (1998) Celebrating America's real heroes: Three months to the second century. Available at: http://www.naswnyc.org/p16.html. Accessed on January 7, 2004

Haustein KO (2003) What can we do in secondary prevention of cigarette smoking? Journal of Cardiovascular Risk 10(6):476–485

Hawkins JD, Catalano RF Jr. (1992) Communities that Care: Action for Drug Abuse Prevention. San Francisco: Jossey-Bass

Heyd JM, Carlin BP (1999) Adaptive design improvements in the continual reassessment method for Phase 1 studies. Statistics in Medicine 18:1307–1321

Holtgrave (2002) Estimating the effectiveness and efficiency of US HIV prevention efforts using scenario and cost-effectiveness analysis. AIDS 6(17):2347–2349

Jana S, Basu I, Rotheram-Borus MJ, Newman PA. The Sonagachi Project: A Sustainable Community Intervention Program. AIDS Educ Prev (in press).

Jolicoeur DG, Richter KP, Ahluwalia JS, Mosier MC, Resnicow K (2003) Smoking cessation, smoking reduction, and delayed quitting among smokers given nicotine patches and a self-help pamphlet. Subst Abus 24(2):101–106

Kobor P, Wurtz S, Johnson D (2002) Behavioral and Social Sciences Research in the FY 2003 Budget. Washington DC: American Association for the Advancement of Science. Available at: http://www.aaas.org/spp/rd/03pch20.htm. Accessed on January 7, 2004

Leverett M, Ashe M, Gerard S, Jenson J, Woollery T (2002) Tobacco use: the impact of prices. Journal of Law and Medical Ethics 30(3 Suppl):88–95

Marlow SP, Stoller JK (2003) Smoking cessation. Respiratory Care 48(12):1238–1254; discussion 1254–1256

Meichenbaum D (1993) Changing conceptions of cognitive behavior modification: retrospect and prospect. J Consult Clin Psychol 61(2):202–204

MMWR (1999) Achievements in Public Health, 1900–1999: Tobacco Use – United States, 1900–1999. Available at: http://www.cdc.gov/mmwr/preview/mmwrhtml/mm4843a2.htm#fig2. Accessed on December 12, 2003

The National Advisory Mental Health Council Workgroup on Child and Adolescent Mental Health Intervention Development and Deployment. (2001). Blueprint for Change: Research on Child and Adolescent Mental Health. Washington DC. http://www.nimh.nih.gov/child/blueprin. pdf

National Institutes of Health (NIH), Office of Extramural Research (2003) Small Business Innovation Research (SBIR) and Small Business Technology Transfer (STTR) Programs. Available at: http://grants.nih.gov/grants/funding/sbirsttr_programs. htm. Accessed on: January 7, 2004

National Library of Medicine (2003) Visual culture and public health posters: anti-smoking campaigns. Available at: http://www.nlm.nih.gov/exhibition/visualculture/anti-smoking.html. Accessed on: January 6, 2004

NIMH Intervention Workgroup (Bellack A, Elkin I, Flay B et al.) (2001) An integrated framework for preventive and treatment interventions. Presented at the National Institute of Mental Health Intervention Workgroup Meeting, Washington DC, November 12–14

NIMH (2002) Psychotherapeutic Interventions: How and Why they Work. Available at: http://www.nimh.nih.gov/research/interventions.cfm. Accessed on: December 5, 2003

Office of State Attorney General Elliot Spitzer (2003, February) State Suit Targets Illegal Pricing Scheme for Cancer Drugs: Spitzer Cites Bribery, Kickbacks and False Statements by Leading Drug Companies. Available at: http://www.oag.-state.ny.us/press/2003/feb/feb13a_03.html. Accessed on: December 22, 2003

Olds D, Henderson CR, Jr, Kitzman H (1994) Does prenatal and infancy nurse home visitation have enduring effects on qualities of parental caregiving and child health at 25 to 50 months of age? Pediatrics 93:89–98

Olds DL, Robinson J, O'Brien R, et al. (2002) Home visiting by paraprofessionals and by nurses: a randomized, controlled trial. Pediatrics 110:486–496

Oyserman D (2001) Self and Identity. In: A Tesso, N Schwarz, eds. Blackwell Handbook of Social Psychology, Oxford University Press, pp. 499–517

Paikoff RL (1995) Early heterosexual debut: situations of sexual possibility during the transition to adolescence. Am J Orthopsychiat 65:389–401

Pequegnat W, Stover E (1994) Strategies to improve research on behavioral issues in HIV vaccine trials. Int Conf AIDS, Aug 7–12;10(2):402 (abstract no. PD0790)

Pharmaceutical Research and Manufacturers Association (1999) Leading the Way in the Search for Cure. Available at: http://www.phrma.org/publications/publications/brochure/leading/. Accessed on January 8, 2004

Public Health Service (2003) PSC Form 398. Available at: http://forms.psc.gov/forms/PHS/phs.html. Accessed on January 2, 2004

Rabkin R, Rabkin J (1995) Management of depression in patients with HIV infection. Caring 14:28–30, 32, 34

Riedl BM (2003) The Quiet Earthquake in Spending. Press Room Commentary. The National Heritage Foundation. Available at: http://www.heritage.org/Press/Commentary/ed112403b.cfm. Accessed on January 2, 2004

Rotheram-Borus MJ, Duan N (2003) Next generation of preventive interventions. JAm Acad Child Psy 42(5):518–26.

Rotheram-Borus MJ, Cantwell SM, Newman PA (2000). HIV prevention programs with heterosexuals. AIDS, 14:1–9

Rotheram-Borus MJ, Lee MB, Gwadz M, Draimin B (2001a) An intervention for parents with AIDS and their adolescent children. Am J Public Health 91:1294–1302

Rotheram-Borus MJ, Stein JA, Lin YY (2001b) Impact of parent death and an intervention on the adjustment of adolescents whose parents have HIV/AIDS. J Consult Clin Psych 69:763–773

Sandler IN, Wolchik SA, Braver SL, Fogas BS (1991) Stability and quality of life events and psychological symptomatology in children of divorce [Special Issue]: Preventive Intervention Research Centers. Am J Commun Psychol 19:501–520

Schwitzgebel RL, Schwitzgebel RK (1980) Law and psychological practice. New York: Wiley

Shapiro MF, Morton SC, McCaffrey DF, Andersen RM, Berk ML, Bing EG, Cleary PD, Cunningham WE, Fleishman JA, Kanouse DE, Senterfitt JW, Bozzette SA (1999) HTV/AIDS Care in the United States II. Variations in Receipt of Care: Initial Results from the HIV Cost and Services Utilization Study. J Am Med Assoc 281(24):2305–2315

Spivack G, Platt JJ, Shure MB (1976) The problem solving approach to adjustment. San Francisco: Jossey-Bass

Tebb S (2002) Overworked child welfare workers need proper training. Available at: http://www.slu.edu/readstory/newsinfo/2037.html

US Department of Health and Human Services (2002, October 3) Press Release: HHS Awards $30 Million to Help Level Playing Field for Faith-Based and Community Institutions. Available at: http://www.hhs.gov/news/press/2002pres/20021003a.html. Accessed on: January 6, 2004

US General Accounting Office (GAO) (2003) Child Welfare: HHS Could Play a Greater Role in Helping Child Welfare Agencies Recruit and Retain Staff. GAO-03–357 March 31, 2003.

Wolpe J (1953) Learning theory and abnormal fixations. Psychol Rev 60(2):111–116

Prevention of Risks for Mental Health Problems: Lessons Learned in Examining the Prevention of Depression in Families

William R. Beardslee, Tracy R.G. Gladstone

18.1   Key Concepts   – 245
18.1.1   The Preventive Intervention Research Cycle   – 245
18.1.2   Developmental Plasticity   – 246
18.1.3   The Ecological Framework   – 246
18.1.4   Focus on the Long-Term Futures of Children   – 246
18.1.5   Developmental Perspective   – 246
18.1.6   Prevention and Treatment   – 247

18.2   Risks and Protective Factors   – 247
18.2.1   Risk Factors   – 247
18.2.1.1 Adult Depression   – 247
18.2.1.2 Childhood Depression   – 247
18.2.1.3 Children of Depressed Parents   – 248
18.2.2   Protective Factors   – 248
18.2.3   How Risk/Protective Factors Work Together –
          The Example of Families Facing Adversity   – 249

18.3   Examples of Preventive Intervention
          Programs   – 250
18.3.1   Clarke's Preventive Intervention   – 250
18.3.2   Seligman's Penn Preventive Intervention   – 251
18.3.3   Boston Preventive Intervention Project   – 252

18.4   Healthcare Policy Perspectives: Systems Support
          and Reform for Prevention   – 252

18.5   Summary and Conclusions   – 253

          References   – 254

The understanding of risks and outcome for psychopathology in children and adolescents has advanced dramatically over the past 20 years. Correspondingly, so has the understanding of protective factors. The development and evaluation of preventive intervention programs are informed by such advances. Indeed, in some ways, the scientific basis for the development of preventive interventions is the understanding of normal development and its vicissitudes. The purpose of this chapter is to discuss some recent developments in our understanding of risk and protective factors in youth, and to illustrate how such understanding has been used in the design of preventive interventions. We will use the example of empirical prevention approaches for adolescent depression, as a discussion of prevention programs for other diagnoses is beyond the scope of this chapter.

We will begin with a review of several key concepts that will guide our discussion of risk and prevention. We will then discuss current research on risks and protective factors for mental health problems. We will review studies that have applied this research on risk and protective factors to the development of prevention programs for adolescent depression. Finally, we will offer some overall conclusions and recommendations.

18.1   Key Concepts

In any discussion of preventive intervention approaches, a number of key concepts provide an important background.

18.1.1   The Preventive Intervention Research Cycle

Preventive interventions typically move through a series of phases (IOM 1994). Following public health traditions, the first stage is the identification of the problem. The second stage is the understanding of risk factors and protective factors and the mechanisms underlying these. The third stage is the design of theoretically driven preventive interventions to address reduction of risk, and enhancement of the protective capacities primarily through pilot studies and efficacy trials. The fourth stage involves taking findings from successful efficacy studies to large-scale effectiveness trials. Finally, large-scale programs are developed. More recently, investigators have come to understand that this is not a simple progression but, indeed, that understandings at different stages can mutually inform one another. For example, consideration of how programs can be taken to scale should be built into the design of efficacy studies. Furthermore, effectiveness and programmatic investigations may indeed suggest new preventive interventions for testing in efficacy studies and may even help to uncover basic mechanisms of risk and protective processes (Blueprint for Change, NIMH 2002).

18.1.2   Developmental Plasticity

Central to advances in a variety of scientific inquiries has been increasing awareness of the concept of developmental plasticity (Beardslee 2002). Whereas in earlier models, fixed deficits were expected in response to risks or indeed actual injury to the developing nervous system of a growing child, investigators are increasingly aware of a variety of pathways that emerge across development and allow children to overcome both risks and episodes of illness (Beardslee 2002). The finding of resilience across a wide array of studies of youngsters who are faced with unusual adversities is one example of the phenomenon of developmental plasticity (Luthar et al. 2000). As another, it is evident that the expression even of genetic endowment is heavily influenced by the environment surrounding the child. A strong positive caregiver-infant bond facilitates the development of the infant in multiple domains including the development and myelinization of the nervous system. The bond as it evolves also influences the caregivers. Dr. Leon Eisenberg emphasized environmental influences in a recent and important paper with the apt title »The Social Construction of the Human Brain« (1995).

18.1.3   The Ecological Framework

Another key concept is awareness of the »ecological framework« surrounding the child (Bronfenbrenner 1979). A child's development is profoundly influenced by multiple factors at multiple levels including the child's caregivers, siblings, school, neighborhood, home, community, health care system, and State and Federal political systems. The direct influence of these factors changes across the span of childhood with peers, schools, and neighborhoods gaining greater influence as the child matures. In

conceptualizing the various domains that present opportunities for preventive intervention, understanding the ecological framework is important. For example, in fostering a strong bond between parents and the developing infant in the first year of life, family leave policies, health insurance, the attitudes and perspectives of religious and community organizations, and the availability of extended family support all exert measurable and powerful influences in addition to what goes on in the developmental transactions between the infant and his or her caregivers. Each could be the target of a prevention strategy; indeed, several could be targeted simultaneously (Beardslee and Knitzer 2003).

18.1.4   Focus on the Long-Term Futures of Children

Preventive intervention inevitably focuses resources on the long-term future of children and their families. Prevention involves considering what the child or family will need one, two, five, and ten years from the time of initial contact. By considering multiple frames of influence, prevention scientists aim to put into place supports, opportunities, and the encouragement of capacities that will increase the likelihood of a healthy development.

18.1.5   Developmental Perspective

The study and implementation of preventive interventions inevitably involves a developmental perspective. Preventive intervention trials enroll individuals who are not ill; thus, considerable time is required to evaluate the effects of interventions. This is in contrast to clinical trials in which subjects are enrolled when they are acutely ill and the expected outcome is recovery within a relatively short period of time. Preventive interventions aim to influence processes and mechanisms that, in the end, will foster long-term positive development. Moreover, the evaluation of preventive intervention programs involves following youngsters over long periods of time as they undergo various phases of development in the building of self-sustaining resources.

18.1.6   Prevention and Treatment

Preventive interventions aim to build resources and capacities in individuals, families, and social systems that will eventually become self-sustaining. In our experience, preventive intervention and treatment are inseparable, but there needs to be both administrative support for prevention and recognition of the differences between prevention and treatment (Beardslee 1998). As one example, the clinician doing treatment often sees the family in the midst of an acute episode of illness and is regarded as the expert. The preventionist performs much of his or her work not at a time of crisis and is regarded more as a partner than an expert (Beardslee 1998).

18.2   Risks and Protective Factors

An understanding of the risk factors for mental illness, and how these risk factors interact, is essential to the design, evaluation, and implementation of successful preventive intervention programs. In addition, an understanding of the protective factors associated with mental health is equally important. Below, we will outline research on risk and protective factors, again with a focus on the example of depression.

18.2.1   Risk Factors

18.2.1.1   Adult Depression

The list below presents the well-identified risk factors for depression in adulthood (Institute of Medicine 1994):
1. Having a parent or other close biological relative with a mood disorder
2. Experiencing a severe stressor such as a loss, divorce, marital separation, unemployment, job dissatisfaction, a physical disorder such as a chronic medical illness, a traumatic experience, or in children, a learning disorder
3. Experiencing low self-esteem, a sense of low self-efficacy, and a sense of helplessness and hopelessness
4. Being female
5. Living in poverty.

Many of these are also potent risk factors for depression in children. What is striking is that the risk factors cluster in two main areas: family history, and

living in chronic difficult life circumstances or undergoing negative life events. It is worth noting that many of the factors associated with negative life circumstances and adverse life events are nonspecific, although potent for depression. That is, exposure to trauma is a risk factor for many negative outcomes, not just depression. The same is true for poverty. For example, in the Epidemiological Catchment Area (Bruce et al. 1991) study of the New Haven site, poverty accounted for 10% of the onsets of new episodes of depression in a one-year period, and it was also a risk factor for other disorders.

Interventions could be designed to approach each of these risk factors. In addressing risk factors, preventionists inevitably think about both the larger nonspecific risks and the specific risks associated with the targeted disorder. In the case of depression, in addition to the nonspecific risk factors, the specific risk factors of family history, experiences of loss, and persistent feelings of helplessness and hopelessness have emerged as particularly powerful.

Also, a preventive intervention designed to address a nonspecific risk factor may have important consequences for the prevention of a specific disorder. Thus, the Jobs Retraining Program, developed by Rick Price and associates (1992), has been shown to be effective in helping people become reemployed. In a two-year follow-up, this intervention has also been shown to reduce episodes of depression.

18.2.1.2   Childhood Depression

Turning specifically to children at risk for depression, two kinds of studies are most useful: large studies of systematically chosen youth, some of whom become depressed, and studies of the children of depressed parents. As regards the former, Lewinsohn and colleagues (1994) used diagnostic rating scales and questionnaires to assess over 1,500 high school students at two points in time. They found that 17.4% of the participants had a history of depression. Diagnoses of the parents were not ascertained. Past psychopathology of suicide attempts, a depressogenic cognitive style, negative body image, low self esteem, emotional dependence, self consciousness, less effective coping, less support, and cigarette smoking were associated with depression at the time of interview, while a history of depression was associated with internalizing problem behaviors, reduced coping skills, and low self esteem. Thus, in terms of thinking about preventive interventions, negative cognitions, low social support, and ineffective coping are particularly important.

A long-term study of youngsters enrolled when they were 5 years old (Reinherz et al. 1989, 1999, 2000) identified a range of risk factors for depression including anxious and depressed feelings and a lack of peer acceptance. Specific risk factors were also identified for boys and for girls. For boys, neonatal problems and poor health development were risk factors for depression; for girls, risk factors included family composition, death of a parent, and difficulties in school. In older adolescents, career difficulties, financial stress, poor relationships with parents, lack of support, and negative life events predicted outcome. Reinherz's elegant work following a sample over decades emphasizes two points often found in risk studies: (a) the risk factors for a particular disorder are somewhat different for boys and girls, and (b) risk factors are different at different developmental epochs, i.e., young childhood versus adolescence.

18.2.1.3 Children of Depressed Parents

Numerous studies have documented increased rates of depression and related disorders in children from homes with parents with mood disorders, relative to children who live with parents who are not ill (Beardslee et al. 1998). There is a considerable variability in rates, but in general the diagnosis of depression occurs at least 2–4 times more often in children of depressed parents than in children whose parents are not depressed. Risk factors for depression in this group may include genetic factors in some depressions, although little is known at present about the genetics of childhood and adolescent depression. A genetic influence is suggested by the clustering of depressions in some families, although this is not definitive evidence. Clearly, as we understand the complexities of the sequencing of the human genome and the multiple ways in which the environment influences gene expression across development, we will be better able to identify those at highest risk and also ways to develop prevention strategies to specifically address these high risk groups. It is likely that there is considerable heterogeneity in the genetic factors in depression. As we understand heterogeneity better, we will also be better able to understand the delicate and multiple ways that genes influence environment and environment influences genes. As one example, recently, investi-

gators in Dunedin, New Zealand were able to isolate a functional polymorphism in a serotonin transporter gene (Caspi et al. 2003). Individuals who had the short allele had more depression and symptoms of depression in response to difficult life events than those who had the long allele. This provides evidence of a gene environment interaction. A recent discussion by Drs. Rutter and Silberg is illuminating in providing a useful perspective on the various kinds of interactions between genes and environment that may occur in adolescent depression (Silberg and Rutter 2002).

18.2.2 Protective Factors

The study of protective factors for mental illness is frequently overlooked. Yet, research indicates that many individuals who have risk factors for illness actually do quite well. For example, despite the high risk for depression and other forms of psychopathology in children of depressed parents, a number of researchers have demonstrated that many youngsters who grow up with ill parents actually remain healthy. These »resilient« individuals exhibit the ability to adapt successfully despite the presence of significant adversity. Understanding such qualities offers important opportunities for preventive intervention (Garmezy 1985; Rutter 1987).

Luthar, Cicchetti, and Becker (2000) define resilience as a »dynamic developmental construct« that leads to competence in the face of adversity. For understanding both risk and resilience, Sameroff and Chandler (1987) and Cicchetti and Shneider-Rosen (1986) have argued that a developmental transactional framework is the most useful perspective. In this, although risk factors for depression or other diseases may be stable and static, the processes that lead either to psychopathology or health are dynamic and are profoundly influenced by changes across the life span. Moreover, across development, systems and individuals mutually influence one another. The temperament of a particular child may call for a particular response from a caregiver. That same temperament in another child may call forth a different response from a different caregiver. The interaction between caregiver and child early in life may influence the child's development and indeed the caregiver's development later. The successful accomplishment of a particular stage in childhood, be that learning to speak or walk or learning to read, may in and of itself influence the caregivers or the teacher in positive ways.

Garmezy (1985) has argued that resilience can best be understood in three domains: the child, the family, and the community. Werner and Smith's (1982) study on the Island of Hawaii provides an important illustration of the complexity of protective factors and opportunities for preventive intervention and also shows factors in each of the three domains. They found that for youngsters growing up exposed to multiple adversities (e.g., poverty, sometimes ill health, victimization by racism), strong relationships with the mother and the father and living in a relatively small family served as protective factors in infancy and young childhood. Relationships were protective in general across the span of childhood and adolescence. During childhood, strong relationships with siblings and parents also proved to be protective; later, peer relationships served a protective function. Moreover, early in life, a match between parental expectations and the particular temperament that the child displayed was adaptive. In addition, high quality parenting was important both in expressing support, and also in providing structure, rule setting, and expectations. As the youngsters progressed into the developmental phase of adolescence, community, religious organizations, schools, and peers were more important. As they approached young adulthood, the availability of employment, education, mentoring, and social support were vital.

In terms of protective factors for adolescent depression, in a study of resilient youth with depressed parents, Beardslee and Podorefsky (1988) found that resilient youngsters were activists, deeply involved in school and extracurricular activities, and deeply committed to interpersonal relationships. Resilient youngsters also were found to have considerable self-understanding. Self-understanding involved recognizing the parents' illness, the youngsters' believing that they were not to blame, and understanding that they were free to go on with their own lives. These domains have been identified in a variety of other studies of resilience (Masten et al. 1990; Kupfer and DeMarsh 1985). Related work by Carbonell and colleagues (2002), using the data from the Reinherz longitudinal study showed that youngsters who were resilient had higher levels of family cohesion, higher self concept and self appreciation, a more positive outlook on life, more positive peer relationships, and they enjoyed spending time in the company of others.

18.2.3 How Risk/Protective Factors Work Together – The Example of Families Facing Adversity

A number of researchers have found that risk and protective factors work in concert to produce their effects. Rutter and Quinton (1977) examined the effect of the assembly of risk factors on the Isle of Wright and later in inner city London looking at outcomes in 10-year-old children. The factors they examined were severe marital discord, low social status, overcrowding, large family size, paternal criminality, maternal psychiatric disorder, and admission into the care of local authorities (foster care). Those youngsters with a single risk factor were no more likely to present with a psychiatric disorder than children with no risk factors. However, as the number of risk factors increased, the likelihood of childhood psychopathology increased as well. The risk was significantly greater than the simple sum of the effects.

Looking at younger children and focusing on maternal illness, Sameroff and colleagues (1998) found similar effects on the cumulative impact of risk factors on child outcome by enrolling mothers with four types of psychiatric disorder and examining their youngsters shortly after birth and then over a ten-year period. They found that a range of risk factors (e.g., severity of mental illness, minority status, the presence of adverse life events, large family size, lack of social support) working in combination led to greater risk than any single factor alone. They similarly found that the presence of a single risk factor did not lead to major developmental problems, but when the number of risk factors increased, competence decreased. Moreover, it was not the diagnostic category of the parents but the level of impairment that led to poor outcome. Perhaps most importantly, children who came from homes where parents were poor and uneducated but non-ill fared less well than did children living in more well-to-do circumstances, even when their parents had a serious psychiatric illness. This emphasizes the importance of social class and neighborhood in examining risk.

In the case of children of depressed parents, it is the assembly of adversities that predicts who becomes depressed or develops other difficulties, rather than any one factor alone (Beardslee et al. 1996).

It is important to note that the presence of family history in leading to psychopathology in children does not imply necessarily a genetic mechanism and certainly not entirely a genetic mechanism. To begin with, children experience the same adversities as their parents, and there may be a direct effect (e.g., in a family, the loss of bereavement may have an effect on the child directly as well as on the parent, or in a job loss, diminished economic status). Also, it is often difficult to separate genetic and psychosocial influences and almost impossible to weigh the relative balance because the parenting and social functioning of parents is impaired by their depression.

Large scale epidemiologic studies have identified factors that produce general, negative influences on children's development and have shown how these factors work together. Also, just as an assembly of adversities is most likely to cause a poor outcome in these children, an assembly of protective resources in multiple domains is most likely to protect them (Aarons et al. 1999). This is the place where the opportunities for preventive intervention reside and, indeed multiple preventative interventions across developmental epochs of childhood may have a cumulative effect. (Yoshikawa 1994).

18.3 Examples of Preventive Intervention Programs

Although there is a dearth of research focused on prevention programs for depression, a few such programs have been developed. Specifically, Clarke and colleagues (2001) have studied prevention in adolescents at risk for depression, Seligman and colleagues (Jaycox et al. 1994) have examined the prevention of depression in a school-based program, and Beardslee and colleagues (2003) have examined a family-based approach to the prevention of depression in youth. These programs have in common an emphasis on empirical evaluation through randomized trial designs, strong links to cognitive behavioral traditions, the targeting of specific risk by well-identified risk processes and, above all, an emphasis on building strengths and resources. Each of these programs will be reviewed below.

18.3.1 Clarke's Preventive Intervention

Based on the social learning model of depression, and on research by Lewinsohn and colleagues examining risk for depression in adolescents (1994), Clarke and Lewinsohn (1995) developed the Coping with Stress (CWS) course, a manual-based psycho-

educational group program that targets adolescents who are at risk for the development of significant depressive disorders. CWS is a modification of the Coping with Depression Course for Adolescents (CWDA; Clarke et al. 1990), which was developed for use with clinically depressed adolescents. It aims to assist vulnerable adolescents in gaining control over negative moods, resolving conflicts that arise at home and with peers, and altering maladaptive thought patterns. The basic premise is to help youngsters return to normal functioning. The program also encourages resilience by teaching teens the importance of positive thinking, and by reviewing ways to plan for stressful situations that may arise and to deal with them successfully. This program, which targets adolescents aged 13–18, was designed to be administered by mental health professionals (e.g., psychologists, psychiatrists, social workers) with prior experience with cognitive behavioral treatments. A group rather than an individual format was used because it is more cost effective, it provides opportunities for modeling and role-playing of interpersonal behaviors, and research suggests that the group setting may be beneficial during mid to late adolescence when peer relations are primary (e.g., Moreau et al 1991). Fifteen 1-h sessions are conducted over an 8-week period in which adolescents are instructed in self-help and cognitive restructuring techniques and then role-playing and modeling exercises are used to help adolescents apply new information to real world situations. In addition, sessions include time to review and assign homework exercises, and each session concludes with unstructured sharing time.

In the most recent report, Clarke and colleagues (2001) recruited adolescents with depressed parents who were enrolled in a program maintained by a health maintenance organization. Prospective adults (aged 30–65 with dependents aged 13–18 years) were identified if they had received two dispensations of an antidepressant medication in the past year, or if they had two mental health visits within the past year.

Adolescents enrolled in the project were divided into three groups based on the severity of depressive symptoms they endorsed. Adolescents labeled demoralized were the focus of the prevention study, as they presented with subdiagnostic levels of depressive symptoms or had an elevated score on a self-report measure of depressive symptoms. Adolescents labeled depressed met criteria for a diagnosis of major depressive disorder or dysthymia, and they participated in a separate treatment study.

Likewise, resilient adolescents presented with no significant depressive symptoms and no history of depressive disorder, and they were not investigated further. Demoralized youth and their parents completed a battery of extensive assessments, including interview and self-report measures, at intake, post-treatment, and at follow-up assessments approximately 1 and 2 years later. Demoralized youth were then randomized to the experimental (n = 45) or to a usual care condition (n = 49).

In the experimental condition, adolescents participated in 15 1-h sessions in groups of 6–10 people; each group was led by a masters level therapist trained in CWS, as described above. Adolescents assigned to both groups were permitted to continue any non-study-related mental health services, and information regarding those services was collected from usual care participants as a representation of the comparison group. Parents of children in both groups were invited to three separate informational and psychoeducational meetings during the early, middle, and later sessions of the youth groups. Parents were informed about the general topics covered in the youth groups and were able to ask questions specific to their children. Parent groups did not address parental illness, and no individual or family sessions were conducted.

On measures of self-report depressive symptoms and on interview diagnostic assessments, adolescents assigned to the experimental condition generally reported less depression than did adolescents assigned to the usual care condition. Survival analysis over a 15-month period indicated that there was a rate of 9% in the experimental group, versus 28% in the usual care condition. No significant effects of the parent groups were reported. Clarke and his colleagues have concluded that participation in their group intervention program brought the rate of depressive illness in demoralized offspring of depressed parents to a level consonant with the general rate of depression in community samples (i.e., in samples with no particular risk for illness). Currently, Clarke and his associates are conducting a four-site effectiveness study using this preventive intervention. From the point of view of the Institute of Medicine's diagram, this is moving to the effectiveness stage. Clarke's work illustrates another principle that runs throughout the work with individuals and families with depression. That is, prevention and treatment are inseparable; in recruiting for a prevention study, the investigator is bound to also identify a number of youngsters who need treatment.

18.3.2 Seligman's Penn Preventive Intervention

In the Penn Prevention Program, Seligman and his colleagues (Jaycox et al. 1994) developed and evaluated a district-wide, school-based indicated prevention program targeting 10- to 13-year-old children at risk for depression based on elevated, self-reported depressive symptomatology, self-reported parental conflict, or both. This prevention program was based on a model of explanatory style introduced by Seligman and his colleagues (Nolen-Hoeksema et al. 1992) and on research identifying core cognitive deficits associated with youth depression, including negative self-evaluation, dysfunctional attitudes, poor interpersonal problem solving, and low expectations for self-performance (Garber et al. 1993; Kaslow et al. 1984; Quiggle et al. 1992). Participants recruited for the treatment group were assigned to one of three treatment programs: a cognitive training program, a social problem-solving program, or a combined program. Eighty-eight students were recruited for the no-participation control group. Assessments included child self-report, teacher-report, and parent-report questionnaires.

Results indicated that relative to control subjects, children who participated in any of the treatment groups reported significantly fewer depressive symptoms immediately following the program and at the 6-month follow-up, even controlling for initial levels of symptomatology. Moreover, teacher reports at follow-up revealed better classroom behavior in treatment participants relative to control participants. Finally, overall treatment effects were more significant for children who, at the screening phase of the study, reported more significant depressive symptomatology and more significant parental conflict at home.

Seligman has expanded this approach and has taken it from efficacy into effectiveness. They have examined the next phase effectiveness trials by studies in China (which found reduced symptomatology at 6-months old follow-up) and through a program with African-American youth (Seligman and Yu 2002; Cardemil et al 2002). In the public health domain, Seligman and his colleagues have also written a volume, »The Optimistic Child« (1995), for use directly by parents, another programmatic translation of data from an efficacy study.

18.3.3   Boston Preventive Intervention Project

In Boston, William Beardslee and associates developed public health interventions for families where parents are depressed based on Rutter's assertion (1990) that the transmission of risk occurs through negative interactions between parents and children. Beardslee's approach emphasized a strong cognitive orientation, included the family as a whole, and emphasized building strengths and resilience in youngsters. His approach came directly from studies of resilience, and was designed from the beginning to be used by a wide range of practitioners from a large group of disciplines. The three specific areas of resilience encouraged in youth were (1) activities outside the home, (2) involvement in relationships, and (3) the capacity for self-understanding. The preventive intervention approach directly incorporated information about resilience that was presented to parents. Two interventions incorporated these principles and were manual based: public health lectures, and a six-session, stepwise clinician-based family intervention program. The latter intervention included a family meeting. Regularly scheduled follow-ups occurred at 6–9 month intervals.

Over a period of time, it has become clear that families in the clinician-based group made more substantial gains, but that families in both groups have made substantial changes in parental behaviors and attitudes, and these changes have been sustained over time. Specifically, at the 4th assessment point two and one half years after enrollment, when following over 100 families with very little sample loss, Beardslee and associates showed that there were sustained behavior and attitude changes towards the illness on the parents' part and, more importantly, that there were also sustained changes in understanding of parental depression and related issues on the children's part (Beardslee et al. 2003). Perhaps most strikingly, regardless of the intervention group to which they were assigned, those families that showed the most change had youngsters who increased the most in understanding. Thus, the intervention did improve family interactions about understanding parental depression substantially. Also, both groups showed a reduction in depressive symptomatology, arguing for the value of the preventive interventions on a core area related to the actual occurrence of depression.

Beardslee and associates have followed these families for about 8 years and have used qualitative narrative analyses in addition to quantitative findings. The sustained behavior and attitude changes described by objective measurement reflected the family's continued conversations about depression, and the family's application of problem solving skills learned to new problems that emerged over time. Families reported that they understood depression better and were more likely to seek care in the early stages of a depressive episode (Beardslee 2002).

Beardslee and colleagues found that as the children matured, they expressed a need for more complex explanations of depression and related family adversities. Similarly, the reoccurrence of illness in the parents also required further conversations. In this sense, depression had to be understood anew as youngsters went through developmental epochs. Beardslee and associates believe this is a manifestation of a more general process in which families' making meaning of adversity needs to be revisited and reunderstood both because of the processes of development within children and the continued adversities families face. They also found that as families used prevention principles over several years, parents came to see depression in perspective and were able to make peace, move on, and indeed return to usual functioning (Beardslee 2002).

At the present time, the empirical evidence for the prevention of depression is robust but small in scope. The three approaches illustrate the specific applications of the general principles outlined earlier in this chapter. Each targets empirically identified risk factors in groups at high risk for depression. Each aims to enhance adaptive capacities over the long term, not just reduce risk. Each has a strong cognitive orientation, and consideration of eventually being able to be used in effectiveness trials and large-scale programs were included from the beginning. Other examples of prevention approaches for childhood and adolescent psychiatric disorders are offered throughout this volume and have much in common with these initial efforts for depression prevention.

18.4   Healthcare Policy Perspectives: Systems Support and Reform for Prevention

Systematic support for preventive interventions vary widely across health districts, and indeed are quite different in different countries. For example, in Holland, there is a network of preventionists and a substantial portion (10%) of the budget of community mental health center must be devoted to preventive intervention. Hence, there is a ready vehicle for the delivery of the intervention in place and what is required is simply training people to do it. Moreover, there is a large and extensive program of other preventions and interventions for children of mentally ill parents; hence new programs can be easily introduced. In settings where there is no tradition of preventive intervention and no requirement to focus on it (e.g., in the USA), prevention requires a great deal more attention to systems support and funding mechanisms in order to introduce and sustain these prevention programs.

As another example, in Finland there is a strong tradition of adopting evidence-based prevention approaches, and considerable experience in how to both implement with fidelity to the investigator's original approach, and how to translate approaches to large scale country-wide programmatic initiatives. This makes the adoption of any particular new prevention program much easier.

Consideration of systems failures and systems reform is an essential part of preventive interventions. Beardslee and associates examined what the preventionists in their study were actually doing and found that they were investing a great deal of time engaging in the health care system and trying to get treatment for parents. In fact, many parents experienced systematic discrimination and systems difficulties in obtaining their health care. As a result, Beardslee and colleagues argue that an essential part of the preventive interventionist's role is to advocate for health care reform for better coverage for mental illness, parity, and extending coverage to those who don't have it (Beardslee 1998, 2002).

18.5 Summary and Conclusions

1. There is great promise for future prevention efforts because the scientific understanding of the multiple influences on development is expanding rapidly. As we come to know more about how systems interact with individual lives and how systems reform at the local, city, state, and national levels can affect individual lives, we will have multiple opportunities to design more effective and comprehensive prevention programs. Similarly, as basic advances in neuroscience, developmental epidemiology, and genetics evolve, these will offer many opportunities for the development of preventive intervention programs. Consideration of preventive in-

terventions should be built in from the beginning of these investigations.
2. From a clinical point of view, treatment and prevention are inseparable. Preventive interventions are often not considered either by clinicians or by health care systems that often become preoccupied with treatment. However, clearly an evidence base is emerging for the value of preventive interventions. The example of preventive intervention in adolescent depression has been cited, but many other examples exist as well. Systematic attention needs to be devoted to preventive intervention by countries, health care districts, and clinical practitioners. Both clinicians and health care policy makers need to recognize that prevention and clinical care require somewhat different orientations (Beardslee 1998). Support for both is necessary.
3. Approaches that have a strong cognitive orientation and build strengths and resources are likely to be most effective. A recent book by the American Psychological Association on strength-based programs (Maton et al. 2003) emphasizes a wide array of evidence-based preventions or systems programs that can improve care.
4. An approach to risk suggests two major ways of preventing difficulties. Early in life, programs that support the general development of the child and are not specific for a particular mental illness such as high quality daycare or high quality schools are in order. Later in the life of children and their families, more specific approaches for those at highest risk can be employed.
5. From the point of view of prevention and youngsters, consideration of the family as a whole is absolutely essential. Far more efforts need to be directed to family care and prevention as opposed to individual care and prevention.
6. While some treatments and prevention programs have been tested in different countries and different cultural settings, very little work has been done on understanding either resilience differently in different cultures or the delicate, unfolding interplay of risk and protective factors and how this evolves in different cultures and different countries. Understanding the vicissitudes in risk and resilience in different cultural and national contexts is an important goal in and of itself and will also substantially advance the development and evaluation of preventive interventions. Similarly, understanding the impacts of different kinds of health care sys-

tems, those that incorporate prevention and those that do not, for example, would aid a great deal in understanding how to be most effective in mounting preventive interventions. As a complement to this, of course, is the need for much further work on understanding cultural competence and developing prevention programs that reflect such competence.

7. Much more consideration needs to be given to mounting multiple preventive interventions simultaneously that address a single condition but using multiple strategies working in concert. These approaches have been used successfully in combating smoking and risks for cardiovascular disease (IOM Report 1994) and some comprehensive community-wide interventions exist (Hawkins et al. 1992). More effort to coordinate and integrate approaches in mental health is needed.

References

Aarons B, Kumpfer KL, Johnson J, Windle M, Beardslee WR, Flynn B, English MJ, Masten A, Rolf J (1999) Resilience Working Group proceedings. Proceedings of the Center for Mental Health Services, pp 1–38

Beardslee WR (1998) Prevention and the clinical encounter. American Journal of Orthopsychiatry 68:521–533

Beardslee WR (2002) Out of the darkened room: When a parent is depressed: Protecting the children and strengthening the family. Little, Brown and Company, New York

Beardslee WR, Knitzer J (2003) Strengths-based family mental health services: A family systems approach. In: Maton K, Schellenbach C, Leadbeater B, Solarz A (eds) Investing in children, youth, families, and communities: Strengths-based research and policy. American Psychological Association, Washington DC, pp 157–171

Beardslee, WR, Podorefsky D (1988) Resilient adolescents whose parents have serious affective and other psychiatric disorders: The importance of self-understanding and relationships. American Journal of Psychiatry 145:63–69

Beardslee WR, Keller MB, Seifer R, Lavori PW, Staley D, Podorofsky D, Shera D (1996) Prediction of adolescent affective disorder: Effects of prior parental affective disorders and child psychopathology. Journal of the American Academy of Child and Adolescent Psychiatry 35:279–288

Beardslee WR, Versage EM, Gladstone TRG (1998) Children of affectively ill parents: A review of the past ten years. Journal of the American Academy of Child and Adolescent Psychiatry 37:1134–1141

Beardslee WR, Gladstone TRG, Wright EJ, Cooper AB (2003) A family-based approach to the prevention of depressive symptoms in children at risk: Evidence of parental and child change. Pediatrics 112:119–131

Bronfenbrenner U (1979) The ecology of human development: Experiments by nature and design. Cambridge, MA: Harvard University Press

Bruce ML, Takeuchi DT, Leaf PJ (1991) Poverty and psychiatric status: Longitudinal evidence from the New Haven Epidemiologic Catchment Area Study. Archives of General Psychiatry 48:470–474

Carbonell DM, Reinherz HZ, Giaconia RM, Stashwick CK, Paradis AD, Beardslee WR (2002) Adolescent protective factors promoting resilience in young adults at risk for depression. Child and Adolescent Social Work Journal 19:393–412

Cardemil EV, Reivich KJ, Seligman MEP (2002) The prevention of depressive symptoms in inner-city middle school students. Prevention & Treatment 5:np

Caspi A, Sugden K, Moffitt TE, Taylor A, Craig IW, Harrington HL, McClay J, Mill J, Martin J, Braithwaite A, Poulton R (2003) Influence of life stress on depression: Moderation by a polymorphism in the 5-HTT gene. Science 301:386–389

Cicchetti D, Schneider-Rosen K (1986) An organizational approach to childhood depression. In Rutter M, Izard CE, Read PB (eds) Depression in young people: Developmental and clinical perspectives. Guilford Press, New York, pp 71–134

Clarke GN, Hawkins W, Murphy M, Sheeber LB, Lewinsohn PM, Seeley JR (1995) Targeted prevention of unipolar depressive disorder in an at-risk sample of high school adolescents: A randomized trial of a group cognitive intervention. Journal of the American Academy of Child and Adolescent Psychiatry 34:312–321

Clarke GN, Hornbrook M, Lynch F, Polen M, Gale J, Beardslee WR, O'Conner E, Seeley J (2001) A randomized trial of a group cognitive intervention for preventing depression in adolescent offspring of depressed parents. Archives of General Psychiatry 58:1127–1134

Clarke GN, Lewinsohn PM, Hops H (1990) Instructor's manual for the Adolescent Coping with Depression course. Castalia Press, Eugene, OR

Eisenberg L (1995) The social construction of the human brain. American Journal of Psychiatry 152:1563–1575

Focht L, Beardslee WR (1996) »Speech after long silence«: The use of narrative therapy in a preventive intervention for children of parents with affective disorder. Fam Process, pp 407–422

Garber J, Weiss B, Shanley N (1993) Cognitions, depressive symptoms, and development in adolescents. Journal of Abnormal Psychology 102:47–57

Garmezy N (1985) Stress-resistant children: The search for protective factors. In Stevenson JE (ed) Recent research in developmental psychology. Pergamon Press, Oxford, pp 213–233

Hawkins JD, Catalano RF, Morrison DM, O'Donnell J, Abbott RD, Day LE (1992) The Seattle Social Development Project: Effects of the first four years on protective factors and problem behaviors. In McCord J, Tremblay RE (eds) Preventing antisocial behavior: Interventions from birth through adolescence. New York, Guilford Press, pp 139–161

Institute of Medicine (1994) Reducing risks for mental disorders: Frontiers for preventive intervention research. National Academy Press, Washington DC

Jaycox LH, Reivich KJ, Gillham J, Seligman MEP (1994) Prevention of depressive symptoms in school children. Behavior Research and Therapy 32:801–816

Kaslow NJ, Rehm LP, Siegel AW (1984) Social-cognitive and cognitive correlates of depression in children. Journal of Abnormal Child Psychology 12:605–620

Kumpfer KL, DeMarsh J (1985) Family, environmental, and genetic influences on children's future chemical dependency. Journal of Children in a Contemporary Society 18:49–91

Lewinsohn PM, Roberts RE, Seeley JR, Rohde P, Gotlib IH, Hops H (1994) Adolescent psychopathology: II. Psychosocial risk factors for depression. Journal of Abnormal Psychology 103:302–315

Luthar SS, Cicchetti D, Becker B (2000) The construct of resilience: A critical evaluation and guidelines for future work. Child Development 71:543–562

Masten AS, Best KM, Garmezy N (1990) Resilience and development: Contributions from the study of children who overcome adversity. Development and Psychopathology 2:425–444

Maton K, Schellenbach C, Leadbeater B, Solarz A, eds (2003) Investing in children, youth, families, and communities: Strengths-based research and policy. American Psychological Association, Washington DC

Moreau D, Mufson L, Weissman MM, Klerman GL (1991) Interpersonal psychotherapy for adolescent depression: Description of modification and preliminary application. Journal of the American Academy of Child and Adolescent Psychiatry 30:642–651

National Advisory Mental Health Workgroup on Child and Adolescent Mental Health Intervention Development and Deployment (2001) Blueprint for change: Research on child and adolescent mental health. Washington DC

Nolen-Hoeksema S, Girgus JS, Seligman MEP (1992) Predictors and consequences of childhood depressive symptoms: A 5-year longitudinal study. Journal of Abnormal Psychology 101:405–422

Price RH, van Ryn M, Vinokur AD (1992) Impact of a preventive job search intervention on the likelihood of depression among the unemployed. Journal of Health and Social Behavior 33:158–167

Quiggle NL, Garber J, Panak WF, Dodge KA (1992) Social information processing in aggressive and depressed children. Child Development 63:1305–1320

Reinherz HZ, Giaconia RM, Hauf AMC, Wasserman MS, Silverman AB (1999) Major depression in the transition to adulthood: Risks and impairments. Journal of Abnormal Psychology 108:500–510

Reinherz HZ, Giaconia RM, Hauf AMC, Wasserman MS, Paradis BA (2000) General and specific childhood risk factors for depression and drug disorders by early adulthood. Journal of the American Academy of Child And Adolescent Psychiatry 39:223–231

Reinherz HZ, Stewart-Berhauer G, Pakiz B, Frost AK, Moeykens BA, Holmes WM (1989) The relationship of early risk and current mediators to depressive symptomatology in adolescence. Journal of the American Academy of Child and Adolescent Psychiatry 28:942–947

Rutter M (1987) Psychosocial resilience and protective mechanisms. American Journal of Orthopsychiatry 57:316–331

Rutter M (1990) Commentary: Some focus and process considerations regarding effects of parental depression on children. Developmental Psychology 26:60–67

Rutter M, Quinton D (1977) Psychiatric disorder: Ecological factors and concepts of causation. In: McGurk H (ed) Ecological factors in human development. North-Holland, Amsterdam, pp 173–187

Sameroff AJ, Chandler MJ (1975) Reproductive risk and the continuum of caretaking casualty. In: Horowitz FD, Hetherington M, Scarr-Salopatek S (eds) Review of child developmental research, vol. 4. University of Chicago Press, Chicago, pp 187–244

Sameroff AJ, Bartko WT, Baldwin A, Baldwin C, Seifer R (1998) Family and social influences on the development of child competence. In: Lewis M, Feiring C (eds) Families, risk and competence. Erlbaum, Mahwah, NJ, pp 161–185

Seligman MEP, Reivich K, Jaycox L, Gillham J (1995) The Optimistic Child: A proven program to safeguard children against depression and build lifelong resilience. Harper-Perennial, New York

Yu DL, Seligman MEP (2002) Preventing depressive symptoms in Chinese children. Prevention & Treatment 5:np

Silberg J, Rutter M (2002) Nature-nurture interplay in the risks associated with parental depression. In: Goodman SH, Gotlib IH (eds) Children of depressed parents: Mechanisms of risk and implications for treatment. American Psychological Association, Washington DC, pp 13–36

Werner EE, Smith RS (1982) Vulnerable but invincible: A study of resilient children. McGraw-Hill, New York

Yoshikawa H (1994) Prevention as a cumulative protection: Effects of early support and education on chronic delinquency and its risks. Psychological Bulletin 115:28–54

Prevention and Early Detection of Developmental Disorders

Sophie Willemsen-Swinkels, Herman van Engeland

19.1 Early Detection and Prevention, General Remarks – 256
19.1.1 Introduction – 256
19.1.2 Clinical Observations and Review of Milestones – 257
19.1.3 Standardized Developmental Screening Tests – 257
19.1.4 Parental Concerns – 257
19.1.5 Prevention – 257

19.2 Autism Spectrum Disorder – 257
19.2.1 Introduction – 257
19.2.2 Relevance for Further Development – 258
19.2.3 Early Detection – 258
19.2.4 Prevention – 259
19.2.4.1 Primary Prevention – 259
19.2.4.2 Secondary Prevention – 259
19.2.4.3 Tertiary Prevention – 259

19.3 Attachment Disorder – 261
19.3.1 Introduction – 261
19.3.2 Relevance for Future Development – 261
19.3.3 Early Detection – 261
19.3.4 Prevention – 262
19.3.4.1 Primary Prevention – 262
19.3.4.2 Secondary Prevention – 262
19.3.4.3 Tertiary Prevention – 262

19.4 Language Disorder – 262
19.4.1 Introduction – 262
19.4.2 Relevance for Future Development – 262
19.4.3 Early Detection – 263
19.4.4 Prevention – 263
19.4.4.1 Primary Prevention – 263
19.4.4.2 Secondary and Tertiary Prevention – 264

19.5 Mental Retardation – 264
19.5.1 Introduction – 264
19.5.2 Relevance for Future Development – 265
19.5.3 Early Detection – 265
19.5.4 Prevention – 266
19.5.4.1 Primary Prevention – 266
19.5.4.2 Secondary Prevention – 266
19.5.4.3 Tertiary Prevention – 266

19.6 Concluding Remarks – 267

References – 267

19.1 Early Detection and Prevention, General Remarks

19.1.1 Introduction

This chapter focuses on developmental disorders. The term »developmental« implies that individuals with these conditions suffer from disturbances in the normal sequence of developmental milestones in terms of skills and competencies, with possible important implications throughout the life span. The developmental problems of young children are attracting increasing interest because it is now possible to achieve an early diagnosis. This, in turn, makes it possible to provide timely medical care, educational planning, and family support and instruction, which will reduce the stress and anguish experienced by the families of these children.

The early detection of developmental disorders calls for two different levels of investigation. Level 1 screening, which should be applied to all children, relies on the health care professional's ability to identify children at risk of developmental disorders, based on clinical observation and a review of milestones (Glascoe 1999), screening tests, and parental concerns. Level 2 involves a more in-depth investigation of children identified as being at risk of a developmental disorder. This diagnostic assessment aims at differentiating between the different developmental disorders and determining the best intervention based on the child's behavioral abilities and deficiencies.

19.1.2 Clinical Observations and Review of Milestones

Regular monitoring of a child's development during early life may facilitate the early detection of developmental problems. The monitoring system used varies between countries. Some countries have well-baby clinics, in which trained doctors see children at regular intervals during the first years of life, with the aim of detecting developmental problems in an early stage and of referring children on to appropriate centers. Some well-baby clinics use specific well-child clinical forms with preprinted developmental milestones that are appropriate for each routine visit. The use of these forms, together with assessment of age-appropriate skills in various developmental domains, increases the probability of accurately identifying a child at risk. In other countries, general practitioners (GPs) provide all primary care services for young children. Some general practices have specialized nurses to monitor and supervise the development and health of under 5-year-olds (Garralda 2002). Yet other health care systems have specially trained nurses who carry out home visits, either on request or routinely. Regardless of the type of organization or health care system, most fail to allocate sufficient time for a thorough examination of the child.

19.1.3 Standardized Developmental Screening Tests

Screening activities are crucial to early diagnosis. The purpose of screening is to identify children at risk so that they can be referred for full diagnostic assessment. The most important obstacles to the routine use of developmental screening tests are their length, their expense, and the difficulty managing children's behavior during testing (Glascoe 1999).

19.1.4 Parental Concerns

Physicians and nurses should listen to the concerns parents may voice about the development of their child. Several studies by Glascoe have shown that parental concerns about speech and language development, behavior, or other developmental issues are highly sensitive (i.e., 74–83%) in detecting global developmental problems (Glascoe 1994, 1997,

1999). Parents are usually correct in their concerns about their child's development. They may not be accurate regarding the qualitative and quantitative parameters surrounding the developmental abnormality, but usually if there is a concern, there is indeed a problem in some aspect of the child's development. Under some circumstances, parental concern is a better predictor than the result of a screening test. Two or more concerns voiced by parents was found to be a significant predictor of disabilities, whereas additional screening resulted in underdetection of disabilities (Glascoe 2000).

19.1.5 Prevention

Prevention initiatives can be classified as primary, secondary, or tertiary (Offord and Bennett 2002; Caplan 1964; Cowen 1983). Primary prevention seeks to reduce the incidence or number of new cases of a disorder or illness. Secondary prevention aims to lower the prevalence of the disorder or illness by early identification and effective treatment, and tertiary prevention aims to reduce the severity of the impairment associated with an existing disorder or illness.

19.2 Autism Spectrum Disorder

19.2.1 Introduction

Social interaction is a bidirectional process in which each interacting member adapts his or her behavior to correspond with that of the other. It is the overall ability of a person to initiate interactions and to respond to another person's behavior (Ghuman et al. 1998). Impairments of socialization are the core-defining feature of autism. Other important features of autism are impairments in verbal and nonverbal communication and restricted and repetitive patterns of behaviors. The impairments in these domains go beyond simple immaturity, with children showing behaviors that would be abnormal at any age. Autism was first reported in 1943, but in recent years the construct has been broadened and it is now considered to be a spectrum of related disorders: the autism spectrum disorders (ASD).

19.2.2 Relevance for Further Development

Autism is a lifelong disorder and it is unlikely that the affected individual will be able to live independently. Individuals with both autism and severe mental retardation require supervised living and working situations throughout their lives. But even the large majority of individuals with average or higher intelligence require help in finding and keeping jobs and with coping with responsibilities and social demands throughout their lives (Rutter et al. 1992).

The ASD are not rare. Large systematic epidemiological studies conducted since 1987 suggest a prevalence of 6–9 per 10,000 people (Fombonne 1999). An additional 12.25 cases per 10,000 individuals was estimated for atypical autism, giving an overall rate for ASD of 20 per 10,000. Recent studies reported rates for ASD of 45.8 per 10, 000 (Charkrabarti and Fombonne 2001), and 30.8 per 10,000 (Baird et al. 2000). These prevalence rates are significantly higher than those reported in the early 1970s and further emphasize the need for improved early screening and diagnosis.

19.2.3 Early Detection

Autism is usually considered to start in infancy but is rarely diagnosed before 3 years, which is considered unacceptably late (Bristol-Power and Spinella 1999). Typically, social interaction is assessed as part of routine developmental monitoring procedures. Further evaluation is required if a parent expresses concern about delayed socialization because parents rarely complain about the social development of their children (Filipek et al. 1999). The problems noticed by parents are usually not specific features of autism, but rather reflect difficulties in talking (even before the child might normally be expected to speak) or difficulties in settling, eating, or sleeping; the child may throw tantrums (Dahlgren and Gillberg 1989). Since we have currently no biological marker for ASD, screening must focus on behavior.

It is particularly difficult to diagnose ASD in very young children. This may be due to several factors. For instance, there is a considerable heterogeneity among people with ASD. Moreover, social and language deficits and delays can be identified only after the child is of an age to interact with other children,

and the developmental level or intelligence of the child may affect symptom expression. The low incidence of autism leads to low index of suspicion, and the disorder appears to have a gradual onset without clear evidence of sensorimotor impairment. Children with ASD typically sit, crawl, and walk at the expected age. Many even produce a few words at developmentally appropriate times, although these words seldom develop into useful early language (Filipek et al. 1999). Symptoms and signs that may be present during infancy (serious facial expression, increased irritability, sleep and eating difficulties, placidity, stereotypies) are behaviors commonly seen in otherwise typically developing young children.

Despite these difficulties, retrospective and prospective studies have shown evidence not only for the early occurrence of autistic symptoms, but also for the continuity between some early manifestations and later disorders (Adrien et al. 1993; Osterling and Dawson 1994). This has led to the development of screening instruments for autism in young children. Baron-Cohen and colleagues have been influential in this, with the development of the Checklist for Autism in Toddlers (CHAT Baron-Cohen et al. 1992). This short checklist, which assesses joint attention and pretend play behaviors, is intended for use in children aged about 18 months. In England, health visitors and general practitioners screened over 16,000 children with the CHAT (Baron-Cohen et al. 1996). The CHAT was found to have a sensitivity of 38% and a specificity of 98% for identifying autism. Repeated screening 1 month later reduced the sensitivity to 20%, although the specificity was close to 100% (Baird et al. 2000).

Robins et al. (2001) made several modifications to the CHAT in an attempt to improve its sensitivity. They extended the checklist to 23 items, changed the age of screening to 24 months instead of 18 months, and used a structured telephone interview as an intermediate screening step. The revised instrument, the modified-CHAT (M-CHAT), was primarily designed to act as a level 1 screening instrument. When used to screen a nonselected population of 1,122 children, 3 children with autism/ASD were identified. These results are promising although the sample size was too small to draw definite conclusions about the use of the M-CHAT as a level 1 screening instrument. In another study, the M-CHAT identified 36 children with autism/ASD from a population of 171 children referred for early intervention.

The Autism Screening Questionnaire is a 40-item scale based on a diagnostic interview, the

ADI-R (Berument et al. 1999). It was designed by Michael Rutter and Cathy Lord to be completed by the primary caregiver of individuals who might have an ASD. The instrument was found to have good discriminative validity with respect to distinguishing ASD from other diagnoses in children older than 4 years.

The Screening Tool for Autism in 2-year-old infants (STAT) consists of 12 items that are administered within a play-like interaction with the child (Stone et al. 2001). It was developed to assist community professionals in identifying young children with possible autism. The instrument was tested in an outpatient multidisciplinary evaluation center; however, its utility in other community-based settings remains to be determined.

The Pervasive Developmental Disorders Screening Test [PDDST (Siegel 1996)] is a clinically derived parent questionnaire that consists of three versions, each version being targeted at a different level of screening. No information has been published on its utility in young children.

Our research group has worked on the development of a screening questionnaire that can be used to test infants at about 14 months of age (Willemsen-Swinkels, submitted). The screening instrument ESAT (Early Screening of Autistic Traits) was tested in a random population of 31,724 toddlers via a two-staged method (Dietz et al., submitted a). Items of the ESAT are answered by parents as well as by trained psychologists, during a home visit. Although 17 very young children with ASD could be adequately identified with this screening method, many cases were missed. Moreover, the differentiation from other childhood psychiatric disorders was poor, resulting in a high number of false-positive results for related disorders such as language disorder and mental retardation without ASD. Another problem was that many parents refused to cooperate with in-depth clinical assessments at this very young age. Overall, the results suggested that a suitable age to be extra alert to the presence of autistic disorders is about the second birthday. Post hoc analyses of 44 parent-response items for more than 350 preschool children (over 40 with ASD) will be used to develop the final version of this screening instrument to be used in infants of about 2 years (Dietz et al., submitted b).

In the absence of a medical test to unequivocally diagnose ASD, definitions of autism and related conditions are based on behavioral manifestations, with all the unreliability this entails. To minimize this unreliability as much as possible, the diagnostic process for ASD should include the use of a diagnostic observation instrument like the Autism Diagnostic Observation ScheduleGeneric (ADOS-G; Lord et al. 1998). Furthermore, sufficient time should be planned for a standardized parent interview, such as the Autism Diagnostic Interview-revised (ADI-R; Le Couteur et al. 1989; Lord et al. 1994).

19.2.4   Prevention

19.2.4.1   Primary Prevention

There is a growing interest in the genetics of ASD. Several research groups have identified chromosomal regions that appear to be strongly linked with ASD (Szatmari et al. 1998; Shastry 2003; Yonan et al. 2003; International Molecular Genetic Study of Autism Consortium 1998). It is very likely that in the next decade susceptibility genes will be identified. Susceptibility genes, or genes of minor effect, increase the risk of disease but they are neither necessary nor sufficient for its development. Therefore, the identification of susceptibility genes is a long way from preimplantation diagnosis and prenatal diagnosis. Primary prevention by means of genetics is not a real option in the immediate future.

19.2.4.2   Secondary Prevention

Overall, there is consensus that autism is a lifelong disorder that, on the basis of current knowledge, cannot be cured. A study of the application of Applied Behavioral Analysis (ABA) to very young preschool-aged children with autism reported extraordinary results (Lovaas 1987). However, numerous studies in the 1990s used the original ABA techniques or modified versions and reported smaller improvements. All failed to replicate the complete restoration of »normal« functioning reported in the original study (Leaf and McEachin 1999; Smith et al. 2000).

19.2.4.3   Tertiary Prevention

With the current state of knowledge, tertiary prevention (e.g., reducing the severity of the impairment) is the only realistic aim of interventions for autism. In 2001 the National Research Council of the USA considered the state of scientific evidence of the effects of early educational intervention on young children with ASD. The Council concluded:

»A large body of research has demonstrated substantial progress in response to specific intervention techniques in relatively short periods of time (e.g., several months) in many specific areas, including social skills, language acquisition, nonverbal communication, and reduction in challenging behaviors. Longitudinal studies over longer periods of time have documented changes in IQ scores and in core deficits (e.g., joint attention), in some cases related to treatment, that are predictive of longer term outcomes. However, children's outcomes are variable, with some children making substantial progress and others showing very slow gains. Although there is evidence that interventions lead to improvements, there does not appear to be a clear, direct relationship between any particular intervention and children's progress. Thus while substantial evidence exists that treatment can reach short-term goals in many areas, gaps remain in addressing larger questions of the relationship between particular techniques and specific changes.«

Different types of early treatment, which differ in their focus, approach, setting, and especially intensity, have been described. Below, we briefly review the literature about early intervention for autism.

A distinction can be made between interventions that target special features and more comprehensive programs (Rogers 1998). While there is extensive evidence that targeted interventions, such as those focused on aspects of communication, are effective, there is less evidence that comprehensive educational programs result in general gains (Lord 2000). A likely candidate for a targeted intervention is joint attention behaviors. In typical development, joint attention behaviors emerge between 6 months and 12 months and involve the triadic coordination or sharing of attention between the infant, another person, and an object or event. The term encompasses a complex of behavioral forms including gaze and point following, showing, and pointing. Numerous observations suggest that joint attention disturbances reflect a fundamental component of the etiology of autism (Mundy and Neal 2001; Leekam et al. 2000). For example, an impairment in joint attention skills is specific to children with autism, is characteristic of the majority of young children with autism, and is associated with later developmental outcome (see for review Kasari et al. 2001; Charman 2003). Interventions that focused on joint attention skills resulted in significant gains in responding to

joint attention and joint attention initiation (Whalen and Schreibman 2003) or language development (Drew et al. 2002) after treatment.

Two contrasting treatment approaches have received much attention in the literature: the traditional, discrete trial approach and the contemporary behavioral approach. Contemporary behavioral approaches use systematic teaching trials that are initiated by the child and focus on the child's interest. The trials are embedded in the natural environment and natural reinforcers are used that follow what the child is trying to communicate. The few studies that have compared the traditional discrete trial approach with naturalistic approaches report that naturalistic approaches are more effective at leading to generalization of gains to natural contexts (Koegel 1998, 2000; Krantz 2000). Lack of generalization across stimuli, settings, and people has been noted as the most important limitation of the discrete trial approach (National Research Council 2001).

It has been suggested that clinic-based, professionally directed treatment approaches provide the optimal setting for early intervention. However, in practice, in most countries the facilities for this, such as specialized clinics and professionals with sufficient training, experience, and expertise, are not available. For this reason, treatment programs tend to involve the child's parents as a (partial) substitute for professionals. However, the demands associated with having a child with disabilities are often stressful to parents, and this stress could be aggravated by the need to designate certain times to work on one-to-one with their child. Yet, programs designed to fit into the family lifestyle and routine, so that teaching can occur on an ongoing basis throughout the day in natural settings, have been shown to actually decrease family stress because of increased feelings of competence and success (Koegel 2000). An additional advantage of involving parents is that they provide support and assistance throughout the child's life (Ozonoff and Cathcart 1998).

An extreme example of parental involvement are the so-called workshop programs, in which the parents themselves initiate, manage, and direct a treatment program with a minimum of professional consultancy. Preliminary results for the use of parent-managed treatment approaches are not very encouraging. Research to date suggests that although parent-managed programs may bring about gains in language, adaptive, and intellectual functioning, the gains are much smaller than those reported for clinic-based programs (Bibby et al. 2001; Smith et al. 2000).

Parent training approaches represent an intermediate form between the two extremes of purely professional-based and purely parent-based treatment settings. In parent training approaches, parents are extensively trained to provide at least part of the behavioral intervention. In this approach, parental treatment delivery and the number of hours of intervention are closely monitored and backed up by the constant availability of professional advice and support.

An issue that has generated heated controversy in recent years concerns how often interventions should be given (Koegel 2000). Some investigators have claimed that a very intensive behavioral intervention (minimum 25 h per week) is needed for maximum therapeutic effect (Lovaas 1987; Pelios and Lund 2001; Schreibman 2000; Gill 2001). Others have protested against intensive behavioral interventions (Marcus et al. 2000; Rapin 2001; Boyd and Corley 2001), arguing that the value of these treatments is far from scientifically proven and does not exceed the burden that intensive treatment places on the family and community resources. Sheinkopf and Siegel analyzed the effect of treatment intensity in a study of home-based behavioral treatment and found that treatment intensity was not related to therapeutic response (Sheinkopf and Siegel 1998). They advanced two possible explanations. The minimum number of treatment hours per week needed for a therapeutic effect may have been overestimated, and the involvement of parents and the implementation of treatment at home may have helped parents generalize their skills to instructive interactions outside the formal treatment sessions.

The treatment studies performed so far have shown that even the most effective treatment has a very variable response. Thus, while some children may improve substantially, even achieving normal and near-normal functioning, the majority improve to a lesser degree or not at all. This variability in treatment outcome suggests that there are variables affecting outcome that have not yet been identified (Ingersoll et al. 2001). Given the heterogeneity in the autism population in terms of symptom presentation, it is likely that important child variables are involved. Other possible moderators of the efficacy of interventions, especially caregiver-involved interventions, are caregiver sensitivity, motivation, stress, depression level, socio-economic status, education, and child's attachment security to the caregiver.

19.3   Attachment Disorder

19.3.1   Introduction

According to attachment theory, there is a biologically based bond between the child and the caregiver that assures the protection and survival of the child. This theory is widely accepted with regard to social and emotional development, and there is considerable theoretical and empirical evidence that the quality of this child-parent bond significantly influences the development of psychopathology.

Besides attachment theory, interest is emerging in the much less well-understood Reactive Attachment Disorder. The first diagnostic definition of Reactive Attachment Disorder appeared in 1980. Nowadays, two forms of Reactive Attachment Disorder are recognized. The core of the »disinhibited« form is »indiscriminate« sociability or a lack of selectivity in the choice of attachment figures. In the second subtype, the »inhibited« form, the predominant disturbance in social relatedness is »the persistent failure to initiate and to respond to most social interactions in a developmentally appropriate way« (American Psychiatric Association 1994). The connection between attachment theory and reactive attachment disorder is unresolved (O'Conner 2002).

19.3.2   Relevance for Future Development

Attachment status is a reflection of a child's level of social competence in settings beyond the caregiver-child dyad and in later phases of development. Infant attachment status predicts a child's socio-emotional functioning in at least three domains: interacting with siblings, developing relationships with friends, and dealing with peers who are not close friends. Insecure attachment patterns are not seen as being abnormal in themselves, but rather as a risk factor, while security is viewed as a protective factor. The rate of attachment disorder is thought to be very low, but its actual prevalence is unknown.

19.3.3   Early Detection

There is no established protocol or assessment strategy for measuring attachment disorders in a clinical or research context. This stresses the need for collecting information from a variety of sources and with a variety of methods. At the very least, this should include a clinical interview with caregivers and an observation of the child interacting with a stranger (O'Conner 2002).

19.3.4   Prevention

19.3.4.1   Primary Prevention

Primary prevention can take the form of minimizing separation from parents. Nowadays, in hospitals it is less common for parents and infants to be separated than in the past. Another aspect is the prevention or early detection of emotional separation caused by serious parental mental illness, particularly depression.

19.3.4.2   Secondary Prevention

According to the attachment theory, care-giving styles play a causal role in attachment status. Studies of infants have shown that several indices of maternal sensitivity are associated with security. For example, experimental studies have shown that when infants have to undergo medical interventions, the care-giving sensitivity of their mothers increases, which in turn increases the probability that the mothers and infants form a strong attachment (van IJzendoorn et al. 1995). However, a meta-analysis revealed that dimensions of maternal behavior accounted for only a modest-to-moderate portion of the variance in attachment status (DeWolff and van IJzendoorn 1997). Care-giving sensitivity can therefore not be regarded as the sole determinant of attachment status.

Intervention can also focus on parent education (Marvin 2003). The goal of this type of intervention is to make explicit the parents' knowledge of normal ordered patterns of the attachmentcare-giving interaction and to help them understand the cause and logic of disordered behavior.

More needs to be learned of the mechanisms underlying these interventions and whether beneficial effects of attachment-based interventions are comparable to or greater than those found with alternative approaches, such as individual thematic play therapy. Nevertheless, there is strong and growing empirical support for attachment-based interventions (O'Conner 2002).

19.3.4.3   Tertiary Prevention

Very little is known about the form and effectiveness of interventions for children with attachment disturbances severe enough to warrant the term attachment disorder. It seems natural to suppose that interventions developed for attachment disorder would build on existing knowledge about effective attachment-based interventions, but this is not the case (O'Conner 2002). »Alternative« approaches, such as so-called holding therapies (Hughes 1999), have attracted attention but have not been adequately evaluated (O'Conner 2002).

19.4   Language Disorder

19.4.1   Introduction

In general, children are born with an astonishing facility to learn languages. A typical child can, by 4 years of age, produce long and complex sentences, speak clearly and intelligibly, and understand a vocabulary of tens of thousands of words. However, there are children whose communicative development does not proceed in such a straightforward fashion. There are several possible causes of language delay, such as mental retardation, craniological disorders, cerebral palsy, autism, traumatic brain injury, and hearing loss (Downey et al. 2002).

A diagnosis of specific developmental language disorder (DLD) is appropriate when the child's language lags well behind that of children of a similar age although the child's development is proceeding normally in other respects. The Diagnostic and Statistical Manual of Mental Disorders fourth edition (DSM-IV; American Psychiatric Association 1994) draws a distinction between expressive DLD and mixed receptive-expressive DLD. There have been suggestions that the two subtypes are qualitatively distinct (Lahey and Edwards 1995), but most evidence justifies treating them as points on a continuum of severity (Bishop 2002).

19.4.2   Relevance for Future Development

Speech and language impairments are among the most common handicapping conditions of childhood. Two epidemiological surveys, in the USA and Canada, estimated the prevalence of these impairments to be about 7% in 5-year-old children (Tomblin et al. 1997; Johnson et al. 1999).

The existence of language impairments in a young child is highly prognostic of a relatively low level of language performance in the adult (Johnson et al. 1999). In particular, children with significantly impaired receptive language skills experience language difficulties that often increase with age (Rutter and Mawhood 1991). Furthermore, there is a strong co-occurrence of spoken and written language difficulties, probably because both stem from deficiencies in the underlying speech processing system. In addition, children with a DLD have more social problems and psychiatric disorders.

19.4.3   Early Detection

A hallmark of DLD appears to be the late appearance of first words, with a protracted period of lexical development thereafter. Word combinations also appear at a later age than expected.

Middle-class children with slow expressive language development as toddlers have a real chance of performing within the normal range in terms of language and academic achievement by the time they reach school age, even in the absence of intensive intervention. Follow-up studies have found that approximately half of the toddlers who display a late onset of talking at age 2 years catch up with their peers by 3 years and exhibit no further language problems (Paul 1991; Rescola and Schwartz 1990; Roberts et al. 1998). This has led some to recommend the policy of monitoring rather than direct intervention (Paul 2000), at least for children from stable, relatively advantaged families with no additional risk factors. Others have argued that every late talker should be treated, to increase the chance that their language skills will fall within the normal range. This argument is based on the need to take advantage of the critical period for brain development and the optimal degree of neural plasticity that is present before 3 years of age. The benefits of starting an intervention early, before secondary impairments develop, needs to be balanced against the risk of wasting intervention resources on children whose difficulties are likely to resolve spontaneously. The question is how to identify young children with serious language impairments who are unlikely to spontaneously »outgrow« their delay. Bishop offered the following guidelines (Bishop 1994, 2002): children whose expressive vocabularies consist of fewer than 50 words at the age of 24 months should be carefully monitored, whereas long-term problems are unlikely in children with vocabularies of more than eight words who have good comprehension.

The conventional way to assess and identify children with language impairments is to use traditional standardized omnibus tests, using the criterion that the standard score on a language test and a nonverbal IQ test differ by at least 1 SD. This omnibus test approach has several limitations. First, there are no intrinsic criterion for where to draw the line between »normal« and »affected«, and the choice of 1 SD is arbitrary. Secondly, there is no clear indication of how to translate a child's score into particular linguistic competencies that may or may not be affected. Knowledge of a child's standardized test score does not indicate which aspects of language development require supplementary training. Thirdly, it is not possible to interpret a child's performance relative to the expected adult level of language, or a child's level of progress toward that level (Rice 2000).

Rice argues that instead of trying to encompass all dimensions of language competence in a single identification instrument, it would be of more value to target those dimensions that accurately identify affected children (i.e., show high levels of sensitivity). She suggests that it might be possible to identify young children with language impairments based on certain grammatical morphemes. Children with specific language impairments are very late in acquiring grammatical morphemes, a characteristic symptom that is thought to be a hallmark of the condition (Bishop 1997; Leonard 1998; Rice 2000). The use of a clinical grammatical marker for identification purposes could improve the »hit« rate in determining which children have a specific language impairment and which can be considered to be developing in a typical manner.

19.4.4   Prevention

19.4.4.1   Primary Prevention

Twin and adoption studies consistently suggest that heritance has a strong influence on measures of verbal ability. Indeed, a case could be made that verbal measures are among the most heritable behavioral traits (Plomin and Dale 2000). This offers the hope of early gene-based detection or prediction of children at risk of language impairments in the future. This would enable the use of preventive interventions instead of treatment interventions when language problems are full blown and cast a long and broad shadow over a child's cognitive and social development.

Preventive interventions are sometimes used for children from more deprived backgrounds. Children raised in economic poverty have a below average development of language and are over-represented among children with reading difficulties. This has led to the development of intervention programs providing »enrichment« or »compensatory education«. The idea is to compensate for the children's supposed deprivation. These types of programs are discussed in the section on overall level of cognitive functioning.

19.4.4.2 Secondary and Tertiary Prevention

Somewhat surprisingly, children with specific language impairments who are acquiring a language with a rich inflectional morphology seem less impaired in the use of grammatical inflections than their counterparts who are acquiring a language with a sparse inflectional morphology, such as English. This suggests that certain characteristics render grammatical morphemes more (or less) accessible. This finding has implications for intervention because it means that one could try to provide optimal input (Leonard 2000). Stories and conversations with young infants and children could be adjusted to include more inflected forms of words. Other investigators have suggested that increasing the duration of pauses separating speakers' utterances may be another way to promote linguistic processing (Ellis Weismer 2000).

A related theory suggests that children with specific language impairments have a limited processing capacity. This theory suggests that one should try to reduce the processing demands of the language learning task for these children, for instance by lowering the rate of speech, vocal stress, or by using visual cues accompanying spoken language (Ellis Weismer 2000). Another suggestion is the use of scripts, familiar routines for common events such as bath-time, bedtime, and birthday parties. The assumption is that an intervention given during a familiar routine will reduce a child's cognitive load so he or she can focus on language targets (McCormick 1997).

Other procedures that are widely used to facilitate language development in children are sentence recasting (a child's utterance is immediately repeated by the adult with some modifications, often correcting errors in the child's utterance); elicited

imitation (presentation of a nonverbal stimuli along with a request for a specific verbal response from the child); and modeling (presentation of a set of training stimuli, and asking the child to respond in the same manner; Frey and Proctor-Williams 2000).

In general, there has been a move away from a focus solely on grammar and phonology toward interventions that develop the social use of language (Bishop 2002). Speech and language therapists usually carry out the interventions. Clinician-implemented early language intervention programs have significant facilitating effects on language development (Ellis Weismer and Schraeder 1993; Robertson and Ellis Weismer 1999). Moreover, professional intervention can often prevent the development of additional behavioral, learning, reading, and social development disorders (Downey et al. 2002).

It can be especially attractive to involve parents in interventions for preschool-aged children. In these approaches, parents are trained to promote their children's language development at home, so that the intervention can be interwoven into natural episodes of communication. These programs are generally effective (Whitehurst et al. 1991; Girolametto et al. 1997, 1999).

A third way is to use computer programs to promote language development. Several studies suggest that children with DLD have difficulty processing brief or rapidly presented stimuli. This inspired Tallal and colleagues to develop a special computer-based training exercise called »Fast Forward«, which attempts to speed up the neural processing of rapidly successive acoustic stimuli (Merzenich et al. 1996; Tallal et al. 1996).

19.5 Mental Retardation

19.5.1 Introduction

People who have a level of cognitive functioning significantly below the average are called mentally retarded (preferred in USA) or learning disabled (preferred in UK). Cognitive functioning, or the general capacity for judgment, comprehension, and reasoning, is referred to as intelligence. In general, intelligence is viewed as the capacity to lead one's life, to cope with and to master the external environment. In practice, intelligence has been defined in rather different ways, with some definitions emphasizing more abstract cognitive abilities and others more practical »real world« capacities for solving problems. The current approach to the diagnosis of mental retardation is a compromise: an individual is considered to be mentally retarded if he or she fulfills the following three criteria: (a) a significant subaverage general intellectual functioning, (b) deficits or impairments in present adaptive functioning, and (c) onset before age 18 months (American Psychiatric Association 1994). The intelligence quotient (IQ) is often used to express the level of cognitive disability.

19.5.2 Relevance for Future Development

The rate of mental retardation is somewhere between 1% and 3%, depending on the criterion used. The use of IQ < 70 as the sole criterion for mental retardation results in a prevalence rate of between 2% and 3%. The use of IQ < 70 in combination with significant adaptation impairment as criterion results in a prevalence rate of about 1% (Volkmar and Dykens 2002).

Given the heterogeneous nature of mental retardation, it is not surprising that its natural history and course vary considerably depending on the severity of mental retardation and on underlying biomedical, psychological, and environmental factors. In general, mild mental retardation has the best outcome. But even when special services are not apparently required, the individual may still be vulnerable, and the presence of a supportive environment may be of particular importance. The prognosis for adult self-sufficiency and independence is more guarded for individuals with moderate mental retardation. However, many individuals can live semi-independently with partial support. Individuals with severe or profound retardation require high levels of supervision and support throughout life (Volkmar and Dykens 2002).

19.5.3 Early Detection

Genetic tests exist for some disorders associated with mental retardation, allowing prenatal or newborn screening. In general, women wish to be given the choice whether or not to participate in screening tests. However, in some countries and centers prenatal screening may not be available or may not be voluntary and women may not be given sufficient information to make informed decisions (Al Jader et al. 2000).

In many countries, monitoring of a child's cognitive development is one of the key functions of well-baby clinics, pediatric nurses, or health visitors. Accurate identification of children at risk of developmental delay requires knowledge of whether a child shows age-appropriate skills in various developmental domains. At the in-depth clinical investigation, the level of functioning is assessed by means of standardized tests of intelligence.

Galton was one of the first to attempt to measure intelligence with a series of tests. He considered intelligence, like the physical variables of height and weight, to be distributed systematically in the general population (Kelley and Surbeck 2000). In the decades that followed, a driving force for the development of intelligence tests was the need to evaluate school-aged children for appropriate school placement. The first intelligence test to be used widely was the Stanford-Binet Intelligence Scale (Binet and Simon 1905). The main objective of this test was to distinguish the retarded from the normal – to differentiate between those who were failing at school and those who were successful. Many revised versions followed. By 1910, testing of school-age children was well-established (Kelley and Surbeck 2000). At that time, the general theoretical approach viewed intelligent activity as passive and stable.

In the 1930s, factor analytic studies reported a number of recognizable group factors in terms of intelligence. This led to the introduction of subtests to measure the various components of intelligence, such as verbal ability, numerical ability, mechanical ability, and attention. Tests such as the Wechsler Intelligence Scales for Children (WISC) have both verbal and performance scales.

In the late 1940s and early 1950s, an alternative view of development altered the nature of tests. Intelligence was no longer considered a general unitary ability. Instead, a child's personal variables and socio-cultural environment were viewed as important components of an individual's level of functioning in addition to primary mental abilities. Piaget (Piaget 1952), among others, stressed the importance of experience. To Piaget the quality of the environment and the nature of the organism's activity were of vital importance. Many research studies confirmed that the quality of the environment was an important factor in development. As a result, educators called for preschool intervention and early education for the economically disadvantaged and those »at risk of school failure« (Kelley and Surbeck 2000).

19.5.4   Prevention

19.5.4.1   Primary Prevention

With respect to mental retardation, primary prevention often takes the form of preconceptional counseling, to minimize the risk factors associated with specific conditions. Examples are genetic counseling, dietary advice, and the use of preconceptional folic acid to reduce the risk of neural tube defect, and immunization to prevent congenital rubella (Bernard 2002).

A genetic cause has been identified in some disorders associated with mental retardation, for example, fragile X and Down syndrome. This makes primary prevention possible. First, it enables preconception genetic counseling for couples at risk, to allow couples to make informed reproductive decisions. Secondly, the option of preimplantation diagnosis makes possible the selection of unaffected fetuses for implantation (Simonoff 2002). Thirdly, prenatal diagnosis offers parents the option of terminating pregnancies of affected fetuses.

19.5.4.2   Secondary Prevention

Lack of exposure to appropriate opportunities for learning is known to result in impaired intellectual performance, due to psychosocial or sensory deprivation. The effect of psychosocial deprivation in lowering mean intellectual performance was demonstrated in the highly contentious issue of relative IQ levels among different ethnic groups in the same society. When adopted into more privileged families, children from a socially deprived group showed a 15-point higher mean IQ than children from their original social milieu (Scarr and Weinburg 1976).

In the years following the Second World War, most Western societies embraced the philosophy of »equality of opportunity« – all children should have an equal opportunity for acquiring intelligence and for developing their talents and abilities to the fullest (the Newsom report, Central Advisory Council for Education 1963). In many countries, the notion that some children are reared in a deprived or impoverished environment led to the implementation of preschool programs for economically disadvantaged children. The aims of such programs usually reflect one of three philosophies: an emphasis on maturational principles that stress a nurturant social-emotional environment; a behavioristic approach that emphasizes highly structured didactic methods; or a cognitive-interactionist approach that focuses on the child's construction of knowledge.

The general idea behind these programs is that »enrichment« or »compensatory education« may compensate for the supposed deprivation. In certain circumstances, for example, in institutions such as children's homes, enrichment programs can have very substantial effects. In general, however, the outcome of compensatory education programs has been modest at best. Early evaluation studies reported disappointing results (Oliver and Head 1990; Richmond 1990). These disappointing results have been explained in several ways. One explanation is that schools are essentially white, middle-class institutions in terms of their values, language used by teachers, and content of course. It can therefore be expected that children from different backgrounds do not fit in and therefore achieve less. Another explanation is that compensatory education programs do not deal with the underlying social and material inequalities, such as lower income, poor housing, and difficult family circumstances. As long as these underlying inequalities remain, interventions will not have a large effect. Finally, it has been argued that children from a lower social class background have, on average, a genetically lower potential for intelligence (Smith and Cowie 1992).

Later evaluation studies concluded that early compensatory education programs for economically disadvantaged children could have significant long-term effects. A meta-analysis of 167 interventions for children from 0 to 6 years showed that these programs affected health and social outcomes, although their effects were variable (Brown et al. 2000).

19.5.4.3   Tertiary Prevention

Children with special needs are usually those who are failing within the normal educational system or who are, in some way, performing below the average that can be expected of children of their age. How the educational needs of these children should be met is controversial. If children with special needs continue within the normal school system, they have the advantages of sports facilities, laboratories, libraries, and other school resources, as well as the possibility of choosing from the full range of school subjects; there are also opportunities to mix with ordinary children and to learn the social skills they will need in adult life. There are also disadvantages: lessons may not always be designed to cater for these children's needs; children may have a sense of failure and inadequacy; and other children may not always be tolerant. Resentment may arise from the extra time and tuition that children with special needs require.

The twentieth century has witnessed massive changes in the attitude toward people with mental retardation, and with these changes has come a shift from institutionalized and custodial care to individualized and community-based care. Some educationalists maintain that there are still strong arguments in favor of special schools staffed by people trained to meet the social emotional, physical, and educational needs of these children (Smith and Cowie 1992).

19.6   Concluding Remarks

Much progress has been made in the early detection and prevention of developmental disorders, with emphasis on the characteristics of the disorders in very young children and on the development of screening instruments and early intervention programs. There seems to be consensus that the success of an intervention is determined by the age at which it is started. Developmental principles support the notion of »earlier is better«. One could argue that an earlier intervention means a smaller developmental gap that has to be closed. Another argument for early intervention is that neurological plasticity decreases with age. Moreover, age at the start of intervention has been shown to be correlated with treatment outcome: children who start behavioral intervention earlier achieve a better prognosis (Bibby et al. 2001; Fenske et al. 1985; Harris and Handleman 2000). However, the pursuit of very early identification of a disability may lead to misdiagnosis and inappropriate use of services. Furthermore, an inherent danger of premature labeling is unnecessary stigmatization of the infant.

It is likely that in the next decades the focus will shift from behavior-based screening and intervention to genetics. It is likely that susceptibility genes for a number of developmental disorders will be identified. As a result, gene-based early identification of children at risk of developmental disorders will become more and more important for primary prevention.

We would like to conclude with some recommendations. With respect to level 1 screening, primary care providers must change their approach to well-child care and proactively screen for developmental disorders (Filipek et al. 1999). The time

allowed for well-child appointments should be increased, to make routine developmental surveillance and screening possible. As standard practice, parents should be encouraged to voice their concerns. In the next phase, in-depth investigations must include appropriate standardized diagnostic instruments (Filipek et al. 1999). Screening and assessment instruments should be valid, reliable, standardized, and easy to use. Equally important is the relevance of these instruments to planning, monitoring, and evaluating human services and educational programs for children and families.

Often, it is not one specific risk factor but rather the accumulation and interplay of several risk factors and the absence of sufficient protective factors that lead to a developmental disorder. The probability of a specific developmental disorder may increase as a function of the number, the duration, and the impact of risk factors as well as the number, the duration, and the impact of protective factors. To gain insight in this developmental process longitudinal studies of representative populations are needed that start early in life and follow up into adulthood. Effective prevention programs are likely to be those that address a combination of malleable risk and protective factors (Jane-Llopis 2002).

Finally, our own studies have shown that compliance can be a troublesome issue. Many children at high risk are not enrolled in screening or intervention programs by their parents, even if these programs are widely available (Cunningham et al. 1995, 2000; O'Donnell et al. 1995; Offord and Bennett 2002). Families who begin the process sometimes withdraw prematurely (Kazdin and Alan 1996). More research is needed to determine the factors that influence parental compliance.

References

Adrien JL, Lenoir P, Martineau J, Perrot A, Hameury L, Larmande C, Sauvage D (1993) Blind ratings of early symptoms of autism based upon family home movies. Journal of the American Academy of Child and Adolescent Psychiatry 32:617–626

Al Jader LN, Parry-Langdon N, Smith RJ (2000) Survey of attitudes of pregnant women towards Down syndrome screening. Prenatal Diagnosis 23:779–783

American Psychiatric Association (1994) Diagnostic and Statistical Manual of Mental Disorders, fourth edition, DSM-IV. APA, Washington

Baird G, Charman T, Baron CS, Cox A, Swettenham J, Wheelwright S, Drew A (2000) A screening instrument for autism at 18 months of age: a 6-year follow-up study. Journal of the American Academy of Child and Adolescent Psychiatry 39:694–702

Baron-Cohen S, Allen J, Gillberg C (1992) Can autism be detected at 18 months? The needle, the haystack and the CHAT. British Journal of Psychiatry 161:839–843

Baron-Cohen S, Cox A, Baird G, Swettenham J, Nightingale N, Morgan K, Drew A, Charman T (1996) Psychological markers in the detection of autism in infancy in a large population. British Journal of Psychiatry 168:158–163

Bernard SH (2002) Services for children and adolescents with severe learning disabilities (Mental Retardation). In: Rutter M, Taylor E, (eds) Child and Adolescent Psychiatry. Blackwell Science, Oxford, pp 1114–1127

Berument SK, Rutter M, Lord C, Pickles A, Bailey A (1999) Autism screening questionnaire: diagnostic validity. British Journal of Psychiatry 175:444–451

Bibby P, Eikeseth S, Martin NT, Mudford OC, Reeves D (2001) Progress and outcomes for children with autism receiving parent-managed intensive interventions. Research in Developmental Disabilities 22:425–447

Binet A, Simon T (1905) New methods for diagnosis of the intellectual level of subnormals. L'Annee Psychologique 14:1–90

Bishop DVM (1994) Developmental Disorders of Speech and Language. In: Rutter M, Taylor E, (eds) Child and Adolescent Psychiatry. Blackwell Scientific, Oxford, pp 546–568

Bishop DVM (1997) Uncommon understanding: Development and disorders of language comprehension in children. Psychology Press, Howe

Bishop DVM (2002) Speech and Language Difficulties. In: Rutter M, Taylor E (eds) Child and Adolescent Psychiatry. Blackwell Science, Oxford, pp 664–681

Boyd RD, Corley MJ (2001) Outcome survey of early intensive behavioral intervention for young children with autism in a community setting. Autism 5:430–441

Bristol-Power MM, Spinella G (1999) Research on screening and diagnosis in autism: a work in progress. Journal of Autism and Developmental Disorders 29:435–438

Brown CH, Brendt D, Brinales J, Zong X, Bhagwat D (2000) Evaluating the evidence of effectiveness for preventive interventions: using a registry system to influence policy through science. Additive Behaviours 25:955–964

Caplan G (1964) Principles of Preventive Psychiatry. Basic Books, New york

Central Advisory Council for Education (1963) Newson Report: Half Our Future. HSMO, London

Chakrabarti S, Fombonne E (2001) Pervasive developmental disorders in preschool children. Journal of the American Medical Association 285:3141–3142

Charman T (2003) Why is joint attention a pivotal skill in autism? Philosophical Transactions of the Royal Society of London Series B Biological sciences 358:315–324

Cowen EL (1983) Primary prevention in mental health: past present and future. In: Felner RD, Jason A, Moritsugu JN, Farber SS (eds) Preventive Psychology: Theory, Research, and Practice. Pergamon Press, New York, pp 11–25

Cunningham CE, Bremner R, Boyle M (1995) Large group community-based parenting programs for families of pre-schoolers at risk for disruptive behaviour disorders: utilization, cost effectiveness and outcome. Journal of Child Psychology and Psychiatry 36:1141–1159

Cunningham CE, Boyle M, Offord DR (2000) Correlates of school-based parenting course utilization. Journal of Consulting and Clinical Psychology 68:928–933

Dahlgren SO, Gillberg C (1989) Symptoms in the first two years of life. A preliminary population study of infantile autism. European Archives of Psychiatry and Neurological Sciences 238:169–174

DeWolff MS, van IJzendoorn MH (1997) Sensitivity and attachment. A meta-analysis on parental antecedents of infant-attachment. Child Development 68:571–591

Dietz C, Willemsen-Swinkels SHN, Van Daalen E, Van Engeland H, Buitelaar J (Submitted a) Population screening for Autism Spectrum Disorders at 14 months. Design and general findings

Dietz C, Willemsen-Swinkels SHN, Van Daalen E, Van Engeland H, Buitelaar J (Submitted b) The development of a screening instrument for Autism Spectrum Disorders in Pre-schoolers

Downey D, Mraz R, Knott J, Knutson C, Holte L, Van Dyke D (2002) Diagnosis and evaluation of children who are not talking. Infants and Young Children 15:38–48

Drew A, Baird G, Baron-Cohen S, Cox A, Slonims V, Wheelwright S, Swettenham J, Berry B, Charman T (2002) A pilot randomised control trial of a parent training intervention for per-school children with autism: preliminary findings and methodological challenges. European Child and Adolescent Psychiatry 11:266–272

Ellis Weismer S (2000) Intervention for children with developmental language delay. In: Bishop DVM, Leonard LB (eds) Speech and Language Impairments in Children. Causes, Characteristics, Intervention and Outcome. Psychology Press LTD, Hove, pp 157–176

Ellis Weismer S, Schraeder T (1993) Discourse characteristics and verbal reasoning: Wait time effects on the performance of children with language learning disabilities. Exceptionality Education Canada 3:71–92

Fenske EC, Zalenski S, Krantz PJ, Mcclannahan LE (1985) Age at intervention and treatment outcome for autistic children in a comprehensive intervention program. Analysis and Intervention in Developmental Disabilities 5:49–58

Filipek PA, Accardo PJ, Baranek GT, Cook-EH J, Gordon B, Gravel JS, Johnson CP, Kallen RJ, Levy SE, Minshew NJ, Prizant BM, Rapin I, Rogers SJ, Stone WL, Teplin S, Tuchman RF, Volkmar FR (1999) The screening and diagnosis of autistic spectrum disorders. Journal of Autism and Developmental Disorders 29:439–484

Fombonne E (1999) The epidemiology of autism: a review. Psychological Medicine 29:769–786

Frey ME, Proctor-Williams K (2000) Recasting, elicited imitation and modelling in grammar intervention for children with specific language impairments. In: Bishop DVM, Leonard LB (eds) Speech and Language Impairments in Children. Causes, Characteristics, Intervention and Outcome. Psychology Press LTD, Hove, pp 177–194

Garralda ME (2002) Primary Health Care Psychiatry. In: Rutter M, Taylor E (eds) Child and Adolescent Psychiatry. Blackwell Science, Oxford, pp 1090–1100

Ghuman JK, Freund L, Reiss A, Serwint J, Folstein S (1998) Early detection of social interaction problems: development of a social interaction instrument in young children. Journal of Developmental and Behavioral Pediatrics 19:411–419

Gill AR (2001) Letter: Interventions for Autism. Journal of the American Medical Association 286

Girolametto L, Pearce P, Weitzman E (1997) Effects of lexical intervention on the phonology of late talkers. Journal of Speech, Language, and Hearing Research 40:378–388

Girolametto L, Pearce P, Weitzman E (1999) Interactive focused stimulation for toddlers with expressive vocabulary delays. Journal of Speech, Language, and Hearing Research 39:1274–1283

Glascoe FP (1994) It's not what it seems. The relationship between parents' concerns and children with global delays. Clinical Pediatrics 33:292–296

Glascoe FP (1997) Parents' concerns about children's development: prescreening technique or screening test? [see comments]. Pediatrics 99:522–528

Glascoe FP (1999) Using parents' concerns to detect and address developmental and behavioral problems. Journal of the Society of Pediatric Nurses 4:24–35

Glascoe FP (2000) Evidence-based approach to developmental and behavioural surveillance using parents' concerns. Child: Care, Health and Development 26:137–149

Harris SL, Handleman JS (2000) Age and IQ at intake as predictors of placement for young children with autism: a four- to six-year follow-up. Journal of Autism and Developmental Disorders 30:137–142

Hughes DA (1999) Adopting children with attachment problems. Child Welfare 78:541–560

Ingersoll B, Schreibman L, Stahmer A (2001) Brief report: Differential treatment outcome for children with autism spectrum disorder based on level of peer social avoidance. Journal of Autism and Developmental Disorders 31:343–349

International Molecular Genetic Study of Autism Consortium (1998) A full genome screen for autism with evidence for linkage to a region on chromosome 7q. Human Molecular Genetics 7:571–578

Jane-Llopis E (2002) What makes the ounce of prevention effective? Dissertation, Nijmegen, The Netherlands

Johnson CJ, Beitchman JH, Young A, Escobar M, Atkinson L, Wilson B, Brownlie EB, Douglas L, Taback N, Lam I, Wang M (1999) Fourteen year follow-up of children with and without speech/language impairment. Journal of Speech and Hearing Research 42:744–760

Kasari C, Freeman SFN, Paparella T (2001) Early intervention in autism: joint attention and symbolic play. International Review of Research in Mental Retardation 23:207–237

Kazdin AE, Alan E (1996) Dropping out of child psychotherapy: issues for research and implications for practice. Clinical Child Psychology and Psychiatry 1:133–156

Kelley MF, Surbeck E (2000) History of preschool assessment. In: Bracken BA (ed) The psychoeducational assessment of preschool children. Allyn and Bacon, Boston, pp 1–18

Koegel LK (2000) Intervention to facilitate communication in autism. Journal of Autism and Developmental Disorders 30:383–391

Koegel LK, Camarata SM, Valdez-Menchaca M, Koegel RL (1998) Setting generalization of question-asking by children with autism. American Journal on Mental Retardation 102:346–357

Krantz PJ (2000) Commentary: interventions to facilitate socialization. Journal of Autism and Developmental Disorders 30:411–413

Lahey M, Edwards M (1995) Specific language impairment: preliminary investigation of factors associated with family history and with patterns of language performance. Journal of Speech and Hearing Research 38:643–657

Le Couteur A, Rutter M, Lord C, Rios P, Robertson S, Holdgrafer M, McLennan JD (1989) Autism Diagnostic Interview: a semi-structured interview for parents and caregivers of autistic persons. Journal of Autism and Developmental Disorders 19:363–387

Leaf R, McEachin J (1999) A work in progress: Behavioral Management Strategies and a Curriculum for Intensive Behavioral Treatment of Autism. Different Roads to Learning, New York

Leekam S, Lopez B, Moore C (2000) Attention and joint attention in preschool children with autism. Developmental Psychology 39:261–273

Leonard LB (1998) Children with specific language impairment. MIT Press, Cambridge

Leonard LB (2000) Specific language impairments across languages. In: Bishop DVM, Leonard LB (eds) Speech and Language Impairments in Children. Causes, Characteristics, Intervention and Outcome. Psychology Press LTD, Hove, pp 115–129

Lord C (2000) Commentary: Achievements and future directions for intervention in communication and autism spectrum disorders. Journal of Autism and Developmental Disorders 30:393–398

Lord C, Rutter M, Le Couteur A (1994) Autism Diagnostic Interview-Revised: a revised version of a diagnostic interview for caregivers of individuals with possible pervasive developmental disorders. Journal of Autism and Developmental Disorders 24:659–685

Lord C, Rutter M, DiLavore P (1998) Autistic Diagnostic Observation Schedule-Generic. University of Chicago, Chicago, Illinois

Lovaas OI (1987) Behavioral treatment and normal educational and intellectual functioning in young autistic children. Journal of Consulting and Clinical Psychology 55:3–9

Marcus LM, Rubin JS, Rubin MA (2000) Benefit-cost analysis and autism services: a response to jacobson and mulick. Journal of Autism and Developmental Disorders 30:595–598

Marvin RS (2003) Implications of Attachment Research for the Field of Family Therapy. In: Erdman P, Caffery T (eds) Attachment and Family Systems. Conceptual, Empirical, and Therapeutic Relatedness. Brunner-Routledge, New York Hove, pp 3–27

McCormick L (1997) Language intervention and support. In: McCormick L, Frome Loeb D, Schiefelbusch R (eds) Supporting children with communication difficulties in inclusive settings: school-based language intervention. Allyn & Bacon, Needham Heights, pp 257–306

Merzenich MM, Jenkins WM, Johnston P, Schreiner C, Miller SL, Tallal P (1996) Temporal processing deficits of language-learning impaired children ameliorated by training. Science 271:77–81

Mundy P, Neal R (2001) Neural Plasticity, Joint attention, and a transactional social-orienting model of autism. International Review of Research in Mental Retardation 23: 139–168

National research council (2001) Educating children with autism. National Academy of Sciences, Washington DC

O'Conner TG (2002) Attachment Disorders of Infancy and Childhood. In: Rutter M, Taylor E (eds) Child and Adolescent Psychiatry. Blackwell Science, Oxford, pp 776–792

O'Donnell, Hawkins JD, Catalano RF, Abbott RD, Day LE (1995) Preventing school failure, drug abuse, and delinquency among low-income children: long-term intervention in elementary schools. American Journal of Orthopsychiatry 65:87–100

Offord DR, Bennett KJ (2002) Prevention. In: Rutter M, Taylor E, (eds) Child and Adolescent Psychiatry. Blackwell Science, Oxford, pp 881–899

Oliver C, Head D (1990) Self-injurious behaviour in people with learning disabilities: recent advances in assessment and intervention. Journal of Child and Adolescent Psychiatrie 30:909–927

Osterling J, Dawson G (1994) Early Recognition of Children with Autism – A Study of First Birthday Home Videotapes. Journal of Autism and Developmental Disorders 24:247–257

Ozonoff S, Cathcart K (1998) Effectiveness of a home program intervention for young children with autism. Journal of Autism and Developmental Disorders 28:25–32

Paul R (1991) Profiles of toddlers with slow expressive language disorders. Topics in Language Disorders 11:1–13

Paul R (2000) Predicting outcomes of early expressive language delay: Ethical implications. In: Bishop DVM, Leonard LB (eds) Speech and Language Impairments in Children. Causes, Characteristics, Intervention and Outcome. Psychology Press LTD, Hove, pp 195–211

Pelios LV, Lund SK (2001) A selective overview of issues on classification, causation, and early intensive behavioral intervention for autism. Behavior Modification 25:678–697

Piaget J (1952) The origins of intelligence in children (M. Cook, trans.). Holt, New York

Plomin R, Dale P (2000) Genetics and early language development: A UK study of twins. In: Bishop DVM, Leonard LB (eds) Speech and Language Impairments in Children. Causes, Characteristics, Intervention and Outcome. Psychology Press LTD, Hove, pp 35–51

Rescola L, Schwartz E (1990) Outcomes of toddlers with specific expressive language delay. Applied Psycholinguistics 11:393–407

Rice ML (2000) Grammatical symptoms of specific language impairment. In: Bishop DVM, Leonard LB (eds) Speech and Language Impairments in Children. Causes, Characteristics, Intervention and Outcome. Psychology Press LTD, Hove, pp 17–34

Richmond J (1990) Low birth weight infants: can we enhance their development? Journal of the American Medical Association 263:3069–3070

Roberts J, Rescola L, Giroux J, Stevens L (1998) Phonological skills of children with specific expressive language impairment (SLI-E): Outcome at age 3. Journal of Speech, Language, and Hearing Research 41:374–384

Robertson SB, Ellis Weismer S (1999) Effects of treatment on linguistic and social skills in toddlers with delayed language development. Journal of Speech, Language, and Hearing Research 42:1234–1248

Robins DL, Fein D, Barton ML, Green JA (2001) The modified Checklist for autism in toddlers: an initial study investigating the early detection of autism and pervasive developmental disorders. Journal of Autism and Developmental Disorders 2001:131–144

Rogers SJ (1998) Empirically supported comprehensive treatments for young children with autism. Journal of Clinical Child Psychology 27:168–179

Rutter M, Mawhood L (1991) The long-term psychosocial sequelae of specific developmental disorders of speech and language. In: Rutter M, Casaer P (eds) Biological Risk Factors for Psychosocial Disorders. Cambridge University Press, Cambridge, pp 233–259

Rutter M, Mawhood I, Howlin P (1992) Language delay and social development. In: Fletcher P, Hall D (eds) Specific Speech and Language Disorders in Children: Correlates, Characteristics, and Outcome. Whurr, London, pp 63–78

Scarr S, Weinburg RA (1976) IQ test performance of black children adopted by white families. American Psychologist 31:726–739

Schreibman L (2000) Intensive behavioral/psychoeducational treatment for autism: Research needs and future directions. Journal of Autism and Developmental Disorders 30:373–378

Shastry BS (2003) Molecular genetics of autism spectrum disorders. Journal of Human Genetics 48:495–501

Sheinkopf SJ, Siegel B (1998) Home-based behavioral treatment of young children with autism. Journal of Autism and Developmental Disorders 28:15–23

Siegel B (1996) Pervasive Developmental Disorders Screening test. Unpublished Work

Simonoff E (2002) Genetic Counseling. In: Rutter M, Taylor E (eds) Child and Adolescent Psychiatry. Blackwell Science, Oxford, pp 1101

Smith PK, Cowie H (1992) Understanding children's development. Blackwell Publishers, Oxford

Smith T, Buch GA, Gamby TE (2000) Parent-directed, intensive early intervention for children with pervasive developmental disorder. Research in Developmental Disabilities 21:297–309

Stone WL, Coonrod EE, Ousley OY (2001) Brief report: Screening Tool for Autism in two-year-olds (STAT): Development

19

and Preliminary Data. Journal of Autism and Developmental Disorders 30:607–612

Szatmari P, Jones MB, Zwaigenbaum L, MacLean JE (1998) Genetics of Autism: Overview and new directions. Journal of Autism and Developmental Disorders 28:351–368

Tallal P, Miller SL, Bedi G, Byma G, Wang X, Nagarajan SS, Schreiner C, Jenkins WM, Merzenich MM (1996) Language comprehension in language-learning impaired children improved with acoustically modified speech. Science 271:81–84

Tomblin JB, Records NL, Buckwalter P, Zhang X, Smith E, O'Brien M (1997) Prevalence of specific language impairment in kindergarten children. Journal of Speech and Hearing Research 40:1245–1260

Van IJzendoorn M, Juffer F, Duyvesteyn MGC (1995) Breaking the intergenerational cycle of insecure attachment: A review of the effects of attachment-based interventions on maternal sensitivity and infant security. Journal of Child Psychology and Psychiatry 36:225–248

Volkmar FR, Dykens E (2002) Mental Retardation. In: Rutter M, Taylor E (eds) Child and Adolescent Psychiatry. Blackwell Science, Oxford, pp 697–710

Whalen C, Schreibman L (2003) Joint attention training for children with autism using behavior modification procedures. Journal of Child Psychology and Psychiatry 44:456–468

Whitehurst GJ, Fischel JE, Lonigan CJ, Valdez-Menchaca MC, Arnolds DS, Smith M (1991) Treatment of early expressive language delay: if, when, and how. Topics in Language Disorders 11:55–68

Willemsen-Swinkels SHN, Dietz C, Van Daalen E, Kerkhof GA, Van Engeland H, Buitelaar J (submitted) Screening instrument for Autism Spectrum Disorder in children younger than 18 months

Yonan AL, Alarcon M, Cheng R, Magnusson PK, Spence SJ, Palmer AA, Grunn A, Juo SH, Terwilliger JD, Liu J, Cantor RM, Geschwind DH, Gilliam TC (2003) A genomewide screen of 345 families for autism-susceptibility loci. American Journal of Human Genetics 73:886–897

Prevention and Early Detection of Emotional Disorders

Andreas Dick-Niederhauser, Wendy K. Silverman

20.1 Introduction – 272

20.2 Why Prevention Is Necessary – 272

20.3 Identification of Preventive Factors – 273

20.4 Principles, Strategies, and Methods of Intervention – 275

20.5 Implementation and Outcome – 277
20.5.1 Universal Prevention – 278
20.5.2 Selective Prevention – 279
20.5.3 Indicated Prevention – 280

20.6 Conclusions and Further Research Directions – 281

References – 283

20.1 Introduction

The terms »emotional disorders« and »internalizing disorders« are traditionally used interchangeably for a group of mental disorders in childhood and adolescence that are primarily experienced in the form of internal distress. Although they might often affect a young person's functioning in important life areas such as family, friends, and school, they are usually less recognized by and less visible to parents and teachers than »conduct disorders« or »externalizing disorders« (see Chap. 21).

In terms of psychiatric diagnoses, according to the **Diagnostic and Statistical Manual of Mental Disorders, 4th revision** (DSM-IV; American Psychiatric Association 1994), emotional (or internalizing) disorders in childhood and adolescence comprise two major categories of disorders: mood disorders (with the diagnoses of major depressive disorder, dysthymic disorder, bipolar disorder, and cyclothymic disorder as the major subcategories) and anxiety disorders (with the diagnoses of panic disorder, agoraphobia, specific phobia, social phobia, obses-

sive-compulsive disorder, generalized anxiety disorder, and posttraumatic stress disorder as the major subcategories) plus separation anxiety disorder, an anxiety disorder that is grouped under »Disorders Usually First Diagnosed In Infancy, Childhood, Or Adolescence«.

This chapter focuses on the prevention and early detection of these mood and anxiety disorders. Suicide and suicidal behavior or ideation are not considered in this chapter, since suicide prevention in childhood and adolescence reaches beyond the scope of preventing emotional disorders (for review, cf. Gould and Kramer 2001). Moreover, this chapter focuses on prevention of emotional disorders in childhood and adolescence as a means to reduce the incidence of new cases through intervention before the onset of the initial episode of the disease as well as on early detection of problems or mild disorders and early intervention before the disorder becomes severe. This chapter does not include, however, prevention as a means of reducing the prevalence of emotional disorders that have already become manifest by reducing their duration, which involves treatment and relapse prevention.

20.2 Why Prevention Is Necessary

Taken together, mood and anxiety disorders represent the most common forms of psychopathology among children and adolescents. For mood disorders, community studies show that approximately 0.4%–2.5% of children and 0.4%–8.3% of adolescents experience clinically significant episodes of major depression, and approximately 0.6%–1.7% of children and 1.6%–8.0% of adolescents meet criteria for dysthymic disorder (Fristad et al. 2002). The prevalence of any anxiety disorder has been found to be approximately 10% in the general population among children and adolescents. In clinic-referred samples, prevalence rates of emotional disorders are considerably higher. Comorbidity among mood and anxiety disorders in children and adolescents is common (Verhulst 2001).

Significant progress has been made in developing efficacious treatment approaches for child and adolescent anxiety (cf. Silverman and Berman 2001) and depression (cf. Kazdin and Marciano 1998). Although efficacious for the majority of youths, there are several reasons why it would be preferable to prevent the development of child anxiety disorders before they become well established.

First, many adult anxiety disorders have their origins in childhood and adolescence (Keller et al. 1992). Unless successfully treated, anxiety disorders in childhood frequently persist or develop into some other form of anxiety disorder (Dadds et al. 1999). Recent evidence suggests child anxiety may play a causal role in the development of depression among young people (Cole et al. 1998). Childhood depression is a significant risk factor for depression and other disorders during adulthood, and earlier age of onset has been found to be associated with more frequent recurrence of depressive episodes and greater likelihood of conversion to bipolar disorder (Kovacs 1996; Rao et al. 1995). In a number of investigations, up to 40% of children originally identified with depressive symptoms remained symptomatic years later (e.g., DuBois et al. 1995; Lewinsohn et al. 1994).

Second, in addition to the personal suffering of children and their families, the costs of treatment for anxiety and mood disorders by mental health professionals are high. If emotional disorders persist to adulthood, additional expenses are incurred (e.g., cost of unemployment, days lost from work, lost productive work time, hospitalization, medication, and pension payments). Estimates from the recent Burden of Disease Project (Murray and Lopez 1996) suggest that mood and anxiety disorders represent one of the most significant health problems in terms of global burden of disease, exceeding the vast majority of physical health problems. Globally, the ten leading causes of disability account for 40% of all years lived with a disability (YLD) and include five psychiatric conditions: unipolar major depression, alcohol use, bipolar disorder, schizophrenia, and obsessive-compulsive disorder. Major depression alone accounts for 11% of global YLD.

Third, by the time children are referred for treatment, the disorder is often well established and many of the adverse effects on school perfor-

mance and peer relationships have occurred and are difficult to reverse. Finally, current treatments have been found to be ineffective for a significant proportion of anxious and depressive children, with approximately 30%–40% still meeting diagnostic criteria for a clinically significant anxiety disorder or mood disorder at posttreatment (Kendall 1994; Michael and Crowley 2002; Silverman et al. 1999).

There is thus a strong case for the development of programs that aim to reduce the prevalence of children's emotional problems. If we could prevent the onset of childhood depression and anxiety, the benefits in terms of costs savings and reductions in personal suffering by children and their families would be enormous. Not surprisingly, government and mental health agencies have started to emphasize the prevention of mental health problems (cf. Barrett and Turner 2004). This interest is reflected as well by the growing number of papers in academic journals on the topic (e.g., Albee 1996; Coie et al. 1993).

20.3 Identification of Preventive Factors

Programs that aim to prevent the development of emotional disorders typically make use of approaches that manipulate the risk factors involved in the development and/or maintenance of anxiety and mood disorders. Risk factors refer to variables predicting the onset, severity, and duration of psychopathology (Coie et al. 1993). Risk factors for mood and anxiety disorders may be related to (a) general features of the environment (e.g., parents' socioeconomic status), (b) specific environmental influences and learning experiences (e.g., home and school violence, parental attitudes and care-giving, parental psychopathology), and (c) individuals' characteristics (e.g., temperamental factors, coping skills).

Risk factors may be nonspecific and applicable to several mental health problems; others may specifically impact on internalizing disorders only. Of those risk factors that only relate to internalizing disorders, some may be specific to anxiety and depression, others to either anxiety or depression, others only to a specific anxiety or mood disorder. ◘ Table 20.1 summarizes the risk factors that have been found to be associated with mood and anxiety disorders in previous research (for reviews see Beardslee and Gladstone 2001; McWhirter et al. 2000; Silverman and Treffers 2001; Vasey and Dadds 2001).

⬛ **Table 20.1.** Risk factors increasing the probability of developing an anxiety disorder or a mood disorder in childhood and adolescence

Type of risk factor	Anxiety disorders	Mood disorders
Living conditions and social support	Low socioeconomic status, poor housing; large family size; family stress and high daily hassles	Living in poverty, poor housing, poor educational resources; poor social support; lack of care after early loss of parent; family stress and high daily hassles
Parenting, parent-child relationship, attachment	Parental anxiety and overprotection; over-controlling and critical parenting style; parental support of avoidant coping; parental cueing to threat; insecure-disorganized attachment associated with unresolved trauma or loss	Conflict with parents; low family cohesion
Parental psychopathology	Parental anxiety disorder; general parental psychopathology	Parental depression; general parental psychopathology
Peer relationships	Avoidance of peer interactions	Hostility to peers at early age; feeling of lack of peer acceptance
Exposure to traumatic and stressful life-events	Natural disasters; physical and sexual abuse; life transitions (e.g., entering and changing school)	Early loss of a loved one; conflict with parents; poor academic performance; presence of a learning disorder; neonatal health problems, poor health development
Learning processes	Aversive experiences with feared stimulus (classical conditioning); reinforcement of avoidance (operant conditioning); vicarious learning through parent's reactions to feared stimulus (modeling)	Inadequate or insufficient positive reinforcement; avoidance of the depressed person by others; excess in punishment; further reinforcement of depressive symptoms by others' concern or sympathy
Biological and temperamental factors	Heritability approximately 40–50% for anxiety symptoms in children; behavioral inhibition; anxiety sensitivity; abnormalities in neurotransmitter metabolism	Heritability approximately 50% for mood disorders (based on adult twin and adoption research); abnormalities in neurotransmitter metabolism
Coping skills, cognitive style, and emotional processing	Avoidant/emotion-focused coping style; pessimistic/threat-bias thinking and information processing; feeling of lack of control	Negative, self-devaluative appraisal of events; negative view of self, world, and future; automatic cognitive errors (negativistic, categorical, absolute, judgmental thinking); self-defeating attributions (internal, stable, global attributions for failure); negative body image; low self-esteem, emotional dependence, low self-efficacy, sense of helplessness and hopelessness; loss of meaning, feelings of emptiness and loss

In addition to identifying and reducing risk factors, emotional disorders may be prevented by identifying and promoting factors that have been found to protect individuals from developing an anxiety or mood disorder and improve individuals' resilience to both risk factors and psychopathology (Coie et al. 1993). Similar to risk factors, protective factors may be general features of an individual's environment, specific to his or her environment and learning experiences, or internal characteristics of a person. The search for protective factors in the development of emotional disorders has not been as intensive as the search for risk factors and is mainly limited to the areas of social support and coping skills.

With respect to social support, the risk of developing an emotional disorder is reduced when stressful or traumatic life events occur in the presence of positive social support (Murray 1992). White et al. (1998), for example, found a strong negative relation between anxiety level and family social support in a longitudinal study investigating the effects of family social support on anxiety in 11–14-year-olds exposed to community violence.

Coping skills refer to a variety of methods individuals employ in an attempt to cope with negative or aversive situations and may be categorized as (a) problem-focused, (b) emotion-focused, or (c) avoidant. Problem-focused coping refers to strategies that directly address or minimize the effect of the problem. Emotion-focused coping is directed towards the subjective level of distress associated with the problem; avoidant coping strategies focus on avoiding or escaping the problem.

Problem-focused methods such as actively seeking out information, positive self-talk, diversion of attention, relaxation, and thought-stopping have been found to be associated with lower levels of anxiety and distress in 8–18 year-old youths (Brown et al. 1986). Generally, adolescents' use of problem-focused coping strategies is associated with more positive psychological adjustment than their use of emotion-focused coping strategies (Compas et al. 2001), and specifically, avoidant coping has been found to be associated with higher levels of depression in adolescence (Ebata and Moos 1991).

As noted, the identification and investigation of protective factors in youths' lives is a new and developing research approach. Much is to be expected from the area of »positive psychology« and »positive prevention« devoted to creating a science of human strengths that act as buffers against mental illness (Seligman 2002; Snyder and Lopez 2002). This approach assumes that individuals are capable of developing positive human traits such as courage, optimism, interpersonal skill, hope, and honesty, which will make them more resilient against developing emotional and other disorders.

Dick-Niederhauser and Silverman (2004) have explored the usefulness of this approach in understanding the development of anxiety resilience. Specifically, hope and the active pursuit of goals seem to facilitate the manifestation of courage, which in turn increases optimistic cognitive processing, a sense of self-efficacy, and skillful coping. Optimism and self-efficacy reduce the likelihood of threat-biased information processing and avoidant coping associated with anxiety disorders. Based on current knowledge about the risk factors of emotional disorders (see ◘ Table 20.1), other positive psychological concepts that may be important in preventing anxiety and mood disorders include self-esteem, positive affectivity, emotional approach, personal control, problem-solving appraisal, mindfulness, toughness, and social support (cf. Snyder and Lopez 2002).

20.4 Principles, Strategies, and Methods of Intervention

Before preventive measures can be applied to reduce either the incidence of an emotional disorder or the severity of internalizing symptoms in children and adolescents, decisions need to be made regarding general principles and strategies of prevention and early intervention. These concern the timing of the interventions, the systemic level of where the preventive efforts are to be applied (individual child; family; organizations and institutions), and the targets of prevention (e.g., all individuals within a community or only certain selected ones considered to be »at risk«).

The timing of preventive strategies is an important consideration in the implementation of prevention programs for youths with anxiety and mood disorders. Some risk and protective factors such as the parent-child relationship influence a child over an extended period of his or her life; others may occur only at one specific time such as exposure to traumatic or negative life events. Certain risk factors are more likely to occur in certain developmental stages than in others. For example, a behaviorally inhibited child might be at heightened risk of developing an anxiety disorder when confronted with entering school in middle childhood and with having to make the transition to high school in adolescence. For both continual and time-specific risk factors, it

◼ Table 20.2. Prevention and early intervention methods for emotional disorders in children and adolescents

Child focused methods	
Targeting learning processes	Positive reinforcement of approach behavior; imaginal and in-vivo exposure to potentially stressful situations; nontraumatic pre-exposure; scheduling pleasant activities
Targeting inadequate coping skills and information processing	Modeling of non-avoidant coping skills (live or videotaped); teaching coping strategies such as relaxation, positive self statements, problem-solving, and attention distraction; behavioral rehearsal, role-play and practice of coping skills for dealing with the stressful situation; providing information about feared situations (verbally or filmed); identifying automatic negative cognitions, examining evidence related to distorted automatic cognition, substituting more realistic interpretations for distorted cognitions
Targeting peer relationships	Social skills training; self-assertiveness training; anger management training
Targeting trauma exposure	Education about danger; anticipation and prevention of trauma exposure; enhancement of peer and self-protective behaviors; stress inoculation training
Targeting social support	Teaching children how to gain access to social support
Parent focused methods	
Targeting parenting, parent-child relationship, and attachment	Reduction of over-protective and critical child-rearing responses; avoiding focusing on, and communicating, the potentially threatening aspects of the child's environment; parent effectiveness training (training parents in healthy confrontations, conflict resolution, active listening skills)
Targeting vicarious learning through parent	Encouraging and reinforcing their child's use of coping skills; encouraging their child to expose himself/herself to appropriate situations; ignoring and preventing avoidance of situations by their child, where avoidance is not appropriate
Targeting parental psychopathology	Reduction of parent's own anxious behavior; modeling of appropriate coping behavior
Targeting temperamental factors	Education about nature of withdrawal and anxiety; anxiety management strategies for parent; information about importance of promoting child's independence; instructing parents in helping children expose themselves to avoided situations
Environmental restructuring methods	
Targeting traumatic and stressful life-events	Reducing the risk involved in high risk situations (e.g., reducing the inherent stressfulness of high school transition by reorganizing the school structure); attempting to reduce the risk factor (e.g., prevention of divorce, car accidents, etc.)
Targeting living conditions and social support	Providing children with school- and community-based support and activities, e.g. classroom enrichment, homework help, summer tutoring, holiday activities, play groups, cultural programs

is necessary to tailor the presentation of the prevention strategy to the developmental level of the child for the strategy to be effective (cf. Spence 2001).

Most prevention studies on youths' internalizing problems have focused primarily on factors relating to the individual, such as cognitions and behaviors. Winnett (1998) argued that multilevel prevention strategies are necessary to encourage lasting change. He suggested that adequate prevention requires strategies aimed at four levels: (1) personal, (2) interpersonal, (3) organizational and environmental, and (4) institutional. Within each of these four levels, prevention strategies require the appropriation of (a) adequate competencies (knowledge and skills), (b) tangible and intangible resources, and (c) settings in which prevention strategies may be implemented.

Much of the recent literature regarding prevention distinguishes among universal, selected, and indicated prevention (Mrazek and Haggerty 1994), which differ in terms of their target populations. Universal prevention strategies apply to all individuals within a community with the aim of reducing the probability that a disorder will develop. Whole classes or schools may be involved in a prevention program, or whole communities may be targeted through media communications or community programs. Selective prevention strategies are targeted at specific groups or individuals who are considered to be at risk for the development of particular problems as the result of exposure to some risk factor(s) in the past or in the imminent future. For example, children who have experienced a traumatic event, or whose parents experience a mental disorder, may be viewed as more likely to develop certain psychological problems in comparison to the general population. The same is true for children who will undergo medical or dental procedures. The aim is to reduce the negative psychological reactions during the procedure as well as future occurrences of the procedures. Finally, indicated prevention strategies target high-risk individuals who demonstrate minimal but detectable symptoms of a mental disorder.

After making decisions about the timing, level, and target population of prevention and early intervention, experts interested in reducing the occurrence of emotional disorders in youths need to choose an early detection strategy (screen) that reliably identifies at risk youth. In addition, an access point where children can be identified needs to be available such as a school, health-care institution, or the internet using web-based surveys. The types of early detection and screening strategies are likely to vary with the type of preventive intervention program being implemented. In the case of an indicated prevention strategy targeting individuals already demonstrating minimal symptoms, youth, parent, and teacher rating scales are available that offer moderate accuracy in identifying children with, or at risk for anxiety and mood problems (for review see Silverman and Rabian 1999).

Once the target population has been selected, an intervention procedure needs to be implemented without major cost to the clientele or the mental health system. Experts can choose from a variety of preventive methods. Donovan and Spence (2000) distinguish three general types of prevention methods: (1) child focused methods, (2) parent focused methods, and (3) environmental restructuring methods. ◘ Table 20.2 provides a summary of these preventive methods for childhood emotional disorders as found in the literature (Beardslee and Gladstone 2001; Donovan and Spence 2000; Dusenbury and Albee 1988; Rapee 2002; Spence 1994, 2001; McWhirter et al. 2000), grouped according to the risk factors described in ◘ Table 20.1.

20.5 Implementation and Outcome

Prevention research with emotionally disturbed children and adolescents is in its »infancy«. There is a marked absence of empirical data to permit evaluation of the effectiveness of prevention programs for emotional problems in youths. As Spence (1994) pointed out, large-scale studies are needed that assess the long-term impact of preventive interventions, in comparison to no intervention and placebo approaches. These studies should use reliable and valid outcome measures that provide information from a variety of sources (e.g., parent, child, teacher) and across a range of settings (e.g., home, school). Moreover, to permit evaluation of the long-term impact of any preventive effort, follow-ups should be of adequate duration (e.g., 5–10 years).

Well-controlled experimental studies of this type have yet to be designed and evaluated. Most reviews of childhood prevention programs report that few prevention studies have been adequately designed, particularly for children younger than 7 or 8 years old (Durlak and Wells 1997; Mrazek and Brown 2002). However, some insights into the implementation and the effectiveness of prevention and early intervention of emotional disorders in children can be gained by reviewing existing findings from universal, selective, and indicated preventive approaches aiming to reduce the incidence and severity of children's anxious and depressive symptoms.

20.5.1   Universal Prevention

Only a small number of studies have attempted to prevent the incidence of childhood internalizing disorders by targeting an entire population that has not been identified on the basis of any risk factor. One of them is the »I CAN DO« program by Dubow et al. (1993). This study aimed to provide fourth-grade children with protective factors for dealing with stressful situations and consisted of thirteen 45-min sessions, presented by researchers within a classroom setting. The first three sessions focused on teaching children general coping skills, such as problem-solving, social-support seeking, and strategies to increase positive affect in uncontrollable situations. The remaining sessions were devoted to the practice of these coping skills within each of five stressful experiences that are likely to occur to a significant number of children: parental separation/divorce, loss of a loved one, move to a new home/school, spending time in self-care, and being different (e.g., ethnically, physically). Students also were instructed in ways to assist peers experiencing these negative life events and problematic feelings.

Children participating in the »I CAN DO« program demonstrated significantly greater abilities to generate a repertoire of effective solutions to the stressful situations, as well as significantly higher levels of self-efficacy to implement effective solutions than children not receiving the program. Most of these effects were either maintained or strengthened at 5-month follow-up. The study did not include measures of stress, anxiety, or depression, and it does not allow any conclusions on how children would react when faced with real-life events.

Lowry-Webster, Barrett, and Dadds (2001; see also Barrett and Turner 2001) developed and evaluated a program designed to prevent the development of anxiety and depressive symptoms in children aged 10–13 years using a universal prevention approach. Five hundred ninety-four children were randomly assigned on a class-by-class basis to either a 10-session family group cognitive-behavioral program called »FRIENDS« routinely implemented as part of the school curriculum, or to a comparison group. Pre-post intervention changes were exam-

ined universally, and for children who scored above the clinical cut-off for anxiety at pretest. Results revealed that children in the FRIENDS intervention group reported significantly fewer anxiety symptoms, regardless of their risk status, than the comparison group at posttest. The high anxiety group who completed FRIENDS also showed significant reductions in self-ratings of depression at posttreatment.

In addition, the FRIENDS program was conducted and evaluated with culturally diverse migrant high school students of non-English-speaking background in Australia (Barrett, Sonderegger, and Sonderegger 2001) and with children aged 8–18 in Germany (Essau et al. 2001). Both studies found significant reductions in anxiety scores for the intervention group at posttest. The long-term effectiveness of FRIENDS in reducing anxious and depressed symptoms, however, is yet to be determined.

Australian researchers have dominated the field of universal depression prevention, some of them using the Penn Prevention Project (see Sect. 20.5.3) by Jaycox et al. (1994) as a universal intervention with differing levels of success (e.g., Cunningham, Brandon, and Frydenberg 1999; Pattison and Lynd-Stevenson 2001; Quayle et al. 2001; Shochet et al. 2001). About half of these studies found significant improvements in coping skills, attributional style, and perceived control at posttest. Significant reductions in depressive symptoms were only found by Shochet et al. (2001) at posttest and by Quayle et al. (2001) at 6-months follow-up.

One of the most comprehensive and most thoughtfully designed large-scale universal prevention studies is currently being conducted in Ontario, Canada. Peters, Petrunka, and Arnold (2003) published preliminary findings from this government-funded »Better Beginnings, Better Futures Project« based on 554 children (aged 4 years at baseline) and their families living in three disadvantaged neighborhoods in Ontario. The program aims at preventing emotional and behavioral problems and promoting general development in young children, while also attempting to improve family and neighborhood characteristics. The project is intended to run for 25 years and mainly consists of school- and community-based support and activities such as classroom enrichment, homework help, summer tutoring, play groups, social skills training for children, parent-child drop-in, craft activities, and cultural programs. Longitudinal analyses of changes over the first 5 years of project operation indicated significantly larger and more widespread improvements in children's emotional problems, behavioral problems, and social skills in the two sites that provided in-classroom support to all children continuously from pre-kindergarten to 2nd grade than in the one site that mainly based its intervention programs on community activities.

20.5.2 Selective Prevention

Selective prevention targeting specific groups or individuals considered to be at risk for the development of particular problems due to exposure to some risk factor is the most common type of strategy employed in prevention research. With regard to the prevention of emotional disorders, the most common risk factors upon which populations at risk are being selected for intervention are the occurrence of traumatic or stressful life-events such as parental divorce, transition to a new school, and medical and dental procedures.

Several programs have been designed to teach children coping skills for effectively dealing with parental divorce (e.g., Hightower and Braden 1991; Zubernis et al. 1999). These programs are typically conducted in school settings and, in addition to teaching coping skills, attempt to facilitate the identification and expression of divorce-related feelings, to promote understanding of parental divorce and common misconceptions, and to enhance positive self and family perceptions. Prevention programs for children dealing with parental divorce have been found to be effective in enhancing problem-focused coping and self-esteem and in reducing anxiety, depressive symptoms, and behavioral problems at posttreatment. However, Hightower and Braden (1991) found that at 3-year follow-up only one-half of the children continued to demonstrate the gains evident at posttreatment and 2-year follow-up, and in Zubernis et al. (1999) a significant group X time interaction was found, indicating that for children of divorce, the effectiveness of the prevention program may diminish over time.

An example of a program that has been developed to facilitate the transition between primary and secondary school, which can be associated with emotional and behavioral difficulties (e.g., peer relationship problems, school refusal) is the School Transition Environment Project (STEP; Felner and Adan 1988). The STEP program directed its preventive strategy toward an environmental setting by reducing the large school environment into smaller units by creating »home-rooms«, in which students are instructed in their core academic subject. Students involved in the program demonstrated significantly higher levels of academic performance and self-esteem, better school attendance and lower school dropout rates than student nonparticipants.

The prevention of anxiety and emotional distress induced through medical procedures represents another example of selective prevention using a stressful life event as a selection factor. Not only the medical procedure itself may induce fear or pain in children, but also the related circumstances such as separation from parents and the unfamiliar surroundings. Strategies for helping children cope with injections, bone marrow aspirations, and changing of burn dressings are now widely used (Melamed 1998). A related area is the prevention of excessive dental fears, which has been estimated to affect 10%–20% of children and adolescents (Milgrom et al. 1992). Providing youths with as much control over the procedure as possible, providing youths with nontraumatic pre-exposure prior to invasive treatment, and allowing youths to view a videotaped coping model all have been found helpful (Weinstein 1990).

Although exposure to parental divorce, school transition, and medical and dental procedures constitute stressful life-events, some events in youths' lives can be so traumatic that these events usually directly result in some form of stress reaction in otherwise healthy youths. Such traumatic experiences include interfamilial violence, sexual abuse, community violence, war-related uprooting, terrorism, natural disasters, fatal road accidents, terminal illness, and death of a loved one. Many children and adolescents recover from these traumatic life-events under favorable conditions. However, in some instances, children show persistent emotional reactions for many months after the trauma (Terr 1981). There is thus a strong case for rapid intervention following exposure to trauma to prevent the development of persistent emotional problems.

Children who have difficulties integrating the traumatic experience are viewed to be unable to cope effectively with the trauma due to its overwhelming effect (Van der Kolk et al. 1996). From a preventive perspective, these children are required to work through the issues of regaining a sense of safety in their life, and of completing the unfinished past event (e.g., by giving it meaning, reframing it, and dealing with avoidance of specific triggers of trauma-related emotions; Klingman 2001). Two types of traumatic events have been distinguished (Terr 1991): (1) a short-term event, which is usually unexpected and more amenable to quick recovery (e.g., a natural disaster); and (2) a series of exposures to prolonged traumatic events that are likely to lead to complex reactions and poor recovery (e.g., sexual abuse). Preventive interventions can be applied to both types, either using one-to-one or group approaches, in home or community settings.

Given that children rely on adults' appraisals of the traumatic situation (McFarlane 1987), parents and significant others should be included in preventive efforts aimed at reducing posttraumatic stress reaction in children. It is important that parents and other significant adults communicate to the children that the situation, or part of it, is (at least partially) under control; that the child's response is proper under such circumstances; that the child is not alone in the world; that the parents/significant others are available and empathic companions; and, that the adult is coping. In particular, the adults are expected to show confidence that things will improve, and precrisis roles should be gradually resumed. In large-scale disasters that affect whole communities, preventive efforts also should include community counseling and crisis-oriented group approaches in order to provide mutual support, decrease isolation, and provide a larger perspective for the individual (Klingman 2001).

Approximately 4% of children younger than 18 years of age in the USA have experienced the death of one of their parents (Social Security Administration 2000). Sandler et al. (2003) conducted and evaluated their Family Bereavement Program (FBP), a group intervention for parentally bereaved children and their caregiver aiming at improving children's self-esteem and coping skills and at decreasing relationship problems between children and their caregivers as well as possible health problems of the caregiver. Results with 244 children and adolescents (aged 8–16 years) from 156 families indicated that the FBP led to significantly improved parenting, coping, and caregiver mental health and to reductions in the number of stressful events experienced at posttest. At 11-months follow-up, the FBP led to significantly reduced internalizing and externalizing problems, but only for girls who had higher problem scores at baseline.

Stressful and traumatic life-events are not the only risk factors of emotional disorders that can be used as criteria for selective prevention. Rapee (2002) developed a selective prevention program for anxiety disorders based on early behavioral inhibition. In the Macquarie University Preschool Intervention Program, children with an inhibited temperament, aged 3.5–4.5 years, were recruited mainly via questionnaires distributed to preschools. The screening procedure was based on mothers' rating of their child's temperament and on laboratory observation of behavioral inhibition. Intervention was conducted with parents only, with the main aim of educating them in techniques to help their child to become more confident and outgoing. Data at 12-month follow-up with 78 children showed that the program was effective in preventing new cases of anxiety disorders from developing. (No posttreatment data was reported for this study.)

Another risk factor in the development of anxiety and mood disorders is the presence of parental psychopathology. Beardslee et al. (1997) developed and evaluated a family-based selective prevention program targeting nonsymptomatic early adolescents at risk for future depression due to the presence of an affective disorder in one or both parents. The study's findings indicated that providing parents with factual information regarding risk and resilience in adolescents, and linking this information to family members' illness experiences, can result in behavioral and attitudinal changes among parents that ultimately translate into improved functioning among adolescents.

In considering the findings presented in ◘ Table 20.1 (see above), it is clear that other risk factors, in addition to those used in the above studies, could potentially serve as criteria in selecting at risk children for preventive interventions. For example, interventions in early childhood have been found to be successful in enhancing parental sensitivity and infant attachment security (Bakermans-Kranenburg et al. 2003). Effective prevention programs have been developed for reducing child maltreatment and improving parenting skills (e.g., Peterson et al. 2003). Even though it has yet to be empirically demonstrated that these kinds of interventions actually reduce the risk of developing an emotional disorder in childhood, trying to reduce risk factors and to enhance protective factors in the area of parent-child relationships seems a promising approach to the prevention of mood and anxiety disorders.

20.5.3   Indicated Prevention

Indicated prevention involves targeting those individuals who exhibit subclinical symptoms of a disorder. Drawing on data from the Great Smoky Mountains Study (Costello et al. 2003) in which

1,420 youths (ages 9–16) and their parents were interviewed annually, children and adolescents with an anxiety disorder but no other psychiatric diagnoses were twice as likely to show functional impairment as those with no disorder. Further, children and adolescents who were going to develop an anxiety disorder in the following year, these youths reported at least two clinically significant symptoms of anxiety in the previous year. Subclinical levels of anxiety can thus be an indicator of the subsequent development of a full-blown anxiety or mood disorder.

An example of an indicated prevention study relating to childhood anxiety is the Queensland Early Intervention and Prevention of Anxiety Project by Dadds et al. (1997, 1999). A total of 1,786 children (aged 7–14 years) were screened for anxiety problems using teacher nominations and children's self-report. After initial diagnostic interviews, 128 children were selected and assigned either to a 10-week school-based child- and parent-focused psychosocial intervention or to a monitoring group. Given that 55% of the selected children met diagnostic criteria for at least one anxiety disorder at baseline while the remaining children demonstrated subclinical symptomatology, the study represents a combination of early intervention and indicated prevention.

The intervention was based on a cognitive-behavioral approach teaching children strategies for coping with anxiety within a group format and was conducted over 10 weekly, 1- to 2-h sessions at each intervention school. Children who initially had a moderate to severe severity rating by the clinician benefited most from the intervention with approximately 50% of these children retaining a clinical diagnosis at the 2-year follow-up if they did not receive the intervention. For those children who initially showed symptoms of anxiety, but did not actually have a clinically significant anxiety disorder, there was no significant difference between the preventive intervention and the monitoring-only conditions at 2-year follow-up, with 11% showing an anxiety disorder in the intervention group and 16% in the monitoring group. Thus, children with subclinical anxiety problems did not appear to be at a high risk of developing a more severe anxiety disorder if left untreated and benefited only minimally from the intervention.

In the area of childhood mood disorders, several controlled indicated prevention studies have been conducted, most of them finding significantly fewer depressive symptoms in the intervention children than in controls at posttest, at follow-up, or at both

(cf. Barrett and Turner 2004). For example, Clarke et al. (1995) adapted their successful depression treatment program for use as an indicated preventive intervention program targeting adolescents at risk for future depressive disorder. After screening 1,652 adolescents, a final sample of 150 youths (mean age 15.3 years) was selected for the study. The intervention program, »Coping with Stress Course«, consisted of fifteen 45-min group sessions and was based on a cognitive distortion model of depression. In the treated as usual care condition, adolescents were free to either continue with pre-existing treatment or seek new treatment opportunities. Results showed a significant difference in the incidence of major depressive disorder or dysthymia in the treated as usual care group (25.7%) versus the active intervention group (14.5%) at 12-months follow-up.

In the Penn Prevention Program, Jaycox et al. (1994) developed a district-wide, school-based indicated prevention program consisting of cognitive and social problem solving techniques targeting 10–13-year old youths at risk for depression based on elevated depressive symptoms, parental conflict, or both, as reported by the youths themselves. Depressive symptoms were significantly reduced and classroom behavior was significantly improved in the treatment group as compared to controls at posttest. Six-months follow-up showed continued significant reductions in depressive symptoms, as well as significantly fewer externalizing conduct problems, as compared to controls. Reduction in symptoms was most pronounced in children who were most at risk. Results from the 2-year follow-up study showed that the prevention program produced enduring relief of depressive symptoms, and the prevention effect grew over time. The program also improved the participants' explanatory style, making them more optimistic. Authors suggested that change in the explanatory style for negative events was a mediator of the prevention program's effect on depressive symptoms.

20.6 Conclusions and Further Research Directions

As this chapter has made clear, there is a paucity of research conducted on early detection and prevention of emotional disorders in youth. As this chapter has also made clear, research progress on prevention corresponds considerably with research progress in the area of developmental psychopathology, including issues relating to the longitudinal course of disorders, the role of specific risk and protective factors, and the complex interrelations that likely exist among risk and protective factors, including possible additive, if not multiplicative effects of these factors. Filling the gaps in these critical developmental psychopathology areas will help a great deal in improving the theoretical foundation upon which to develop effective prevention intervention programs. The need for such programs is an issue of much public health significance given the personal and societal damages that anxiety and mood disorders in youths accrue.

Practical constraints have further served to limit the development and evaluation of preventive intervention programs. Prevention efforts are costly, as they necessarily involve collection of data from large samples over a lengthy time period. Large samples are needed because of the relatively low base rates of emotional disorders in the population of interest, and because it is unknown which individuals will develop an anxiety disorder, a mood disorder, or both. Further, because the relevant outcome is the future development of these disorders and perhaps of other comorbid conditions (e.g., substance abuse), prevention studies require data collection years after the intervention. The need for longitudinal follow-ups for long periods of time renders implementation and evaluation of prevention programs exceedingly difficult, especially when most external funding of mental health studies is typically for brief time intervals (5 years maximum in the USA), which also are required to yield tangible outcomes. Thus, alternative or new mechanisms of funding are needed if knowledge is to be developed in this area.

Much of the prevention research on children's emotional problems has adopted a targeted or high-risk approach. A major issue facing programs targeting high-risk children is the relative strength of the risk factors selected. Of importance here is the concept of the population attributable fraction (Levin 1953), which indicates the maximum reduction in the incidence of a disorder that could be expected if the effects of the risk factor(s) could be eliminated. A study by Offord, Boyle, and Racine (1989) showed that even if it were possible to eliminate the five family risk factors they targeted, the reduction in children's mental health problems would only be from 14% to 18%. It is thus of major importance for prevention studies to identify and modify factors that account for a large proportion of the incidence of the targeted disorder(s).

It has been shown that a focus on the most high-risk individuals is unlikely to have a large impact on rates of disorders within a population, since most cases of a disorder come from the large population that is at low or modest risk (Davis et al. 2003; Scott 2003). The sensitivity and specificity of early detection methods are well below what is needed to make individual risk predictions. Prevention programs targeting the higher proportion of people who have a more moderate level of risk has a much greater impact on the population than targeting people with the largest cumulative risk. Yale et al. (2003) have recently shown that one way to maximize the prevention of new cases of a disorder is to select the target population by residence in a certain high-risk neighborhood, based on epidemiological data, rather than by internal or interpersonal risk factors. Thus, although many existing prevention programs have a positive effect on the development of individual children, they do not have much effect on the incidence of emotional problems in the population as a whole.

There are other methodological and conceptual issues that make prevention research a challenging field of study. For universal prevention programs, a main issue of concern is finding an optimal way to prompt youths, parents, or both to participate in a study for a condition that the youth probably does not even have. Selective and indicated prevention programs, on the other hand, hold the challenge of trying to recruit and select a sample of young people from a population, who will be encouraged to participate in some type of intervention. Potential deleterious effects of such identification and the ethical issues involved, including issues relating to confidentiality in programs involving groups require careful consideration. Overall, issues such as these have been insufficiently discussed in the prevention literature.

As the field moves forward in developing and evaluating preventive intervention programs, it will become increasingly important that outcome be assessed not only at postintervention, but also as mentioned above, at longitudinal follow-ups that even extend into early adulthood. A related question is whether booster sessions are needed to retain the gains from prevention programs since the fairly predictable stressful life events that face young people might compromise long-term maintenance.

It also will be important for future research to move beyond symptoms and diagnosis and pay increased attention to whether youths' functional impairment has improved. For example, are there improvements in the youth's grades or in his or her peer relationships? Such outcomes should be seriously considered in the design and evaluation of future prevention studies. As also noted in this chapter, the potential of the positive psychology movement has yet to be seriously considered in the context of developing prevention programs and in determining targets of outcome. For example, rather than only asking whether anxiety or depression, or both, have decreased, researchers might ask whether courage or hopefulness, or both, have increased. Research questions of this type will require further measurement development so that instruments that assess constructs relevant to positive psychology exist for use with youths.

In addition, future prevention studies should begin to incorporate cost-benefit analyses into their evaluations. One explanation for the lack of government funding is the absence of cost-benefit data from psychologically based prevention studies. In the area of physical health, convincing evidence is available regarding the savings involved (Mrazek and Haggerty 1994). The benefits of prevention in mental health are harder to estimate. However, there are indicators that could be used in cost-benefit analyses, such as reductions in mental health consultations, time off work, lost productive work time, hospitalizations, and pension payments.

The few prevention intervention studies that have been conducted thus far have not shed light on the mechanisms and mediators of change. The lack of attention paid to mediators of change is understandable in any new, emerging area. However, as researchers continue to design and evaluate prevention intervention studies, they might consider a priori potential key mediators of change, and thus design studies so that these potential mediators can at least begin to be evaluated. Future efforts also are needed that more carefully consider issues relating to development, gender, and ethnicity in both the development of emotional disorders in young people and in understanding how these issues may inform the development of preventive intervention programs. It is known for example that rates of emotional disorders show dramatic increases in females compared to males over the course of development (Silverman and Carter, in press). More careful attention to the particular biopsychosocial challenges that females face over the course of development would go a long way in improving current prevention efforts. Similarly, given that during adolescence social and peer pressures magnify, prevention programs should carefully consider the role of peers

and how peers may be used to help promote positive youth functioning. In contrast, for younger children, the effect of including parents in the intervention relative to not including parents requires further study.

Finally, and maybe most importantly – in order for prevention of emotional disorders in youths to have a significant impact not only on individual cases but also on the population as a whole – nothing less than a »paradigm shift« in prevention research seems necessary. This would involve a shift away from short-term, individual- or family-focused interventions based on highly-selected at-risk samples with the aim of modifying a single risk factor whose population attributable fraction remains unexplored, to large-scale, long-term, community-based interventions that are rooted in epidemiological knowledge about the incidence of the disorder in different areas. These interventions should target as many children within the population as possible in an attempt to modify those risk factors or enhance those protective factors whose impact on the incidence of the disorder has been found to be considerable. If mental health experts want to make a significant difference on the epidemiology of disorders, preventive measures need to be based either on a universal prevention strategy or on a selective prevention strategy targeting not those few with the highest risk but the larger amount of youths with a more moderate level of risk.

Acknowledgements. Support for the writing of this chapter was funded in part by fellowship #8210-064757 from the Swiss National Research Foundation (SNF) awarded to Andreas Dick-Niederhauser and grant #63977 from the National Institute of Mental Health (NIMH) awarded to Wendy K. Silverman.

References

Albee, G. W. (1996) Revolutions and counterrevolutions in prevention. American Psychologist, 51, 1130–1133.

American Psychiatric Association (1994) Diagnostic and Statistical Manual of Mental Disorders, 4th ed. Washington, DC: American Psychiatric Association.

Bakermans-Kranenburg, M. J., van Ijzendoorn, M. H., and Juffer, F. (2003) Less is more: Meta-analyses of sensitivity and attachment interventions in early childhood. Psychological Bulletin, 129, 195–215.

Barrett, P. M., and Turner, C. T. (2001) Prevention of anxiety symptoms in primary school children: Preliminary results from a universal school-based trial. British Journal of Clinical Psychology, 40, 399–410.

Barrett, P.M., and Turner, C.M. (2004) Prevention of childhood anxiety and depression. In P. M. Barrett and T. H. Ollendick (Eds.), Handbook of interventions that work with children and adolescents: Prevention and treatment (pp. 429–474). New York: Wiley.

Barrett, P.M., Sonderegger, R., and Sonderegger, N.L. (2001) Evaluation of an anxiety-prevention and positive-coping program (FRIENDS) for children and adolescents of non-English-speaking background. Behaviour Change, 18, 78–91.

Beardslee, W.R., and Gladstone, T.R.G. (2001) Prevention of childhood depression: Recent findings and future prospects. Biological Psychiatry, 49, 1101–1110.

Beardslee, W.R., Versage, E.M., Wright, E., and Salt, P. (1997) Examination of preventive interventions for families with depression: Evidence of change. Developmental Psychopathology, 9, 109–130.

Brown, J.M., O'Keeffe, J., Sanders, S.H., and Baker, B. (1986) Developmental changes in children's cognition to stressful and painful situations. Journal of Pediatric Psychology, 11, 343–357.

Clarke, G.N., Hawkins, W., Murphy, M., Sheeber, L.B., Lewinsohn, P. M., and Seeley, J.S. (1995) Targeted prevention of unipolar depressive disorder in an at-risk sample of high schol adolescents: A randomized clinical trial of a group cognitive intervention. Journal of the American Academy of Child and Adolescent Psychiatry, 34, 312–321.

Coie, J.D., Watt, N.F., West, S.G., Hawkins, J.D., Asarnow, J.R., Markman, H.J., Ramey, S.L., Shure, M.B., and Long, B. (1993) The science of prevention: A conceptual framework and some directions for a national research program. American Psychologist, 48, 1013–1022.

Cole, D.A., Peeke, L.G., Martin, J.M., Truglio, R., and Serocynski, A.D. (1998) A longitudinal look at the relation between depression and anxiety in children and adolescents. Journal of Consulting and Clinical Psychology, 66, 451–460.

Compas, B.E., Connor-Smith, J.K., Saltzman, H., Thomsen, A.H., and Wadsworth, M.E. (2001) Coping with stress during childhood and adolescence: Problems, progress, and potential in theory and research. Psychological Bulletin, 127, 87–127.

Costello, E.J., Mustillo, S., Erkanli, A., Keeler, G., and Angold, A. (2003) Prevalence and development of psychiatric disorders in childhood and adolescence. Archives of General Psychiatry, 60, 837–844.

Cunningham, E.G., Brandon, C.M., and Frydenberg, E. (1999) Building resilience in early adolescence through a universal school-based prevention program. Australian Journal of Guidance and Counselling, 9, 15–23.

Dadds, M.R., Spence, S.H., Holland, D.E., Barrett, P. M., and Laurens, K.R. (1997) Prevention and early intervention for anxiety disorders: A controlled trial. Journal of Consulting and Clinical Psychology, 65, 627–635.

Dadds, M.R., Holland, D.E., Laurens, K.R., Mullins, M., Barrett, P., and Spence, S.H. (1999) Early intervention and prevention of anxiety disorders in children: Results at 2-year follow-up. Journal of Consulting and Clinical Psychology, 67, 145–150.

Davis, C.H., MacKinnon, D.P., Schultz, A., and Sandler, I. (2003) Cumulative risk and population attributable fraction in prevention. Journal of Clinical Child and Adolescent Psychology, 32, 228–235.

Dick-Niederhauser, A., and Silverman, W.K. (2004) Courage and fearlessness: A positive approach to the etiology and treatment of anxiety disorders. Manuscript submitted for publication.

Donovan, C.L., and Spence, S.H. (2000) Prevention of childhood anxiety disorders. Clinical Psychology Review, 20, 509–531.

DuBois, D.L., Felner, R.D., Bartels, C.L., and Silverman, M.M. (1995) Stability of self-reported depressive symptoms in a community sample of children and adolescents. Journal of Clinical Child Psychology, 24, 386–396.

Dubow, E.F., Schmidt, D., McBride, J., Edwards, S., and Merck, F. L. (1993) Teaching children to cope with stressful experiences: Implementation and evaluation of a primary prevention program. Journal of Clinical Child Psychology, 22, 428–440.

Durlak, J.A., and Wells, A.M. (1997) Primary prevention mental health programs for children and adolescents: A meta-analytic review. American Journal of Community Psychology, 25, 115–152.

Dusenbury, L., and Albee, G.W. (1988) Primary prevention of anxiety disorders. In C.G. Last and M. Hersen (Eds.), Handbook of anxiety disorders (pp. 571–583). Elmsford, NY: Pergamon Press.

Ebata, A.T., and Moos, R.H. (1991) Coping and adjustment in distressed and healthy adolescents. Journal of Applied Developmental Psychology, 12, 33–54.

Essau, C.A., Conradt, J., Kuhle, R., and Low, R. (2001) Feasibility and efficacy of the FRIENDS program for the prevention of anxiety in children. Manuscript submitted for publication.

Felner, R.D., and Adan, A.M. (1988) The School Transition Environment Project: An ecological intervention and evaluation. In R.H. Price, E.L. Cowen, R.P. Lorion, and J. Ramos-McKay (Eds.), Fourteen ounces of prevention: A case book for practitioners (pp. 111–122). Washington, DC: American Psychological Association.

Fristad, M.A., Shaver, A.E., and Holderle, K.E. (2002) Mood disorders in childhood and adolescence. In D.T. Marsh and M.A. Fristad (Eds.), Serious emotional disturbance in children and adolescents (pp. 228–265). New York: John Wiley and Sons.

Gould, M.S., and Kramer, R.A. (2001) Youth suicide prevention. Suicide and Life-Threatening Behavior, 31, 6–31.

Hightower, A.D., and Braden, J. (1991) Prevention. In T.R. Kratochwill and R. J. Morris (Eds.), The practice of child therapy (pp. 410–440). New York: Pergamon.

Jaycox, L.H., Reivich, K.J., Gillham, J., and Seligman, M.E.P. (1994) Prevention of depressive symptoms in school children. Behaviour Research and Therapy, 32, 801–816.

Kazdin, A.E., and Marciano, P.L. (1998) Childhood and adolescent depression. In E.J. Mash and R.A. Barkley (Eds.),

Treatment of childhood disorders, 2nd ed. (pp. 211–248). New York: Guilford Press.

Keller, M. B., Lavori, P. W., Wunder, J., Beardslee, W R., Schwartz, P., and Roth, T. (1992) Chronic course of anxiety disorders in children and adolescents. Journal of the American Academy of Child and Adolescent Psychiatry, 31, 595-599.

Kendall, P.C. (1994) Treating anxiety disorders in children: Results of a randomized clinical trial. Journal of Consulting and Clinical Psychology, 62, 100–110.

Klingman, A. (2001) Prevention of anxiety disorders: The case of posttraumatic stress disorder. In W. K. Silverman and P. D. A. Treffers (Eds.), Anxiety disorders in children and adolescents: Research, assessment, and intervention (pp. 368–391) Cambridge, UK: Cambridge University Press.

Kovacs, M. (1996) The course of childhood-onset depressive disorders. Psychiatric Annals, 26, 326–330.

Levin, M. L. (1953) The occurrence of lung cancer in man. Acta Union International Contra Cancrum, 9, 531–541.

Lewinsohn, P. M., Clarke, G. N., Seeley, J. R., and Rohde, P. (1994) Major depression in community adolescents: age at onset, episode duration, and time to recurrence. Journal of the American Academy of Child and Adolescent Psychiatry, 33, 809–818.

Lowry-Webster, H. M., Barrett, P. M., and Dadds, M. R. (2001) A universal prevention trial of anxiety and depressive symptomatology in childhood: Preliminary data from an Australian study. Behaviour Change, 18, 36–50.

McFarlane, A. C. (1987) Posttraumatic phenomena in a longitudinal study of children following a natural disaster. Journal of the American Academy of Child and Adolescent Psychiatry, 26, 764–769.

McWhirter, B. T., McWhirter, J. J., Hart, R. S., and Gat, I. (2000) Preventing and treating depression in children and adolescents. In D. Capuzzi and D. R. Gross (Eds.), Youth at risk: A prevention resource for counselors, teachers, and parents (pp. 137–165) Alexandria, Va.: American Counseling Association.

Melamed, B. G. (1998) Preparation for medical procedures. In R. T. Ammerman and J. V. Campo (Eds.), Handbook of pediatric psychology and psychiatry, vol. 2: Disease, injury, and illness (pp. 16–30). Boston, Ma.: Allyn and Bacon.

Michael, K. D., and Crowley, S. L. (2002) How effective are treatments for child and adolescent depression? A meta-analytic review. Clinical Psychology Review, 22, 247–269.

Milgrom, P., Vignehsa, H., and Weinstein, P. (1992) Adolescent dental fear and control: Prevalence and theoretical implications. Behaviour Research and Therapy, 30, 367–375.

Mrazek, P. J., and Brown, C. H. (2002) An evidence-based literature review regarding outcomes in psychosocial prevention and early intervention in young children. In C. C. Russel (Ed.), The state of knowledge about prevention/early intervention (pp. 42–144). Toronto, Canada: Invest in Kids Foundation.

Mrazek, P. J., and Haggerty, R. J. (Eds.) (1994) Reducing the risks for mental disorders: Frontiers for preventive intervention research. Washington, DC: National Academy Press.

Murray, C. J. L., and Lopez, A. D. (1996) The global burden of disease. Boston: Harvard University Press.

Murray, J. (1992) Prevention and identification of high risk groups. International Review of Psychiatry, 4, 281–286.

Offord, D. R., Boyle, M. H., and Racine, Y. A. (1989) Children at risk. Toronto, Canada: Ontario Ministry of Community and Social Services.

Pattison, C., and Lynd-Stevenson, R. M. (2001) The prevention of depressive symptoms in children: The immediate and long-term outcomes of a school-based program. Behaviour Change, 18, 92–102.

Peters, R. D., Petrunka, K., and Arnold, R. (2003) The Better Beginnings, Better Futures Project: A universal, comprehensive, community-based prevention approach for primary school children and their families. Journal of Clinical Child and Adolescent Psychology, 32, 215–227.

Peterson, L., Tremblay, G., Ewigman, B., and Saldana, L. (2003) Multilevel selected primary prevention of child maltreatment. Journal of Consulting and Clinical Psychology, 71, 601–612.

Quayle, D., Dziurawiec, S., Roberts, C., Kane, R., and Ebsworthy, G. (2001) The effect of an optimism and lifeskills program on depressive symptoms in preadolescence. Behaviour Change, 18, 1–10.

Rao, U., Ryan, N. D., Birmaher, B., and Dahl, R. E. (1995) Unipolar depression in adolescents: Clinical outcome in adulthood. Journal of the American Academy of Child and Adolescent Psychiatry, 34, 566–578.

Rapee, R. M. (2002) The development and modification of temperamental risk for anxiety disorders: Prevention of a lifetime of anxiety? Biological Psychiatry, 52, 947–957.

Sandler, I. N., Ayers, T. S., Wolchik, S. A., Tein, J.-Y., Kwok, O.-M., Haine, R. A., Twohey-Jacobs, J., Suter, J., Lin, K., Padgett-Jones, S., Weyer, J. L., Cole, E., Kriege, G., and Griffin, W. A. (2003) The Family Bereavement Program: Efficacy evaluation of a theory-based prevention program for parentally bereaved children and adolescents. Journal of Consulting and Clinical Psychology, 71, 587–600.

Scott, K. G. (2003) Commentary: Individual risk prediction, individual risk, and population risk. Journal of Clinical Child and Adolescent Psychology, 32, 243–245.

Seligman, M. E. P. (2002) Positive psychology, positive prevention, and positive therapy. In C. R. Snyder and S. J. Lopez (Eds.), Handbook of positive psychology (pp. 3–9). New York: Oxford University Press.

Shochet, I. M., Dadds, M. R., Holland, D., Whitefield, K., Harnett, P., and Osgarby, S. M. (2001) The efficacy of a universal school-based program to prevent adolescent depression. Journal of Clinical Child Psychology, 30, 525–535.

Silverman, W. K., and Berman, S. L. (2001) Psychosocial interventions for anxiety disorders in children: status and future directions. In W. K. Silverman and P. D. A. Treffers (Eds.), Anxiety disorders in children and adolescents. Research, assessment, and intervention (pp. 313–334). Cambridge, UK: University Press.

Silverman, W. K., and Carter, R. (in press) Anxiety disturbance. In J. Worell and C. Goodheart (Eds.), Handbook of girls' and women's psychological health: Gender and well-being across the life span. New York: Oxford University Press.

Silverman, W. K., and Rabian, B. (1999) Rating scales for anxiety and mood disorders. In D. Shaffer, C. P. Lucas, and J. E. Richters (Eds.), Diagnostic assessment in child and adolescent psychopathology (pp. 127–166). New York: Guilford Press.

Silverman, W. K., and Treffers, P. D. A. (2001) (Eds.) Anxiety disorders in children and adolescents: Research, assessment, and intervention. Cambridge, UK: Cambridge University Press.

Silverman, W. K., Kurtines, W. M., Ginsburg, G. S., Weems, C. F., Rabian, B., and Serafini, L. T. (1999) Contingency management, self-control, and education support in the treatment of childhood phobic disorders: A randomized clinical trial. Journal of Consulting and Clinical Psychology, 67, 675–687.

Snyder, C. R., and Lopez, S. J. (Eds.) (2002) Handbook of positive psychology. New York: Oxford University Press.

Social Security Administration (2000) Intermediate assumptions of the 2000 trustees report. Washington, DC: Office of the Chief Actuary of the Social Security Administration.

Spence, S. H. (1994) Preventive strategies. In T. H. Ollendick, N. J. King, and W. Yule (Eds.), International handbook of phobic and anxiety disorders in children and adolescents (pp. 453–474). New York: Plenum Press.

Spence, S. H. (2001) Prevention strategies. In M. W. Vasey and M. R. Dadds (Eds.), The developmental psychopathology of anxiety (pp. 325–351) New York: Oxford University Press.

Terr, L. C. (1981) Psychic trauma in children: Observations following the Chowchilla school-bus kidnapping. American Journal of Psychiatry, 138, 14–19.

Terr, L. C. (1991) Childhood trauma: An outline and overview. American Journal of Psychiatry, 148, 10–20.

Van der Kolk, B. A., McFarlane, A. C., and Weiseath, L. (Eds.) (1996) Traumatic stress: The effect of overwhelming experience on mind, body and society. New York: Guilford Press.

Vasey, M. W., and Dadds, M. R. (2001) (Eds.) The developmental psychopathology of anxiety. New York: Oxford University Press.

Verhulst, F. C. (2001) Community and epidemiological aspects of anxiety disorders in children. In W. K. Silverman and P. D. A. Treffers (Eds.), Anxiety disorders in children and adolescents. Research, assessment, and intevention (pp. 273–292). Cambridge, UK: University Press.

Weinstein, P. (1990) Breaking the worldwide cycle of pain, fear and avoidance: Uncovering risk factors and promoting prevention for children. Annals of Behavioral Medicine, 12, 141–147.

White, K. S., Bruce, S. E., Farrell, A. D., and Kliewer, W. (1998) Impact of exposure to community violence on anxiety: A longitudinal study of family social support as a protective factor for urban children. Journal of Child and Family Studies, 7, 187–203.

Winnett, R. A. (1998) Prevention: A proactive developmental-ecological prespective. In T. H. Ollendick and M. Hersen (Eds.), Handbook of child psychopathology, 3rd ed. (pp. 637–671). New York: Plenum Press.

Yale, M. E., Scott, K. G., Gross, M., and Gonzalez, A. (2003) Using developmental epidemiology to choose the target population for an intervention program in a high-risk neighborhood. Journal of Clinical Child and Adolescent Psychology, 32, 236–242.

Zubernis, L. S., Cassidy, K. W., Gillham, J. E., Reivich, K. J., and Jaycox, L. H. (1999) Prevention of depressive symptoms in preadolescent children of divorce. Journal of Divorce and Remarriage, 30, 11–36.

20

Prevention and Early Detection of Conduct Disorder and Delinquency

David P. Farrington, Brandon C. Welsh

21.1   Introduction   – 287

21.2   Risk Factors   – 287
21.2.1   Temperament and Personality   – 287
21.2.2   Impulsiveness   – 288
21.2.3   Low IQ and Low Educational Achievement   – 288
21.2.4   Child Rearing and Child Abuse   – 289
21.2.5   Parental Conflict and Disrupted Families   – 289
21.2.6   Antisocial Parents and Large Families   – 290
21.2.7   Socio-Economic Factors   – 290
21.2.8   Peer Influences   – 291
21.2.9   School and Community Influences   – 291

21.3   Successful Interventions   – 291
21.3.1   Early Home Visiting   – 291
21.3.2   Preschool Programs   – 292
21.3.3   Parent Training   – 292
21.3.4   Skills Training   – 293
21.3.5   Peer Programs   – 293
21.3.6   School Programs   – 294
21.3.7   Anti-Bullying Programs   – 294
21.3.8   Multi-Modal Programs   – 295

21.4   Discussion and Conclusions   – 295

References   – 296

21.1   Introduction

This chapter has two main aims. First, it summarizes the major risk factors for conduct problems and delinquency and, second, it reviews the scientific evidence on the effectiveness of interventions to prevent conduct disorder and delinquency. The chapter focuses on risk factors discovered in prospective longitudinal surveys and on successful interventions demonstrated in randomized controlled experiments. (For descriptions of longitudinal surveys, see Kalb et al. 2001; for reviews of risk factors, see Hawkins et al. 1998; for reviews of intervention studies, see Farrington and Welsh 2003.) It also focuses mainly on young people aged 10–17 and relies

on research carried out in North America, Great Britain, or similar Western countries. Most research has been carried out with males, but studies of females are included where applicable (e.g., Moffitt et al. 2001). The focus is on substantive results rather than methodological and theoretical issues.

In general, all types of antisocial behavior tend to coexist and are intercorrelated. Conduct disorder (CD) and delinquency are among the most important types of adolescent antisocial behaviors. These behaviors are logically and empirically related, so that risk factors and successful interventions that apply to one of these types of antisocial behavior are also likely to apply to the other.

21.2   Risk Factors

Risk factors – identified in prospective longitudinal studies – for conduct problems and delinquency will be discussed one by one; additive, interactive, independent, or sequential effects will not be exhaustively reviewed, although these are important issues. Also not discussed are protective factors and resilience (see Masten and Reed 2002). Because of limitations of space, and because of their limited relevance for psychosocial interventions, biological factors are not reviewed (see Rowe 2002). There is also little space to review theories of the causal mechanisms by which risk factors might have their effects on antisocial behavior (see, e.g., Juby and Farrington 2001).

21.2.1   Temperament and Personality

Personality traits such as sociability or impulsiveness describe broad predispositions to respond in certain ways, and temperament is basically the childhood equivalent of personality. Temperament is clearly influenced by biological factors but is not itself a biological variable like heart rate (in our view). Important results on the link between childhood temperament and later offending have been obtained in the Dunedin longitudinal study in New Zealand (Caspi 2000). Temperament at age 3 years was rated by observing the child's behavior during a testing session. The most important dimension of temperament was being undercontrolled (restless, impulsive, with poor attention), and this predicted aggression, self-reported delinquency, and convictions at age 18–21.

In the Cambridge Study, which is a prospective longitudinal survey of 400 London boys, those high on both Extraversion and Neuroticism tended to be juvenile self-reported delinquents, adult official offenders, and adult self-reported offenders, but not juvenile official delinquents (Farrington et al. 1982). Furthermore, these relationships held independently of other variables such as low family income, low intelligence, and poor parental child-rearing behavior. However, when individual items of the personality questionnaire were studied, it was clear that the significant relationships were caused by the items measuring impulsiveness (e.g., doing things quickly without stopping to think).

21.2.2   Impulsiveness

Impulsiveness is the most crucial personality dimension that predicts antisocial behavior (Lipsey and Derzon 1998). Unfortunately, there are a bewildering number of constructs referring to a poor ability to control behavior. These include impulsiveness, hyperactivity, restlessness, clumsiness, not considering consequences before acting, a poor ability to plan ahead, short time horizons, low self-control, sensation-seeking, risk-taking, and a poor ability to delay gratification.

Many studies show that hyperactivity predicts later offending. In the Copenhagen Perinatal project, hyperactivity (restlessness and poor concentration) at age 11–13 significantly predicted arrests for violence up to age 22, especially among boys experiencing delivery complications (Brennan et al. 1993). Similarly, in the Orebro longitudinal study in Sweden, hyperactivity at age 13 predicted police-recorded violence up to age 26. The highest rate of violence was among males with both motor restlessness and concentration difficulties (15%), compared to 3% of the remainder (Klinteberg et al. 1993).

In the Cambridge Study, boys nominated by teachers as lacking in concentration or restless, those nominated by parents, peers, or teachers as the most daring or taking most risks, and those who were the most impulsive on psychomotor tests at age 8–10, all tended to become offenders later in life. Daring, poor concentration and restlessness all predicted both official convictions and self-reported delinquency, and daring was consistently one of the best independent predictors (Farrington 1992b). Interestingly, Farrington et al. (1990) found that hyperactivity predicted juvenile offending independently of conduct problems. Lynam (1996) proposed that boys with both hyperactivity and CD were most at risk of chronic offending and psychopathy, and Lynam (1998) presented evidence in favor of this hypothesis from the Pittsburgh Youth Study.

21.2.3   Low IQ and Low Educational Achievement

Low IQ and low school achievement are important predictors of CD, delinquency, and adolescent antisocial behavior (Moffitt 1993). In an English epidemiological study of 13-year-old twins, low IQ of the child predicted conduct problems independently of social class and of the IQ of parents (Goodman et al. 1995). Low school achievement was a strong correlate of CD in the Pittsburgh Youth Study (Loeber et al. 1998). In both the Ontario Child Health Study (Offord et al. 1989) and the New York State longitudinal study (Velez et al. 1989), failing a grade predicted CD. Under-achievement, defined according to a discrepancy between IQ and school achievement, is also characteristic of CD children, as Frick et al. (1991) reported in the Developmental Trends Study.

Low IQ and low school achievement also predict youth violence. In the Philadelphia Biosocial project (Denno 1990), low verbal and performance IQ at ages 4 and 7, and low scores on the California Achievement test at age 13–14 (vocabulary, comprehension, mathematics, language, spelling) all predicted arrests for violence up to age 22. In Project Metropolitan in Copenhagen, low IQ at age 12 significantly predicted police-recorded violence between ages 15 and 22. The link between low IQ and violence was strongest among lower class boys (Hogh and Wolf 1983).

21.2.4   Child Rearing and Child Abuse

In the Pittsburgh Youth Study, poor parental supervision was an important risk factor for CD (Loeber et al. 1998). Poor maternal supervision and low persistence in discipline predicted CD in the Developmental Trends Study (Frick et al. 1992), but not independently of parental Antisocial Personality Disorder. Rothbaum and Weisz (1994) carried out a meta-analysis and concluded that parental reinforcement, parental reasoning, parental punishments, and parental responsiveness to the child were all related to externalizing child behavior.

Of all child rearing factors, poor parental supervision is the strongest and most replicable predictor of delinquency (Smith and Stern 1997), and harsh or punitive discipline (involving physical punishment) is also an important predictor (Haapasalo and Pokela 1999). The classic longitudinal studies by McCord (1979) in Boston and Robins (1979) in St. Louis show that poor parental supervision, harsh discipline, and a rejecting attitude all predict delinquency. Similar results were obtained in the Cambridge Study. Harsh or erratic parental discipline, cruel, passive, or neglecting parental attitudes, and poor parental supervision, all measured at age 8, all predicted later juvenile convictions and self-reported delinquency (West and Farrington 1973). Generally, the presence of any of these adverse family background features doubled the risk of a later juvenile conviction.

There seems to be significant intergenerational transmission of aggressive and violent behavior from parents to children, as Widom (1989) found in a study of abused children in Indianapolis. Children who were physically abused up to age 11 were significantly likely to become violent offenders in the next 15 years (Maxfield and Widom 1996). Similarly, in the Rochester Youth Development Study, Smith and Thornberry (1995) showed that recorded child maltreatment under age 12 predicted self-reported violence between ages 14 and 18, independently of gender, ethnicity, SES, and family structure. The extensive review by Malinosky-Rummell and Hansen (1993) confirms that being physically abused as a child predicts later violent and nonviolent offending.

21.2.5   Parental Conflict and Disrupted Families

There is no doubt that parental conflict and interparental violence predict adolescent antisocial behavior, as the meta-analysis of Buehler et al. (1997) shows. Also, parental conflict is related to childhood externalizing behavior, irrespective of whether the information about both comes from parents or children (Jenkins and Smith 1991). In the Pittsburgh Youth Study, CD boys tended to have parents who had unhappy relationships (Loeber et al. 1998). Parental conflict also predicts delinquency (West and Farrington 1973).

In the Christchurch Study in New Zealand, children who witnessed violence between their parents were more likely to commit both violent and property offenses according to their self-reports (Fergusson and Horwood 1998). Witnessing father-initiated violence was still predictive after controlling for other risk factors, such as parental criminality, parental substance abuse, parental physical punishment, a young mother, and low family income.

Parental separation and single parent families predict CD children. In the Christchurch Study, separations from parents in the first 5 years of a child's life (especially) predicted CD at age 15 (Fergusson et al. 1994). In the New York State longitudinal study, CD was predicted by parental divorce, but far more strongly by having a never-married lone mother (Velez et al. 1989). In the Ontario Child Health Study, coming from a single-parent family predicted CD, but this was highly related to poverty and dependence on welfare benefits (Blum et al. 1988).

In the Dunedin Study in New Zealand, boys from single parent families disproportionately tended to be convicted; 28% of violent offenders were from single parent families, compared with 17% of nonviolent offenders and 9% of unconvicted boys (Henry et al. 1996). Based on analyses of four surveys (including the Cambridge Study), Morash and Rucker (1989) concluded that the combination of teenage child-bearing and a single-parent female-headed household was especially conducive to the development of offending in children. Later analyses of the Cambridge Study showed that teenage child-bearing combined with a large number of children particularly predicted offending by the children (Nagin et al. 1997).

Many studies show that broken homes or disrupted families predict delinquency (Wells and Rankin 1991). In the Newcastle (England) Thousand-Family Study, Kolvin et al. (1988) reported that marital disruption (divorce or separation) in a boy's first 5 years predicted his later convictions up to age 32. Similarly, in the Dunedin study in New Zealand, Henry et al. (1993) found that children who were exposed to parental discord and many changes of the primary caretaker tended to become antisocial and delinquent. In the Cambridge Study, Juby and Farrington (2001) showed that boys who remained with their mother after a family break had the same delinquency rate as boys from intact low conflict families, but boys who remained with their fathers, with relatives, or with others (e.g., foster parents) had high delinquency rates.

21.2.6   Antisocial Parents and Large Families

It is clear that antisocial parents tend to have antisocial children (Lipsey and Derzon 1998). In the Developmental Trends Study, parental APD was the best predictor of childhood CD (Frick et al. 1992) and parental substance use was an important predictor of the onset of CD (Loeber et al. 1995). Similarly, in the New York State longitudinal study, parental APD was a strong predictor of externalizing child behavior (Cohen et al. 1990). In the Pittsburgh Youth Study, parents with behavior problems and substance use problems tended to have CD boys (Loeber et al. 1998).

In their classic longitudinal studies, McCord (1977) and Robins et al. (1975) showed that criminal parents tended to have delinquent sons. In the Cambridge Study, the concentration of offending in a small number of families was remarkable. Less than 6% of the families were responsible for half of the criminal convictions of all members (fathers, mothers, sons, and daughters) of all 400 families (Farrington et al. 1996). Having a convicted mother, father, brother, or sister significantly predicted a boy's own convictions. Same-sex relationships were stronger than opposite-sex relationships, and older siblings were stronger predictors than younger siblings. Furthermore, convicted parents and delinquent siblings were related to a boy's self-reported as well as official offending (Farrington 1979). CD symptoms also tend to be concentrated in families, as shown in the Ontario Child Health Study (Szatmari et al. 1993).

Many studies show that large families predict delinquency (Fischer 1984). For example, in the British National Survey of Health and Development, Wadsworth (1979) found that the percentage of boys who were officially delinquent increased from 9% for families containing one child to 24% for families containing four or more children. The Newsons in their Nottingham study also concluded that large family size was one of the most important predictors of delinquency (Newson et al. 1993). Large family size also predicts adolescent self-reported violence (Farrington 2000).

In the Cambridge Study, if a boy had four or more siblings by his tenth birthday, this doubled his risk of being convicted as a juvenile (West and Farrington 1973). Large family size predicted self-reported delinquency as well as convictions (Farrington 1979), and adult as well as juvenile convictions (Farrington 1992 a). Also, large family size was the most important independent predictor of convictions up to age 32 in a logistic regression analysis (Farrington 1993). Large family size was similarly important in the Cambridge and Pittsburgh studies, even though families were on average smaller in Pittsburgh in the 1990s than in London in the 1960s (Farrington and Loeber 1999).

21.2.7   Socio-Economic Factors

It is clear that antisocial children disproportionately come from low SES families. In the Ontario Child Health Study, CD children tended to come from low income families, with unemployed parents, living in subsidized housing and dependent on welfare benefits (Offord et al. 1986). In the New York State longitudinal study, low SES, low family income, and low parental education predicted CD children (Velez et al. 1989). In the Developmental Trends Study, low SES predicted the onset of CD (Loeber et al. 1995), and, in the Pittsburgh Youth Study, family dependence on welfare benefits was characteristic of CD boys (Loeber et al. 1998).

Low SES is a less consistent predictor of delinquency. However, a lot depends on whether it is measured by income and housing or by occupational prestige. In the Cambridge Study, low family income and poor housing predicted official and self-reported, juvenile and adult delinquency, but low parental occupational prestige predicted only self-reported delinquency (Farrington 1992 a, b). Low family income was a strong predictor of self-reported violence (Farrington 2000), and having an unemployed father was one of the strongest predictors of convictions for violence (Farrington 1994).

21.2.8   Peer Influences

It is well established that having delinquent friends is an important predictor of delinquency (Lipsey and Derzon 1998). What is less clear is how far antisocial peers encourage and facilitate adolescent antisocial behavior, or whether it is merely that »birds of a feather flock together«. Delinquents may have delinquent friends because of co-offending, which is particularly common under age 21 (Reiss and Farrington 1991). Elliott and Menard (1996) in the U.S. National Youth Survey concluded that delinquent friends influenced an adolescent's own delinquency and that the reverse was also true: more delinquent adolescents were more likely to have delinquent friends. In the Pittsburgh Youth Study, Keenan et al. (1995) discovered that having antisocial friends predicted the later onset of a boy's antisocial behavior.

21.2.9   School and Community Influences

It is also well established that delinquents disproportionately attend high delinquency rate schools, which have high levels of distrust between teachers and students, low commitment to the school by students, and unclear and inconsistently enforced rules (Graham 1988). In the Cambridge Study, attending a high delinquency-rate school at age 11 significantly predicted a boy's own delinquency (Farrington 1992b). However, what is less clear is how far the schools themselves influence antisocial behavior, by their organization, climate, and practices, and how far the concentration of offenders in certain schools is mainly a function of their intakes. In the Cambridge Study, most of the variation between schools in their delinquency rates could be explained by differences in their intakes of troublesome boys at age 11 (Farrington 1972). However, reviews of American research show that schools with clear, fair, and consistently enforced rules tend to have low rates of student misbehavior (Gottfredson 2001; Herrenkohl et al. 2001).

It is difficult to determine how far communities themselves influence antisocial behavior and how far it is merely the case that antisocial people tend to live in deprived areas (e.g., because of their poverty or public housing allocation policies). Interestingly, both neighborhood researchers such as Gottfredson et al. (1991) and developmental researchers such as Rutter (1981) have concluded that neighborhoods have only indirect effects on antisocial behavior via their effects on individuals and families. However, Sampson et al. (1997) argued that a low degree of »collective efficacy« in a neighborhood (a low degree of informal social control) caused high crime rates.

21.3   Successful Interventions

This section reviews successful interventions in preventing conduct disorder and delinquency. The focus here is on results obtained in randomized controlled experiments with reasonably large samples, since the effect of any intervention on antisocial behavior can be demonstrated most convincingly in such experiments (Farrington 1983). For more extensive reviews of the effects of interventions, see Wasserman and Miller (1998) and Catalano et al. (1998). Most interventions target risk factors and aim to prevent antisocial behavior. However, it is equally important to strengthen protective factors and promote healthy adolescent development (Catalano et al. 2002).

21.3.1   Early Home Visiting

Adolescent delinquency can be prevented by intensive home visiting programs. For example, in New York state, Olds et al. (1986) randomly allocated 400 mothers either to receive home visits from nurses during pregnancy, or to receive visits both during pregnancy and during the first 2 years of life, or to a control group who received no visits. The home visitors gave advice about prenatal and postnatal care of the child, about infant development, and about the importance of proper nutrition and avoiding smoking and drinking during pregnancy.

The results of this experiment in New York state showed that the postnatal home visits caused a decrease in recorded child physical abuse and neglect during the first 2 years of life, especially by poor unmarried teenage mothers; 4% of visited versus 19% of nonvisited mothers of this type were guilty of child abuse or neglect. This last result is important because children who are physically abused or neglected tend to become violent offenders later in life. In a 15-year follow-up, the main focus was on lower class unmarried mothers. Among these high-risk mothers, those who received prenatal and postnatal home visits had fewer arrests than those who received prenatal visits or no visits (Olds et al. 1997). Also, children of these mothers who received prenatal and/or postnatal home visits had less than half as many arrests as children of mothers who received no visits (Olds et al. 1998). According to Aos et al. (2001a), the benefit-to-cost ratio for high risk mothers was 3.1, based on savings to crime victims and the criminal justice system.

21.3.2 Preschool Programs

One of the most successful early prevention programs has been the Perry preschool project carried out in Michigan by Schweinhart and Weikart (1980). This was essentially a »Head Start« program that targeted disadvantaged African-American children. The experimental children attended a daily preschool program, backed up by weekly home visits, usually lasting 2 years (covering ages 3–4). The aim of the »plan-do-review« program was to provide intellectual stimulation, to increase thinking and reasoning abilities, and to increase later school achievement.

As demonstrated in several other Head Start projects, the experimental group showed gains in intelligence that were rather short-lived. However, they were significantly better in elementary school motivation, school achievement at age 14, teacher ratings of classroom behavior at ages 6–9, self-reports of classroom behavior at age 15, and self-reports of offending at age 15. A later follow-up of the Perry sample (Berrueta-Clement et al. 1984) showed that, at age 19, the experimental group was more likely to be employed, more likely to have graduated from high school, more likely to have received college or vocational training, and less likely to have been arrested. By age 27, the experimental group had accumulated only half as many arrests on average as the controls (Schweinhart et al. 1993). Also, they had significantly higher earnings and were more likely to be home owners. Hence, this preschool intellectual enrichment program led to decreases in school failure, to decreases in delinquency, and to decreases in other undesirable outcomes. For every $1 spent on the program, $7 were saved in the long run.

Like the Perry project, the Child Parent Center (CPC) in Chicago provided disadvantaged children with a high-quality, active learning preschool supplemented with family support (Reynolds et al. 2001). However, unlike Perry, CPC continued to provide the children with the educational enrichment component into elementary school, up to age 9. Just focusing on the effect of the preschool intervention, it was found that, compared to a control group, those who received the program were less likely to be arrested for both nonviolent and violent offenses by the time they were 18. The CPC program also produced other benefits for those in the experimental compared to the control group, such as a higher rate of high school completion.

21.3.3 Parent Training

Parent training is also an effective method of preventing delinquency. Many different types of parent training have been used (Kazdin 1997), but the behavioral parent management training developed by Patterson (1982) in Oregon is one of the most hopeful approaches. His careful observations of parent-child interaction showed that parents of antisocial children were deficient in their methods of child rearing. These parents failed to tell their children how they were expected to behave, failed to monitor their behavior to ensure that it was desirable, and failed to enforce rules promptly and unambiguously with appropriate rewards and penalties. The parents of antisocial children used more punishment (such as scolding, shouting, or threatening), but failed to make it contingent on the child's behavior.

Patterson attempted to train these parents in effective child rearing methods, namely noticing what a child is doing, monitoring behavior over long periods, clearly stating house rules, making rewards and punishments contingent on behavior, and negotiating disagreements so that conflicts and crises did not escalate. His treatment was shown to be effective in reducing child stealing and antisocial behavior over short periods in small-scale studies (Dishion et al. 1992; Patterson et al. 1982, 1992).

Another parenting intervention, termed functional family therapy, was evaluated in Utah by Alexander and Parsons (1973). This aimed to modify patterns of family interaction by modeling, prompting, and reinforcement, to encourage clear communication of requests and solutions between family members, and to minimize conflict. Essentially, all family members were trained to negotiate effectively, to set clear rules about privileges and responsibilities, and to use techniques of reciprocal reinforcement with each other. This technique halved the recidivism rate of minor delinquents in comparison with other approaches (client-centered or psychodynamic therapy). Its effectiveness with more serious delinquents was confirmed in a replication study using matched groups (Gordon 1995).

The Multidimensional Treatment Foster Care (MTFC) program, evaluated in Oregon by Chamberlain and Reid (1998), also produced desirable results. Participants (young males with a history of serious and chronic offending and their parents) in the MTFC program received individual (e.g., skills in problem solving) and family (e.g., parent management training) therapy, while controls went to the usual community-based group care facility. One year after the completion of the program, MTFC cases were less likely than controls to have engaged in further criminal activity, as measured by police arrests.

21.3.4   Skills Training

The set of techniques variously termed cognitive-behavioral interpersonal social skills training have proved to be successful (Lipsey and Wilson 1998). For example, the »Reasoning and Rehabilitation« program developed by Ross and Ross (1995) in Ottawa, Canada, aimed to modify the impulsive, egocentric thinking of delinquents, to teach them to stop and think before acting, to consider the consequences of their behavior, to conceptualize alternative ways of solving interpersonal problems, and to consider the impact of their behavior on other people, especially their victims. It included social skills training, lateral thinking (to teach creative problem solving), critical thinking (to teach logical reasoning), values education (to teach values and concern for others), assertiveness training (to teach nonaggressive, socially appropriate ways to obtain desired outcomes), negotiation skills training, interpersonal cognitive problem-solving (to teach thinking skills for solving interpersonal problems), social perspective training (to teach how to recognize and understand other people's feelings), role-playing, and modeling (demonstration and practice of effective and acceptable interpersonal behavior). This program led to a large decrease in reoffending by a small sample of delinquents.

Jones and Offord (1989) implemented a skills training program, known as Participate and Learn Skills (PALS), in an experimental public housing complex in Ottawa and compared it with a control complex. The program centered on nonschool skills, both athletic (e.g., swimming and hockey) and nonathletic (e.g., guitar and ballet). The aim of developing skills was to increase self-esteem, to encourage children to use time constructively, and to provide desirable role models. Participation rates were high; about three-quarters of age-eligible children in the experimental complex took at least one course in the first year. The program was successful; delinquency rates decreased significantly in the experimental complex compared to the control complex. The benefit-to-cost ratio, based on savings to taxpayers, was 2.5.

21.3.5   Peer Programs

There are no outstanding examples of effective intervention programs for antisocial behavior targeted on peer risk factors. The most hopeful programs involve using high-status conventional peers to teach children ways of resisting peer pressure; this is effective in reducing drug use (Tobler et al. 1999). Also, in a randomized experiment in St. Louis, Feldman et al. (1983) showed that placing antisocial adolescents in activity groups dominated by prosocial adolescents led to a reduction in their antisocial behavior (compared with antisocial adolescents placed in antisocial groups). This suggests that the influence of prosocial peers can be harnessed to reduce antisocial behavior.

The most important intervention program whose success seems to be based mainly on reducing peer risk factors is the Children at Risk program (Harrell et al. 1997), which targeted high risk adolescents (average age 12) in poor neighborhoods of five cities across the USA. Eligible youths were identified in schools, and randomly assigned to experimental or control groups. The program was a comprehensive community-based prevention strategy targeting risk factors for delinquency, including case management and family counseling, family skills training, tutoring, mentoring, after-school activities, and community policing. The program was different in each neighborhood.

The initial results of the program were disappointing, but a 1-year follow-up showed that (according to self-reports) experimental youths were less likely to have committed violent crimes and used or sold drugs (Harrell et al. 1999). The process evaluation showed that the greatest change was in peer risk factors. Experimental youths associated less often with delinquent peers, felt less peer pressure to engage in delinquency, and had more positive peer support. In contrast, there were few changes in individual, family, or community risk factors, possibly linked to the low participation of parents in parent training and of youths in mentoring and tutoring (Harrell et al. 1997, p. 87). In other words, there were problems of implementation of the program, linked to the serious and multiple needs and problems of the families.

21.3.6   School Programs

An important school-based prevention experiment was carried out in Seattle by Hawkins et al. (1991). This combined parent training, teacher training, and skills training. About 500 first grade children (aged 6) were randomly assigned to be in experimental or control classes. The children in the experimental classes received special treatment at home and school, which was designed to increase their attachment to their parents and their bonding to the school, based on the assumption that delinquency was inhibited by the strength of social bonds. Their parents were trained to notice and reinforce socially desirable behavior in a program called »Catch them being good«. Their teachers were trained in classroom management, for example, to provide clear instructions and expectations to children, to reward children for participation in desired behavior, and to teach children prosocial (socially desirable) methods of solving problems.

In an evaluation of this program, known as the Seattle Social Development Project, 18 months later, when the children were in different classes, Hawkins et al. (1991) found that the boys who received the experimental program were significantly less aggressive than the control boys, according to teacher ratings. This difference was particularly marked for white boys rather than African-American boys. The experimental girls were not significantly less aggressive, but they were less self-destructive, anxious and depressed. At age 18, Hawkins et al. (1999) found that the full intervention group (those receiving the intervention from grades 1–6) admitted less violence, less alcohol abuse, and fewer sexual partners than the late intervention group (grades 5–6 only) or the controls. The benefit-to-cost ratio of this program according to Aos et al. (2001a) was 4.3. Other school-based programs have also been successful in reducing antisocial behavior (Catalano et al. 1998).

21.3.7   Anti-Bullying Programs

Several school-based programs have been designed to decrease bullying. The most famous of these was implemented by Olweus (1994) in Norway. It aimed to increase awareness and knowledge of teachers, parents, and children about bullying and to dispel myths about it. A 30-page booklet was distributed to all schools in Norway describing what was known about bullying and recommending what steps schools and teachers could take to reduce it. Also, a 25-minute video about bullying was made available to schools. Simultaneously, the schools distributed to all parents a four-page folder containing information and advice about bullying. In addition, anonymous self-report questionnaires about bullying were completed by all children.

The program was evaluated in Bergen. Each of the 42 participating schools received feedback information from the questionnaire, about the prevalence of bullies and victims, in a specially arranged school conference day. Also, teachers were encouraged to develop explicit rules about bullying (e.g., do not bully, tell someone when bullying happens, bullying will not be tolerated, try to help victims, try to include children who are being left out) and to discuss bullying in class, using the video and role-playing exercises. Also, teachers were encouraged to improve monitoring and supervision of children, especially in the playground. The program was successful in reducing the prevalence of bullying by half.

A similar program was implemented in England in 23 Sheffield schools by Smith and Sharp (1994). The core program involved establishing a »whole-school« anti-bullying policy, raising awareness of bullying and clearly defining roles and responsibilities of teachers and students, so that everyone knew what bullying was and what they should do about it. In addition, there were optional interventions tailored to particular schools: curriculum work (e.g., reading books, watching videos), direct work with students (e.g., assertiveness training for those who were bullied), and playground work (e.g., training lunch-time supervisors). This program was successful in reducing bullying (by 15%) in primary schools, but had relatively small effects (a 5% reduction) in secondary schools.

21.3.8   Multi-Modal Programs

Multimodal programs including both skills training and parent training are more effective than either alone (Wasserman and Miller 1998). An important multimodal program was implemented by Tremblay et al. (1995) in Montreal, Canada. They identified about 250 disruptive (aggressive/hyperactive) boys at age 6 for a prevention experiment. Between ages 7 and 9, the experimental group received training to foster social skills and self-control. Coaching, peer modeling, role playing, and reinforcement contingencies were used in small group sessions on such topics as »how to help«, »what to do when you are angry«, and »how to react to teasing«. Also, their parents were trained using the parent management training techniques developed by Patterson (1982).

This prevention program was quite successful. By age 12, the experimental boys committed less burglary and theft, were less likely to get drunk, and were less likely to be involved in fights than the controls. Also, the experimental boys had higher school achievement. At every age from 10 to 15, the experimental boys had lower self-reported delinquency scores than the control boys. Interestingly, the differences in antisocial behavior between experimental and control boys increased as the follow-up progressed.

Intervention programs that tackle several of the major risk factors for CD and delinquency are likely to be particularly effective. Henggeler et al. (1993) in South Carolina evaluated multisystemic therapy (MST) for juvenile offenders, tackling family, peer, and school risk factors simultaneously in individualized treatment plans tailored to the needs of each family. MST was compared with the usual Department of Youth Services treatment, involving out-of-home placement in the majority of cases. In a randomized experiment with delinquents, MST was followed by fewer arrests, lower self-reported delinquency, and less peer-oriented aggression. Borduin et al. (1995) also showed that MST was more effective in decreasing arrests and antisocial behavior than was individual therapy. According to Aos et al. (2001 b), MST has one of the highest benefit-to-cost ratios of any program. For every $1 spent on it, $13.45 was saved in victim and criminal justice costs.

The results were somewhat less favorable in a real world implementation of MST using therapists recruited and trained in each site. Previous experiments had been implemented and closely monitored by MST experts. Henggeler et al. (1997) randomly allocated chronic and violent juvenile offenders either to MST or to the usual services (which in this case mainly involved probation and restitution). MST led to a decrease in arrests, self-reported delinquency, and antisocial behavior, but only when treatment fidelity was high. The researchers concluded that, in real world applications, therapist adherence to MST principles was a crucial factor. Worrying results were also obtained in a large-scale independent evaluation of MST in Canada by Leschied and Cunningham (2002). Over 400 youths who were either offenders or at risk of offending were randomly assigned to receive either MST or the usual services (typically probation supervision). Six months after treatment, 28% of the MST group had been reconvicted, compared with 31% of the control group, a nonsignificant difference.

21.4   Discussion and Conclusions

A great deal is known about the key risk factors for adolescent antisocial behavior, which include impulsiveness, low IQ and low school achievement, poor parental supervision, child physical abuse, punitive or erratic parental discipline, cold parental attitude, parental conflict, disrupted families, antisocial parents, large family size, low family income, antisocial peers, high delinquency-rate schools, and high crime neighborhoods. However, the causal mechanisms linking these risk factors with antisocial outcomes are less well established. Larger developmental theories that explain all the results need to be formulated and tested (Lahey et al. 2003). More research is needed on risk factors for persistence or escalation of antisocial behavior. How far risk factors are the same for males and females, for different ethnic groups, or at different ages needs to be investigated. More cross-cultural comparisons of risk factors, and more studies of protective factors, are needed.

The comorbidity and versatility of antisocial behavior poses a major challenge to understanding. It is important to investigate how far all results are driven by a minority of multiple problem adolescents or chronic delinquents. Often, multiple risk factors lead to multiple problem boys (Loeber et al. 2001). How far any given risk factor generally predicts a variety of different outcomes (as opposed to specifically predicting one or two outcomes) and how far each outcome is generally predicted by a variety of different risk factors (as opposed to being specifically predicted by only one or two risk factors) is unclear. An increasing number of risk factors seems to lead to an increasing probability of antisocial outcomes, almost irrespective of the particular risk factors included in the prediction measure, but more research is needed on this. There was insufficient space in this chapter to review theories explaining the links between risk factors and antisocial outcomes, but these have to be based on knowledge about the additive, independent, interactive, and sequential effects of risk factors.

There are many examples of successful intervention programs, including general parent education in home visiting programs, preschool intellectual enrichment programs, parent management training, cognitive-behavioral skills training, anti-bullying programs, and multimodal programs including individual and family interventions. However, many experiments are based on small samples and short follow-up periods. The challenge to researchers is to transport carefully monitored small-scale programs implemented by high quality university personnel into routine large-scale use, without losing their effectiveness. Often, multimodal programs are the most successful, making it difficult to identify the active ingredient. Successful multimodal programs should be followed by more specific experiments targeting single risk factors, which could be very helpful in establishing which risk factors have causal effects.

More efforts are needed to tailor types of interventions to types of adolescents. Ideally, an intervention should be preceded by a screening or needs assessment to determine which problems need to be rectified and which adolescents are most likely to be amenable to treatment. It is important to establish how far interventions are successful with the most antisocial adolescents, in order to identify where the benefits will be greatest in practice. Also, more cost-benefit analyses are needed, to show how much money is saved by successful programs. Saving money is a powerful argument to convince policy-makers and practitioners to implement intervention programs.

A great deal has been learned about adolescent antisocial behavior in the last 25 years, especially from longitudinal and experimental studies. More investment in these kinds of studies is needed in the next 25 years in order to advance knowledge about and decrease these troubling social problems.

References

Alexander, J.F. and Parsons, B.V. (1973) Short-term behavioral intervention with delinquent families: Impact on family process and recidivism. Journal of Abnormal Psychology, 81, 219–225.

Aos, S., Phipps, P., Barnoski, R. and Lieb, R. (2001 a) The Comparative Costs and Benefits of Programs to Reduce Crime (version 4.0). Olympia, WA: Washington State Institute for Public Policy.

Aos, S., Phipps, P., Barnoski, R., and Lieb, R. (2001 b) The comparative costs and benefits of programs to reduce crime: A review of research findings with implications for Washington State. In B. C. Welsh, D. P. Farrington and L.W. Sherman (Eds.) Costs and benefits of preventing crime (pp. 149–175). Boulder, CO: Westview Press.

Berrueta-Clement, J.R., Schweinhart, L.J., Barnett, W.S., Epstein, A.S. and Weikart, D.P. (1984) Changed lives. Ypsilanti, MI: High/Scope.

Blum, H.M., Boyle, M.H. and Offord, D.R. (1988) Single-parent families: Child psychiatric disorder and school performance. Journal of the American Academy of Child and Adolescent Psychiatry, 27, 214–219.

Borduin, C.M., Mann, B.J., Cone, L.T., Henggeler, S.W., Fucci, B.R., Blaske, D.M. and Williams, R.A. (1995) Multisystemic treatment of serious juvenile offenders: Long-term prevention of criminality and violence. Journal of Consulting and Clinical Psychology, 63, 569–578.

Brennan, P.A., Mednick, B.R. and Mednick, S.A. (1993) Parental psychopathology, congenital factors, and violence. In S. Hodgins (Ed.) Mental disorder and crime (pp. 244–261). Newbury Park, CA: Sage.

Buehler, C., Anthony, C., Krishnakumar, A., Stone, G., Gerard, J. and Pemberton, S. (1997) Interparental conflict and youth problem behaviors: A meta-analysis. Journal of Child and Family Studies, 6, 233–247.

Caspi, A. (2000) The child is father of the man: Personality continuities from childhood to adulthood. Journal of Personality and Social Psychology, 78, 158–172.

Catalano, R.F., Arthur, M.W., Hawkins, J.D., Berglund, L. and Olson, J.J. (1998) Comprehensive community and school based interventions to prevent antisocial behavior. In R. Loeber and D.P. Farrington (Eds.) Serious and violent juvenile offenders: Risk factors and successful interventions (pp. 248–283). Thousand Oaks, CA: Sage.

Catalano, R.F., Hawkins, J.D., Berglund, L., Pollard, J.A. and Arthur, M.W. (2002) Prevention science and positive youth development: Competitive or cooperative frameworks? Journal of Adolescent Health, 31, 230–239.

Chamberlain, P. and Reid, J.B. (1998) Comparison of two community alternatives to incarceration for chronic juvenile offenders. Journal of Consulting and Clinical Psychology, 66, 624–633.

Cohen, P., Brook, J.S., Cohen, J., Velez, C.N. and Garcia, M. (1990) Common and uncommon pathways to adolescent psychopathology and problem behavior. In L.N. Robins and M. Rutter (Eds.) Straight and devious pathways from childhood to adulthood (pp. 242–258). Cambridge: Cambridge University Press.

Denno, D. W. (1990) Biology and violence: From birth to adulthood. Cambridge: Cambridge University Press.

Dishion, T. J., Patterson, G. R. and Kavanagh, K. A. (1992) An experimental test of the coercion model: Linking theory, measurement and intervention. In J. McCord and R. Tremblay (Eds.) Preventing antisocial behavior (pp. 253–282). New York: Guilford.

Elliott, D. S. and Menard, S. (1996) Delinquent friends and delinquent behavior: Temporal and developmental patterns. In J. D. Hawkins (Ed.) Delinquency and crime: Current theories (pp. 28–67). Cambridge: Cambridge University Press.

Farrington, D. P. (1972) Delinquency begins at home. New Society, 21, 495–497.

Farrington, D. P. (1979) Environmental stress, delinquent behavior, and convictions. In I. G. Sarason and C. D. Spielberger (Eds.) Stress and anxiety, vol. 6 (pp. 93–107). Washington, DC: Hemisphere.

Farrington, D. P. (1983) Randomized experiments on crime and justice. In M. Tonry and N. Morris (Eds.) Crime and justice, vol. 4 (pp. 257–308). Chicago: University of Chicago Press.

Farrington, D. P. (1992 a) Explaining the beginning, progress and ending of antisocial behavior from birth to adulthood. In J. McCord (Ed.) Facts, frameworks and forecasts: Advances in criminological theory, vol. 3 (pp. 253–286). New Brunswick, NJ: Transaction.

Farrington, D. P. (1992 b) Juvenile delinquency. In J. C. Coleman (Ed.) The school years, 2nd ed. (pp. 123–163). London: Routledge.

Farrington, D. P. (1993) Childhood origins of teenage antisocial behavior and adult social dysfunction. Journal of the Royal Society of Medicine, 86, 13–17.

Farrington, D. P. (1994) Childhood, adolescent and adult features of violent males. In L. R. Huesman (Ed.) Aggressive behavior: Current perspectives (pp. 215–240). New York: Plenum.

Farrington, D. P. (2000) Adolescent violence: Findings and implications from the Cambridge Study. In G. Boswell (Ed.) Violent children and adolescents: Asking the question why (pp. 19–35). London: Whurr.

Farrington, D. P. and Loeber, R. (1999) Transatlantic replicability of risk factors in the development of delinquency. In P. Cohen, C. Slomkowski, and L. N. Robins (Eds.) Historical and geographical influences on psychopathology (pp. 299–329). Mahwah, NJ: Lawrence Erlbaum.

Farrington, D. P. and Welsh, B. C. (2003) Family-based prevention of offending: A meta-analysis. Australian and New Zealand Journal of Criminology, 36, 127–151.

Farrington, D. P., Barnes, G. and Lambert, S. (1996) The concentration of offending in families. Legal and Criminological Psychology, 1, 47–63.

Farrington, D. P., Biron, L. and LeBlanc, M. (1982) Personality and delinquency in London and Montreal. In J. Gunn and D. P. Farrington (Eds.) Abnormal offenders, delinquency, and the criminal justice system (pp. 153–201). Chichester, England: Wiley.

Farrington, D. P., Loeber, R. and van Kammen, W. B. (1990) Long-term criminal outcomes of hyperactivity-impulsivity-attention deficit and conduct problems in childhood. In L. N. Robins and M. Rutter (Eds.) Straight and devious pathways from childhood to adulthood (pp. 62–81). Cambridge: Cambridge University Press.

Feldman, R. A., Caplinger, T. E. and Wodarski, J. S. (1983) The St. Louis conundrum. Englewood Cliffs, NJ: Prentice-Hall.

Fergusson, D. M. and Horwood, L. J. (1998) Exposure to interparental violence in childhood and psychosocial adjustment in young adulthood. Child Abuse and Neglect, 22, 339–357.

Fergusson, D. M., Horwood, J. and Lynskey, M. T. (1994) Parental separation, adolescent psychopathology, and problem behaviors. Journal of the American Academy of Child and Adolescent Psychiatry, 33, 1122–1131.

Fischer, D. G. (1984) Family size and delinquency. Perceptual and Motor Skills, 58, 527–534.

Frick, P. J., Kamphaus, R. W., Lahey, B. B., Loeber, R., Christ, M. A. G., Hart, E. L. and Tannenbaum, L. E. (1991) Academic underachievement and the disruptive behavior disorders. Journal of Consulting and Clinical Psychology, 59, 289–294.

Frick, P. J., Lahey, B. B., Loeber, R., Stouthamer-Loeber, M., Christ, M. A. G. and Hanson, K. (1992) Familial risk factors to oppositional defiant disorder and conduct disorder: Parental psychopathology and maternal parenting. Journal of Consulting and Clinical Psychology, 60, 49–55.

Goodman, R., Simonoff, E. and Stevenson, J. (1995) The impact of child IQ, parent IQ and sibling IQ on child behavioral deviance scores. Journal of Child Psychology and Psychiatry, 36, 409–425.

Gordon, D. A. (1995) Functional family therapy for delinquents. In R. R. Ross, D. H. Antonowicz and G. K. Dhaliwal (Eds.) Going straight: Effective delinquency prevention and offender rehabilitation (pp. 163–178). Ottawa, Canada: Air Training and Publications.

Gottfredson, D. C. (2001) Schools and delinquency. Cambridge: Cambridge University Press.

Gottfredson, D. C., McNeil, R. J. and Gottfredson, G. D. (1991) Social area influences on delinquency: A multilevel analyses. Journal of Research in Crime and Delinquency, 28, 197–226.

Graham, J. (1988) Schools, disruptive behaviour and delinquency. London: Her Majesty's Stationery Office.

Haapasalo, J. and Pokela, E. (1999) Child-rearing and child abuse antecedents of criminality. Aggression and Violent Behavior, 1, 107–127.

Harrell, A. V., Cavanagh, S. E., Harmon, M. A., Koper, C. S. and Sridharan, S. (1997) Impact of the Children at Risk program: Comprehensive final report, vol. 2. Washington, DC: The Urban Institute.

Harrell, A. V., Cavanagh, S. E. and Sridharan, S. (1999) Evaluation of the Children at Risk program: Results one year after the program. Washington, DC: U.S. National Institute of Justice.

Hawkins, J. D., Herrenkohl, T., Farrington, D. P., Brewer, D., Catalano, R. F. and Harachi, T. W. (1998) A review of predictors of youth violence. In R. Loeber and D.P. Farrington (Eds.) Serious and violent juvenile offenders: Risk factors and successful interventions (pp. 106–146). Thousand Oaks, CA: Sage.

Hawkins, J.D., Catalano, R.F., Kosterman, R., Abbott, R. and Hill, K.G. (1999) Preventing adolescent health risk behaviors by strengthening protection during childhood. Archives of Pediatrics and Adolescent Medicine, 153, 226–234.

Henggeler, S.W., Melton, G.B., Smith, L.A., Schoenwald, S.K. and Hanley, J.H. (1993) Family preservation using multisystemic treatment: Long-term follow-up to a clinical trial with serious juvenile offenders. Journal of Child and Family Studies, 2, 283–293.

Henggeler, S.W., Melton, G.B., Brondino, M.J., Scherer, D.G. and Hanley, J.H. (1997) Multisystemic therapy with violent and chronic juvenile offenders and their families: The role of treatment fidelity in successful dissemination. Journal of Consulting and Clinical Psychology, 65, 821–833.

Henry, B., Moffitt, T., Robins, L., Earls, F. and Silva, P. (1993) Early family predictors of child and adolescent antisocial behavior: Who are the mothers of delinquents? Criminal Behavior and Mental Health, 2, 97–118.

Henry, B., Caspi, A., Moffitt, T.E. and Silva, P.A. (1996) Temperamental and familial predictors of violent and nonviolent criminal convictions: Age 3 to age 18. Developmental Psychology, 32, 614–623.

Herrenkohl, T.I., Hawkins, J.D., Chung, I.-J., Hill, K.G. and Battin-Pearson, S. (2001) School and community risk factors and interventions. In R. Loeber and D.P. Farrington (Eds.) Child delinquents: Development, intervention and service needs (pp. 211–246). Thousand Oaks, CA: Sage.

Hogh, E. and Wolf, P. (1983) Violent crime in a birth cohort: Copenhagen 1953–1977. In K.T. van Dusen and S.A. Mednick (Eds.) Prospective studies of crime and delinquency (pp. 249–267). Boston: Kluwer-Nijhoff.

Jenkins, J.M. and Smith, M.A. (1991) Marital disharmony and children's behavior problems: Aspects of a poor marriage that affect children adversely. Journal of Child Psychology and Psychiatry, 32, 793–810.

Jones, M.B. and Offord, D.R. (1989) Reduction of antisocial behavior in poor children by non-school skill-development. Journal of Child Psychology and Psychiatry, 30, 737–750.

Juby, H. and Farrington, D.P. (2001) Disentangling the link between disrupted families and delinquency. British Journal of Criminology, 41, 22–40.

Kalb, L.M., Farrington, D.P. and Loeber, R. (2001) Leading longitudinal studies on delinquency, substance use, sexual behavior, and mental health problems with childhood samples. In R. Loeber and D.P. Farrington (Eds.) Child delinquents: Development, intervention, and service needs (pp. 415–423). Thousand Oaks, CA: Sage.

Kazdin, A.E. (1997) Parent management training: Evidence, outcomes and issues. Journal of the American Academy of Child and Adolescent Psychiatry, 36, 1349–1356.

Keenan, K., Loeber, R., Zhang, Q., Stouthamer-Loeber, M. and van Kammen, W.B. (1995) The influence of deviant peers on the development of boys' disruptive and delinquent

behavior: A temporal analysis. Development and Psychopathology, 7, 715–726.

Klinteberg, B.A., Andersson, T., Magnusson, D. and Stattin, H. (1993) Hyperactive behavior in childhood as related to subsequent alcohol problems and violent offending: A longitudinal study of male subjects. Personality and Individual Differences, 15, 381–388.

Kolvin, I., Miller, F.J.W., Fleeting, M. and Kolvin, P.A. (1988) Social and parenting factors affecting criminal-offence rates: Findings from the Newcastle Thousand Family Study (1947–1980). British Journal of Psychiatry, 152, 80–90.

Lahey, B.B., Moffitt, T.E. and Caspi, A. (Eds.) (2003) The causes of conduct disorder and serious juvenile delinquency. New York: Guilford Press.

Leschied, A. and Cunningham A. (2002) Seeking effective interventions for serious young offenders: Interim results of a four-year randomized study of multisystemic therapy in Ontario, Canada. London, Canada: London Family Court Clinic.

Lipsey, M.W. and Derzon, J.H. (1998) Predictors of violent or serious delinquency in adolescence and early adulthood: A synthesis of longitudinal research. In R. Loeber and D.P. Farrington (Eds.) Serious and violent juvenile offenders: Risk factors and successful interventions (pp. 86–105). Thousand Oaks, CA: Sage.

Lipsey, M.W. and Wilson, D.B. (1998) Effective intervention for serious juvenile offenders: A synthesis of research. In R. Loeber and D.P. Farrington (Eds.) Serious and violent juvenile offenders: Risk factors and successful interventions (pp. 313–345). Thousand Oaks, CA: Sage.

Loeber, R., Farrington, D.P., Stouthamer-Loeber, M. and van Kammen, W.B. (1998) Antisocial behavior and mental health problems: Explanatory factors in childhood and adolescence. Mahwah, NJ: Lawrence Erlbaum.

Loeber, R., Green, S.M., Keenan, K. and Lahey, B.B. (1995) Which boys will fare worse? Early predictors of the onset of conduct disorder in a six-year longitudinal study. Journal of the American Academy of Child and Adolescent Psychiatry, 34, 499–509.

Loeber, R., Farrington, D.P., Stouthamer-Loeber, M., Moffitt, T.E., Caspi, A. and Lynam, D. (2001) Male mental health problems, psychopathy, and personality traits: Key findings from the first 14 years of the Pittsburgh Youth Study. Clinical Child and Family Psychology Review, 4, 273–297.

Lynam, D. (1996) Early identification of chronic offenders: Who is the fledgling psychopath? Psychological Bulletin, 120, 209–234.

Lynam, D.R. (1998) Early identification of the fledgling psychopath: Locating the psychopathic child in the current nomenclature. Journal of Abnormal Psychology, 107, 566–575.

Malinosky-Rummell, R. and Hansen, D.J. (1993) Long-term consequences of childhood physical abuse. Psychological Bulletin, 114, 68–79.

Masten, A. and Reed, M.-G.J. (2002) Resilience in development. In C.R. Snyder and S.J. Lopez (Eds.) The handbook of positive psychology (pp. 74–88). Oxford: Oxford University Press.

Maxfield, M. G. and Widom, C. S. (1996) The cycle of violence revisited six years later. Archives of Pediatrics and Adolescent Medicine, 150, 390–395.

McCord, J. (1977) A comparative study of two generations of native Americans. In R. F. Meier (Ed.) Theory in criminology (pp. 83–92). Beverly Hills, CA: Sage.

McCord, J. (1979) Some child-rearing antecedents of criminal behavior in adult men. Journal of Personality and Social Psychology, 37, 1477–1486.

Moffitt, T. E. (1993) The neuropsychology of conduct disorder. Development and Psychopathology, 5, 135–151.

Moffitt, T. E., Caspi, A., Rutter, M. and Silva, P. A. (2001) Sex differences in antisocial behavior. Cambridge: Cambridge University Press.

Morash, M. and Rucker, L. (1989) An exploratory study of the connection of mother's age at childbearing to her children's delinquency in four data sets. Crime and Delinquency, 35, 45–93.

Nagin, D. S., Pogarsky, G. and Farrington, D. P. (1997) Adolescent mothers and the criminal behavior of their children. Law and Society Review, 31, 137–162.

Newson, J., Newson, E. and Adams, M. (1993) The social origins of delinquency. Criminal Behavior and Mental Health, 3, 19–29.

Offord, D. R., Alder, R. J. and Boyle, M. H. (1986) Prevalence and sociodemographic correlates of conduct disorder. American Journal of Social Psychiatry, 6, 272–278.

Offord, D. R., Boyle, M. H. and Racine, Y. (1989) Ontario Child Health Study: Correlates of disorder. Journal of the American Academy of Child and Adolescent Psychiatry, 28, 856–860.

Olds, D. L., Henderson, C. R., Chamberlain, R. and Tatelbaum, R. (1986) Preventing child abuse and neglect: A randomized trial of nurse home visitation. Pediatrics, 78, 65–78.

Olds, D. L., Eckenrode, J., Henderson, C. R., Kitzman, H., Powers, J., Cole, R., Sidora, K., Morris, P., Pettitt, L. M. and Luckey, D. W. (1997) Long-term effects of home visitation on maternal life course and child abuse and neglect. Journal of the American Medical Association, 278, 637–643.

Olds, D. L., Henderson, C. R., Cole, R., Eckenrode, J., Kitzman, H., Luckey, D., Pettitt, L., Sidora, K., Morris, P. and Powers, J. (1998) Long-term effects of nurse home visitation on children's criminal and antisocial behavior: 15-year follow-up of a randomized controlled trial. Journal of the American Medical Association, 280, 1238–1244.

Olweus, D. (1994) Bullying at school: Basic facts and effects of a school based intervention program. Journal of Child Psychology and Psychiatry, 35, 1171–1190.

Patterson, G. R. (1982) Coercive family process. Eugene, OR: Castalia.

Patterson, G. R., Chamberlain, P. and Reid, J. B. (1982) A comparative evaluation of a parent training program. Behavior Therapy, 13, 638–650.

Patterson, G. R., Reid, J. B. and Dishion, T. J. (1992) Antisocial boys. Eugene, OR: Castalia.

Reiss, A. J. and Farrington, D. P. (1991) Advancing knowledge about co-offending: Results from a prospective longitudi-

nal survey of London males. Journal of Criminal Law and Criminology, 82, 360–395.

Reynolds, A. J., Temple, J. A., Robertson, D. L. and Mann, E. A. (2001) Long-term effects of an early childhood intervention on educational achievement and juvenile arrest: A 15-year follow-up of low-income children in public schools. Journal of the American Medical Association, 285, 2339–2346.

Robins, L. N. (1979) Sturdy childhood predictors of adult outcomes: Replications from longitudinal studies. In J. E. Barrett, R. M. Rose and G. L. Klerman (Eds.) Stress and mental disorder (pp. 219–235). New York: Raven Press.

Robins, L. N., West, P. J. and Herjanic, B. L. (1975) Arrests and delinquency in two generations: A study of black urban families and their children. Journal of Child Psychology and Psychiatry, 16, 125–140.

Ross, R. R. and Ross, R. D. (Eds.) (1995) Thinking straight: The reasoning and rehabilitation program for delinquency prevention and offender rehabilitation. Ottawa, Canada: Air Training and Publications.

Rothbaum, F. and Weisz, J. R. (1994) Parental caregiving and child externalizing behavior in nonclinical samples: A meta-analysis. Psychological Bulletin, 116, 55–74.

Rowe, D. C. (2002) Biology and crime. Los Angeles, CA: Roxbury.

Rutter, M. (1981) The city and the child. American Journal of Orthopsychiatry, 51, 610–625.

Sampson, R. J., Raudenbush, S. W. and Earls, F. (1997) Neighborhoods and violent crime: A multilevel study of collective efficacy. Science, 277, 918–924.

Schweinhart, L. J. and Weikart, D. P. (1980) Young children grow up. Ypsilanti, MI: High/Scope.

Schweinhart, L. J., Barnes, H. V. and Weikart, D. P. (1993) Significant benefits. Ypsilanti, MI: High/Scope.

Smith, C. A. and Stern, S. B. (1997) Delinquency and antisocial behavior: A review of family processes and intervention research. Social Service Review, 71, 382–420.

Smith, C. A. and Thornberry, T. P. (1995) The relationship between childhood maltreatment and adolescent involvement in delinquency. Criminology, 33, 451–481.

Smith, P. K. and Sharp, S. (1994) School bullying: Insights and perspectives. London: Routledge.

Szatmari, P., Boyle, M. H. and Offord, D. R. (1993) Familial aggregation of emotional and behavioral problems of childhood in the general population. American Journal of Psychiatry, 150, 1398–1403.

Tobler, N. S., Lessard, T., Marshall, D., Ochshorn, P. and Roona, M. (1999) Effectiveness of school-based drug prevention programs for marijuana use. School Psychology International, 20, 105–137.

Tremblay, R. E., Pagani-Kurtz, L., Vitaro, F., Masse, L. C. and Pihl, R. D. (1995) A bimodal preventive intervention for disruptive kindergarten boys: Its impact through mid-adolescence. Journey of Consulting and Clinical Psychology, 63, 560–568.

Velez, C. N., Johnson, J. and Cohen, P. (1989) A longitudinal analysis of selected risk factors for childhood psychopathology. Journal of the American Academy of Child and Adolescent Psychiatry, 28, 861–864.

Wadsworth, M. (1979) Roots of delinquency. London: Martin Robertson.

Wasserman, G. A. and Miller, L. S. (1998) The prevention of serious and violent juvenile offending. In R. Loeber and D. P. Farrington (Eds.) Serious and violent juvenile offenders: Risk factors and successful interventions (pp. 197–247). Thousand Oaks, CA: Sage.

Wells, L. E. and Rankin, J. H. (1991) Families and delinquency: A meta-analysis of the impact of broken homes. Social Problems, 38, 71–93.

West, D. J. and Farrington, D. P. (1973) Who becomes delinquent? London: Heinemann.

Widom, C. S. (1989) The cycle of violence. Science, 244, 160–166.

Early Detection and Prevention of Attention Deficit/Hyperactivity Disorders

Eric Taylor

22.1   Introduction   – 301

22.2   **Primary Prevention**   – 302
22.2.1 Genetic and Environmental Influences   – 302
22.2.2 Changes in Society   – 303

22.3   **Early Detection: What to Detect?**   – 304
22.3.1 Genetic Risks   – 304
22.3.2 Neurobiological Factors   – 305
22.3.3 Cognitive Changes   – 305
22.3.4 Behavioral Measures   – 307

22.4   **When to Detect**   – 307

22.5   **How to Detect**   – 308
22.5.1 Rating Scales   – 308
22.5.2 Interviews   – 308
22.5.3 Observation   – 308

22.6   **Interventions**   – 308

22.7   **Outstanding Problems**   – 310
22.7.1 Is Prevention Needed at All?   – 310
22.7.2 Should Interventions Be Universal Rather Than
        in High-Risk Groups?   – 310
22.7.3 Could Interventions Do Harm?   – 310

22.8   **Conclusions**   – 311

        References   – 311

22.1 Introduction

Attention deficit/hyperactivity disorder (ADHD) should in theory be a good candidate for prevention programs.

1. ADHD is readily recognized, being based on overt and salient behaviors. Overactivity, impulsiveness, and inattentiveness are recognized problems for children's development in most cultures.
2. The behavior problems are common. This greatly facilitates the accuracy of detection in screening programs, and suggests that intervention in high-risk groups could be feasible in lo-

cal communities. It is true that clinical practice varies in different places, and the entity recognized varies from mild ADHD with a prevalence of 5% or more to severe hyperkinetic disorder with a point prevalence around 1.5% (Swanson et al. 1998). But this is not necessarily a key problem for prevention. The behavior problems are distributed continuously in the population (Taylor et al. 1991), and diagnostic disagreements are essentially about the cut-offs that should be imposed on this distribution.

3. Considerable knowledge has been gathered about developmental course. There is, for instance, reasonable consensus that hyperactivity is persistent throughout childhood (at least from the early social years), and predicts an adverse outcome in early adult life for mental health, academic qualification, occupational success, substance abuse and »accidental« injury (Schachar and Tannock 2002). It is therefore entirely possible that early interventions could be cost-effective even if they had to be applied to a large fraction, or even the whole, of the population.
4. Effective treatments are available. Stimulant medication given during the school years is one of the most successful therapies in mental health (Santosh and Taylor 2000) and behavioral therapies are well established as home- and school-based interventions (Herbert 2002).
5. Knowledge is advancing rapidly about the etiology of the disorder, and many associations are now known with factors in the environment that could be targeted in prevention (Schachar and Tannock 2002).

These factors are all encouraging to those considering developing prevention programs. There are also some formidable obstacles in their way:

1. The problems comprised in ADHD are complex and may be heterogeneous. Inattentiveness may

22

have different antecedents from hyperactivity (Taylor et al. 1991). There are often coexistent problems – especially, oppositional-defiant behaviors and anxiety; together with autism spectrum disorders and, in older children, tics, affective disorders, and disorders of conduct. This leaves uncertainty about what should most efficiently be targeted in prevention, and whether ADHD itself is a good target or should be subsumed within generally based programs for the improvement of child mental health.

2. The research on etiology has stressed the power of genetic influences and their polygenic nature. This has probably discouraged investigators from seeking primary prevention by removal of the causes, even though there may still be important environmental factors and even though early interventions can still be appropriate.

3. The most effective treatments may not be appropriate for use in prevention. Stimulant medication is not licensed below the age of 6 years in most European countries (though in some countries dexamfetamine – unlike methylphenidate – is licensed down to the age of 3 years). Even if it were licensed, there would be a serious lack of evidence base for its safety and efficacy in preschool children, let alone in children young enough that the initial development of hyperactivity might be halted.

4. ADHD is a controversial topic in most European countries. While clinical professionals may think that they have a reasonable consensus, educational and media professionals do not. Objections to the use of the idea come from many sources, some of which are deep-rooted in social values. Sometimes the fear of genetic determination leads the public to reject the idea that a common type of behavior could be a genetic phenomenon. Sometimes the fear of collapsing family values leads the public to think that failures of parents are being blamed on individual pathology in the child. Sometimes the fear of scapegoating children leads the public to wish to avoid stigmatizing labels. Of course, all these fears misrepresent the views of psychological and medical science. But they are likely to be practical obstacles to the enactment of any program with the avowed purpose of reducing ADHD.

For all these reasons, prevention programs specifically for ADHD have not developed. This chapter will consider the scope for developing them. It begins with the possibility of primary prevention, reviewing what we know of the contribution made by avoidable causes in early development. It proceeds to issues about early detection: what to detect and when and how to do it most efficiently. It then goes on to consider the effects of early interventions; and to make recommendations about future research and development.

22.2　Primary Prevention

22.2.1　Genetic and Environmental Influences

Genetic influences are known to be strong. A succession of comparisons between monozygotic and dizygotic twins has indicated heritabilities in the region of 70% to 90% (Thapar 1995). This is a high level of genetic influence, but it falls short of demonstrating that it amounts to an inherited illness. In present knowledge, the genetic effects do not seem to be bringing about a specific disorder of ADHD: Rather, the genes act across the whole range of hyperactivity in the population, influencing a trait rather than an illness.

The presence of strong genetic influences in no way implies that environmental influences do not matter, or that primary prevention by manipulating the environment is pointless. The environment in which children live can be associated in several ways with the genetic effects: the child's environment can be shaped by any hyperactivity there may be in the parents, and the expression of genes may be different in different environments. Several of the epidemiological associations of ADHD are likely to be of causal importance.

In the prenatal environment these associations include exposure to maternal alcohol drinking and cigarette smoking. Hyperactive behavior is a common association of fetal alcohol syndrome, yet the presence of this risk factor is all too seldom detected even when it is there. Lead exposure, both in utero and in childhood is an association of hyperactivity. Prenatal exposure to certain drugs, including benzodiazepines and anticonvulsants, also predict later hyperactive behavior.

Low birth weight can be an index of prenatal adversity, and there is a known association with Attention Deficit Hyperactivity Disorder. A good deal of this association, however, is likely to be mediated by other factors, such as social adversity, that influence intellectual performance quite generally and not just attention. Brain injury at this time usually has diffuse rather than specific effects on mental development. The direct role of birth trauma should not be exaggerated. It is true that severe brain damage, usually of a kind causing neurological signs at the time, can cause organic syndromes including hyperactivity; but this is, happily, uncommon enough that it does not contribute to many cases of ADHD. Minor degrees of obstetric complications probably have little direct causative role on hyperactive behavior unless they occur in children who are already at risk because of serious family or social disadvantage.

In the early environment, major disruptions of attachment – such as those seen in children in depriving institutions – are a known association of hyperactive behavior and are likely to be a causative influence; but no evidence yet links ADHD to subtler and commoner degrees of relationship failure. But factors in the psychological environment can be important in determining the later course of children with hyperactivity.

Factors in children's diet may exert some influence on behavior: probably not a direct toxic effect of certain foods (such as additives) on behavior; but rather an idiosyncratic reaction of some children to certain foods (Committee on Toxicity 2000). The most conclusive way of determining children's reactions is for them to adopt a few-food diet for an assessment period, and add in one at a time the foods that are likely to be responsible (Carter et al. 1993); but this is an expensive and troublesome procedure that cannot be recommended for routine use on a population basis.

All of these causes are of rather small effect, either because the effect on each individual is small (e.g., low-level lead) or because the cause is rare and affects a few individuals (e.g., severe neglect). The abolition of none of them would by itself make much difference to the prevalence of ADHD. Further, they are all causes with general effects on brain function rather than specifically on ADHD: IQ, for example, is often sensitive to the same causes. The case for ameliorating all of them is strong: Improved pre- and perinatal care, for example, is of great importance but the case does not rest primarily on the evidence from ADHD work.

Some more specific recommendations, however, could be taken up by child health services. Environmental stresses should be asked about in the assessment of children with ADHD. The detection of fetal alcohol exposure, for example, may not give much benefit to the individual child; but advice to the mother may well prevent another child in the family from being affected in the same way.

High-risk groups can be identified from their history. Children at risk, for example, those who have survived a very low birth weight, will be candidates for cognitive and social enrichment programs. These may not detectably influence the population prevalence of children with ADHD, but they could have cost-effective results for the children at risk.

Recommendations about diet await further scientific evidence about the nature of the mechanisms. If, as I suggest, the key process in dietary influences is the idiosyncratic reaction of individual children to any of a wide range of substances, then the major public health consideration is that foods designed for young children should have ingredients clearly labeled so that parents can be vigilant regarding possibly harmful ingredients. If, on the other hand, the main mechanism is a toxic effect of substances such as synthetic food dyes, then the public health conclusion would be that those substances should be banned unless the alternatives prove to be more toxic.

Child health teams – mental and physical – should inform themselves of any specific risks in their locality: is there, for instance, an industrial source of lead pollution? If so, blood lead may well be justified as a routine test in clinic practice or even – depending on the extent – in routine surveillance.

22.2.2 Changes in Society

Many, perhaps most, lay people think that the whole child population is becoming steadily less attentive and more impulsive over time. In this view, the effect of the television as a constant companion to the child is detrimental to habits of sustained thought and reflection. No attention is required to enjoy the sensational and titillating pleasures of the box, so attention does not develop. By the same token, children are said to become accustomed to, and to demand, instant gratification. If they are not shown how to wait and control themselves they will not learn how to do so.

These ideas are very popular, and fit with an increased concern about the development of children in societies where both parents, or the only parent, work outside the home. They are very relevant to the question of prevention, because they would be targets for universal prevention programs. But testing them rigorously is difficult, partly because the ideas themselves are not rigorously worked out. Is it the case that television induces less attention than other activities; or that delaying gratification is learned better in traditional family structures? We do not know the answers.

Some circumstantial predictions can be tested. Is it true that ADHD is increasing over time? Epidemiological surveys of prevalence have not indicated a rising trend – but most of these are based on ratings by parents or teachers so may not be relevant. If, as suggested, the effect of changing society is on the mean levels of inattention and impulse control in the population, then it might not be demonstrated in ratings that could be subject to an »adaptation level« effect. Teachers, for example, might rate each child on the basis of an implicit judgment of how far they are from current norms rather than by any absolute standard. Even when more objective measures are used, however, there is little evidence of secular change. Two studies in the UK surveyed school-age children with measures that included behaviorally oriented interviews with parents – i.e., interviews covering the details of actions shown by the child rather than an overall rating of their »abnormality«. One was carried out in the early 1980s in London (Taylor et al. 1991), the other was a national survey some 20 years later (Meltzer et al. 2000); both produced point prevalence figures of about 1.5% for hyperkinetic disorder.

A clearer secular change is in cognitive function generally. A steady rise in the abilities measured by the IQ tests has been found in many developed countries and is well known. Every few years the IQ tests have to be restandardized to allow for this. This is not a rigorous measure of attention, but does suggest that whatever is happening to attention over time is at any rate not leading to an inability to cope with new intellectual challenges.

Another argument against societal changes being responsible can be applied to many other putative causes that affect the population as a whole. It comes from the genetic twin studies that have already been cited to indicate the strength of genetic influences. The remaining environmental influence in these researches can be partitioned between that which is shared between twins (i.e., those that affect all children in a family) and those that are nonshared, but affect one twin rather than another. Nearly all the environmental influence comes in the latter, nonshared category. Society as a whole, the absence of fathers, and the availability of computers are therefore unlikely to be good targets for prevention campaigns.

22.3 Early Detection: What to Detect?

During early development, one can seek both to detect the early signs of ADHD itself (hyperactivity/impulsiveness, inattention) and the risks for its development (which could be genetic, e.g., alterations of DNA structure; cognitive, e.g., poor attention in infancy; or social, e.g., neglectful parenting). In present knowledge, the strongest continuities between early childhood and school age seem to be behavioral.

22.3.1 Genetic Risks

Two genetic variants – in the dopamine (4) receptor and the dopamine transporter molecules – have been robustly associated with ADHD by several independent groups of researchers. Other genes, including one coding for a synaptosomal protein (SNAP-25) and one for the dopamine (5) receptor, have had variant forms associated with ADHD by more than one research group. Even so, some competent studies have failed to find their presence: a likely explanation is that there is heterogeneity within the populations investigated. Meta-analysis has indicated that some DNA changes are associated with ADHD at a very high level of significance; but the effect size is small. It is doubtful whether any of the molecular genetic variants can account for as much as 5% of the variance in hyperactivity. Most children with DNA variants do not have ADHD; and many children with ADHD do not have any of the known DNA variants.

One of the reasons for gene-hunting is the hope that it will be possible one day to identify infants who are at such high risk for developing attention deficits or hyperactivity that it becomes feasible to provide treatment for them. The day has not yet come. Indeed, many genetic investigators are increasingly thinking that no DNA variant will in itself be necessary or sufficient, that genetic influences will interact with and modify each other, and that many different combinations of genes may be involved in groups of children with ADHD. If this is so, then very much more research will be needed to reach a working understanding of how the genetic influences work. More optimistically, however, clinicians and educators can hope for the near future: that, even in the absence of a full understanding, the knowledge of DNA constitution may let high-risk groups be screened.

The alternative strategy for genetic screening is identifying young children whose parents themselves have, or have had, ADHD. The increase of risk for those with an affected parent is approximately fivefold; however, most of the offspring will not be at risk, so the economics of prevention would need careful assessment before investing resources.

22.3.2   Neurobiological Factors

ADHD is a descriptive and not an explanatory category. It describes children with alterations in attentive behavior and activity control; it does not automatically mean a brain etiology except in the unhelpful sense that all mental events are dependent upon brain activity. It is true that research has indicated a number of significant neurobiological associations in studies of groups of children with carefully diagnosed ADHD (Schachar and Tannock 2002). Imaging studies concur that there are associations with reduced brain size, with disproportionate volumetric changes (e.g., in frontal and caudate areas), and there is some evidence for reduced perfusion of brain areas, including those with structural abnormalities, during the performance of »inhibitory« tasks (Rubia et al. 2001). These changes are reliable, but quite small, and there is considerable overlap between ADHD subjects and normal controls. None of these changes yet gives a clear identification of individuals; so they are of slight relevance to therapeutic questions. Even if they reach the stage of good classification of individuals, their expense will be a deterrent to population screening. Even if they become affordable, there will still be possible misidentification. It would be unfortunate if scarce therapeutic resources were rationed by the markers of brain dysfunction rather than the actual problems known to impose impairment.

22.3.3   Cognitive Changes

Early cognitive changes are present, and could well become grounds for early identification in an objective way; however, predictive value so far is rather low. They were reviewed by Taylor (1995), and documentation for the following conclusions can be found there. It has been hard to give a clear developmental account of the very early stages of development of children who will eventually be identified as showing ADHD. Babies are seldom identified as inattentive, and the earliest manifestations of brain dysfunction may be rather different from what will later be a disorder of attention or impulsiveness. There may be a discontinuity in activity level between the neonatal period and later infancy (Bell et al. 1971): the least active babies during the first days of life become the most active by the age of 4 months. Even in the second and third years of life, there is rather little information on the development of abnormalities of attention and motor impulse control. The neuropsychological deficits associated with ADHD may be different at different stages of life; if so, the recognition of disordered attention will require the examiner to focus on different abilities at different ages.

The early course of development of attention has been charted in normal children. It is clear that even in the first days of life babies use plans to sample information systematically. There is order in the way that neonates scan with their eyes, depending on whether they are in the light or the dark and whether or not a sound is also present. It is not entirely necessary to learn what one must examine: some strategies of examination are innate. Neonates look at moving stimuli with high contrast in preference to those that are still and homogenous. Their eyes fixate on the edges of contours; if there are no edges in the visual field then their eyes continue to search. There is a corresponding set of preferences in auditory attention. An intermittent tone produces more behavioral quietening than does a continuous tone, and an intense tone produces more cardiac deceleration than does a quiet one.

This kind of process is sometimes summarized by saying that the neonate's attention is passively captured by qualities of the stimuli. This, however, does not take into account the extent to which the neonate is actively following strategies and modifying its dispositions of visual gaze according to the circumstances that it encounters. The distribution of attention is from the start an active process. The active contribution of the baby is also emphasized by the finding that novel stimuli attract gaze preferentially over familiar stimuli; for the difference between a novel and a familiar stimulus depends upon the infant's memory of its previous experience. The same phenomenon, of a novel stimulus creating a greater internal effect than a familiar one, can be detected with other means of assessing the response of the child. The extent to which the stimulus will interrupt an ongoing activity such as sucking has been used in some laboratories; the autonomic orienting response of changes in heart rate, skin resistance, and other peripheral measures is also useful. Physiological measures such as these have shown that the enhanced effect of a novel stimulus cannot be dependent upon experience after birth, for it is detectable even during embryonic life.

A large amount of developmental research has therefore focused upon the visual preference for unfamiliar stimuli. Could this be a means of detecting early abnormalities in the development of attention? A standardized test has been developed by Fagan and Shepherd (1987) but the significance of individual differences on this test are not yet entirely clear. It may well be an index of infant intelligence rather than of specific processes of attention. Even for this purpose, much caution is needed in the application of the Fagan test (Benasich and Bejar 1992): some 40% of infants were misclassified into low- or high-risk status on the basis of the test, and the much higher base rate of low-risk status implies that most children identified as high-risk on this basis are not in fact at high risk at all.

The stability of infant tests of attention is also quite low. Even when children are tested only a couple of weeks apart, the correlations are modest; and when tests of habituation are taken, measures performed on the same children at 3 months and at 8 months have a correlation of about zero. There is an interesting paradox here: these measures of low stability are also quite highly predictive. The preference for a novel over a familiar stimulus predicts the later IQ quite strongly: indeed it is a better predictor of IQ in later childhood than are infant tests of general development. The association is at its strongest when the predicting assessments are made between 2 and 8 months of age – the period in which stability in individual differences is very low (McCall and Carriger 1993). The implication appears to be – not that measures of visual attention are inherently unreliable – but that they are determined by different factors at different stages of development. A similar lesson comes from the inspection time literature. A short inspection time in a baby predicts high IQ later; but, by contrast, the tendency to inspect new stimuli briefly is, by the age of about 7 years, a problem: it is associated with hyperactivity, and accounts for at least some of the cognitive impairment in hyperactivity.

During later childhood, there is an increasing preference for more complex patterns. This goes hand in hand with a decrease in the average time which any given stimulus holds the attention. Because any one stimulus is inspected for a shorter period, it is possible to look at more things in a given period and correspondingly to extract more information about the world. Visual attention becomes more active and varied; it is correspondingly important that the distribution of attention is governed by efficient rules. The possibilities for exploration are dramatically increased with the ability to link auditory and visual information together and especially with the ability to explore manually and therefore to learn the properties of the outside world by experiment.

The importance of knowledge and theory in guiding the distribution of attention increases during later childhood. Stimuli previously associated with reward come to evoke longer gazes than do novel stimuli. Ruff and Lawson (1990a,b) made longitudinal descriptions of children's orienting behavior. Children's focused attention (involving intent facial expression and manipulation) increases from one to 5 years. Casual attention – the mere tendency to look at toys – did not increase over this period. However, the focused attention nearly always followed a period of casual attention. They suggested that a first, casual exploration of the world set in motion a set of ideas and the full deployment of active and focused orientation followed upon that. This is a readily observed behavior that could well become a basis for early screening.

Wright and Vlietstra (1975) reviewed a wide range of observational studies about the direction of attention during childhood. They concluded that there was a developmental line in which an early form of perceptual **exploration** of the most salient and novel aspects of the world gradually gave rise to an active, logically organized **search**. Older children are more capable than younger ones at adapting their strategy to the changing demands of a task. Older children will explore more dimensions of an object (e.g., shape, texture, size) if they are not given any information about which is relevant; on the other hand, if the important and relevant dimension of the stimulus is made clear in advance then older children will explore that dimension only and will therefore orient themselves to fewer stimulus dimensions than a younger child. Their strategy of exploration has been more successfully adapted to the changing demands of the task.

In short, we should not necessarily be expecting to find isomorphic continuity of attention from early to later childhood. Better longitudinal evidence is needed on the early antecedents of attention problems before cognitive testing becomes a realistic contender as a detector of early risk. Inhibition of prepotent responses looks like a stronger associate of »attention deficit« than does inattentiveness. By the age of 3, hard-to-manage preschoolers can already be distinguished from their more normal peers on the basis of poor performance on tests where a correct response requires the child not to make the obvious and immediate response but to pause, or detour round an obstacle in order to reach the goal. Tests such as these could indeed become the basis of identifying high-risk groups in the future. At present it is not clear how they will perform in terms of sensitivity and specificity. It is not enough to show that they discriminate significantly between groups: they have to be good enough to classify individual children with reasonable accuracy. This is not yet achieved, and there is much overlap between groups.

22.3.4 Behavioral Measures

Behavioral measures in early childhood are more promising.

1. If the presence of **overactive-impulsive behavior** is detected, then it is very probable that oppositional behaviors will also be present, and not unlikely that other problems will coexist. We do not know which of them will carry the major hazard for development, so broad-spectrum interventions are likely to be called for. It does, however, seem – for example, from preschool surveys in the New Forest (Sonuga-Barke et al. 2001) – that parental interviews focusing on impulsiveness and restlessness identify groups of children at considerably enhanced risk for behavior problems in later childhood. This suggests that hyperactive behavior should be a part of a screen for high-risk groups.

2. If **inattentiveness** is present without overactivity/impulsiveness, then there is much less of an evidence base to guide practice. In older children – from, say, the age of 7 – there is reasonable knowledge (Warner-Rogers et al. 2000). »Pure inattentiveness« is more closely linked even than hyperactivity to motor clumsiness, language delays, and educational failure. Their scores on attention tests are indeed less accomplished than those of normal controls; but this deficit can be accounted for by overall ability measured by IQ – or, to put it another way, their attention problems are pervasive enough to impair other aspects of cognitive development. They are at educational risk, but not at the same risk of conduct disorders as the hyperactive.

If one applies this conclusion to the first 3 years of life, then one might argue that pure deficits of attention at that time would require a different kind of goal for intervention. It could well do children a disservice if a unitary concept of »ADHD« led to the same sort of help being offered to both.

3. Self-regulation of affectivity is another component of ADHD, though not included in the diagnostic criteria. Intensity and volatility of mood are so often described that they seem clinically to be part of a single symptom complex. Research could well focus on the nature of problems in this domain that should enter into early detection.

22.4 When to Detect

Infants vary greatly in their activity levels, but individual differences are not very strongly predictive: in one study there was actually a negative correlation between activity at the age of 3 days and at 2.5 years (Bell et al. 1971). Detection at this age is likely to be of risk factors rather than the early signs of disorder.

In the preschool period, overactivity is a very common complaint made by parents. This is the period during which the problem typically becomes established; retrospective accounts show that the more severe and pervasive forms of hyperactivity are often apparent by the age of 2 years and nearly always noted by the fifth birthday. It is often hard to evaluate because activity is very high in normal children, there are few demands upon sustained concentration, and so it is difficult to determine whether the complaint is a valid comment on a deviation of development or whether it reflects a parent's reduced tolerance of a developmentally unremarkable level of demandingness. Sometimes »hyperactivity« is used by caretakers to refer to quite different problems from those in this chapter – such as sleeplessness and oppositionality.

Nevertheless, the complaint of overactivity at 3 years is a predictor of the presence of behavior problems, including conduct disorder, in later childhood. After the age of 3 the normal course of development involves a reduction of the general level of activity in some settings but not others. Many children will develop impulse control and attentiveness after the age of 3. The possible advantages of early intervention at or before the age of 3 would therefore need to be set against the numbers of screened-positive children who will grow out of their problems without intervention.

Starting at school makes prolonged attention more necessary. Some children – especially the most intelligent – cope with this transition well and meet all the requirements even if they are still distressingly uncontrolled at home. The persistence of unmodulated and inattentive behavior beyond this age becomes more and more of a problem as schooling proceeds. It carries risks for failing to learn, and other children are antagonized and begin to withdraw from them. One major outcome is the development of aggressive and antisocial behavior and delinquency (Farrington et al. 1990). Affected children also tend to remain inattentive and impulsive, become isolated and unpopular among their peers, and do not achieve academically as they should (Hinshaw 1994). Conduct disorder, once it has developed, is expensive and difficult to treat; so detection of hyperactivity early in the school career should be cost-effective.

22.5   How to Detect

22.5.1   Rating Scales

A wide variety of parent and teacher rating scales is available. In general, instruments developed for the specific purpose of assessing ADHD are more accurate than general-purpose psychopathological instruments. The sensitivity and specificity of such instruments often appear to be very good; yet even then the classification obtained can be inadequate. Measures such as Conners' rating scales show an effect size for children with ADHD, compared to normal controls, of around three standard deviations; and this level of discrimination could well correspond roughly to 80% levels of sensitivity and specificity, or even better.

While this sounds very impressive, it is still such a broad screen that interventions will have to be done on many children in order to prevent a case of ADHD. The difference in base rates implies that nonhyperactive children, although they show a much lower rate of hyperactivity as detected by rating scales, will still be wrongly identified as ADHD so often that they will outnumber the true cases. (The 20% wrongly identified come from 95% of the children, so the resulting 18% false positives outweigh the 4% of cases correctly detected and

add greatly to the cost of a prevention program.) Causes of false positives include raters without sufficient appreciation of the developmental norms for that age, raters who bring qualities of their relationship with the child to bear on making their rating of behavior, and contrast effects in which children are implicitly rated against other members of the family, or other members of the subculture.

22.5.2   Interviews

Detailed clinical interview with the parent (or other caregiver) is the most valuable single measure. In this context it is possible to go, beyond the request for a rating of whether a child's impulsiveness is abnormal, to the descriptions of the behavior on which that description is based. The interviewer can then apply a clinically informed judgment as to whether that level of behavior is in fact abnormal for the child. This is a more expensive process than a rating scale, but greater accuracy of discrimination could be enough to make intervention cost-effective.

22.5.3   Observation

Observations of the child's behavior are especially valuable in younger children. It may be possible to witness directly the overactivity, the disinclination to wait and the choice of immediate rather than delayed gratification. These can often be seen directly in younger children, for example by setting up a waiting situation in which the children will have a larger reward if they refrain from grabbing an immediate one. By the time of school entry, however, much of this overt behavior will be modified – at least in the artificial circumstances of clinic assessment. The novelty of the situation, the focused adult attention and the structured nature of the situation all militate against hyperactivity being readily observable. The diagnosis should therefore not be dismissed for the sole reason that the child appears well controlled during assessment. Nevertheless, when abnormality is seen, then direct observation is invaluable for detecting its pattern, its antecedents, and its consequences.

22.6   Interventions

The evidence base for choosing treatments in children of school age is extensive (Jadad et al. 1999).

The best evidence relates to stimulant medication. There is no doubt that it is more effective than a placebo, and comparisons of effect size have suggested that it is more potent than behavioral therapy in reducing the symptoms of ADHD (Santosh and Taylor 2000).

There is also evidence for the effectiveness of some psychological approaches. Cognitive therapy directly with children has not yet worked well (Abikoff and Gittelman 1985) but behavioral modification delivered by parents or teachers is an effective and widely used treatment (Barkley 1990).

A large-scale trial has made a systematic comparison of medication management, behaviorally oriented therapy, the combination of both these treatments, and a control group who received routine intervention in the community (MTA Cooperative Group 1999). For most kinds of outcome, medication was more effective than either behavior therapy or community treatment; and the combination of medication and behavior therapy added little to medication alone – provided that the medication was given with the intensive monitoring of the research program.

The application of these findings to high-risk groups would need careful examination. Interventions with hazards are unattractive when applied preventively to children who do not (yet) have any impairment from their symptoms. The treatment could indeed be considered for those who have already reached school age and been screened positive as described above – though awkward issues about consent would be raised, communities might well not tolerate it, and the need for physician supervision will mean that the therapy can never be cheap.

By contrast, there has been little systematic research about treatment in younger children. The few studies of the stimulants in this age group suggest that they can indeed reduce impulsiveness and improve general social adjustment more effectively than a placebo. They may also improve the quality of mother-child relationships. To set against this, there are some indications that adverse effects such as mood changes and lack of spontaneity do occur, and may be more common than in school-aged children. Furthermore, we simply do not know about the longer-term brain changes that could be induced by stimulant medication in the first 3 years. Much more research knowledge would be required about the treatment of established cases in the preschool period before one could responsibly plan for the treatment of those who are merely at-risk.

There is a much larger literature about programs designed for young children to prevent antisocial behavior; they are reviewed by Offord and Bennett (2002). Programs typically involve psychological interventions including parent training, academic tutoring, and social skills training for the children. Some of them are encouraging, at least for high-risk groups during elementary school years, but not yet well enough evaluated to convince many of those who fund services. The cost-effectiveness of universal interventions (such as television programs encouraging good child rearing) is even less clear. These programs have not included interventions specifically targeting inattention or hyperactivity, so are only relevant to this chapter in that they encourage the idea that psychological prevention is possible.

Recently there has been a beginning of randomized controlled trials of psychological therapies for hyperactivity in the preschool period. The most promising intervention is parent training. Sonuga-Barke et al. (2001) made a comparison between this, a program of parent counseling and support, and a waiting list control. Parent training was more effective than the other interventions in reducing the symptoms of ADHD and of oppositional defiant disorder; and it also increased the mother's sense of general well being. The gains in the parent training group were not entirely transient: they were still present at a 15-week follow up. The investigators in another trial compared behavioral family intervention (in both standard and enhanced forms) with a waiting list control and again found that the experimental groups showed reduced levels of behavior problems and greater competence shown by the parents (Bor et al. 2002). In this study also, gains were maintained at follow up, and this time the follow-up period was for 1 year.

There are plainly many questions left unanswered. What are the most effective and cost-effective components of the interventions? What are the effects upon other important aspects of a young child's life, such as the ability to cope with the environment of school and to initiate and maintain satisfying peer relationships? Can the benefits be obtained in ordinary clinical practice rather than the favored circumstances of a clinical trial? Research to answer these questions should be undertaken because of the real promise that current knowledge could deliver effective schemes of early detection and treatment.

22.7   Outstanding Problems

The argument of the chapter so far has been for a rather limited role of primary prevention, but a strong potential place for behavioral interventions, based at home, in the second to fourth year of life; and/or at both home and school to be timed soon after entry into the kind of schooling that requires attention and impulse control (typically, around age 7 in many school systems).

This leaves a number of objections unconsidered, and problems unresolved.

22.7.1   Is Prevention Needed at All?

A counter-argument would point out that many children with ADHD are already referred for treatment in primary or specialist health care. Why should this not just continue? It has the advantages that powerful therapies can be given because the young people already have evident impairment; and that one does not waste resources on treating at-risk children whose difficulties will settle down eventually in the natural course of events.

This is an important economic issue, and deserves a randomized trial of routine therapy against prevention (with routine therapy if still needed), using health economic measures as one of the outcomes.

The argument assumes that the right children are referred and treated. The issue of »who are the 'right' children to be referred?« is a deep one, but need not be considered deeply here. From the perspective of this chapter, the right children to be referred are those who: (a) will, if untreated, have an adverse outcome, and (b) will, if treated, benefit from treatment. By this definition, referral practices are imperfect. For example, girls are under-represented in the community by about 2: or 3:1; but in clinics by more than 8:1 (Heptinstall and Taylor 2002). Yet they seem to be no less at risk, and no less likely to respond to therapy. They are probably under-referred. As another example, Sayal et al. (2002) followed a group of children (found by screening to have high hyperactivity scores) through their contacts with a health system. Parents' perception that there was a problem was governed more by whether the family was suffering financial loss than by their ratings of symptoms. Physician's recognition that there was a problem was governed more by parental pressure for referral than by severity of symptoms.

Yet severity of symptoms will predict better both a poor, untreated outcome and a large change with medication.

The implication is that the cost-effectiveness of screening by symptoms, rather than awaiting referral because of adult distress, could be high.

22.7.2   Should Interventions Be Universal Rather Than in High-Risk Groups?

It is often difficult for universal interventions – i.e., those applied to all children of a certain age – to prove their effect. To take a crude example: – If the risk of ADHD is 5%, then an intervention producing a halving of that rate will have to be given to 40 unselected children if it is to prevent 1 case; but only to 4 children for the same effect if applied to a high-risk group in which half the children would develop ADHD. Therefore, a universal intervention must be 10 times cheaper to be able to compete with one given to a well-selected high-risk group.

Some universal programs could well be worth evaluating. Television courses to encourage understanding about how to react to hyperactive children have much intuitive appeal. As a speculation, effective attention training programs might become available on the Internet. But any of these would need a substantial research investment before they could be recommended.

The advantages of a high-risk approach include the possibility of enhancing the accessibility and appeal of a program to burdened and vulnerable families. They may find themselves stigmatized in community-based groups, or marginalized by lack of telephone or internet access. In one trial of behavior therapy for preventing behavior problems in children with severe learning disabilities, immigrant families from Africa were less likely than others to attend group sessions but equally likely to profit from individual therapy (Chadwick et al. 2001).

22.7.3   Could Interventions Do Harm?

The safety of medication for children less than 4 years old is – as considered above – unknown. This does not seem to have deterred many USA physicians from using it in this age group, but it would need much more understanding before it could be the basis of intervention. The monoamines that are influenced by the drugs determine the growth of the brain as well as synaptic transmission. Conceivably there is scope for long-term benefit by giving drugs at this time – but if so there is also scope for long-term harm. Much more information is needed, and a good start would simply be an adequately sized trial of stimulant against placebo in children under 4 who show established ADHD.

Less obviously, psychological interventions might do harm. On the face of it, parent training is a benign intervention; but it could have unexpected effects. Educators often dislike the idea of stigmatizing children with a label. On the whole, the evidence does not support this in any simple sense. Labeling is a powerful force both for good or ill: much depends on how it is done. We need trials of screening in which subjects are randomized to being informed of the results or not.

22.8 Conclusions

The treatment of established ADHD in schoolchildren is well developed – though more knowledge about factors mediating course would be helpful to guide a fuller understanding of how best to intervene for the longer term. The treatment of referred cases, and the education of referrers in recognition, can be important in tertiary prevention, to reduce the complications of ADHD.

The early detection of symptoms, and initiation of treatment before impairment has developed, has a strong rationale from developmental studies. Research is needed about the acceptability, cost, hazards, and effectiveness of early intervention. There is enough encouraging knowledge, for instance about the value of behavioral approaches in high-risk children before they enter school, to justify the research being supported.

The scope for primary prevention is at present limited because the etiology seems to involve a multiplicity of risks, each of small effect. Basic knowledge about causes, however, is advancing rapidly and the scope for useful applications of the knowledge should be kept under continuing review.

References

Abikoff H, Gittelman R (1985) Hyperactive children treated with stimulants. Is cognitive training a useful adjunct? Arch Gen Psychiatry 42:953–961.

Barkley RA (1990) Attention Deficit Hyperactivity Disorder: A Handbook for Diagnosis and Treatment. New York: Guilford.

Bell RQ, Weller GM, Waldrop MF (1971) Newborn and preschooler: organization of behavior and relations between periods. Monographs of the Society for Research in Child Development 36, 1–145.

Benasich AA, Bejar II (1992) The Fagan Test of Infant Intelligence: A Critical Review. Journal of Applied Developmental Psychology 13, 153–171.

Bor W, Sanders MS, Markie-Dadds C (2002) The effects of the Triple-P Positive Parenting Program on preschool children with co-occurring disruptive behavior and attentional/hyperactive difficulties. Journal of Abnormal Child Psychology, 30, 571–589.

Carter CM, Urbanowicz M, Hemsley R, Mantilla L, Strobel S, Graham PJ, Taylor E (1993) Effects of a few food diet in attention deficit disorder. Archives of Disease in Childhood 69, 564–568.

Chadwick O, Momcilovic N, Rossiter R, Stumbles E, Taylor E (2001) A randomized trial of brief individual versus group parent training for behavior problems in children with severe learning disabilities. Behavioral and Cognitive Psychotherapy 29, 151–167.

Committee on Toxicity (2000) Adverse Reactions to Food and Food ingredients. COT Secretariat, Food Standards Agency, London.

Fagan JF, Shepherd PA (1987) Fagan Test of Infant Intelligence: Training Manual. Cleveland, OH, Infantest Corporation.

Farrington DP, Loeber R, van Kammen WB (1990) Long-term criminal outcomes of hyperactivity-impulsivity-attention deficit and conduct problems in childhood. In: Straight and Devious Pathways from Childhood to Adulthood, Robins LN, Rutter M, eds. Cambridge: Cambridge University Press, pp 62–81.

Heptinstall E, Taylor E (2002) Sex differences and their significance. In Sandberg S (ed.): Hyperactivity and Attention Disorders of Childhood. Cambridge University Press.

Herbert M (2002) Behavioral Therapies; In Child and Adolescent Psychiatry: Fourth Edition, Rutter M, Taylor E eds. Oxford: Blackwell Science, p. 900.

Hinshaw SP (1994) Attention Deficits and Hyperactivity in Children. Vol. 29 Developmental Clinical Psychology and Psychiatry. London, Sage Publications Ltd.

Jadad AR, Booker L, Gauld M, Kakuma R, Boyle M, Cunningham CE, Kim M, Schachar R (1999) The treatment of attention-deficit hyperactivity disorder: an annotated bibliography and critical appraisal of published systematic reviews and metaanalyses. Can J Psychiatry 44, 1025–1035.

McCall RB, Carriger MS (1993) A meta-analysis of infant habituation and recognition memory performance as predictors of later IQ. Child Development 64, 57–79.

Meltzer H, Gatward R, Goodman R, Ford T (2000) Mental health of children and adolescents in Great Britain. London: The Stationery Office.

MTA Cooperative Group (1999) A 14-month randomized clinical trial of treatment strategies for attention-deficit/hyperactivity disorder. Multimodal Treatment Study of Children with ADHD. Arch Gen Psychiatry 56:1073–1086.

Offord D and Bennett KJ (2002) Prevention; In Child and Adolescent Psychiatry: Fourth Edition, Rutter M, Taylor E eds. Oxford: Blackwell Science, p. 881.

Rubia K, Taylor E, Smith AB, Oksanen H, Overmeyer S, Newman S, Oksannen H (2001) Neuropsychological analyses of impulsiveness in childhood hyperactivity. Br J Psychiatry 179, 138–143.

Ruff HA, Lawson KR (1990a) Development of sustained, focused attention in young children during free play. Developmental Psychology 26, 85–93.

Ruff HA, Lawson KR, Parrinello R, Weissberg R (1990b) Long-term stability of individual differences in sustained attention in the early years. Child Development 61, 60–75.

Santosh PJ, Taylor E (2000) Stimulant drugs. Eur Child Adolesc Psychiatry 9 Suppl 1, I27–143.

Sayal K, Taylor E, Beecham J, Byrne P (2002) Pathways to care in children at risk of attention-deficit hyperactivity disorder. Br J Psychiatry 181, 43–48.

Schachar R, Tannock R (2002) Syndromes of Hyperactivity and Attention Deficit In Child and Adolescent Psychiatry: Fourth Edition, Rutter M, Taylor E eds. Oxford: Blackwell Science, pp 399–418

Sonuga-Barke EJ, Daley D, Thompson M, Laver-Bradbury C, Weeks A (2001) Parent-based therapies for preschool attention-deficit/hyperactivity disorder: a randomized, controlled trial with a community sample. J Am Acad Child Adolesc Psychiatry 40, 402–408.

Swanson JM, Sergeant J, Taylor E, Sonuga-Barke E, Jensen PS, Cantwell D (1998) The Lancet 351, 429–433

Taylor E (1995) Dysfunctions of attention. In Developmental Psychopathology, Vol. 2: Risk, Disorder, and Adaptation (eds. D. Cicchetti and D.J. Cohen). John Wiley and Sons, Inc., New York, 243–273.

Taylor E, Sandberg S, Thorley G, Giles S (1991) The Epidemiology of Childhood Hyperactivity, Maudsley Monographs No. 33. Oxford: Oxford University Press

Taylor E, Chadwick O, Heptinstall E, Danckaerts M (1996) Hyperactivity and conduct problems as risk factors for adolescent development. J Am Acad Child Adolesc Psychiatry 35, 1213–1226.

Thapar A (1995) Childhood hyperactivity scores are highly heritable and show sibling competition effects: Twin study evidence. Behavior Genetics 25, 537–543.

Warner-Rogers J, Taylor A, Taylor E, Sandberg S (2000) Inattentive Behavior in Childhood: Epidemiology and Implications for Development. Journal of Learning Disabilities 33, 520–536.

Wright JC, Vlietstra AG (1975) The development of selective attention: From perceptual exploration to logical search. In Reese HW (ed.) Advances in Child Development and Behavior, Vol. I0. New York, Academic Press.

Prevention and Intervention in Primary Care

Kelly Kelleher

23.1   Introduction   – 313

23.2   Defining Primary Care   – 314

23.3   Burden of Emotional and Behavioral Disorders in Primary Care   – 314

23.4   Assessment and Evaluation of Emotional and Behavioral Disorders in Primary Care   – 316

23.5   Treatment and Interventions for Emotional and Behavioral Disorders in Primary Care   – 317

23.6   Improving the Quality of Primary Care Mental Health Services   – 318

23.6.1   Enhancing Identification, Diagnosis and Evaluation   – 318

23.6.2   Improving Management   – 320

23.7   Conclusions   – 322

References   – 322

23.1 Introduction

International appreciation of the tremendous burden placed on individuals, families, and societies as a result of mental disorders increased greatly in the last decade. This appreciation extends to the heavy burden that pediatric emotional disorders comprise as well. Unfortunately, specialty mental health services will never be adequate to address the pandemic of pediatric mental disorders even in countries with the greatest healthcare resources. This is in large part because of the global shortage of pediatric mental health clinicians (Mechanic 1996; Deva 1981). In addition, many if not most cultures do not have a history of using specialty mental health services. Such services may be associated with negative stereotypes and stigma. In addition, mental health care may be paid almost completely out of pocket (Maingay 2002).

In response, many countries focused their mental health delivery prevention and intervention efforts on primary care settings (Murthy 1998). Eighty-nine percent of the world's countries provide mental health services in primary care settings and more than half train primary care workers in mental health evaluation and treatment (Jenkins 2002). This is especially important for children and adolescents since youths are even less likely than adults to receive specialty services. In this Chapter, we (a) define primary care, (b) present information on the burden of pediatric emotional and behavioral disorders in primary care settings for children and adolescents, (c) consider current evaluation and diagnostic practices in primary care settings for children and adolescents, (d) report on existing treatments and interventions, and (e) discuss changes in assessment, treatment, and delivery systems likely to improve outcomes of children with emotional and behavioral disorders and their families in primary care settings.

Because of space limitations, we aim to demonstrate the range of issues rather than provide a comprehensive review of this broad topic. In addition, we do not address the complex issues of primary care medical services for severely mentally ill youth, the unique issues of alcohol and drug services to youth in primary care settings, the large volume of mental health services delivered in emergency rooms or other acute medical settings that do not make up the primary care system, nor the special issues of youth with developmental and cognitive disabilities. Instead, we focus on the delivery of mental health services to school-age children suffering from emotional and behavioral disorders and their families in primary care settings that are the points of access to the health system for young children and adolescents. Complicating this discussion further are the many terms used to refer to pediatric conditions of emotions and behaviors in the primary care research literature. These terms include psychosocial problems, mental disorders, psychiatric disorders, and emotional and behavioral disorders among others. We resort to the last for consistency in this manuscript.

23.2 Defining Primary Care

Primary care settings are those locations, institutions, and providers offering first contact care for personal health services that are community-based, comprehensive, and longitudinal (Donaldson 1996). They are distinguished from specialty providers in the comprehensiveness of the services offered and from urgent care or emergency services by the longitudinal and coordinated nature of services that they provide (Rowan 2002). Primary care clinicians have established relationships with the communities they serve.

Greater density and availability of primary care services are associated with improved health care access, decreased hospital use for certain conditions, better population health indicators and longevity (Macinko 2003). Countries with higher investment in primary care services as compared to specialty services have lower morbidity and mortality than countries with higher proportionate levels of investment in specialty care services (Starfield 2002). Primary care services are more patient and family-focused than corresponding specialty services and provide greater efficiency for most conditions than similar patients treated in specialty settings (Shi 1999; Starfield 2002). In short, primary care services are known to have a salutary effect on population health status and are efficient.

Because primary care services are in part a reflection of their community, they are extremely diverse. In some countries, primary care health services employ comprehensive health records, are linked to public health systems, use standardized instruments, and conduct longitudinal research (Holm 1999; Galan 1995). At the other extreme, primary care services may be staffed by poorly trained village health workers with inadequate supplies and resources (Abas 2003; Abiodun 1990). These disparate situations are linked by being the initial point of contact and the place of medical care coordination for their respective populations. Between these two extremes are an almost infinite variation in levels of resource investment, linkage between public health systems and primary care, and primary care coordination across sites. The variation in availability of specialty mental health services, training in

emotional and behavioral disorders, and demand for such services is tremendous from place to place.

Because of the integration of primary care clinicians within their community, they are ideally positioned to address chronic conditions like emotional and behavioral disorders in childhood and adolescence both because of their knowledge of the family and patient as well as their access to health and human services in the community (The National Academies Press 1996). In addition, primary care clinicians and services are likely to be less stigmatizing than visits to mental health centers and oft-times primary care clinicians are considered an integral part of the community. In surveys of patients, many prefer to be seen in primary care sites for pediatric emotional and behavioral disorders as compared to mental health specialty clinics (Flisher 1997; Roeloffs 2003).

For disenfranchised patients unlikely to use specialty patient services, they are a particularly important source of services. For example, several authors in the USA and Europe note that minority and immigrant children are more likely to use primary care services for emotional and behavioral disorders than specialty mental health services when compared to majority populations (Cooper-Patrick 1999). This accessibility and preference, especially among the disenfranchised has encouraged the development of mental health services within primary care settings in many parts of the world.

23.3 Burden of Emotional and Behavioral Disorders in Primary Care

Emotional and behavioral disorders impose an enormous burden not only on affected children and their families but also on the general health care system because they are common, disabling, and associated with increased health care utilization. Emotional and behavioral disorders are the most common chronic illnesses confronting primary care clinicians in general medical settings for children and adolescents in developed countries and among the most common in developing countries. Estimates of frank mental disorders in medical settings consistently range from 15% to 30% in pediatric samples from the USA, UK, and western European countries with high levels of persistence over time (Briggs-Gowan 2003). Some of this variability is due to the diversity of methods employed in assessment ranging from behavioral checklists to diagnostic interviews. In addition, these estimates include various levels of impairment. However, this consistent range spans studies and continents. In almost all sites, rates of behavioral and emotional disorders are especially high in youth with chronic illness of various types. Children and adolescents with chronic medical and surgical conditions are one and a half to two times as likely to have emotional and behavioral disorders when compared to those without any chronic medical problems (Mathet 2003; Ortega 2002; Vila 1999; Cadman 1987). Moreover, the risk is multiplicative among those with several medical problems.

Information from developing countries is less clear with very few studies conducted among children and adolescents. However, adult epidemiology studies in primary care studies suggest near universal rates of mental health problems in primary care attenders. For example, 46% of patients presenting to primary care settings in urban India and 33% of primary care presenters in South India screen positive for mental disorders (Patel 1998). Similarly, 46% of primary care patients in Taiwan screened positive for mental disorders with 38% meeting criteria after further review (Liu 2002). In Zimbabwe, 16% of patients originally screened negative were positive for mental disorders after 12 months (Todd 1999). These numbers are almost identical to, or higher than, studies of primary care mental disorder prevalence rates in the USA and Canada (Katz 1995). There is no reason to suspect that children would be much different. In each case, extreme deprivation and poverty are associated with common mental disorders (Patel 1998).

The prevalence of specific emotional and behavioral disorders in primary care is thought to be reflective of their prevalence in community settings. There are some investigators who have employed diagnostic instruments in primary care settings to examine this question. Disorder prevalence estimates are largely dependent on age, gender, and respondent (Wasserman 1999). There is considerable psychiatric comorbidity among children with emotional and behavioral disorders. For example, almost 50% of pediatric patients with Attention Deficit Hyperactivity Disorder (ADHD) present with significant symptoms of internalizing disorders. Similarly, approximately 40% of youth with affective or anxiety conditions present with significant symptoms of externalizing disorders (Wren 2003). These conditions cause significant impairment, and many of those with symptoms not meeting disorder criteria suffer sufficiently to impair their school or family functioning (Angold 1999).

In addition to being common, emotional and behavioral problems may be increasing or at least recognized more often. Higher rates of detection of primary care mental disorders have been noted in the USA (Kelleher 2000). Rates of psychosocial diagnoses among children in primary care settings doubled in the past 20 years (Kelleher 2000). Almost every category of problem increased, with the greatest proportional change in emotional disorders like depression and anxiety problems and the greatest absolute change in attentional and hyperactivity problems. The only condition not to see an increase in this time was mental retardation.

The various emotional and behavioral disorders among children and adolescents are associated with greater use of the healthcare system and especially primary care services (Miranda 1994). Use of primary care is increased among those with emotional and behavioral disorders but affected youth also have higher use of diagnostic services, medications, and treatments of all types. For example, youth with ADHD have higher costs for nonmental health services than youth without ADHD along with much greater use of mental health specialty services (Kelleher 2001). When present with other chronic illnesses, emotional and behavioral disorders are associated with medical costs higher than those with chronic illness alone (Lin 2000). While the association of increased use of healthcare with emotional and behavioral disorders is unmistakable, the mechanism or mechanisms that induce increased healthcare demand among youth with emotional and behavioral disorders are unknown. Recently, it has become clear that emotional and behavioral disorders among youth also increase health care use of other family members as well (Lave 2002).

Emotional and behavioral disorders are also associated with increased visits for unexplained symptoms or »functional complaints« as some have labeled them (Campo 2002). These visits result in low yield medical testing and assessment while increasing the frustration and concerns of health care workers. Fritz and colleagues (1986–1987) noted that primary care clinicians caring for children in the USA found emotional and behavioral disorders to be the most frustrating and challenging of commonly treated conditions they dealt with on a routine basis. Staff time and energy were disproportionately devoted to dealing with parents and affected families, and clinicians perceived few options for effectively treating pediatric emotional and behavioral disorders.

23.4 Assessment and Evaluation of Emotional and Behavioral Disorders in Primary Care

Current primary care assessment practices are little understood although a fair amount is known about their effectiveness, at least in the USA. Primary care clinicians report rarely using routine screening instruments or specific diagnostic criterion in their assessment of children (Gardner 2003). When evaluating children for emotional or behavioral disorders, they do not routinely use information from schools or outside settings and are quite variable in their approach to interviewing both parent and child in making assessments. The wide variability in assessment and diagnostic practices is independent of clinician factors like age, gender, and physician attitudes towards mental health treatment.

In spite of this unstandardized approach, primary care clinicians report increasing number of visits due to emotional and behavioral disorders for children (Kelleher 2000). Although only 3% of children and adolescents present in primary care settings with complaints about emotional or behavioral disorders, many others are symptomatic, and rates of mental health reasons for visits, diagnoses and prescriptions for emotional and behavioral disorders are increasing across the USA and Europe (Garralda 2001). Psychotropic drug prescriptions are proffered to 3.9 per 100 children in the USA (Olfson 2002). This is up from 1.4 per 100 or 1.5% of all visits only 10 years ago (Kelleher 1989). When asked specifically about the presence of behavioral and emotional symptoms and impairment sufficient to warrant medical attention, primary care clinicians identify a growing number of visits with emotional and behavioral disorders. In 1979, such visits accounted for less than 9% of pediatric visits in a sample of 30,000 primary care visits (Kelleher 1989). By 1996, more than 18% of all visits involved a significant emotional and behavioral problem requiring intervention or monitoring (Goldberg 1984). Others note similar numbers in the UK but suggest that when considering the overlay of psychosocial issues on treatment for chronic illness and the importance of visits involving maternal depression or other family psychopathology, up to 65% of all visits to general health care settings are related to psychosocial issues (Rushton 2002; Bailey 1978).

Some emotional and behavioral disorders are more often detected by primary care clinicians than others. In total, primary care clinicians identify between 50% and 65% of parent-reported significant emotional and behavioral symptoms noted on behavioral checklists or diagnostic instruments (Kelleher 1997). Most commonly identified are externalizing problems such as conduct disorders and oppositional-defiant disorder. Less often identified are those with internalizing disorder such as depression or anxiety. Certain youth are also less likely to be identified after controlling for the level of parent-reported symptoms. In particular, girls and younger children with significant levels of emotional and behavioral symptoms are less frequently recognized by primary care clinicians than boys and older children respectively. Minority youth are also less likely to be recognized by primary care clinicians after controlling for parent education and levels of symptoms (Kelleher 1999). For all children and adolescents, more severe cases are likely to be identified.

The growing appreciation for the pandemic of child and adolescent psychosocial problems in primary care settings has led to calls for routine screening of all children in medical clinics (Mathet 2003; Jellinek 1999). These calls note the availability of low-cost, paper and pencil screening tests along with the high prevalence rates of emotional and behavioral disorders. Some of these screening instruments have been translated into several languages, and some are available in the public domain.

Unfortunately, screening instruments are costly to print, store, administer, score, and transcribe. Valenstein (2001) notes that staff costs for depression screening alone in the USA would exceed US$ 6 per visit because of the time involved in administration, scoring, and transcribing, although these costs would obviously be lower where labor is cheaper. Moreover, simple screening instruments could overwhelm already stressed mental health services with real cases and many false positives. In addition, the extremely limited access to specialty mental health services referrals from primary care services makes the identification of mental disorders in primary care problematic (Walders 2003). It is unclear what the appropriate strategies might be given the high cost of screening for mental health problems in such settings and the lack of available treatment services. Nevertheless, as screening instruments get better and effective treatment strategies emerge, institutions with sufficient resources will be called upon to conduct routine assessments.

In general, screening instruments to identify new cases fall into those that are general behavioral checklists [e.g., the Child Behavior Checklist (CBCL; http://www.aseba.org) or the Pediatric Symptom

Checklist (http://psc.partners.org)], or condition specific instruments [e.g., the Child Depression Inventory (http://assessments-stage.ncspearson.com/assessments/tests/cdi), or the Connors Scale for ADHD (http://www.ncbi.nlm.nih.gov)]. The CBCL is one of the most widely used psychopathology instrument in the world and has norms for diverse groups. However, at 128 items it is extremely long for primary care settings, requires computer scoring capacity and can be expensive. Shorter instruments like the Pediatric Symptom Checklist have been better received and are now used in some large prepaid health systems in the USA and some individual practices. Condition-specific instruments like the Conners Scale are not used for screening but may be used for confirming symptoms or monitoring treatment in some primary care settings.

Regardless of which of these might be used, further evaluation is essential to adequately diagnose child psychopathology in primary care settings. Pediatricians and family practitioners employ some measures to validate diagnoses like ADHD, but in general, report that they do not use standardized instruments nor do they use diagnostic standards like the International Classification of Diseases of the World Health Organization or the Diagnostic and Statistical Manual of the American Psychiatric Association (Gardner 2003). They instead rely on their interview with parents and observations of the child and adolescents in the clinic. Similarly, early evidence from the Multimodal Treatment of ADHD study (Arnold 2003; The MTA Cooperative Group 1999) suggests that ongoing assessment and monitoring of cases in any standardized way is infrequent in routine care. They noted that the community comparison group received fewer monitoring visits and few titration trials or increases in doses, in spite of recommendations. This led to lower overall dosages for the community comparison group in their study. It appears that whenever primary care practice has been examined, it does not often involve routine use of standardized instruments, information from multiple sources like schools, or regular monitoring over time.

23.5 Treatment and Interventions for Emotional and Behavioral Disorders in Primary Care

The management of pediatric mental disorders in primary care settings is a complex process. Primary care patients present earlier than those in specialty settings, frequently have undifferentiated symptoms, often have greater medical comorbidity, and have long-standing relationships with their primary care clinicians that may impair discussion of sensitive issues (Gabbay 2003). Thus, the care of patients in primary care settings may unfold slowly over several visits with monitoring or watchful waiting as an integral component of both diagnosis and intervention.

Although complex and sometimes distributed over several visits, a great deal is known about usual care for pediatric mental disorders in primary care settings. This information is often divided into data on psychotropic drug prescribing practices, counseling and referral, although several of these can and do occur simultaneously on some visits. In developed countries generally and the USA in particular, the prescription of psychotropic drugs from primary care has revolutionized the management of common mental disorders. In the USA, the number of persons receiving care for major depressive disorder has doubled in the past quarter of a century and almost all of this increase is a result of pharmacotherapy by primary care clinicians (Olfson 2002). Similar trends are observed with children where diagnosis rates are skyrocketing in primary care and psychotropic medications the most common treatment for these cases (Schirm 2001, Zito 2003, 2002). Moreover, such increases are not only occurring with stimulants for ADHD, the most common prescriptions from pediatric primary care, but also for psychotropic drugs for affective disorders (Zito 2002). Antidepressants are now the second most costly class of pediatric psychotropic drugs in the USA and the most rapidly increasing. The use of these prescriptions has spread from adolescents into early childhood, too (Zito 2002).

Numerous factors affect the likelihood of psychotropic drug prescription in primary care. These include the severity of parent-reported symptoms, how well known the child is to the clinician and whether or not the family agrees with the clinician assessment of the problem (Gabbay 2003). In addition, clinicians are more likely to prescribe drugs for children and adolescents presenting with recurrent symptoms.

In general, primary care clinicians underdose their patients on psychotropic medications (Banazak 1998; Hirschfeld 1997). They also probably treat for insufficient duration. It is likely that such practices decrease the effectiveness of their efforts, at least for conditions like ADHD.

Counseling, support groups, or psychotherapy are also often times provided in primary care settings. Garralda and colleagues note that there is little evidence of effectiveness for such activities (Garralda 2001). Nevertheless, counseling was the most commonly employed strategy among newly recognized behavioral problems in a large national sample of USA patients (Gardner 2000). This counseling with families most often included reassurance, behavioral modification, and supportive listening according to clinicians. Counseling has long been the initial mode of treatment for primary care clinicians confronting pediatric emotional and behavioral disorders (Goldberg 1979). However, some evidence suggests that as medications for these problems increase, office-based counseling is declining (Hoagwood and Kelleher 2000). Similar declines are present in the number of specifically prescribed follow-up visits for youth with ADHD (Hoagwood and Kelleher 2000).

23.6 Improving the Quality of Primary Care Mental Health Services

Recommendations and tools for improving primary care mental health services are almost as old as the appreciation for the burden of pediatric mental disorders in primary care settings. Beginning in 1979 at a World Health Organization conference in Bellagio, investigators and leaders called for new assessment options and nomenclature for improving primary care practice around affected youth and their families (Regier 1982). Until recently, these recommendations have generally been called around specific solutions to improving assessment or treatment or monitoring. Moreover, prevention has generally been ignored in these entreaties.

In considering options for improving care, it is important that the barriers to better primary care mental health service delivery be examined. First and most importantly, the availability of specialty care backup or referral services is essential to provide care for those with comorbidity, severe disease or mitigating social circumstances. For the foreseeable future, this particular problem is unlikely to go away. Declining revenue streams in social service budgets, the lack of adequately trained personnel, and limited expertise in child development and psychopathology suggest that few options will alter the landscape regarding availability of pediatric mental health specialists. Another barrier suggested by numerous authors is the limited training and expertise of primary care clinicians themselves. This training is not only limited in regards to treatment of child and adolescent emotional and behavioral disorders, but also related to patient-clinician communication and ongoing management of chronic illnesses. Of course, this training can only accomplish much if primary care clinicians are committed to improving their care in this area. In the USA, a national survey of pediatricians suggests that they do indeed feel responsible for improving diagnosis and assessment but that most do not feel it is their responsibility to treat conditions like child or adolescent depression (Olson 2001).

While primary care training is likely to be important, several authors note the many other practice issues that are likely to be even more intractable barriers. These include competing time demands on clinicians and staff that place chronic illness issues or time-intensive problems like pediatric emotional and behavioral disorders at the back of the line with regards to reimbursement, practice management, and patient satisfaction. In addition, when psychiatric issues are raised and few resources in the community are available, primary care clinicians will be unlikely to seek out such cases. Purchasers of health and mental health services, at least in the USA and the UK, know little about mental health services, their quality or their provision in primary care, thus creating little demand for improvement efforts (Vanstraelen 1994; Schoenbaum 2004).

23.6.1 Enhancing Identification, Diagnosis and Evaluation

Much of the work around improving primary care mental health services for children and adolescents to date focuses on the process whereby clinicians recognize, diagnose and evaluate children, adolescents, and their families in the primary care setting. While some debate over which children and adolescents with emotional and behavioral disorders should be treated in primary care settings, there is wide consensus that initial identification is a critical role for primary care clinicians. This work includes efforts to increase the relevance of diagnostic systems for the primary care setting, enhancement of measures and their administration, training of clinicians, and attention to communication between primary care clinicians and their patients.

As mentioned previously, the problems of employing psychiatric diagnostic nomenclature in primary care patients were recognized early by the field. Primary care patients present with less differentiated symptoms, greater medical comorbidity and, sometimes, a resistance to a psychiatric diagnosis. The initial response of an international panel of experts was to develop a primary care classification system for persons with mental disorders, including a section specific to children and adolescents (Regier 1982). Later, some of these concepts were incorporated into the International Classification for Primary Care (ICPC), a comprehensive diagnostic nomenclature designed to be more relevant than ICD for primary care (http://www.globalfamilydoctor.com). Since that time, the American Academy of Pediatrics in association with USA psychiatric organizations published the pediatric Diagnostic and Statistical Manual – Primary Care Edition (AAP 1998). This taxonomy developed by psychologists, pediatricians, and psychiatrists considers the range of developmental issues, mental health, and functioning as they present in primary care. In addition, the continuum of normal development is emphasized. While hailed as more useful by primary care clinicians, there is no evidence that any of these systems are used routinely in primary care settings (Kelleher and Wolraich 2001).

The greatest investments in improving primary care practice to date have come by way of attempts to change assessment practices. The majority of these efforts focused on the development or deployment of screening tools. Psychopathology assessment tools for children and adolescents are reviewed extensively elsewhere, but some instruments designed or used extensively in primary care probably merit some discussion. The first instrument designed specifically for the assessment of emotional and behavioral disorders in children and adolescents seen in primary care settings is the Pediatric Symptom Checklist (PSC). Originally a 35-item, forced-choice list of behaviors for parent or caregiver respondents, recent psychometric work identified 17 core items that provide core information for screening (Gardner 1999). The developer and colleagues have extensive experience implementing a paper and pencil version in diverse pediatric settings, including in large health care plans.

Besides parent- or caregiver-completed paper and pencil surveys, clinician-completed interview tools have also been developed for primary care to standardize the psychiatric assessment. These tools are combinations of structured diagnostic questions posed in algorithms for rapid identification of disorders. An example is the Physician Diagnostic Questionnaire by Spitzer (Spitzer 2000). While used in research studies, no information on their use in routine practice exists.

Even more innovative are attempts to employ information technology to enhance recognition and diagnosis. The delivery of computerized psychopathology assessment tools is not new, but consideration of their use in primary care systems is. Suggestions for use include delivery of computerized screeners for primary care assessment (Farvolden 2003) to administration of diagnostic instruments in waiting rooms and schools (DISC 2003). Computerized administration has several advantages. They include portability in diverse settings, numerous options for reporting, and flexibility in administering specific components. In addition, it appears that patients are more likely to report socially undesirable behaviors or attributes on computer-administered tools compared to paper and pencil or interviewer-administered tools.

As computerized administration becomes more feasible, the use of computerized adaptive testing (CAT) will be particularly important for primary care. Using item response theory to identify the highest yield questions, CAT tailors each test to an individual in real time by selecting questions from a bank of relevant items (Gardner 2002). Simulation work with pediatric assessment tools suggests that considerable efficiencies can be gained. Because so many different domains are important for assessment in primary care, CAT will become the standard over time in countries that have access to digital data collection. As adaptive testing becomes more established in the medical field, computerized administration becomes even more flexible.

Initial evaluations of routine screening in primary care settings found results similar to adult trials; that is, screening and providing results of screening to primary care clinicians rarely resulted in improved patient outcomes (Hankin 1978). However, new results suggest that when linked with more effective treatment services, routine screening can improve child and adolescent mental health functioning. These findings will need to be replicated.

Standardized diagnostic assessments in primary care settings and ongoing monitoring with well-validated instruments will be challenging for all but the most sophisticated practices. The increasing use of electronic records and assessment tools will gradually allow their use to become more common. Electronic communications will also allow incorporation of teacher assessments into primary care practice and decision-making about treatment and management of emotional and behavioral disorders in primary care, a practice that is rare today, at least in the USA (Gardner 2003).

Clinician training around identification of behavioral and emotional disorders is often advocated as a way to increase recognition and assessment. The evidence around its effectiveness is mixed. Sharp and colleagues reported on interview and assessment training for pediatric residents (Sharp 1992). They noted that clinicians could be trained to increase their questioning around psychosocial issues and be more open-ended in their inquiries. However, when parents and caregivers reported their concerns, clinicians did not respond favorably or frequently ignored the information. Gardner (2002) did not detect differences in treatment practices by primary care clinicians with more training in child psychiatry, but Horwitz (2002) suggest that training does influence recognition and referral. Some studies document increased recognition over time, but it is not clear if this is related to increased training for primary care clinicians (Kelleher 2000).

Finally, patient-doctor communication or parent-clinician communication is another area of focus for improvement in mental health services in primary care. Early observational studies noted higher recognition rates of emotional and behavioral disorders when certain communication styles were employed by primary care clinicians. Attempts to train patients and families to be more assertive and interactive in primary care visits were focused on adult patients and results were mixed. Some patients seemed to achieve improved clinician-patient communication after training while others did not benefit. In part, these differences may be due to patient and family attitudes and beliefs around illness. Patient and family conceptualizations about the causes and origins of illness are highly related to the types of care they seek and use of treatment services (Brown 2001). Future assessments may also need to take into account patient and family beliefs and willingness to engage in various treatment modalities.

In sum, efforts to improve recognition, diagnosis, and evaluation in primary care largely involve attempts to increase the use of standardized instruments. While useful for research studies, it is not clear that such tools are practical in routine practice without computerized administration. The value of training clinicians and patients to enhance communication is also of uncertain benefit.

23.6.2   Improving Management

Innovations to improve treatment generally focus on specific interventions. Probably the most common internationally is the colocation of mental health specialists in the primary care setting. Colocation of mental health specialty workers for pediatric care is dependent on several factors. First, specialty workers must be available. Space and support are also essential. Also, the need to determine a clear subset of patients for the specialists, the stage of illness at which the specialists will be called upon, and to what extent they will manage and monitor specific interventions all require careful consideration (Bower 2002). In short-term studies, the use of mental health workers in primary care settings increased screening and detection, demonstrated improvements over time, and changed primary care clinician prescribing strategies (Chisholm 2000; Bower 2000). To date, no studies document persistence of such effects (Bower 2002).

Besides colocation, enhanced treatment and intervention training for primary care clinicians is often recommended to improve care for pediatric emotional and behavioral disorders in general health care settings. These recommendations range from broad communication skills training to improve patient interviewing and detection all the way to specific psychotherapy skills. Interventions around communication training suggest that residents and physicians so trained are more likely to detect and elicit family violence and emotional and behavioral symptoms in primary care settings. It is not clear whether such training leads to improved patient or family outcomes.

The literature on training of primary care clinicians around mental health interventions is muddied by the quality, intensity, and type of training proposed. National public relations awareness programs like the Defeat Depression Campaign (Rix 1999) do not appear to have changed practice. More focused interventions such as depression recognition and management training (Gask 1998) or brief family therapy (Real Perez 1996) provide more confidence and skills to the clinicians and improve care for a small set of patients attending these clinicians. However, studies like these usually employ volunteer clinicians interested in the specific topic and intervention. A more broadly designed and stepped intervention like the Positive Parenting Program (Triple P) addresses a wider range of children with emotional and behavioral disorders, provides primary care clinicians with a greater set of skills and intensities of interventions, and addresses prevention issues which are a particularly important aspect of primary care (Sanders 1999). Such flexibility and range should make this program particularly appealing. Early evaluation results report improvements in knowledge, skills, and practice patterns (Sanders 2003).

Besides training clinicians, several attempts to engage patients and their families in or from primary care settings have been considered. In one relatively simple but sophisticated study, Sanders and team examine the impact of a specially prepared, therapeutic television series on families of children with disruptive behaviors. Compared to a wait-list control group, intervention families demonstrated improvements in perceived parental competence and child symptoms that was maintained at 6 months (Sanders 2002).

The use of parent support and psychoeducation groups has also been advocated as a way to engage patients through primary care offices. Adolescents with ADHD and their parents reported such groups to be helpful (McLeary 1998) but no evidence on their effectiveness in primary care settings exist. Similarly, others report on the use of interactive booklets and videotapes distributed from the primary care setting for adults with depression. Patients almost uniformly find such tools useful and suggest they lead to better adherence, but the materials have not been evaluated independently of the larger intervention within which they were embedded (Robinson 1997). It is possible that self-directed or group support programs with behavioral materials may be especially efficient in remote or rural areas where specialty support is lacking, particularly for youth with behavioral disorders (Connell 1997). Among adults, self help materials and family interventions do as well as specialty care, although the implications for pediatric disorders is not clear (Durand 2003).

Because primary care patients with emotional and behavioral disorders frequently drop out of treatment, do not receive adequate follow-up, and struggle with adherence to psychotropic drugs, telephone disease management protocols have been adopted from other disciplines to engage families and patients in aftercare. Although yet to be tested among pediatric patients, three trials in diverse settings all show promising short term results with low-cost telephone follow-up to patients with primary-care-treated depression (Simon 2000; Datto 2003). Patients and families report positive experiences with such supportive aftercare; symptoms were reduced and adherence to treatment regimens increased for intervention groups as compared to controls.

The growing recognition of the chronic and relapsing nature of many emotional and behavioral disorders of children and adolescents forced many to consider the important new chronic care models being discussed in other areas of medicine. Primary care services developed out of an acute care or infectious disease model in many countries. Such services were initiated by patients or their families, were problem based and physician focused. Patients or their proxies sought help for particular complaints in an office setting designed to enhance clinician efficiency. Such a system is an efficient use of resources for the management of acute complaints like exanthems or common infections.

On the other hand, patients with chronic disorders need to prevent relapse and exacerbations, enhance functioning and rehabilitation, and adhere to long term treatment plans (Rothman 2003). Waiting for acute exacerbations to receive care produces worsening of outcomes. Therefore, the ideal chronic care services would engage affected individuals to encourage self care, provide clinicians with up-to-date best practices, track preventive and rehabilitative care over time, and reach out to persons with worsening of symptoms. In theory, chronic care services are patient-focused, community-based, and targeted to treat disease, prevent relapse and improve functioning. Many examples exist in the medical world. These include innovative tuberculosis treatment services with registries, home visitation programs, rehabilitation services and medication monitoring. Similarly, effective diabetes programs in some communities have involved registries, community education, patient motivation, clinician decision support, and routine monitoring (Lim 2002; Berg 2002).

The core elements of chronic care management and prevention are described by several investigators. Central to all these descriptions is the interrelated nature of the various elements since no one of them seems to be sufficient. The core components appear to be (a) specific interventions to engage patients and families in self care, (b) timely assessment and treatment tools and decision support for primary care clinicians in the care of chronic illness, (c) registries and tracking tools to monitor care and adherence over time, (d) information systems to monitor health of the target population and care processes, and (e) organization and financing to support the infrastructure.

Many proposed interventions for improving primary care preventive and treatment services for youth with emotional and behavioral disorders can be considered part of this framework. In fact, evidence-based reviews (Gilbody 2003; Bower 2002) suggest that for both adult depression interventions in primary care and child emotional and behavioral disorders in primary care multifaceted interventions focused on improving practice will be necessary to substantially change outcomes for affected patients and their families. Clinical guidelines and traditional medical education activities are likely to be ineffective, but combinations of patient materials and telephone support combined with standardized assessment tools and training of clinicians have real potential for improving practice.

23.7   Conclusions

The international community is focusing its treatment strategies for mental disorders on primary care settings as the natural point of access to care for most communities. While the evidence for the care of children and adolescents with emotional and behavioral disorders is sparse, two things are apparent. First, emotional and behavioral disorders of youth are common and disabling in primary care settings. Secondly, an examination of current practices suggests many problems with identification, evaluation, and treatment provided in primary care settings. Moreover, the work on prevention in primary care settings is almost nonexistent.

In response, new methods of assessment and intervention have been proposed. In early studies, several of these appear to hold promise but almost none have been subjected to multisite or cost-effectiveness trials. Some require sophisticated technology that is increasingly available, but others are adaptable for almost any setting. The lessons from the adult primary care literature suggests that multifaceted interventions directed at changing patient,

primary care clinician, and system barriers simultaneously may be the most advantageous, especially in light of the growing recognition of the chronic nature of these disorders.

References

Abas M, Baingana F, Broadhead J, Iacoponi E, Vanderpyl J. Common mental disorders and primary health care: current practice in low-income countries. Harv Rev Psychiatry 2003 May-Jun;11(3):166–173.

Abiodun OA. Mental health and primary care in Africa. East Afr Med J. 1990 Apr;67(4):273–278.

Achenbach System of Empirically Based Assessment (ASEBA). http://www.aseba.org/aboutus/origins.html 12/1/03

Angold A, Costello EJ, Farmer EM, Burns BJ, Erkanli A. Impaired but undiagnosed. J Am Acad Child Adolesc Psychiatry 1999 Feb;38(2):129–137.

Arnold LE, Elliot M, Sachs L, Bird H, Kraemer HC, Wells KC, Abikoff HB, Comarda A, Conners CK, Elliott GR, Greenhill LL, Hechtman L, Hindshaw SP, Hoza B, Jensen PS, March JS, Newcorn JH, Pelham WE, Severe JB, Swanson JM, Vitiello B, Wigal T. Effects of ethnicity on treatment attendance, stimulant response/dose, and 14-month outcome in ADHD. J Consult Clin Psychol 2003 Aug;71(4):713–727.

Bailey V, Graham P, Boniface D (1978) How much child psychiatry does a general practitioner do? Journal of the Royal College of General Practitioners, 28, 621–626.

Banazak DA, Wills C, Collins C. Late-life depression in primary care: where do we go from here? J Am Osteopath Assoc. 1998 Sep;98(9):489–497.

Berg GD, S Wadhwa (2002) »Diabetes disease management in a community-based setting.« Manag Care 11(6): 42, 45–50.

Bower P. Primary Care mental health workers: models of working and evidence of effectiveness. Br J Gen Pract 2002 Nov; 52(484):926–933.

Bower P, Sibbald B. On-site mental health workers in primary care: effects on professional practice. Cochrane Database Syst Rev. 2000;(3):CD000532.

Bower P, Garralda E, Kramer T, Harrington R, Sibbald B. The treatment of child and adolescent mental health problems in primary care: a systematic review. Fam Pract 2001 Aug;18(4):373–382.

Briggs-Gowan MJ, Horwitz SM, Schwab-Stone ME, Leventhal JM, Leaf PJ. Mental health in pediatric settings: distribution of disorders and factors related to service use. J Am Acad Child Adolesc Psychiatry 2000 Jul;39(7):841–849.

Briggs-Gowan MJ, Owens PL, Schwab-Stone ME, Leventhal JM, Leaf P, Horwitz SM. Persistence of Psychiatric Disorders in Pediatric Settings. J Am Acad Child Adolesc Psychiatry 2003 Nov;42(11):1360–1369.

Brown C, Dunbar-Jacob J, Palenchar DR, Kelleher KJ, Bruehlman RD, Sereika S, Thase ME. Primary care patients' personal illness models for depression: a preliminary investigation. Journal of Family Medicine 2001;18(3):314–320.

Cadman D, Boyle M, Szatmari P, Offord DR. Chronic illness, disability, and mental and social well-being: findings of the Ontario Child Health Study. Pediatrics 1987 May; 79(5):805–813.

Campo JV, Comer DM, Jansen-McWilliams L, Gardner W, Kelleher KJ. Recurrent pain, emotional distress, and health service use in childhood. J Pediatr 2002 July;141(1):76–83.

Connell S, Sanders MR, Markie-Dadds C. Self-directed behavioral family intervention for parents of oppositional children in rural and remote areas. Behav Modif 1997 Oct; 21(4):379–408.

Cooper-Patrick L, Gallo JJ, Powe NR, Steinwachs DM, Eaton WW, For DE. Mental health service utilization by African Americans and Whites: the Baltimore Epidemiologic Catchment Area Follow-Up. Med Care 1999 Oct;37(10): 1034–1045.

Costello EJ. Psychopathology in pediatric primary care: the new hidden morbidity. Pediatrics 1988 Sep;82(3 Pt 2): 415–424.

Costello EJ. Child psychiatric disorders and their correlates: a primary care pediatric sample. J Am Acad Child Adolesc Psychiatry 1989 Nov;28(6):851–855.

Datto C, Thompson R, Horowitz D, Disbot M, Oslin D. The pilot study of a telephone disease management program for depression. General Hospital Psychiatry 25 (2003):169–177.

Deva MP. Training of psychiatrists for developing countries. Aust N Z J Psychiatry 1981 Dec;15(4):343–347.

Donaldson M, Yordy K, Lohr K, Vanselow N. Front Matter. Primary Care: America's Health in a new Era. Institute of Medicine (1996) pp i-x.

Durand MA, King M. Specialist treatment versus self-help for bulimia nervosa: a randomized controlled trial in general practice. Br J Gen Pract 2003 May;53(490):371–377.

Farvolden P, McBride C, Bagby RM, Ravitz P. A Web-based screening instrument for depression and anxiety disorders in primary care. Journal of Medical Internet Research. 5(3):e23 2003 Jul-Sep.

Flisher AJ, Kramer RA, Grosser RC, Alegria M, Bird HR, Bourdon KH, Goodman SH, Greenwald S, Horwitz SM, Moore RE, Narrow WE, Noven CW. Correlates of unmet need for mental health services by children and adolescents. Psychol Med 1997 Sept;27(5):1145–1154.

Fritz GK, Bergman AS. Child psychiatrists' characteristics, communication, and competence as described by pediatricians in a national survey. Int J Psychiatry Med 1986–87;16(1):91–100.

Gabbay M, Shiels C, Bower P, Sibbald B, King M, Ward E. Patient-practitioner agreement: does it matter? Psychological Medicine 2003, 33, 241–251.

Galan S, Delgado MT, Sanz C, Cordoba R. Family medicine research: analysis of papers accepted at national and international congresses. Aten Primaria 1995 Mar 15;(4):239–42, 244.

Gardner W, Murphy M, Childs C, Kelleher K, Pagano M, Jellinek M, et al. The PSC 17: a brief pediatric symptom checklist with psychosocial problem subscales, A report from PROS and ASPN. Ambulatory Child Health 1999;5(3):225–236.

Gardner W, Kelleher KJ, Wasserman R, Childs G, Nutting P, Lillienfeld H, Pajer K. Primary care treatment of pediatric psychosocial problems: A study from PROS and ASPN. Pediatrics 2000;106(4):e44.

Gardner W, Kelleher KJ,Pajer KA. Multidimensional adaptive testing for mental health problems in primary care. Medical Care 2002;40(9), 812–823.

Gardner W, Kelleher K.J, Page KA,Campo JV. Primary care clinicians' use of standardized tools to assess child psychosocial problems. Ambulatory Pediatrics, July-Aug 2003, 3 (4) 191–195.

Garralda E. Child and adolesecent psychiatry in general practice. Aust N Z J Psychiatry 2001 Jun:35(3):308–314.

Gask L, Usherwood T, Thompson H, Williams B. Evaluation of a training package in the assessment and management of depression in primary care. Med Educ 1998 Mar;32(2): 190–198.

Gilbody S, Whitty P, Grimshaw J, Thomas R. Educational and organizational interventions to improve the management of depression in primary care: a systematic review. JAMA 2003 Jun 18;289(23):3145–3151.

Goldberg ID, Roghmann KJ, McInerny TK, Burke JD Jr. Mental health problems among children seen in pediatric practice: prevalence and management. Pediatrics 1984 Mar; 73(3):278–293.

Hirschfeld RM, Keller MB, Panico S, Arons BS, Barlow D, Davidoff F, Endicott J, Froom J, Goldstein M, Gorman JM, Marek RG, Maurer TA, Meyer R, Phillips K, Ross J, Schwenk TL, Sharfstein SS, Thase ME, Wyatt RJ. The National Depressive and Manic-Depressive Association consensus statement on the undertreatment of depression. JAMA 1997 Jan 22–29;277(4):333–340.

Hoagwood K, Kelleher KJ, Feil M, Comer D. Treatment services for children with ADHD: A national perspective. J Am Acad Child Adolesc Psychiatry 2000; 39(2):198 206.

Holm S, Liss PE, Norheim OF. Access to health care in the Scandinavian countries: ethical aspects. Health Care Anal 1999;7(4):321–330.

Horwitz SM, Kelleher KJ, Boyce T, Jensen P, Murphy M, Perrin E, Stein REK, Weitzman M. Barriers to health care for children and youth with psychosocial problems. JAMA 2002, 288(12):1508–1512.

Jellinek MS, Murphy JM, Little M, Pagano ME, Comer DM, Kelleher KJ. Use of the Pediatric Symptom Checklist to screen for psychosocial problems in pediatric primary care: a national feasibility study. Arch Pediatr Adolesc Med 1999 Mar;153(3):254–260.

Katz R, Stephen J, Shaw BF, Matthew A, Newman F, Rosenbluth M. The East York Health Needs Study. I: Prevalence of DSM-III-R psychiatric disorder in a sample of Canadian women. Br J Psychiatry. 1995 Jan;166(1):100–106.

Kelleher K., Hohmann A, Larson D: Prescription of psychotropic drugs in office based practices. American Journal of Diseases of Children 1989; 143:855–859.

Kelleher KJ, Wolraich ML. Diagnosing psychosocial problems. Pediatrics 1996 June;97(6 Pt 1):899–901.

Kelleher KJ, McInerny TK, Gardner WP, Childs GE, Wasserman RC. Increasing identification of psychosocial problems: 1979–1996. Pediatrics 2000;105(6):1313–1321.

Kelleher KJ, Childs GE, Wasserman RC, McInerny TK, Nutting PA, Gardner WP. Insurance status and recognition of psychosocial problems: A report from PROS and ASPN. Archives of Pediatric & Adolescent Medicine. 1997; 151:1109–1115.

Kelleher KJ, Moore CD, Childs GE, Angelilli ML, Comer DM. Patient race and ethnicity in primary care management of child behavior problems. Medical Care 1999;37(11): 1092–1104.

Kelleher KJ, Childs GE, Harman JS. Health care costs for children with Attention Deficit/Hyperactivity Disorder. The Economics of Neuroscience 2001;3(4)60–63.

Kovacs M. The Children's Depression Inventory. http://assessmentsstage.ncspearson.com/assessments/tests/cdi.htm 12/1/03

Lave JR, Peele PB, Xu Y, Scholle SH, Pincus HA. An exploratory analysis of behavioral health care use within families. Psychiatr Serv 2002 Jun;53(6):743–748.

Lin CJ, Lave JR. Utilization under children's health insurance programs: children with vs. without chronic conditions. J Health Soc Policy 2000;11(4):1–14.

Lim FS, Toh MP, et al (2002) »A preliminary evaluation of a disease management programme for patients with diabetes mellitus and hypertension in a primary healthcare setting.« Ann Acad Med Singapore 31(4):431–439.

Liu SI, Prince M, Blizard B, Mann A. The prevalence of psychiatric morbidity and its associated factors in general health care in Taiwan. Psychol Med 2002 May;32(4):629–637.

Macinko J, Starfield B, Shi L. The contribution of primary care systems to health outcomes within Organization for Economic Cooperation and Development (OECD) countries 1970–1998. Health Serv Res 2003 Jun;38(3):831–865.

Maingay S, Jenkins R, McCulloch A, Friedli L, Parker C. The global response to mental illness– An enormous health burden is increasingly being recognized. BMJ Volume 325 21 September 2002.

Mathet F, Martin-Guehl C, Maurice-Tison S, Bouvard MP. Prevalence of depressive disorders in children and adolescents attending primary care. A survey with the Aquitaine Sentinelle Network. Encephale 2003 Oct;29(5):391–400.

Mattsson S, Stenberg A, Hellstrom AL, Lilja B. The pediatrician's approach to bed-wetting. A survey shows the hospital clinics adhere to current recommendations. Lakartidningen 2003 Jun 26;100(26–27):2300–2302.

McCleary L, Ridley T. Parenting adolescents with ADHD: evaluation of a psychoeducation group. Patient Education and Counseling 38(1999):3–10.

Mechanic D. Emerging issues in international mental health services research. Pscyhiatr Serv 1996 Apr;47(4):371–5.

Miranda J, Hohmann A, Attkisson C, Larson D. Impact of Mental Health Status on Use of Health Services. Mental Disorders in Primary Care ©1994.

The MTA Cooperative Group. A 14-month randomized clinical trial of treatment strategies for attention-deficit/hyperactivity disorder. Multimodal Treatment Study of Children with ADHD. Arch Gen Psychiatry 1999 Dec;56(12):1073–1086.

Murthy RS. Rural Psychiatry in Developing Countries. Psychiatr Serv 49:967–969, July 1998.

Murthy RS. Integration of mental health care into primary care. Demonstration cost-outcome study in India and Pakistan. Br J Psychiatry 2000 June;176:581–588.

The National Academies Press. Institute of Medicine. The Value of Primary Care. Primary Care: America's Health in a New Era (1996) pp.52–75.

Olfson M, Marcus SC, Druss B, Elinson L, Tanielian T, Pincus HA. National trends in the outpatient treatment of depression. JAMA 2002 Jan 9;287(2):203–209.

Olfson M, Marcus SC, Weissman MM, Jensen PS. National trends in the use of psychotropic medications by children. J Am Acad Child Adolesc Psychiatry 2002 May;41(5):514–521.

Olson AL, Kelleher KJ, Kemper KJ, Zuckerman BS, Hammond CS, Dietrich AJ. Primary care pediatrician's roles and perceived responsibilities in the management of depression in children and adolescents. Ambulatory Pediatrics 2001;1:91–92.

Ortega AN, Huertas SE, Canino G, Ramirez R, Rubio-Stipec M. Childhood asthma, chronic illness, and psychiatric disorders. J Nerv Ment Dis 2002 May;190(5):275–281.

Patel V, Pereira J, Coutinho L, Fernandes R, Fernandes J, Mann A. Poverty, psychological disorder and disability in primary care attenders in Goa, India. Br J Psychiatry 1998 Jun;172:533–536.

Pediatric Symptom Checklist (PSC) http://psc.partners.org/ psc_bibliography.htm 12-1-03

Pothen M, Kuruvilla A, Philip K, Joseph A, Jacob KS. Common mental disorders among primary care attenders in Vellore, South India: nature, prevalence and risk factors. Int J Soc Psychiatry 2003 Jun;49(2):119–125.

Real Perez M, Rodriguez-Arias Palomo JL, Cagigas Viadero J, Aparicion Sanz MM, Real Perez MA. Brief family therapy: an option for the treatment of somatoform disorders in primary care. Aten Primaria. 1996 Mar 15:17(4):241–246.

Regier DA, Burke JD, Jr, et al (1982) Proposed classification of health problems. Psychosocial factor affecting health. (eds. Lipkin M, Kupka K) New York, Praeger: 153–184.

Rix S, Paykel ES, Lelliott P, Tylee A, Freeling P, Gask L, Hart D. Impact of a national campaign on GP education: an evaluation of the Defeat Depression Campaign. Br J Gen Pract 1999 Feb;49(439):91–92.

Robinson P, Katin W, Von Korff M, Bush T, Simon G, Lin E, Walker E. The Education of Depressed Primary Care Patients: What Do Patients Think of Interactive Booklets and a Video? The Journal of Family Practice, Vol. 44, No. 6 (June) 1997.

Roeloffs C, Sherbourne C, Unutzer J, Fink A, Tang L, Wells KB. Stigma and depression among primary care patients. Gen Hosp Psychiatry. 2003 Sept-Oct;25(5):311–315.

Rothman A, Wagner E (2003) »Chronic illness management: what is the role of primary care?« Annals of Internal Medicine 138(3):256-261.

Rowan M S, Lawson B, MacLean C, Burge F. Upholding the principles of primary care in preceptors' practices. Fam Med 2002 Nov-Dec;34(10):744–749.

Rushton J, Bruckman D, Kelleher K. Primary care referral of children with psychosocial problems. Arch Pediatr Adolesc Med 2002 Jun;156(6):592–598.

Sanders M R. Triple P-Positive Parenting Program: towards and empirically validated multilevel parenting and family support strategy for the prevention of behavior and emotional problems in children. Clin Child Fam Psychol Rev 1999 Jun;2(2):71–90.

Sanders M R, Montgomery D T, Brechman-Toussaint M L. The mass media and the prevention of child behavior problems: the evaluation of a television series to promote positive outcomes for parents and their children. J Child Psychol Psychiatry 2000 Oct;41(7):939–948.

Sanders M R, Tully L A, Turner K M, Maher C, McAuliffe C. Training GPs in parent consultation skills. An evaluation of training for the Triple P-Positive Parenting Program. Aust Fam Physician 2003 Sep;32(9):763–768.

Schirm E, Tobi H, Zito J M, de Jong-van den Berg LT. Psychotropic medication in children: a study from the Netherlands. Pediatrics 2001 Aug;108(2):E25.

Schoenbaum M., Kelleher K, et al (in Press April 2004) »Exploratory Evidence on the Market for Effective Depression Care in Pittsburgh«. Psychiatr Serv

Sharp L, Pantell R H, et al (1992) »Psychosocial problems during child health supervision visits: eliciting, then what?« Pediatrics 89(4): 619-623.

Shi L, Starfield B, Kennedy B, Kawachi I. Income inequality, primary care, and health indicators. J Fam Pract 1999 Apr;48(4):275–284.

Simon G, VonKorff M, et al (2000) »Randomised trial of monitoring, feedback, and management of care by telephone to improve treatment of depression in primary care.« BMJ 320(7234):550-554.

Sorensen J L, Hargreaves W A, Friedlander S. Child global rating scales: selecting a measure of client functioning in a large mental health system. Eval Program Plann 1982;5(4):337–347. http://www.ncbi.nlm.nih.gov

Spitzer R L, Williams J B, et al (2000) »Validity and utility of the PRIME-MD patient health questionnaire in assessment of 3000 obstetric-gynecologic patients: the PRIME-MD Patient Health Questionnaire Obstetrics-Gynecology Study.« Am J Obstet Gynecol 183(3):759-769.

Starfield B, Shi L. Policy relevant determinants of health: an international perspective. Health Policy. 2002 Jun;60(3): 201–218.

Todd C, Patel V, Simunyu E, Gwanzura F, Acuda W, Winston M, Mann A. The onset of common mental disorders in primary care attenders in Harare, Zimbabwe. Psychol Med 1999 Jan:29(1):97–104.

Valenstein M, Vijan S, Zeber J E, Boehm K, Buttar A. The cost-utility of screening for depression in primary care. Ann Intern Med 2001 Mar 6;134(5):345–360.

Vanstraelen M, Cottrell D. Child and adolescent mental health services: purchasers' knowledge and plans. BMJ 1994 Jul 23;309(6949):259–261.

Vila G, Nollet-Clemencon C, Vera M, Robert J J, de Blic J, Jouvent R, Mouren-Simeoni MC, Scheinmann P. Prevalence of DSM-IV disorders in children and adolescents with asthma versus diabetes. Can J Psychiatry. 1999 Aug; 44(6):562–569.

Walders N, Childs G E, et al (2003) »Barriers to mental health referral from pediatric primary care settings.« Am J Manag Care 9(10): 677-683

Wasserman R C, Kelleher K J, Bocian A, Baker A, Childs G E, Indacochea F, Stulp C, Gardner W P. Identification of attentional and hyperactivity problems in primary care: a report from pediatric research in office settings and the ambulatory sentinel practice network. Pediatrics 1999 Mar; 103(3):E38.

Wren F J, Scholle S H, Heo J, Comer D M. Pediatric mood and anxiety syndromes in primary care: who gets identified? Int J Psychiatry Med 2003;33(1):1–16.

Zito J M, Safer D J, dosReis S, Gardner J F, Boles M, Lynch F. Trends in the prescribing of psychotropic medications to preschoolers. JAMA 2000 Feb 23;283(8):1025–1030.

Zito J M, Safer D J, DosReis S, Gardner J F, Soeken K, Boles M, Lynch F. Rising prevalence of antidepressants among US youths. Pediatrics 2002 May;109(5):721–727.

Zito J M, Safer D J, DosReis S, Gardner J F, Magder L, Soeken K, Boles M, Lynch F, Riddle M A. Psychotropic practice patterns for youth: a 10-year perspective. Arch Pediatr Adolesc Med 2003 Jan;157(1):17–25.

Prevention and Intervention in School Settings

Amira Seif El Din

24.1   Introduction   – 326

24.2   Psychopathology Related
        to School Attendance   – 327
24.2.1 School Mental Health Problems Can Be Divided into
        Two Major Areas: (a) Absenteeism and School
        Refusal, and (b) School Drop Out   – 327
24.2.1.1 Absenteeism and School Refusal   – 327
24.2.1.2 General Characteristics of School Refusal   – 327
24.2.1.3 What Schools Can Do to Address School
        Refusal   – 328
24.2.2 School Drop Out   – 328
24.2.2.1 General Characteristic of School Drop Out   – 328

24.3   School Mental Health Prevention and Intervention
        Programs   – 329
24.3.1 Level I – Primary Prevention   – 330
24.3.1.1 Life Skills Programs   – 330
24.3.1.2 Impact of Life Skills Teaching   – 330
24.3.2 Level II – Secondary Prevention   – 330
24.3.3 Level III – Tertiary Prevention   – 330

24.4   Model Programs   – 331
24.4.1 Program Examples   – 331
24.4.1.1 Norway: Bullying Prevention   – 331
24.4.1.2 United States: Comer Schools   – 331
24.4.1.3 Alexandria, Egypt:
        Comprehensive School Consultation   – 332
24.4.1.4 Rawalpindi, Pakistan: Peer School Support   – 332

24.5   Conclusions   – 333

        References   – 333

If Children live with praise. They learn to appreciate.
If Children live with acceptance and friendship. They learn to find love in the world.

24.1 Introduction

The best place to develop, promote, and intervene to ameliorate child and adolescent mental health problems is the school setting. The following reasons pertain to the importance of the school setting as a venue for care: (1) most children attend school at some time during their lives; (2) schools are often the strongest social and educational institutions available for intervention; (3) schools have a profound influence on children, their families, and the community; (4) schools can act as a safety net, protecting children from hazards that affect their learning, development and psychosocial well being. Schools, in addition to family, may be crucial in building the self esteem and sense of competence of children. On the other hand, the school environment, by its very nature, can cause stresses on children, for example, stress due to examinations, low self esteem in case of failure, and depression in case of bullying (Mohit and Seif El-Din 1998). Lastly, schools are particularly important as a central point of community life, which also can be a factor in supporting positive mental health.

Mental health programs in schools not only contribute to the betterment of mental health of the students, but also tend to improve the image of mental health programs through destigmatization. Globally changes in family structure, rapid urbanization, industrialization, population growth, and migration have had a profound impact on mental health and well being. Schools as a stable structure in communities can help buffer the adverse impact of these changes.

Rutter (1989) found that school variations were systematically associated with characteristics of the school as social organizations. The finding implied casual effects associated with school experiences. However, two alternative explanations needed to be considered; first, that the school variations reflected influences from unmeasured aspects of the child's behavior or family background, and secondly, that the child's characteristics shaped the school rather than the reverse.

Nearly one in five children and adolescents will have an emotional/behavioral disorder at some time regardless of where they live and how well-to-do they are. Children with emotional disturbances exhibit their impairments in a variety of ways. They may fail academically, be socially rejected, and have a poor self-image. They may also have difficulties in relating to peers or adults and may have little respect for the laws of their society. In addition, they may live within financially and emotionally impoverished environments (Bazhenova et al. 1992).

24.2 Psychopathology Related to School Attendance

Clinicians and researchers have commonly divided children who fail to go to school into two groups: those who stay home from school because of fear or anxiety, and those who skip school because of a lack of interest in school and/or defiance of adult authority.(King and Bernstein 2001). The behavior of the first group has variously been called »school refusal«, »anxious school refusal«, school phobia«, or a variant of separation anxiety disorders (SAD), while the behavior of the second group has been called »truancy«. The terms used to describe nontruant school refusal reflect early conceptualizations of the etiology of the behavior (Kearney and Silverman 1996).

24.2.1 The School Mental Health Problems Can Be Divided into Two Major Areas: (a) Absenteeism and School Refusal, and (b) School Drop Out

Because of the uniqueness of these major mental health problems to the school environment and because educators are especially concerned about these groups of problematic students, these two areas will be reviewed as to their etiology.

24.2.1.1 Absenteeism and School Refusal

Definition: School refusal is defined as difficulty attending school associated with emotional distress, especially anxiety and depression. While terms such as separation anxiety and school phobia are often used interchangeably with school refusal, the latter term is preferably used because of its descriptive and comprehensive nature. Kearney and Silverman (1996) defined school refusal behavior as »child-motivated refusal to attend school or difficulties remaining in school for an entire day«. They have argued that descriptive definitions of school refusal, free of assumptions about etiology or associated psychopathology, are critical to understanding the associations between children's refusal to attend school and psychiatric disorders.

24.2.1.2 General Characteristics of School Refusal

School refusal has a strong effect on educational outcomes; some researchers estimate that about half of school refusers underachieve academically (Chazan 1962).

Hersov (1985) suggested that the prevalence of school refusal would be estimated at 5% of all children with psychiatric disorders with a peak period around the beginning of school, at about ages 5–7 (probably associated with separation anxiety), and again at ages 11 and 14 or older (associated with other psychiatric disorders or depressive states). Ollendick and Mayor (1984) concluded that school refusal is more likely to occur between 5–6 years and 10–11 years of age. There is an association of school refusal with separation anxiety disorder or other primary or comorbid disorders such as social phobia, simple phobia, panic disorder, and depressive disorders (Last and Strauss 1989). In other studies it is reported that school refusal occurs in approximately the same percent (5%) of all school age children, although the rate of school absenteeism is much higher in some urban areas (Kearney and Roblek 1997; King et al. 1995).

In relation to educational outcomes, some researchers estimated that about half of school refusers underachieve academically (Chazan 1962). In another research study it was found that in the context of examination stress underachievers develop more school refusal (Ebrahim 1999). Regarding the sex of school refusers, most studies found the phenomenon to be equally common in boys and girls (Egger et al. 2003).

24.2.1.3 What Schools Can Do to Address School Refusal

Stickney and Miltenberger (1998) surveyed 288 schools in North Dakota, including elementary, junior high, and senior high schools, and found that 75% of schools reported having a school refusal identification system in place. Principals were most frequently reported to be responsible for the identification of school refusers. In this study, overall 2.3% of students were identified as »school refusers« (including truants). Almost half presented with somatic complaints in the absence of a medical condition, an important finding from the viewpoint of early identification and treatment. School refusers were most commonly referred to a social worker and least frequently referred to a psychiatrist (Kearney and Beasley 1994; King and Bernstein 2001).

A study of outpatient children and adolescents with anxiety disorders found that those who reported more somatic complaints were more likely to be older and to demonstrate school refusal (Last 1990). Although no known studies of school refusal have looked at school attendance and its relationship to somatic complaints and psychiatric illnesses. Missing school has the attendant consequences of loss of peer relationships and increased academic difficulties (Bernstein et al. 1997). Egger et al. (2003) found that somatic complaints were found in a quarter of pure »anxious« school refusals, and in 42% of the »mixed« school refusers. Very few »pure« truants manifested somatic complaints. Bernstein et al. (1997) found that autonomic and gastrointestinal problems were most commonly endorsed by their sample of outpatient adolescent school refusers. This was in agreement with the findings of Beidel and colleagues (1991).

Egger et al. (2003) reported that nightmares and night terrors were strongly associated with »mixed« school refusal. They also found support for the association between »anxious« school refusal and somatic complaints (Bernstein et al. 1997). A triad of school refusal, sleep difficulties, and somatic complaints might alert pediatricians or family physicians to the presence of associated psychiatric disorders (Bary et al. 1993). In community studies, Egger et al. (2003) found that school refusal was strongly associated with, but not synonymous with, psychiatric disorders.

24.2.2 School Drop Out

Definition: Dropping out of school has several definitions most commonly based on students who are not currently enrolled in school and have not obtained either a high school diploma or a general equivalency diploma (Mattison 2000).

24.2.2.1 General Characteristic of School Drop Out

In a review of high school drop out in the United States, Coley (1995) found the national annual high school dropout rate, that is, the percentage of students aged 15–24 years who leave grades 10–12 in specific years to be 4.5% in 1993, compared with 6.5% in the late 1970s. The high school completion rate for males has increased from 78% in 1972 to a stable 87% from the early 1980s to 1993.

Using National Educational Longitudinal Survey (NELS) data from grade 8 (1988) to grade 10 (1990), Rumberger (1995) found that the most influential, interactive variables (gathered from parent, teacher, and student questionnaires) which determine middle school dropouts were SES, parent attitude toward school (academic support, supervision, and expectations), retention, changing schools, absenteeism, misbehavior, and academic performance. Pearson et al. (2000) found that the causes of school dropout for students before 10th grade were related to poor academic achievement, which was in turn mediated by the effect of other independent factors such as general deviance, bonding to antisocial peers, and socioeconomic status.

Dixon (1999) found that a relationship exists between adolescents at risk for school dropout and peer rejection outcomes. This finding supports the view that variables predictive of students' academic success are not limited to specific academic skills, but involve interpersonal competencies. Other studies correlated the higher proportion of school dropout to early onset cigarette smoking and drug use (Bray et al. 2000; Bates et al. 1997). This was confirmed by the study of Ferguson et al. (1997), where he found a strong association between early onset (prior to 16 years of age) cannabis use and subsequent affiliations with delinquent and substance-using peers, resulting in a move away from home and school dropout.

Most studies have focused on student factors involved in dropping out, and rarely on school factors such as the adequacy of the facilities, leadership,

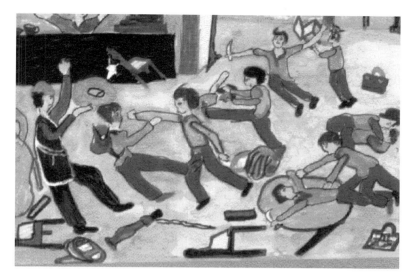

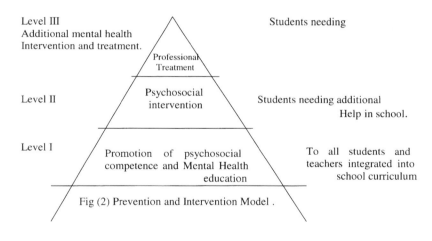

Level III
Additional mental health
Intervention and treatment.

Students needing

◘ Fig. 24.2. Prevention and Intervention Model

Professional
Treatment

Level II

Psychosocial
intervention

Students needing additional
Help in school.

Level I

Promotion of psychosocial
competence and Mental Health
education

To all students and
teachers integrated into
school curriculum

Fig (2) Prevention and Intervention Model .

and teachers (Rumberger 1987). Such variables most likely have a role, as dropout rates do vary among schools. Bryk and Thum (1989) have shown some evidence that dropout rates may be lower in school atmospheres characterized by an emphasis on academic pursuits, orderly environments, active faculty interaction with students, and less differentiation among students in their demographic and academic backgrounds (◘ Fig. 24.1).

24.3 School Mental Health Prevention and Intervention Programs

A comprehensive mental health program should be part of a comprehensive school program, including health instruction at all grade levels, easily accessible health services, a healthful nurturing and safe environment, and interaction with family and community organizations. Hendren el al. (1994) highlighted a model school mental health program. The following diagram can illustrate the prevention and intervention model associated with a positive school intervention (◘ Fig. 24.2).

— **Level I** is primary prevention, targeting the causes of healthy and unhealthy conditions with interventions to promote healthy behaviors and prevent a disorder from developing.

— **Level II** is secondary prevention, targeting a more selected population of high-risk students to protect against the onset of disorder.

— **Level III** is tertiary prevention, targeting students who already have developed a disorder with the intent of treating the disorder, reducing the impairment from the disorder and/or preventing relapse (Rutter 1982).

24.3.1   Level I – Primary Prevention

Primary prevention in school mental health occurs through the promotion of psychosocial competence and mental health education that includes students and teachers. The most significant interventions for the promotion of psychosocial competence in school are those which enhance the child's own coping resources and competencies; this is most often done by the teaching of skills, such as life skills. These skills include: decision making and problem solving, critical and creative thinking, communication and interpersonal relationship skills, self awareness and empathy, and skills for coping with emotions and stressors.

24.3.1.1   Life Skills Programs

Life skills are being taught as part of a wide variety of school-based interventions. Programs with demonstrable effectiveness include those for the prevention of substance abuse (Botvin et al. 1980, 1984; Pentz 1983), adolescent pregnancy (Zabin et al. 1986; Schinke 1984), and the prevention of bullying (Olweus 1990). Educational programs teaching these skills have also been developed for the prevention of AIDS (WHO/GPA 1994), for peace education (Prutzman et al. 1988) and for the promotion of self confidence and self esteem (TACADE 1990). Teaching life skills in this wide range of promotion and prevention programs demonstrates the common value of life skills for health promotion, beyond their value within any specific program (WHO 1997). The introduction of life skills teaching will require input from the school and education authorities for teaching, training and the development of teaching manuals, as well as for the ongoing support of teaching programs, once they are in place.

24.3.1.2   Impact of Life Skills Teaching

— For the student: protecting his health, e.g., by preventing cigarette smoking (Botvin et al. 1980), abuse of alcohol (Botvin et al. 1984) and other drugs (Seif El Din 1993; Botvin et al. 1984), and promoting the child's social interests; e.g., by improving relationship with peers (Venables et al. 1983).

— For the teacher: improved relationship with pupils (Olweus 1990) and fewer classroom behavior problems (Venables et al. 1983).

— For the school: improve academic performance (Wessberg 1983) and possible effects on levels of truancy and school dropout.

24.3.2   Level II – Secondary Prevention

Secondary prevention is useful where mental health problems range from relatively minor and transient disturbances to serious and long-term disorders. Schools are often places where mental health problems are first identified as needing special attention. If children with potential mental health problems are identified early and appropriate interventions made, the problems are more likely to reduce risk-taking behaviors such as smoking and substance abuse. Too early sexual activity may be an early indication of a young person in danger of more serious problems. Early intervention with risk-taking behavior can prevent serious consequences which may need a sophisticated level of intervention.

Psychosocial problems become evident through changes or deviations in emotions and/or behaviors. This may include aggression, decline in academic performance, and failure in school, change in peer groups, fluctuating mood, risk-taking behaviors, and exaggerated or repressed feelings associated with physical illness. Extra care needs to be taken by health professionals in screening for these problems and disorders.

24.3.3   Level III – Tertiary Prevention

Psychosocial and mental health interventions for mental disorders may take place in or out of the classroom. Classroom interventions include health promotion, primary prevention (health education), and early problem identification as mentioned earlier. The intervention may be directed toward the entire classroom or school environment or it may be directed toward an individual child. It is usually desirable to make use of interventions that affect both the school environment and the child.

Assessment and referral for psychiatric treatment can take place out of the classroom, but should be coordinated with the teacher, school nurse, and school administration. When teachers and other school personnel understand the nature of a child's problems they can work effectively with mental health professionals in designing classroom and school programs that provide support and enhance the coping abilities of vulnerable children. Psychological treatment programs for children needing additional help in the classroom have been shown to be of benefit. Shorter-term treatment such as group therapy, play group, and behavior modification have shown promising results in children with psychosocial disorders by enabling them to remain in regular classrooms and advance educationally (Kolvin et al. 1981). Peer counseling, often done by older children and adolescents, has been found to be helpful both for those who give it and for those who receive it. The positive role modeling, problem solving strategies and prosocial behavior are often accepted more readily when they come from peers rather than authority figures.

Schools can be enlisted in crisis management. Parents, teachers and children can be involved in preventively oriented trauma recognition and response (Pynoos et al. 1990). Elements of crisis intervention include consultation with school administrators, training of teachers, and education of parents and children. Identifying and addressing rumors, misconceptions, and fear helps to minimize anxiety in the school community. Classroom drawing exercises and symbolic reconstruction of the crisis can be effective initial interventions with younger children. Special procedures are needed to reintegrate hospitalized or severely traumatized children into classroom, to deal with bereaved children, and to monitor school behavior and performance.

24.4 Model Programs

All over the world several examples of successful school mental health programs exist. Many of these programs are directed to a particular problem or disorder, and others to improve the schools' environment. Some programs dealing with particular problems or disorders are only appropriate for particular cultures and cannot be transferred to other cultures.

The characteristics of effective school mental health programs should take into account the relationship between the school and the community environment. It is important to identify the socio-political conditions and processes likely to be associated with the establishment and survival of a comprehensive mental health program. The involvement of families and community members as active partners in planning, implementation, and ongoing evaluation is key. Hendren et al. (1994) emphasized the need to intervene at multiple levels and focus on teacher and parent trainings (Hendren et al. 1994).

24.4.1 Program Examples

The following are examples of successful prevention and intervention programs.

24.4.1.1 Norway: Bullying Prevention

An example of a successful mental health intervention in the educational environment is one to prevent bullying in Norway (Olweus 1992). Instead of teaching individual children to cope with bullying by aggressive peers, a national campaign was developed and successfully carried out to reduce bullying throughout the entire school system. The intervention consisted of workshops for teachers and parents, booklets, videos, and problem solving and social skills training for students, all with a firm, nonaggressive message that bullying would not be tolerated.

24.4.1.2 United States: Comer Schools

Another example of an environment-centered model is that of Comer (1980) at the Yale Child Study Center. The Comer School Model applies a systems approach to school problems. It focuses on improving the school's social environment by encouraging parent participation through a parent program in support of school activities, and by establishing a multidisciplinary mental health team to provide consultation in the management of student behavior problems. These activities are coordinated by a representative governing body composed of administrators, teachers, support staff, and parents. The governing body identifies and rates problems and opportunities within the school, distributes and promotes resources, establishes mechanisms to solve problems and use the existing opportunities, and monitors and evaluates the outcome, thus providing feedback, so that appropriate modifications can be made to the program. This model is found to improve student academic and behavioral performance over time (Cauce 1987).

24.4.1.3 Alexandria, Egypt: Comprehensive School Consultation

There are parts of the world where the number of child psychiatrists and child mental health professionals are very limited in proportion to the large number of children. In some countries the child population can be about 40% of the total population. In 23 countries of the eastern Mediterranean region there is only one child psychiatrist for every 12 million people and most psychiatric care, if provided at all, is given by general psychiatrists (Seif El Din 1990).

A successful program developed and featured by the World Health Organization is the one developed in Alexandria, Egypt. It offers a strong argument for promoting child psychiatric services in developing countries and providing related mental health training within primary care services. This program overcame strong challenges due to the limited awareness of physicians, teachers, and parents about child mental health. Prior to the program, traditional disciplinary methods were used to manage several child psychiatric problems. Even families were not accepting that child psychiatric problems can develop because they considered childhood as a happy period of human life in which no psychiatric illnesses can develop.

The school mental health program was launched in Alexandria in 1987 by an intersectoral team from the Ministries of Education and Health and the Faculty of Medicine in Alexandria. The goal was to develop a child psychiatric service with the following objectives: train school personnel; orient school children to communicate skillfully with their peers and school staff, with an emphasis on respect and empathy for disadvantage persons; and use school children to convey proper mental health messages to their families. One-week training courses were conducted. This helped most of the personnel working in schools to realize the different school mental health problems they were facing and to manage them, if possible, or to refer them to the proper channels, in addition to their task of promoting school mental health (Seif El-Din et al. 1991).

Two years after the start of this program, with increased awareness of child mental health problems, a question was raised on how to develop more qualified personnel to act as a filter for early detection of children in need of psychiatric services and to manage the detected cases through guidance and counseling for the parents and teachers. The clinical training needs were realized through advanced training courses. An 11 week training course, with intervals of 2–3 months between session groupings to give the trainees a better chance to return back to their schools to apply what they learned during the different training weeks, was initiated.

The advanced training programs conducted from 1990 to 2002 developed about 200 school mental health providers from six advanced training courses. These providers now run school mental health guidance and counseling clinics and will form the core training group for the training of others. The training activities also had the effect of developing the proper referral of needy children and increasing the collaboration between schools and health sectors to promote and intervene properly (Seif El Din 1990; Attia et al. 1991; Seif El Din et al. 1991, 1996; Abou Nazel et al. 1995).

24.4.1.4 Rawalpindi, Pakistan: Peer School Support

Another model school mental health program exists in Rawalpindi, Pakistan. In this program pupils work together to promote their own health as well as that of their families and communities (Mubbashar et al. 1989). The program is reinforced through the use of slogans, essays, and speech contests, mental health committees, parent/teacher associations, and a managerial training workshop for district education officers. Program evaluation indicates improved grades, increased attendance, decreased dropouts, and increased general and mental health case referrals.

In Africa, another innovative mental health education curriculum has been developed in Uganda as part of over all health education for secondary school students. This program is supported by the Ugandan Ministries of Health and Education (1994). The extensive curriculum focuses on the relationship between physical and mental illness; the effect of stress culture on mental disorders; the etiology, prevention and treatment of mental disorders throughout the life cycle; substance abuse; sexual

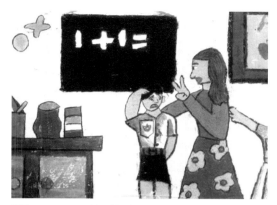

Fig. 24.3. Mental health through children's eyes

disorders, mental retardation, suicide, and mental disorders associated with AIDS (■ Fig. 24.3).

24.5 Conclusions

Schools are one of the most important settings in which to promote the mental health of children. To do so will enhance the possibilities of improved adjustment and health in future generations. The school environment is one of the least stigmatizing and potentially supportive places to intervene properly with needy children.

References

Abou Nazel M, Koura M, Seif El Din A (1995) Impact of mental health knowledge and attitudes of trainees on their school contacts. Bulletin High Institute Public Health 25(2):341–348

Attia M, Abou Nazel M, Guirguis W, et al. (1991) Impact of a mental health program on the utilization of the psychiatric clinic in a sporting student's hospital. J Egyptian Public Health Assn 66(5,6):587–607

Bates S C, Plemons B W, Jumper T P, et al (1997) Volatile solvent use: Patterns by gender and ethnicity among school attenders and dropouts. Drugs and Society 10(1–2):61–78

Bazhenova O, Gorunova A, Kozlovskaya G, Skoblo G (1992) An epidemiological study of mental disorders during early childhood in the Soviet Union. In: Improving children's lives: global perspectives on prevention. Albee GW, Bond LA, Monsey TVC (eds)

Beidel D, Christ M, Long P (1991) Somatic complaints in anxious children. J Abnormal Child Psych 19:659–670

Bernstein G, Massie E, Thuras P, et al. (1997) Somatic symptoms in anxious-depressed school refusers. J Am Acad Child Adolesc Psychiatry 36:661–668

Bools C, Foster J, Brown I, Berg I (1990) The identification of psychiatric disorders in children who fail to attend school: a cluster analysis of a non clinical population. Psychol Med 20:171–181

Botvin G J, Eng A, Williams C L (1980) Preventing the onset of Cigarette smoking through like. Skills Training Preventive Medicine 11:199–211

Botvin G J, Baker E, Renick N L, et al (1984) A cognitive behavioral approach. to substance abuse prevention. Addictive Behaviors 9:137–147

Bray J W, Zarkin G A, Ring W C (2000) The relation between marijuana initiation and dropping out of high school. Health Econ 9(1):9–18

Bryk AS, Thum YM (1989) The effects of high school organization on dropping out: an exploratory investigation. Am Educ Res J 26:353–383

Bryk A S, Thum Y M (1989) The effect of high school organization on dropping out: an exploratory investigation Am Educ Res J 26:353–383

Cauce A M, Comer J P, Schwartz D (1987) Long term effects of a systems-oriented school prevention program. Am J Orthopsychiat 57:127–131

Chazan M (1962) School phobia. Br J Educ Psychol 32:201–207

Coley R(1995) Dreams Deferred: High school Dropouts in the United States. Princeton, New Jersey: Education testing Service

Comer J P (1980) School Power: Implications of an Intervention Project New York. Free Press.

Dixon BJ (1999) Peer acceptance and peer rejection outcomes of adolescents at risk for school dropout. Dissertation Abstract International, Section A: Humanities Soc Sci 59(12-A) 4357

Ebraheim E (1999) Epidemiological study of scholastic underachievement among primary school children in Alexandria: prevalence and causes. Thesis to be submitted for master degree in nursing.

Egger H, Colstello J, Angold A. (2003) School Refusal and Psychiatric Disorders: A community study. J Am Acad Child Psychiatry 42:797–807

Fergusson D M, Horwood L J (1997) Early onset cannabis use and psychological adjustment in young adults. Addiction 92(3):279–296

Gonzalez R (1990) Ministering intelligence: a Venezuelan experience in the promotion of cognitive abilities. International J of Mental Health,18(3):5–19.

Hendren H, Weisen B, Orley J (1994) Mental Health Programmers in School: WHO. MNH. Geneva.

Kearney C, Beasley J (1994) The clinical treatment of school refusal behavior: a survey of referral and practice characteristics. Psychol Schools 31:128–132

Kearney C, Roblekt (1997) Parent training in the treatment of school refusal behavior. In: Handbook of parent training: Parents as co- therapists for children's behavior problems, 2nd ed. Briesmeister J M, Shaefer C D (eds) New York: Wiley.

Kearney C, Silverman W (1996) The evolution and reconciliation of taxonomic strategies for school refusal behavior. Clin Psych School Prac 3:339–354

King N, Bernstein G (2001) School refusal in children and adolescents: a review of the past 10 years. J Am Acad Child Adolesc Psychiatry 40:197–205

King N, Ollendik T, Tonge B (1995) School Refusal: Assessment and treatment Boston: Allyn and Bacon.

Kolvin I, Garside R, Niole A, et al (1981) Help starts here:the maladjusted child in the ordinary school. London, Tavistock Publications

Last, C, Strauss C (1989) School refusal in anxiety disordered children and adolescents. J Am Acad Child Adolesc Psychiatry 29:31–35

Last C, Strauss C (1990) School refusal in anxiety-disordered children and adolescents. J Am Acad Child Adolesc Psychiatry 29:31–35

Mattison R (2000) School consultation: A review of research on issues unique to the school environment. J Am Acad Child Adolesc Psychiatry 39:402–413

Mattison R, (2000) School Consultation: A Review of Research on Issues Unique to the school environment. J Am Acad Child Adolesc Psychiatry 39(4):402–413.

Mohit A, Seif El Din A (1998) Mental Health promotion for school children A manual for school teachers and school mental health workers. WHO- EM/MNH/153/E/L. Regional office for the Eastern Mediterranean, Alexandria, Egypt

Mubbashar M, Saraf T, Afgan S, et al (1989) Promotion of mental health through school health programs. Eastern Mediterranean Region Health Serv J 6:14–19

Ollendick T, Mayer J (1984) School phobia: Behavioral theories and treatment of Anxiety. Turner SM, ed. New York: Plenum, 367–411

Olweus D (1990) A National Campaign in Norway to reduce the prevalence of bulling behavior. Paper presented to the Society for Research on Adolescence Biennial Meeting, Atlanta, December 10–12

Olweus D (1992) Victimization among school children: intervention and prevention. In Improving Children's lives: global perspectives on prevention Ablee GW, Bond CA, Manses TVC (eds). Newbury Park, Sage Publications, 275–295

Pearson B, Newcomb S, Michael D, Hill K, David J (2000) Predictors of early high school dropout: A test of five theories. Journal of Education Psychology 92(3):568–582.

Pentz MA Prevention of adolescent substance through social skills development. In Glym et al (eds) Preventing adolescent drug abuse: Intervention strategies. NIDA Research Monograph No:47 Washington DC:NIDA. 195–235

Prutzman P, Stern L, Burger ML, et al (1988) the Friendly Classroom for a Small Planet Children's Creative Response to conflict program. Santa Cruz:New Society Publishers

Pynoos R, Nader K (1990) Mental health disturbances in children exposed to disaster: preventive intervention strategies. In: Preventing Mental Health Disturbances in Childhood. American Psychiatric Press, Washington DC

Rumberger RW (1987) High school dropouts: a review of issues and evidence. Rev Educ Res 57:121–151

Rutter M (1982) Prevention of Children's Psychosocial disorders: Myth and substance. Pediatrics 70:883–894

Rutter M (1989) Pathways from childhood to adult life. Sixth Jack Tizard Memorial Lecture. J Child Psychol Psychiatry 30:23–51

Schinke SP (1984) Preventing teenage pregnancy. In: Hersen M, Eisler R, Miller P (eds) Progress in behavior modification. New York: Academic Press, 31–64

Seif El-Din A (1990) Evaluation of the training programs for professional working with School Children in Alexandria. Alexandria J Pediatrics 4(1):61–68

Seif El-Din A. (1990) Mental Health training program for school health physician in Alexandria. Bulletin of Public Health 26(1):75–82.

Seif El-Din A, Moustafa A, Mohit A, et al (1993) A multi-sectoral approach to school mental health, Alexandria. Egypt. Part II Health Services Journal Eastern Mediterranean Region WHO 7(2): 34–40

Seif El-Din A, Kamel F, Youssef R, et al. (1996) Evaluation of an educational training program for the development of trainers. In: Child Mental Health in Alexandria. Eastern Mediterranean Health J 2 (3):482–493

TACADE (1990) Skills for primary school child: promoting the protection of children. Salford, UK

Uganda Ministries of Health and Education (1994): Health Education. Syllabus for secondary schools in Uganda. Mental health programs in schools, WHO/MNH

WHO/CPA (1994) School Health Education to Prevent AIDS and STD: A Resource Package for Curriculum Planners. WHO/Global Program on AIDS Geneva.

Zalin LS, Hirsch MB, Smith EA, et al (1986) Evaluation of a pregnancy prevention program urban teenagers. Family Planning Perspectives 18:119–126

Subject Index

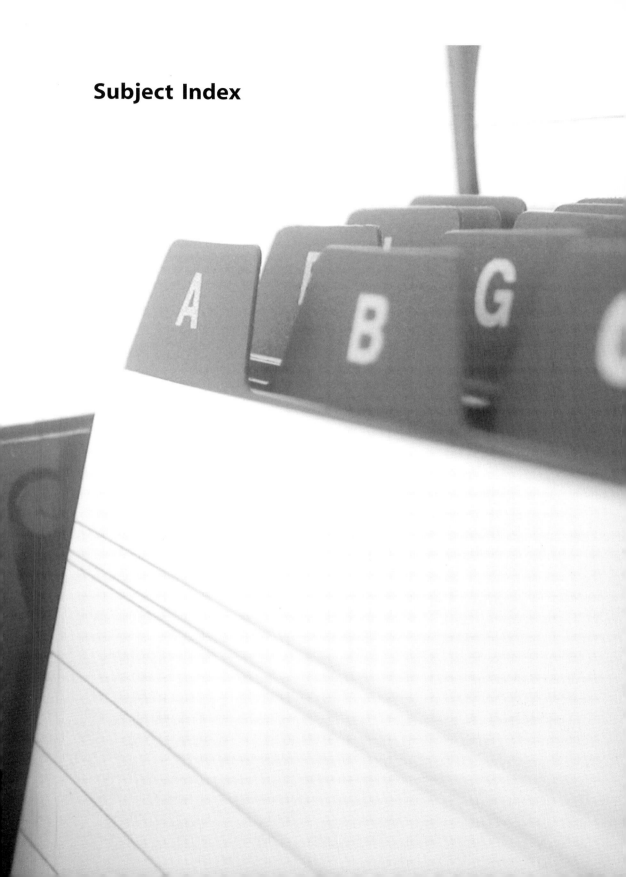

A

aboriginal population   52
accreditation system   61
Achenbach Child Behavior Checklist (CBCL)   59
acute exacerbations   321
ADHD see Attention Deficit/Hyperactivity Disorder
Adolescent Reproductive Health Network   81
advocacy   23
Aggressive Behavior Scale   7
Anger Coping Program   154
anorexia nervosa   30, 128
antipsychotic medication   218
anxiety disorders   120
any anxiety disorder   144
Arab League   71
ASD see autism spectrum disorders
Asperger syndrome   28
assessment procedures   6
assessment tools   319
assessment training   320
ATLAS   23
Attention Deficit/Hyperactivity Disorder (ADHD)   43, 125
Australian Early Intervention Network   56
autism   128, 258
autism spectrum disorders (ASD)   257
Axis   1 disorders   74

B

Background Module   55
baseline medical assessment   210
Baseline-Follow-up Module   55
Beavers/Timberlawn   173
Beck scale   48
behavior management   67
behavioral parent training   151
benzodiazepines   214
beta blockers   217
bio-psycho-social model   43
bipolar disorders   127
birth trauma   303
brain drain   82
bulimia nervosa   129
bullying   294
burden of disease   21

C

CAI see Child Advocacy International
Cambridge-Somerville trial   223
CAP see child adolescent psychiatry
CAPA see Child and Adolescent Psychiatric Assessment
capacity building   239
CAPPI see Child and Adolescent Psychiatrists
   of the Philippines, Inc.
Care Planning Team (CPT)   39
carve-outs   35
CASSP see Child and Adolescent Service Program
CAT see computerized adaptive testing
CBCL see Achenbach Child Behavior Checklist
CBCL see Child Behavior Checklist
CBCL see Child Behavior Checklist
CBT see cognitive-behavioral therapy
CD see conduct disorder
Certificate of Training   54
CGAS see Children's Global Assessment Scale
child adolescent psychiatry (CAP)   27
Child Advocacy International (CAI)   90
Child and Adolescent Psychiatric Assessment (CAPA)   8
Child and Adolescent Psychiatrists of the Philippines, Inc.
   (CAPPI)   64
Child and Adolescent Service System Program (CASSP)   36
child and adolescent mental health   72
Child Behavior Checklist (CBCL)   6, 316
Child Global Assessment Schedule   225
Child Gudiance Movement   32
Child Protection Act   62
child psychiatry   35
Child Rights Councils   23
children protection movement   59
Children's Global Assessment Scale (CGAS)   7
Children's Summer Treatment Program (STP)   152
China Mental Health Association (CMHA)   59
Christian Children's Fund Project   84
cigarette smoking   112
Class Activation Program   195
classroom contingency management   125
classroom interventions   330
clinical significance   108
CMHA see China Mental Health Association
cognitive behavioral family therapy   171
cognitive functioning   264
cognitive psychology   29
cognitive therapy (CT)   114
cognitive-behavioral therapy (CBT)   120
Comer School Model   331
Community Reactivation Program   195
community-based care   267
comorbidity   5
compensatory education   266
computerized adaptive testing (CAT)   319
Concurrent Module   55

conduct disorder (CD)   54, 123
conflict of interest   223
CONSORT criteria   226
constructivism   166
continuity of intent   38
continuum of care   17
Coping Cat   145
Coping with Depression Course for Adolescents
  (CWD-A)   148
Coping with Stress (CWS)   250
corporal punischment   75
cost-benefit analyses   283
cost-effectiveness   47, 229, 237
counseling   318
CPT see Care Planning Team
cross-cultural validation   44
Crowell Prodecure   193
CT see cognitive therapy
cultural competence   85
cultural differences   5, 10
cultural epidemiology   22
cultural validity   89
cultural variables   97
culture-bound syndrome   63
CURRES   237
CWD-A see Coping with Depression Course for Adolescents
CWS see Coping with Stress
cybernetics   165

D

DALYs see disability-adjusted life years
Daphne project   192
DAWBA see Development and Well-Being Assessment
daytime treatment   17
DD see dystymic disorder
Declaration of Venice   85
deinstutionalization   53
delinquency   287
demographic balance   93
depression   147
destigmatization   327
Development and Well-Being Assessment (DAWBA)   44
developmental appropriateness   42
developmental disorders   130, 256
developmental language disorder (DLD)   262
developmental plasticity   246
developmental screening tests   257
Diagnostic Interview Schedule for Children (DISC)   8
disability-adjusted life years (DALYs)   21
disaster intervention   196
DISC see Diagnostic Interview Schedule for Children
disease management   18
disruptive behavior disorders   55
disseminability   229

DLD see developmental language disorder
dopamine   304
double bind therapy   165
DSM   4
DSM-IV   74
dystymic disorder (DD)   122

E

eating disorders   55
EBT see evidence-based treatment
ecological framework   73, 246
effect size   223
effectiveness research   107
efficacy research   106
ehtnic group   9
electroconvulsive therapy   212
Emergency Team   187
emic   172
Empilweni   78
empowerment   197
enuresis   94
epidemiology   3
epilepsy   72
equal right movements   67
ethnographic studies   77
etic   172
evidence-based medicine   45
evidence-based treatment (EBT)   32, 103
externalizing   142
externalizing disorders   272

F

facilitating environment   73
FAM see Family Anxiety Management
Family Anxiety Management (FAM)   146
Family Bereavement Program   280
Family Paradigm   173
family research   173
family therapy   164
FAS see fetal alcohol syndrome
Fast Track Project   239
FDC see Foundation for Community Development
F-E-A-R plan   147
female circumcision   75
fetal alcohol syndrome (FAS)   28
FLAPIA (Latin American Federation of Child and Adolescent
  Psychiatry and Allied Disciplines)   50
fluoxetine   212
forensic child and adolescent psychiatry   32
Fort Bragg   21

Fort Bragg project   223
Foster Care   225
Foundation for Community Development (FDC)   78
functional complaints   315

G

GAD see generalized anxiety disorder
Gatehouse Project   56
gender discrimination   75
general systems theory   165
generalized anxiety disorder (GAD)   120
genetic influences   302
genogram   175
global discrimination   76
global perspective   19
governance   38
Guardianship Councils   23
guidelines   104

H

Hamilton Depression Rating Scale   209
Hanf model   157
Health of the Nation Outcome Scale-Child and Adolescent
   (HONOSCA)   55
high-risk neighborhood   282
hikkigomori   63
HIV/AIDS   75
HOME   44
homeostasis   165
HONOSCA see Health of the Nation Outcome Scale-Child
   and Adolescent
humanitarian intervention   92

I

IACAPAP see International Association of Child and Adolescent
   Psychiatry and Allied Professions
ijime   63
impulsiveness   288
inattentiveness   301
indicated prevention   277
indigenous healers   79
industry-sponsored trials   223
infibulation   75
inpatient unit   43
integrative conceptual model   45
intention-to-treat   226

internalizing   142
internalizing disorders   272
International Association of Child and Adolescent Psychiatry
   and Allied Professions (IACAPAP)   60
Internet addiction   63
interpersonal psychotherapy   123
interpersonal psychotherapy for adolescents (IPT-A)   149
IPT-A see interpersonal psychotherapy for adolescents
IQ   288
IQ test   263
ISO9000   192

J

Japanese Society for Child and Adolescent Psychiatry   60
Japanese Society for Child Psychiatry   60

K

Kanner syndromes   28
Kër Xaleyi (Children's Home)   79
   2 Punkte auf dem ersten e
KFOR (international Kosovo Protection Force)   90
Kids Help Line   55
Korean Academy of Child and Adolescent Psychiatry   62
Kutcher Adolescent Depression Rating Scale   209

L

ladder of empowerment   181
lead pollution   303
level 1 screening   256
life skills   330
literacy rates   81
lithium therapy   211
long-distance parenting   65

M

MacArthur Story Stem Battery (MSSB)   193
magnitude effect   108
mainstreaming   24
major depressive disorder (MDD)   122
malnutrition   42
managed care   18
Maputo transport corridor   78

marijuana   44
marital disruption   290
maternal depression   48
maternal sensitivity   262
McMaster Model   173
MDD see major depressive disorder
mediating mechanisms   227
mediator   114
Medicare   53
mental disorders   18
mental health   18
mental health services   54
Mental Health Services Programs for Youth (MHSPY)   36
Mental Research Institute   165
mental retardation   218
MHSPY see Mental Health Services Programs for Youth
midwife thesis   141
Milan Therapy   167
miracle question   174
Mobile Service   187
modeling   144
moderators of outcome   226
monitoring system   257
Mood Dosorder   54
mortality stratum   72
MSSB see MacArthur Story Stem Battery
MST see multisystemic therapy
MST see Multisystemic Therapy
multiagency intervention   189
multidisciplinary view   32
multisystemic therapy (MST)   125
Multisystemic Therapy (MST)   158

N

narrative model   169
narrative therapy   169
National Health Service   172
National Mental Health Strategy   53
national Policy Guidelines   84
National strategic plan   100
neighborhood socio-economic disadvantage (NSD)   9
neonates   305
neurobiological associations   305
NGOs see nongovernmental organizations
nightmares   328
nongovernmental organizations (NGOs)   18
nonspecific predictors   226
NSD see neighborhood socio-economic disadvantage

O

obsessive-compulsive disorder (OCD)   120
OCD see obsessive-compulsive disorder
ODD see oppositional defiant disorder
Office for Disaster Assistance   91
office-based counseling   318
opposional defiant disorder (ODD)   123
orphans and vulnerable children (OVC)   78
outpatient facility   43
outpatient therapy   17
OVC see orphans ande vulnerable children

P

Pan-American Health Organization   47
paradigm shift   283
parent management training   110
parent training approaches   261
parental concerns   257
parental conflict   289
parental supervision   289
parent-child interaction treatments   156
PCMHC see Professional Commitee of Mental Health for Children
PDD see pervasive developmental disorders
PDDST see Pervasive Developmental Disorders Screening Test
Pediatric Symptom Checklist   317
peer counseling   331
Peer Facilitatiors Training   64
Penn Prevention Program   251
Perry/Highscope study   224
personality traits   287
pervasive developmental disorders (PDD)   61, 218
Pervasive Developmental Disorders Screening Test (PDDST)   259
Philippine Guidance and Counseling Association   63
Philippine Mental Health Association (PMHA)   63
phobia   144
placebo   309
population attributable fraction   281
positive parenting   228
Positive Parenting Program   321
postdisaster support   199
Post-Milan therapy   167
postmodern colloborative therapy   170
posttraumatic stress   280
post-traumatic stress disorder (PTSD)   121
poverty   42
preconceptional counseling   266
predictive factors   12
predictor   289
preimplantation diagnosis   266

prenatal environment   302
prevalence   4
prevention program   236
preventive intervention   245
primary care   313
primary care services   314
primary prevention   257
private sector   18
privatization   18
Problem Solving Skills Training (PSST)   155
problem-focused methods   275
Professional Committee of Mental Health for Children (PCMHC)   59
Professional Development Strategy   55
protective factors   12, 248
PSST see Problem Solving Skills Training
psychiatric morbidity   49
Psychiatry Enquête   200
psychoanalysis   43
psychoanalytic psychotherapy   43
psychodynamic psychotherapy   121
psychoeducation   210
psychoeducation groups   321
psychoeducational interventions   46
PsychoInfo database   143
psychological competence   73
psychological functioning   73
psychopathology   30
psychopathology model   189
psychopharmacologic interventions   43
psychosocial competence   330
psychosocial interventions   119
psychostimulants   217
psychotherapeutic polypragmasy   32
psychotherapy   103, 141
psychotropic drug   316
psychotropics   208
PTSD see post-traumatic stress disorder
puerperal depression   47

R

random allocation model   179
RANZCP see Royal and New Zealand College of Psychiatry
rating scales   308
Reactive Attachment Disorder   261
reactive attachment disorder   61
reactive components   66
real-life conditions   229
reciprocal assistance   73
referral pathways   5
reflecting team conversations   170
regional initiatives   86
relapse rates   224
religion   76

resilience   248
resources for research   49
risk factors   249, 267, 287
Robert Wood Johnson Foundation (RWJF)   21, 37
roots of identity   73
Royal and New Zealand College of Psychiatry (RANZCP)   53
Russian system   93
RWJF see Robert Wood Johnson Foundation

S

SAD see separation anxiety disorder
SAICA   225
SAMHSA see Substance Abuse and Mental Health Services Administration
schizophrenia   127, 214
school achievement   288
school drop out   328
school phobia   327
school setting   326
SDQ see Strengths and Difficulties Questionnaire
secondary prevention   257
selective prevention   277
self worth   73
self-harm   129
self-help manuals   112
senior high disease   63
sentence recasting   264
separation anxiety disorder (SAD)   327
serotonin syndrome   213
service delivery   35
service-user satisfaction   180
SES see socio-economic status
shared mission   38
side effects   211
Sigmund Freud   141
social constructionism   166
social engineering   236
social interaction   257
socio-economic status (SES)   8, 289
Socrates   141
solution-focused therapy   166
somatic-psychic interaction   48
Sonagachi Project   241
special populations   24
specialty providers   314
SSRI   212
Stanford-Binet Intelligence Scale   265
statistical significance   108
stepped care   113
STP see Children's Summer Treatment Program
Strange Situations   193
Strengths and Difficulties Questionnaire (SDQ)   44, 55
stress-related disorders   94
subclinicasl symptomatology   281

sub-Saharan Africa   71
substance abuse   330
Substance Abuse and Mental Health Services Administration
    (SAMHSA)   39
susceptibility genes   259
symptom rating scales   4
synaptosomal protein   304
system of care   16, 39
systemic therapy   164

T

targeted interventions   260
Tel-Aviv Model   198
Telefono Azzurro   187
telemedicine   55
telephone disease management   321
television   310
temperament   287
Tetto Azzurro   187
The Incredible years   157
therapeutic alliance   176
tics   218
Tourette syndrome   127
traditional family systems   67
traumatic life-events   279
treatment manuals   114
tricyclic antidepressants   212
Triple P   321
truancy   327
twins   302

U

United Nations Convention   19
universal prevention   277
urbanization   9

V

Ventura Plan   21
Vienna School   29

W

wang-ta   63
war crime investigator   91
Washington Business Group on Health (WBGH)   37
WBGH see Washington Business Group on Health
Wechsler Intelligence Scales for Children (WISC)   265
well-baby clinics   257
WHO see World Health Organization
WISC see Wechsler Intelligence Scales for Children
World Health Organization (WHO)   20, 4
World Mental Health Day   81
wraparound process   37
wrap-around services   17

Y

YLEP see Youth Life Enrichment Program
Youth Life Enrichment Program (YLEP)   64
Youth Self-Report   7

Printing: Saladruck, Berlin
Binding: Stein+Lehmann, Berlin